Nursing Know-How

Evaluating Signs & Symptoms

Wolters Kluwer | Lippincott Williams & Wilkins
Health

Philadelphia • Baltimore • New York • London
Buenos Aires • Hong Kong • Sydney • Tokyo

STAFF

Executive Publisher
Judith A. Schilling McCann, RN, MSN

Editorial Director
H. Nancy Holmes

Clinical Director
Joan M. Robinson, RN, MSN

Senior Art Director
Mary Ludwicki

Editorial Project Managers
Deborah Grandinetti, Ann Houska

Clinical Project Manager
Beverly Ann Tscheschlog, RN, MS

Editor
Eleanor Levie

Clinical Editor
Pamela Kovach, RN, BSN

Copy Editors
Kimberly Bilotta (supervisor), Scotti Cohn, Amy Furman, Lisa Stockslager, Dorothy P. Terry, Pamela Wingrod

Designers
Deb Moloshok, Joseph John Clark (cover design)

Digital Composition Services
Diane Paluba (manager), Joyce Rossi Biletz, Donald Knauss, Donna S. Morris

Associate Manufacturing Manager
Beth. J. Welsh

Editorial Assistants
Karen J. Kirk, Linda K. Ruhf, Jeri O'Shea

Indexer
Barbara Hodgson

NKHS&S010508

Library of Congress Cataloging-in-Publication Data

Nursing know-how. Evaluating signs & symptoms.
p. ; cm.
Includes bibliographical references and index.
1. Nursing assessment—Handbooks, manuals, etc. 2. Nursing diagnosis—Handbooks, manuals, etc. 3. Symptoms—Handbooks, manuals, etc. I. Title: Evaluating signs & symptoms.
[DNLM: 1. Nursing Assessment—methods—Handbooks. 2. Physical Examination—nursing—Handbooks. WY 49 N97497 2009]
RT48.N89 2009
616.07'5—dc22
ISBN-13: 978-0-7817-9205-9 (alk. paper)
ISBN-10: 0-7817-9205-3 (alk. paper) 2008006526

Contents

Contributors and consultants

Helen C. Ballestas, *RN, MSN, CRRN, PhD (C)*
Instructor – Nursing; New York Institute of Technology; Old Westbury

Julie A. Calvery, *RN, MSN*
Instructor; University of Arkansas; Fort Smith

Kim Cooper, *RN, MSN*
Nursing Department Program Chair; Ivy Tech Community College; Terre Haute, Ind.

Vivian C. Gamblian, *RN, MSN*
Professor of Nursing; Collin County Community College; McKinney, Tex.

Dana Reeves, *RN, MSN*
Assistant Professor; University of Arkansas; Fort Smith

Kendra S. Seiler, *RN, MSN*
Nursing Instructor; Rio Hondo Community College; Whittier, Calif.

Fernisa Sison, RN, MSN, FNP-BC
Medical/Surgical Instructor; San Joaquin Delta College
Registered Nurse; St. Josephs Medical Center; Stockton, Calif.
Family Nurse Practitioner; Lodi (Calif.) Memorial Hospital

A

Abdominal mass

Commonly detected on routine physical examination, an abdominal mass is a localized swelling in one abdominal quadrant. (See *Abdominal masses: Locations and common causes,* page 2.) Typically, this sign develops insidiously and may represent an enlarged organ, a neoplasm, an abscess, a vascular defect, or a fecal mass.

Distinguishing an abdominal mass from a normal structure requires skillful palpation. A palpable abdominal mass is an important clinical sign and usually represents a serious and perhaps life-threatening disorder.

QUICK ACTION ***If the patient has a pulsating midabdominal mass and severe abdominal or back pain, suspect an aortic aneurysm. Don't palpate the mass. Quickly check the patient's vital signs. Because he may require emergency surgery, withhold food or fluids until he's examined. Prepare to give oxygen and to start an I.V. infusion for fluid and blood replacement. Obtain routine preoperative tests, and prepare the patient for computed tomography scan. Frequently monitor blood pressure, pulse, respirations, and urine output.***

Be alert for signs and symptoms of shock, such as altered mental status, tachycardia, hypotension, and cool, clammy skin, which may indicate significant blood loss.

History

- If the mass is painful, ask if the pain is constant or occurs only with palpation, and if it's localized or generalized.
- Ask if the mass has changed size or location.
- Obtain a medical history, noting GI disorders.
- Ask the patient if he's experienced symptoms, such as constipation, diarrhea, rectal bleeding, abnormally colored stools, vomiting, or changes in appetite.
- Ask the female patient to describe her menstrual cycle, noting any abnormalities.

Physical examination

- Auscultate first, listening for bruits or rubs.
- Percuss the mass, noting the sound.
- Lightly palpate and then deeply palpate the abdomen, assessing painful or suspicious areas last.
- Estimate the size of the mass and determine its shape and consistency.
- Note whether the mass is palpable in supine and side-lying positions.
- Determine whether the mass moves with your hand or in response to respiration.
- Note the contour and consistency of the mass.

Causes

Medical causes

Abdominal aortic aneurysm

- This life-threatening disorder produces severe upper abdominal pain or,

Abdominal masses: Locations and common causes

The location of an abdominal mass provides an important clue to the causative disorder. Here are the disorders that are most commonly responsible for abdominal masses in each of the four abdominal quadrants.

Right upper quadrant
- Aortic aneurysm (epigastric area)
- Cholecystitis or cholelithiasis
- Gallbladder, gastric, or hepatic carcinoma
- Hepatomegaly
- Hydronephrosis
- Pancreatic abscess or pseudocysts
- Renal cell carcinoma

Left upper quadrant
- Aortic aneurysm (epigastric area)
- Gastric carcinoma (epigastric area)
- Hydronephrosis
- Pancreatic abscess (epigastric area)
- Pancreatic pseudocysts (epigastric area)
- Renal cell carcinoma
- Splenomegaly

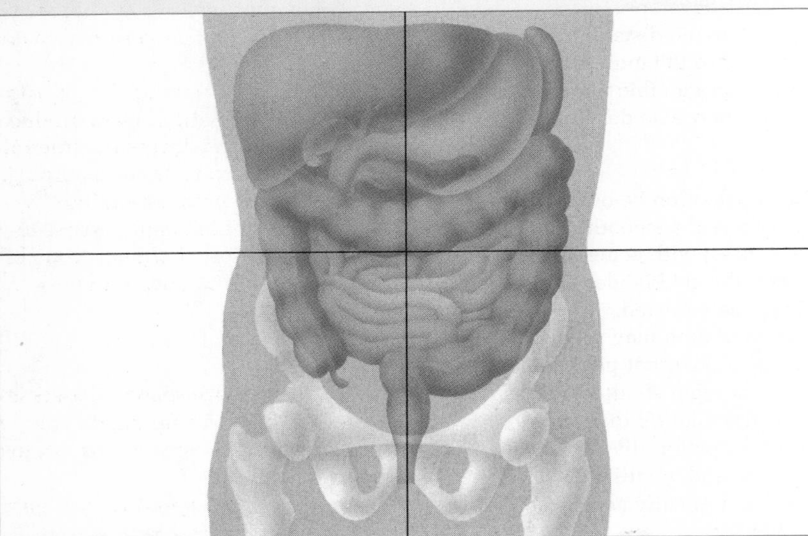

Right lower quadrant
- Bladder distention (suprapubic area)
- Colon cancer
- Crohn's disease
- Ovarian cyst (suprapubic area)
- Uterine leiomyomas (suprapubic area)

Left lower quadrant
- Bladder distention (suprapubic area)
- Colon cancer
- Diverticulitis
- Ovarian cyst (suprapubic area)
- Uterine leiomyomas (suprapubic area)
- Volvulus

less commonly, lower back or dull abdominal pain if rupture occurs.

- The condition may persist for years, producing only a pulsating periumbilical mass with a systolic bruit over the aorta.
- Other signs and symptoms of rupture include mottled skin below the waist, absent femoral and pedal pulses, lower blood pressure in the legs than in the arms, and mild to moderate tenderness with guarding, abdominal rigidity, and shock (with significant blood loss).

Bladder distention

- A smooth, rounded, fluctuant suprapubic mass develops.
- With extreme distention, the mass may extend to the umbilicus.
- Severe suprapubic pain and urinary frequency may also develop.

Cholecystitis

- Deep palpation below the liver border may reveal a smooth, firm, sausage-shaped mass; with acute inflammation, however, the gallbladder may be too tender to be palpated.
- The condition may produce severe right upper quadrant pain that may radiate to the right shoulder, chest, or back; abdominal rigidity and tenderness; fever; pallor; diaphoresis; anorexia; nausea; and vomiting.
- Attacks typically occur 1 to 6 hours after meals.
- Murphy's sign (inspiratory arrest brought on while palpating the right upper quadrant when the patient takes a deep breath) is common.

Cholelithiasis

- A painless, smooth, sausage-shaped mass develops in the right upper quadrant.
- Passage of a calculus through the bile duct or cystic duct may cause severe right upper quadrant pain that radiates to the epigastrium, back, or shoulder blades.
- Other signs and symptoms include anorexia, nausea, vomiting, chills, diaphoresis, restlessness, low-grade fever, jaundice (if the common bile duct is obstructed), fatty food intolerance, and indigestion.

Colon cancer

- If present in the right colon, a right lower quadrant mass may occur with occult bleeding, anemia, and abdominal aching, pressure, or dull cramps.
- Other signs and symptoms of right colon cancer include weakness, fatigue, exertional dyspnea, vertigo and, with intestinal obstruction, obstipation and vomiting.
- If present in the left colon, a palpable left lower quadrant mass produces rectal bleeding and pressure, intermittent abdominal fullness or cramping, and pain relief with defecation.
- Late signs of left colon cancer include obstipation, diarrhea, or pencil-shaped, grossly bloody, or mucus-streaked stools.

Crohn's disease

- Tender, sausage-shaped masses are usually palpable in the right lower quadrant and, at times, in the left lower quadrant.
- Colicky right lower quadrant pain and diarrhea are common.
- Other signs and symptoms include fever, anorexia, weight loss, hyperactive bowel sounds, nausea, abdominal tenderness with guarding, and perirectal, skin, or vaginal fistulas.

Diverticulitis

- A left lower quadrant mass that's usually tender, firm, and fixed may develop.
- Other signs and symptoms may include intermittent abdominal pain that's relieved by defecating or passing flatus,

alternating diarrhea and constipation, nausea, low-grade fever, and a distended and tympanic abdomen.

Gallbladder cancer

- A moderately tender, irregular mass may develop in the right upper quadrant.
- Chronic, progressively severe epigastric or right upper quadrant pain may radiate to the right shoulder.
- Other signs and symptoms include nausea, vomiting, anorexia, weight loss, jaundice, and sometimes hepatomegaly.

Gastric cancer

- An epigastric mass may develop.
- Early findings include chronic dyspepsia and epigastric discomfort.
- Late findings include weight loss, a feeling of fullness, fatigue and, occasionally, coffee-ground vomitus or melena.

Hepatic cancer

- A tender, nodular mass develops in the right upper quadrant or right epigastric area.
- Other signs and symptoms include weight loss, weakness, anorexia, nausea, fever, dependent edema, jaundice, ascites, and a bruit or hum (if the tumor is large).

Hepatomegaly

- A firm, blunt, irregular mass may be present in the epigastric region or below the right costal margin.
- Other signs and symptoms include ascites, right upper quadrant pain and tenderness, anorexia, nausea, vomiting, leg edema, jaundice, palmar erythema, spider angiomas, gynecomastia, testicular atrophy, and splenomegaly.

Hydronephrosis

- A smooth, boggy mass is detected in one or both flanks.
- Severe colicky renal pain or dull flank pain radiates to the groin, vulva, or testes.
- Other signs and symptoms include hematuria, pyuria, dysuria, alternating oliguria and polyuria, nocturia, accelerated hypertension, nausea, and vomiting.

Ovarian cyst

- A smooth, rounded, fluctuant mass may develop in the suprapubic region.
- Mild pelvic discomfort, lower back pain, menstrual irregularities, and hirsutism may occur with large or multiple cysts.
- Abdominal tenderness, distention, and rigidity may occur with twisted or ruptured cysts.

Pancreatic abscess

- Occasionally, a palpable epigastric mass may develop, with accompanying pain and tenderness.
- Other signs and symptoms include nausea, vomiting, diarrhea, tachycardia, hypotension, and an abrupt rise in temperature (although it may also rise steadily).

Renal cell cancer

- A smooth, firm, nontender mass develops near the affected kidney.
- Dull, constant abdominal or flank pain and hematuria occur.
- Other signs and symptoms include elevated blood pressure, fever, and urine retention, and in late stages, weight loss, nausea, vomiting, and leg edema.

Splenomegaly

- The spleen is palpable in the left upper quadrant.
- Other signs and symptoms include a feeling of abdominal fullness, left upper quadrant pain and tenderness, splenic rub, splenic bruits, and low-grade fever.

Uterine leiomyomas (fibroids)

- A round, multinodular mass may develop in the suprapubic region.
- Other signs and symptoms may include menorrhagia, a feeling of heaviness in the abdomen, back pain, constipation, urinary frequency and urgency, and edema and varicosities of the leg.

Nursing considerations

- Offer emotional support to the patient and his family.
- Position the patient comfortably.
- Give drugs for pain or anxiety, as needed.
- If bowel obstruction occurs, watch for indications of peritonitis and shock.
- In neonates, most abdominal masses are caused by renal disorders.
- In older infants and children, abdominal masses are usually caused by enlarged organs.

Patient teaching

- Explain diagnostic tests that are needed.

Abdominal pain

Abdominal pain usually is caused by a GI disorder, but it can be triggered by a reproductive, genitourinary (GU), musculoskeletal, or vascular disorder; drug use; or ingestion of toxins. At times, such pain signals life-threatening complications.

Abdominal pain arises from the abdominopelvic viscera, the parietal peritoneum, or the capsules of the liver, kidney, or spleen. It may be acute or chronic, diffuse or localized. Visceral pain develops slowly into a deep, dull, aching pain that's poorly localized in the epigastric, periumbilical, or lower midabdominal (hypogastric) region. In contrast, somatic (parietal, peritoneal) pain produces a sharp, more intense, and well-localized discomfort that rapidly follows the injury. Movement or coughing aggravates this pain.

Pain may also be referred to the abdomen from another site with the same or similar nerve supply. This sharp, well-localized, referred pain is felt in the skin or deeper tissues and may coexist with skin hyperesthesia and muscle hyperalgesia.

Mechanisms that produce abdominal pain include stretching or tension of the gut wall, traction on the peritoneum or mesentery, vigorous intestinal contraction, inflammation, ischemia, and sensory nerve irritation. (See *Abdominal pain: Types and locations* page 6.)

QUICK ACTION ***If the patient is experiencing sudden and severe abdominal pain, quickly take his vital signs and palpate pulses below the waist. Be alert for signs of hypovolemic shock, such as altered mental status, tachycardia, and hypotension. Obtain I.V. access.***

Emergency surgery may be required if the patient has mottled skin below the waist and a pulsating epigastric mass or rebound tenderness and rigidity.

History

- Obtain a medical history, noting previous abdominal pain; substance abuse; vascular, GI, GU, or reproductive disorders; and menstrual patterns and changes.
- Ask the patient to describe the pain, including quality, quantity, frequency, duration, location, radiation, and what aggravates and alleviates it. Ask the patient to rate the pain on a scale of 0 to 10.
- Ask the patient if he has experienced changes in appetite, increased flatulence, constipation, diarrhea, changes in bowel movements, urinary frequency and urgency, or painful urination.
- If the patient complains of constant, steady abdominal pain, this may suggest

Abdominal pain: Types and locations

AFFECTED ORGAN	VISCERAL PAIN	PARIETAL PAIN	REFERRED PAIN
Appendix	Periumbilical area	Right lower quadrant	Right lower quadrant
Distal colon	Hypogastrium and left flank for descending colon	Over affected area	Left lower quadrant and back (rare)
Gallbladder	Middle epigastrium	Right upper quadrant	Right subscapular area
Ovaries, fallopian tubes, and uterus	Hypogastrium and groin	Over affected area	Inner thighs
Pancreas	Middle epigastrium and left upper quadrant	Middle epigastrium and left upper quadrant	Back and left shoulder
Proximal colon	Periumbilical area and right flank for ascending colon	Over affected area	Right lower quadrant and back (rare)
Small intestine	Periumbilical area	Over affected area	Midback (rare)
Stomach	Middle epigastrium	Middle epigastrium and left upper quadrant	Shoulders
Ureters	Costovertebral angle	Over affected area	Groin: scrotum in men; labia in women (rare)

organ perforation, ischemia, or inflammation or blood in the abdominal cavity.

- If the patient complains of intermittent, cramping abdominal pain, this may suggest an obstruction of a hollow organ.

Physical examination

- Take the patient's vital signs.
- Assess skin turgor and mucous membranes.
- Inspect the patient's abdomen for distention or visible peristaltic waves, and measure his abdomen.
- Auscultate for bowel sounds and characterize their motility.
- Percuss all quadrants, noting the percussion sounds.
- Palpate the entire abdomen for masses, rigidity, and tenderness.
- Check for costovertebral angle (CVA) tenderness, abdominal tenderness with guarding, and rebound tenderness.

Causes

Medical causes

Abdominal aortic aneurysm, dissecting

- This life-threatening disorder is characterized initially by dull lower abdominal, lower back, or severe chest pain.
- Constant upper abdominal pain may worsen when the patient lies down and subside when the patient leans forward or sits up.
- A pulsating epigastric mass may be palpated before rupture but not after it.
- Other signs and symptoms include mottled skin and absent pulses below the waist, lower blood pressure in the legs than in the arms, abdominal ten-

derness with guarding, abdominal rigidity, and signs of shock.

Abdominal trauma

- Generalized or localized abdominal pain occurs with abdominal tenderness, vomiting, and ecchymoses on the abdomen.
- Hemorrhage into the peritoneal cavity causes abdominal rigidity.
- Bowel sounds are decreased or absent.
- Hypovolemic shock may occur.

(See *Responding to abdominal pain,* page 8.)

Adrenal crisis

- Severe abdominal pain appears early.
- Other signs and symptoms include nausea, vomiting, dehydration, profound weakness, anorexia, and fever.
- Late signs and symptoms include progressive loss of consciousness; hypotension; tachycardia; oliguria; cool, clammy skin; and increased motor activity, which may progress to delirium or seizures.

Anthrax, GI

- Early signs and symptoms include loss of appetite, nausea, vomiting, and fever.
- Late signs and symptoms include abdominal pain, severe bloody diarrhea, and hematemesis.

Appendicitis

- In this life-threatening disorder, pain initially occurs in the epigastric or umbilical region and then localizes at McBurney's point in the right lower quadrant.
- Pain is accompanied by abdominal rigidity, tenderness, and rebound tenderness.
- Other signs and symptoms include anorexia, nausea, and vomiting.
- Late signs and symptoms include malaise, constipation (or diarrhea), low-grade fever, and tachycardia.

Cholecystitis

- Severe pain in the right upper quadrant may arise suddenly or increase gradually over several hours, usually after meals.
- Pain may radiate to the right shoulder, chest, or back.
- Murphy's sign—inspiratory arrest brought on by palpating the right upper quadrant while the patient takes a deep breath—is common.
- Other signs and symptoms include anorexia, nausea, vomiting, fever, abdominal rigidity, tenderness, pallor, and diaphoresis.

Cholelithiasis

- Sudden, severe, and paroxysmal pain in the right upper quadrant may radiate to the epigastrium, back, or shoulder blades.
- Other signs and symptoms include anorexia, nausea, vomiting (sometimes bilious), diaphoresis, restlessness, abdominal tenderness with guarding, fatty food intolerance, and indigestion.

Cirrhosis

- A dull abdominal aching occurs early in the disorder's progression, with accompanying anorexia, indigestion, nausea, vomiting, constipation, or diarrhea.
- The pain worsens in the right upper quadrant when the patient sits up or leans forward.
- Other signs and symptoms include fever, ascites, leg edema, weight gain, hepatomegaly, jaundice, severe pruritus, bleeding tendencies, palmar erythema, and spider angiomas.

Crohn's disease

- Acute attacks result in severe cramping pain in the lower abdomen.

CASE CLIP

Responding to abdominal pain

Mr. M. is a 67-year-old male admitted to the medical floor 3 days ago with bilateral pneumonia, fever, productive cough, chest pain, and tachypnea. Since his admission, he has been receiving antibiotics for his pneumonia, but continues to experience frequent coughing episodes.

During tonight's shift, his nurse enters his room to perform her initial assessment of his condition. She finds him sitting upright in a bedside chair. She auscultates his lungs and notes that he continues to have scattered coarse rhonchi throughout both lungs, more so in the bases. He has oxygen available to him at 2 L via nasal cannula, but frequently removes it because he says it is uncomfortable. His current vital signs are:

- heart rate (HR): 92 beats/minute
- respiratory rate (RR): 26 breaths/minute
- blood pressure (BP): 146/88 mm Hg
- oxygen saturation: 92%.

Thirty minutes later, the nurse returns with Mr. M.'s medications and finds him very restless, agitated, and visibly short of breath. He's complaining of a sudden onset of severe left upper abdominal pain that began after a recent coughing spell. He starts to become slightly dusky in color and increasingly agitated, saying he feels like he's dying and that this is the worst pain he has ever had. When asked, he rates the pain as 10 out of 10 on the hospital's pain scale. His vital signs are now:

- HR: 116 beats/minute
- BP: 124/82 mm Hg.

The nurse immediately transfers him back to bed with assistance. As she tries to lower the head of the bed so she can assess his abdomen, he refuses, saying that it increases the pain unbearably. He remains in semi-Fowler's position. She lifts his sheet to check his abdomen and notices a raised area in the left upper quadrant which is very firm to the touch; upon light palpation Mr. M. screams in pain. With this in mind, the nurse activates the Rapid Response Team (RRT).

The RRT arrives within 4 minutes of activation. A stat electrocardiogram is performed, which shows a narrow-complex tachycardia at a current rate of 144 beats/minute. His BP is now 88/54 mm Hg and his oxygen saturation is 87% but he still refuses the oxygen mask. The raised area noted by the nurse earlier has increased markedly in size and rigidity.

An immediate computed tomography (CT) scan is ordered to determine the cause of the newly developing mass. Due to his worsening vital signs, Mr. M. is transferred to the intensive care unit. The CT scan showed a ruptured rectus abdominus muscle on the left, apparently sustained during a particularly violent episode of coughing earlier that evening. Mr. M. was taken to the operating room for an emergency repair of the muscle; he remained intubated for 3 days, but was gradually weaned off the ventilator. He was transferred the next day to the surgical unit for the remainder of his hospitalization.

- Weeks or months of milder cramping pain typically precede an attack.
- Abdominal pain may be relieved by defecation.
- Chronic signs and symptoms include right lower quadrant pain, with diarrhea, steatorrhea, and weight loss.

- Other signs and symptoms include diarrhea, hyperactive bowel sounds, dehydration, weight loss, fever, abdominal tenderness with guarding, and a palpable mass in a lower quadrant.

Cystitis

- Abdominal pain and tenderness are usually suprapubic.
- Other signs and symptoms include malaise, flank pain, low back pain, nausea, vomiting, urinary frequency and urgency, nocturia, dysuria, fever, and chills.

Diverticulitis

- Intermittent, diffuse left lower quadrant pain usually occurs in mild cases.
- The pain may worsen with eating but is relieved by defecation or passage of flatus.
- Rupture causes severe left lower quadrant pain, abdominal rigidity and, possibly, signs and symptoms of shock and sepsis.
- Other signs and symptoms include nausea, constipation or diarrhea, low-grade fever, and a palpable abdominal mass that's usually tender, firm, and fixed.

Duodenal ulcer

- Pain is localized and steady, gnawing, burning, aching, or hungerlike.
- Pain typically occurs 2 to 4 hours after a meal and may cause nocturnal awakening.
- Pain may be high in the midepigastrium and slightly off-center (usually on the right).
- Other symptoms include changes in bowel habits and heartburn or retrosternal burning.

Ectopic pregnancy

- Pain occurs in the lower abdomen and may be sharp, dull, or cramping and constant or intermittent.
- Rupture of the fallopian tube produces sharp lower abdominal pain, which may radiate to the shoulders and neck; signs of shock may also occur.
- Other signs and symptoms include vaginal bleeding, nausea, vomiting, urinary frequency, a tender adnexal mass, and a 1- to 2-month history of amenorrhea.

Endometriosis

- Constant, severe pain in the lower abdomen usually begins 5 to 7 days before the start of menses.
- Pain may be aggravated by defecation.
- Other symptoms include constipation, abdominal tenderness, dysmenorrhea, dyspareunia, and deep sacral pain.

Escherichia coli *O157:H7*

- Abdominal cramping, watery or bloody diarrhea, nausea, vomiting, and fever occur after eating contaminated foods.
- Hemolytic uremia may occur in children younger than age 5 and in elderly patients, possibly leading to acute renal failure.

Gastric ulcer

- Diffuse, gnawing, burning pain in the left upper quadrant or epigastric area occurs 1 to 2 hours after meals.
- Pain may be relieved by ingesting food or antacids.
- Vague bloating and nausea after meals, indigestion, weight change, anorexia, and GI bleeding may also occur.

Gastritis

- The onset of pain is rapid, ranging from mild epigastric discomfort to burning in the left upper quadrant.
- Other signs and symptoms may include belching, fever, malaise, anorexia, nausea, bloody or coffee-ground vomitus, and melena.

Gastroenteritis
- Cramping or colicky pain originates in the left upper quadrant and then radiates or migrates to the other quadrants.
- Pain is accompanied by diarrhea, hyperactive bowel sounds, headache, myalgia, nausea, and vomiting.

Heart failure
- Right upper quadrant pain is common.
- Hallmark signs and symptoms include jugular vein distention, dyspnea, tachycardia, and peripheral edema.
- Other signs and symptoms include nausea, vomiting, ascites, productive cough, crackles, cool extremities, and cyanotic nail beds.

Hepatitis
- Liver enlargement causes discomfort or dull pain and tenderness in the right upper quadrant.
- Other signs and symptoms include dark urine, clay-colored stools, nausea, vomiting, anorexia, jaundice, malaise, and pruritus.

Intestinal obstruction
- This life-threatening disorder produces short episodes of intense, colicky, cramping pain, which alternate with pain-free intervals.
- Accompanying signs and symptoms include abdominal distention, tenderness, and guarding; visible peristaltic waves; high-pitched, tinkling, or hyperactive sounds near the obstruction and hypoactive or absent sounds distally; obstipation; pain-induced agitation; and hypovolemic shock (late sign).
- In jejunal and duodenal obstruction, nausea and bilious vomiting occur early.
- In distal obstruction, nausea and vomiting are commonly feculent.
- Bowel sounds are absent in complete obstruction.

Irritable bowel syndrome
- Lower abdominal cramping or pain is aggravated by ingestion of coarse or raw foods.
- Pain may be alleviated by defecation or passage of flatus.
- Stress, anxiety, and emotional lability intensify the symptoms.
- Other signs and symptoms include abdominal tenderness, diarrhea alternating with constipation or normal bowel function, small stools with visible mucus, dyspepsia, nausea, and abdominal distention with a feeling of incomplete evacuation.

Listeriosis
- Abdominal pain, fever, myalgia, nausea, vomiting, and diarrhea occur after contaminated food is eaten.
- Meningitis may develop if the infection spreads to the nervous system.

Ovarian cyst
- Torsion or hemorrhage causes pain and tenderness in the right or left lower quadrant.
- The pain becomes sharp and severe if the patient suddenly stands or stoops.
- The pain becomes brief and intermittent if torsion self-corrects or dull and diffuse (after several hours) if it doesn't.
- Other signs and symptoms include slight fever, mild nausea and vomiting, abdominal tenderness, a palpable abdominal mass, amenorrhea, and abdominal distention.

Pancreatitis
- In acute pancreatitis (a life-threatening disorder), fulminating, continuous upper abdominal pain may radiate to both flanks and to the back.
- In chronic pancreatitis, severe left upper quadrant or epigastric pain radiates to the back.
- Early findings include abdominal tenderness, nausea, vomiting, fever, pallor, tachycardia, abdominal rigidity, re-

bound tenderness, and hypoactive bowel sounds.

- Turner's sign (ecchymosis of the abdomen or flank) or Cullen's sign (a bluish tinge around the umbilicus) signals hemorrhagic pancreatitis.
- Jaundice may occur as inflammation subsides.

Pelvic inflammatory disease

- Pain occurs in the right or left lower quadrant.
- The extent of pain ranges from vague discomfort to deep, severe, and progressive pain.
- Metrorrhagia may precede or accompany the onset of pain.
- Other signs and symptoms include abdominal tenderness, a palpable abdominal or pelvic mass, fever, chills, nausea, vomiting, urinary discomfort, and abnormal vaginal bleeding or purulent vaginal discharge.

Perforated ulcer

- This life-threatening disorder may cause sudden, severe, and prostrating epigastric pain that radiates through the abdomen to the back or to the right shoulder.
- Other signs and symptoms include abdominal rigidity, tenderness with guarding, generalized rebound tenderness, absent bowel sounds, grunting and shallow respirations, fever, tachycardia, hypotension, and syncope.

Peritonitis

- In this life-threatening disorder, sudden and severe pain can be diffuse or localized.
- Movement worsens the pain.
- Other signs and symptoms include fever; chills; nausea; vomiting; hypoactive or absent bowel sounds; abdominal tenderness, distention, and rigidity; rebound tenderness and guarding; hyperalgesia; tachycardia; hypotension; tachypnea; and psoas and obturator signs.

Prostatitis

- Vague abdominal pain or discomfort may develop in the lower abdomen, groin, perineum, or rectum.
- Scrotal pain, penile pain, and pain on ejaculation may occur in chronic cases.
- Other signs and symptoms include dysuria, urinary frequency and urgency, fever, chills, low back pain, myalgia, arthralgia, and nocturia.

Pyelonephritis, acute

- Progressive lower quadrant pain in one or both sides, flank pain, and CVA tenderness occur.
- Pain may radiate to the lower midabdomen or groin.
- Other signs and symptoms include abdominal and back tenderness, high fever, shaking chills, nausea, vomiting, and urinary frequency and urgency.

Renal calculi

- Depending on the location of calculi, severe abdominal or back pain may occur.
- The classic symptom is severe, colicky pain that travels from the CVA to the flank, suprapubic region, and external genitalia.
- Other signs and symptoms include pain-induced agitation, nausea, vomiting, abdominal distention, fever, chills, hypertension, and urinary urgency.

Sickle cell crisis

- Sudden, severe abdominal pain may accompany chest, back, hand, or foot pain.
- Other signs and symptoms include weakness, aching joints, dyspnea, and scleral jaundice.

Ulcerative colitis

- Initially, vague abdominal discomfort leads to cramping lower abdominal pain.
- Pain may become steady and diffuse, increasing with movement and coughing.
- Recurrent and possibly severe diarrhea with blood, pus, and mucus may relieve pain.
- Other signs and symptoms include a soft, extremely tender abdomen; high-pitched, infrequent bowel sounds; nausea; vomiting; anorexia; weight loss; and mild, intermittent fever.

Other causes

Drugs

- Salicylates and nonsteroidal anti-inflammatory drugs commonly cause burning and gnawing pain in the left upper quadrant or epigastric area.

Nursing considerations

- Have the patient lie in a supine position with his knees slightly flexed.
- Monitor the patient for life-threatening findings, such as tachycardia, hypotension, clammy skin, abdominal rigidity, rebound tenderness, changes in the pain's location or intensity, or sudden relief from pain.
- Withhold food and fluids.
- Prepare for I.V. infusion and insertion of a nasogastric or other intestinal tube.
- Peritoneal lavage or abdominal paracentesis may be required.
- Because children have difficulty describing abdominal pain, pay attention to nonverbal cues.
- A child's complaint of abdominal pain may reflect an emotional need, such as a wish to avoid school or to gain adult attention.
- Advanced age may decrease the signs and symptoms of acute abdominal disease.

Patient teaching

- Explain the diagnostic tests the patient will need.
- Explain which foods and fluids the patient should avoid.
- Tell the patient to report changes in bowel habits.
- Teach the patient how to position himself to alleviate symptoms.

Abdominal rigidity

Detected by palpation, abdominal rigidity refers to abnormal muscle tension or inflexibility of the abdomen. Rigidity may be voluntary or involuntary. Voluntary rigidity reflects the patient's fear or nervousness upon palpation; involuntary rigidity reflects potentially life-threatening peritoneal irritation or inflammation. (See *Recognizing voluntary rigidity.*)

Involuntary rigidity most commonly results from GI disorders but may also be caused by pulmonary and vascular disorders or effects of insect toxins. Usually, involuntary rigidity is accompanied by fever, nausea, vomiting, and abdominal tenderness, distention, and pain.

QUICK ACTION ***After palpating abdominal rigidity, quickly take the patient's vital signs. Although the patient may not appear gravely ill or have markedly abnormal vital signs, abdominal rigidity calls for emergency evaluation and interventions.***

Prepare to give oxygen and to insert an I.V. line for fluid and blood replacement. The patient may require drugs to support blood pressure. Prepare him for urinary catheterization, and monitor intake and output.

A nasogastric tube may have to be inserted to relieve abdominal distention. Because emergency surgery may be needed, the patient should be pre-

pared for laboratory tests and imaging studies.

History

- Ask about the onset of abdominal rigidity.
- Ask if abdominal pain is present and when it began.
- Determine the location of rigidity (localized or generalized).
- Ask about aggravating and alleviating factors, such as position changes, coughing, vomiting, elimination, and walking.

Physical examination

- Inspect the abdomen for peristaltic waves.
- Check for a visibly distended bowel loop.
- Auscultate for bowel sounds.
- Perform light palpation to locate the rigidity and determine its severity.
- Check for signs of dehydration, such as poor skin turgor and dry mucous membranes.

Causes

Medical causes

Abdominal aortic aneurysm, dissecting

- In this life-threatening disorder, mild to moderate abdominal rigidity occurs.
- Constant upper abdominal pain may radiate to the lower back.
- A pulsating mass may be present in the epigastrium with a systolic bruit over the aorta before rupture; after rupture, the mass stops pulsating.
- Significant blood loss causes signs of shock (tachycardia, tachypnea, and cool, clammy skin).
- Other signs and symptoms include mottled skin and absent pulses below the waist, blood pressure lower in the legs than in the arms, and mild to moderate tenderness with guarding.

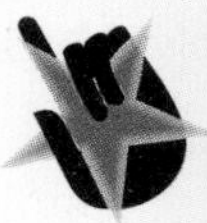

KNOW HOW

Recognizing voluntary rigidity

Distinguishing voluntary from involuntary abdominal rigidity is a must for accurate assessment. Review this comparison so that you can quickly tell the two apart.

Voluntary rigidity

- Usually symmetrical
- More rigid on inspiration (expiration causes muscle relaxation)
- Eased by relaxation techniques, such as positioning the patient comfortably and talking to him in a calm, soothing manner
- Painless when the patient sits up using only his abdominal muscles

Involuntary rigidity

- Usually asymmetrical
- Equally rigid on inspiration and expiration
- Unaffected by relaxation techniques
- Painful when the patient sits up using only his abdominal muscles

Peritonitis

- Rigidity may be localized or generalized, depending on the cause of peritonitis.
- Other signs and symptoms include abdominal tenderness and distention, rebound tenderness, guarding, hyperalgesia, hypoactive or absent bowel sounds, nausea, vomiting, fever, chills, tachycardia, tachypnea, and hypotension.

Other causes

Insect toxins

- Rigidity usually accompanies generalized, cramping abdominal pain.
- Other signs and symptoms include low-grade fever, nausea, vomiting, tremors, burning sensations in the hands and feet, increased salivation, hypertension, paresis, and hyperactive reflexes.

Nursing considerations

- Monitor the patient closely for signs of shock.
- Position the patient in a supine position with knees slightly flexed.
- Withhold analgesics until a tentative diagnosis has been made.
- Withhold food and fluids.
- Give an I.V. antibiotic because emergency surgery may be required.
- Prepare for diagnostic tests, which may include blood, urine, and stool studies; chest and abdominal X-rays; computed tomography; magnetic resonance imaging; gastroscopy; and colonoscopy.
- In a child, voluntary rigidity may be difficult to distinguish from involuntary rigidity if associated pain makes him restless, tense, or apprehensive.
- In a child, abdominal rigidity may stem from gastric perforation, hypertrophic pyloric stenosis, duodenal obstruction, meconium ileus, intussusception, cystic fibrosis, celiac disease, or appendicitis.
- When involuntary rigidity is suspected, monitor the patient for early signs of dehydration and shock, which can rapidly become life-threatening.
- Older patients with weakening abdominal muscles have fewer muscle spasms and decreased rigidity.

Patient teaching

- Explain the diagnostic tests or surgery the patient will need.
- Teach the patient ways to reduce anxiety.

Amenorrhea

The absence of menstrual flow, amenorrhea can be classified as primary or secondary. With primary amenorrhea, menstruation fails to begin before age 16. Secondary amenorrhea begins at an appropriate age, but later stops for 3 or more months in the absence of normal physiologic causes, such as pregnancy, lactation, or menopause.

Pathologic amenorrhea is caused by anovulation or physical obstruction to menstrual outflow, such as from an imperforate hymen, cervical stenosis, or intrauterine adhesions. Anovulation itself may result from hormonal imbalance, debilitating disease, stress or emotional disturbances, strenuous exercise, malnutrition, obesity, or anatomic abnormalities such as a congenital absence of the ovaries or uterus. Amenorrhea may also be caused by drug or hormonal treatments. (See *Understanding disruptions in menstruation.*)

History

- Ask about frequency and duration of the patient's previous menses.
- Obtain the date of her last menses.
- Determine the onset and nature of menstrual pattern changes.
- Ask about related signs (breast swelling or weight changes).
- Obtain a medical history, including illnesses, use of hormonal contraceptives, exercise and eating habits, emotional state, weight changes, and stress levels.
- Obtain family medical and menstrual history.

Physical examination

- Observe for secondary sex characteristics and signs of virilization.

Understanding disruptions in menstruation

A disruption at any point in the menstrual cycle can produce amenorrhea, as illustrated in this flowchart.

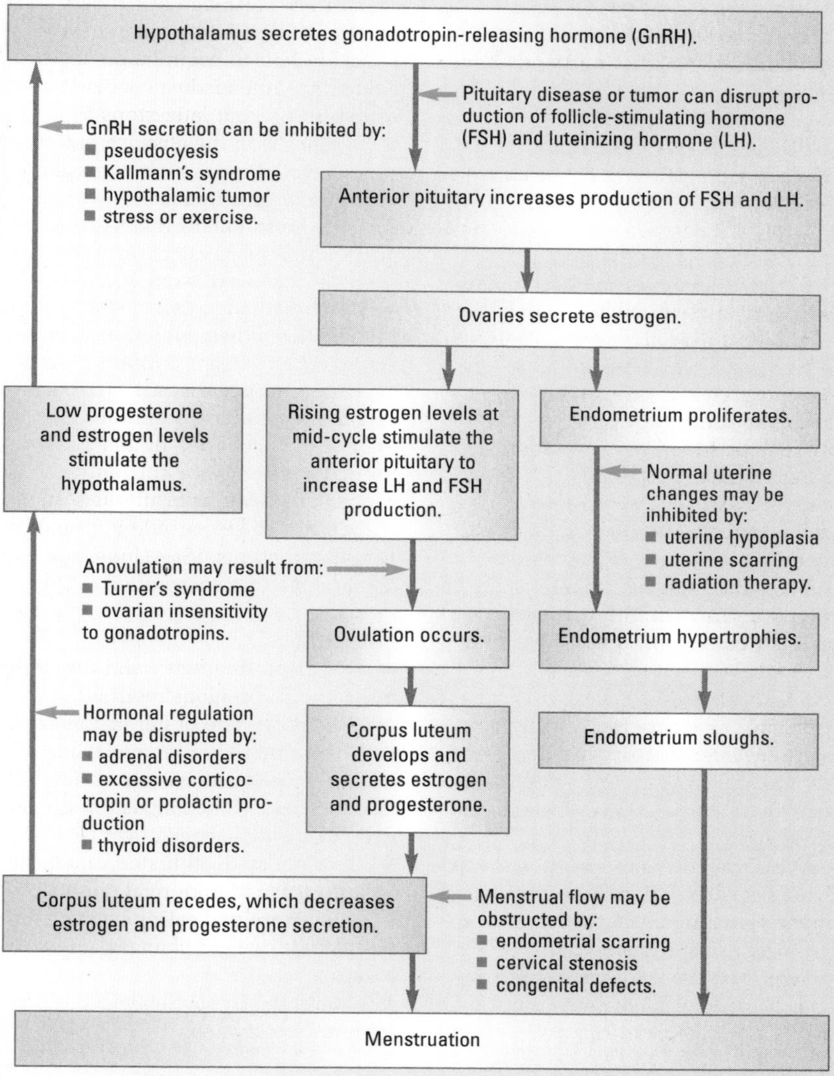

Hypothalamus secretes gonadotropin-releasing hormone (GnRH).

Pituitary disease or tumor can disrupt production of follicle-stimulating hormone (FSH) and luteinizing hormone (LH).

GnRH secretion can be inhibited by:
- pseudocyesis
- Kallmann's syndrome
- hypothalamic tumor
- stress or exercise.

Anterior pituitary increases production of FSH and LH.

Ovaries secrete estrogen.

Low progesterone and estrogen levels stimulate the hypothalamus.

Rising estrogen levels at mid-cycle stimulate the anterior pituitary to increase LH and FSH production.

Endometrium proliferates.

Normal uterine changes may be inhibited by:
- uterine hypoplasia
- uterine scarring
- radiation therapy.

Anovulation may result from:
- Turner's syndrome
- ovarian insensitivity to gonadotropins.

Ovulation occurs.

Endometrium hypertrophies.

Hormonal regulation may be disrupted by:
- adrenal disorders
- excessive corticotropin or prolactin production
- thyroid disorders.

Corpus luteum develops and secretes estrogen and progesterone.

Endometrium sloughs.

Corpus luteum recedes, which decreases estrogen and progesterone secretion.

Menstrual flow may be obstructed by:
- endometrial scarring
- cervical stenosis
- congenital defects.

Menstruation

■ If performing a pelvic examination, check for anatomic aberrations of the outflow tract.

Causes

Medical causes

Adrenal tumor

■ Amenorrhea may be accompanied by acne, thinning scalp hair, hirsutism, increased blood pressure, truncal obesity, and psychotic changes.
■ Asymmetrical ovarian enlargement and the rapid onset of signs of virilizing are key findings.

Adrenocortical hyperplasia

■ Amenorrhea precedes characteristic cushingoid signs, such as truncal obesity, moon face, "buffalo hump," bruises, purple striae, hypertension, renal calculi, psychiatric disturbances, and widened pulse pressure.
■ Thinning scalp hair and hirsutism typically appear.

Adrenocortical hypofunction

■ Amenorrhea, fatigue, irritability, weight loss, increased pigmentation, nausea, vomiting, and orthostatic hypotension may result.

Anorexia nervosa

■ Primary or secondary amenorrhea may occur.
■ Other signs and symptoms include weight loss, emaciated appearance, dry skin, compulsive behavior patterns, blotchy or sallow complexion, constipation, reduced libido, decreased pleasure in once-enjoyable activities, loss of scalp hair, lanugo (downy hair) on the face and arms, skeletal muscle atrophy, and sleep disturbances.

Congenital absence of ovaries and uterus

■ Primary amenorrhea and absence of secondary sex characteristics occur.

Corpus luteum cysts

■ Sudden amenorrhea may occur.
■ Abdominal pain and breast swelling may also occur.

Hypothyroidism

■ Amenorrhea may be primary or secondary.
■ Early signs and symptoms include fatigue, forgetfulness, cold intolerance, weight gain, and constipation.
■ Subsequent signs and symptoms include dry, flaky, inelastic skin; puffy face, hands, and feet; hoarseness; dry, sparse hair; thick, brittle nails; slow mental function; bradycardia; and myalgia.
■ Other common signs and symptoms include anorexia, abdominal distention, decreased libido, ataxia, intention tremor, nystagmus, and delayed reflex relaxation time.

Pituitary tumor

■ Amenorrhea may be the first sign.
■ Other findings include headache, vision disturbances, cushingoid signs, and acromegaly.

Polycystic ovary syndrome

■ Irregular menstrual cycles, oligomenorrhea, and secondary amenorrhea or periods of profuse bleeding may alternate with periods of amenorrhea.
■ Other signs and symptoms include obesity, hirsutism, slight deepening of the voice, and enlarged ovaries.

Pseudoamenorrhea

■ An anatomic anomaly obstructs menstrual flow, causing primary amenorrhea.
■ Examination may reveal a bulging pink or blue hymen.

Testicular feminization

■ Primary amenorrhea may indicate this form of male pseudohermaphroditism.

■ The patient is outwardly female but genetically male, with breast and external genital development but scant or absent pubic hair.

Thyrotoxicosis

■ Overproduction of thyroid hormone may cause amenorrhea.
■ Classic signs and symptoms include an enlarged thyroid gland, nervousness, heat intolerance, diaphoresis, tremors, palpitations, tachycardia, dyspnea, weakness, and weight loss despite increased appetite.

Turner's syndrome

■ Primary amenorrhea and failure to develop secondary sex characteristics may signal this syndrome.
■ Typical features include short stature, webbing of the neck, low nuchal hairline, a broad chest with widely spaced nipples, poor breast development, underdeveloped genitals, and edema of the legs and feet.

Other causes

Drugs

■ Busulfan (Myleran), chlorambucil (Leukeran), injectable or implanted contraceptives, cyclophosphamide (Cytoxan), and phenothiazines may cause amenorrhea.
■ Hormonal contraceptives may cause anovulation and amenorrhea when stopped.

Radiation therapy

■ Irradiation of the abdomen may damage the endometrium or ovaries, causing amenorrhea.

Surgery

■ Surgical removal of the ovaries or uterus produces amenorrhea.

Nursing considerations

■ In patients with secondary amenorrhea, rule out pregnancy before starting diagnostic testing.
■ Provide emotional support because amenorrhea can cause severe emotional distress.
■ Adolescent girls are prone to amenorrhea caused by emotional upsets stemming from school, social, or family problems.
■ In women older than age 50, amenorrhea usually represents the onset of menopause.

Patient teaching

■ Explain treatment and expected outcomes.
■ Encourage the patient to discuss her fears.
■ Refer the patient for psychological counseling, if needed.

Anuria

Clinically defined as urine output of less than 100 ml in 24 hours, anuria indicates either urinary tract obstruction or acute renal failure due to various mechanisms.

Fortunately, anuria is rare; even with renal failure, the kidneys usually produce at least 75 ml of urine daily.

Because urine output is easily measured, anuria rarely goes undetected. Without immediate treatment, it can rapidly cause uremia and other complications of urine retention.

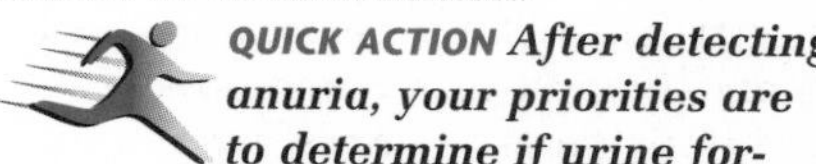

QUICK ACTION ***After detecting anuria, your priorities are to determine if urine formation is occurring and to intervene appropriately. Catheterize the patient to relieve any lower urinary tract obstruction and to check for residual urine. You may find that an obstruction hinders catheter insertion or that urine return is cloudy and foul smelling or bloody. If you collect more***

than 75 ml of urine, suspect lower urinary tract obstruction; if you collect less than 75 ml, suspect renal dysfunction or obstruction higher in the urinary tract.

History

- Ask about changes in voiding pattern.
- Determine the amount of fluid normally ingested and amount ingested in the past 24 to 48 hours.
- Note the time and amount of last urination.
- Ask about drug use.
- Obtain a medical history, noting previous renal or urinary tract disease, prostate problems, congenital abnormalities, and abdominal, renal, or urinary tract surgery.

Physical examination

- Inspect and palpate the abdomen for asymmetry, distention, or bulging.
- Inspect the flank area for edema or erythema.
- Percuss and palpate the bladder.
- Palpate the kidneys and percuss the costovertebral angle.
- Auscultate over the renal arteries for bruits.

Causes

Medical causes

Acute tubular necrosis

- Anuria occurs occasionally; oliguria (diminished urine output) is more common.
- Oliguria precedes the onset of diuresis.
- Other findings reflect the underlying cause and may include signs and symptoms of hyperkalemia, uremia, and heart failure.

Glomerulonephritis, acute

- Anuria or oliguria occurs.
- Other signs and symptoms include mild fever, malaise, flank pain, gross hematuria, edema, elevated blood pressure, headache, nausea, vomiting, abdominal pain, crackles, and dyspnea.

Hemolytic-uremic syndrome

- Anuria occurs in the initial stages and lasts 1 to 10 days.
- Other signs and symptoms include vomiting, diarrhea, abdominal pain, hematemesis, melena, purpura, fever, elevated blood pressure, hepatomegaly, ecchymoses, edema, hematuria, pallor, and signs of upper respiratory tract infection.

Renal artery occlusion, bilateral

- Anuria or severe oliguria is accompanied by severe, continuous upper abdominal and flank pain, nausea and vomiting, decreased bowel sounds, fever, and diastolic hypertension.

Renal vein occlusion, bilateral

- Anuria sometimes develops with lower back pain, fever, flank tenderness, and hematuria.
- Development of pulmonary emboli, a common complication, produces sudden dyspnea, pleuritic pain, tachypnea, tachycardia, crackles and, possibly, hemoptysis.

Urinary tract obstruction

- Acute or total anuria may alternate with or precede burning pain on urination, overflow incontinence or dribbling, urinary frequency and nocturia, voiding in small amounts, or an altered urine stream.
- Other signs and symptoms include bladder distention, pain and a sensation of fullness in the lower abdomen and groin, upper abdominal and flank pain, nausea and vomiting, and signs of secondary infection.

Other causes

Diagnostic tests

- Contrast media can cause nephrotoxicity, producing oliguria and, rarely, anuria.

Drugs

- Nephrotoxic drugs that can cause anuria or oliguria include antibiotics (especially aminoglycosides), adrenergics, anesthetics, anticholinergics, ethyl alcohol, heavy metals, and organic solvents.

Nursing considerations

- If catheterization fails to initiate urine flow, prepare the patient for diagnostic studies, such as ultrasonography, cystoscopy, retrograde pyelography, and renal scan to detect an obstruction higher in the urinary tract.
- If an obstruction is present, prepare the patient for surgery, and insert a nephrostomy tube or ureterostomy tube to drain the urine.
- Monitor the patient's vital signs and measure and record intake and output, saving urine for inspection.
- Restrict daily fluids to 600 ml more than the previous day's total urine output.
- Restrict foods and juices high in potassium and sodium.
- Have the patient maintain a balanced diet and control protein intake.
- Weigh the patient daily.
- In neonates, anuria is the absence of urine output for 24 hours.
- In children, anuria commonly results from loss of renal function.
- Hospitalized or bedridden patients may be unable to generate pressure to void in a supine position.

Patient teaching

- Discuss fluids and foods the patient should avoid.
- Instruct the patient on nephrostomy tube or ureterostomy tube care, if needed.

Anxiety

Anxiety, the most common psychiatric symptom, can cause significant impairment. A subjective reaction to a real or imagined threat, anxiety is a nonspecific feeling of uneasiness or dread that may be mild, moderate, or severe. Mild anxiety may cause slight physical or psychological discomfort. Severe anxiety may be incapacitating or even life-threatening.

Everyone experiences anxiety from time to time—it's a normal response to actual danger, prompting the body (through stimulation of the sympathetic and parasympathetic nervous systems) to action. Anxiety is a normal response to physical and emotional stress, which can be produced by virtually any illness. In addition, anxiety can be precipitated or exacerbated by many nonpathologic factors, including lack of sleep, poor diet, and excessive intake of caffeine or other stimulants. Excessive, unwarranted anxiety may indicate an underlying psychological problem or specific type of anxiety disorder.

History

- Determine the patient's chief complaint.
- Ask about the duration of the anxiety.
- Determine precipitating or exacerbating factors.
- Obtain a medical history, including drug use.

Physical examination

- Perform a physical examination.
- Focus on complaints that trigger or are aggravated by anxiety.
- Assess the patient's level of consciousness (LOC) and observe his behavior.

Causes

Medical causes

Acute respiratory distress syndrome

- Acute anxiety occurs along with tachycardia, mental sluggishness and, in severe cases, hypotension.
- Respiratory symptoms include dyspnea, tachypnea, intercostal and suprasternal retractions, crackles, and rhonchi.

Anaphylactic shock

- Acute anxiety signals the onset of anaphylactic shock.
- Anxiety is accompanied by urticaria, angioedema, pruritus, and shortness of breath.
- Others signs and symptoms include light-headedness, hypotension, tachycardia, nasal congestion, sneezing, wheezing, dyspnea, barking cough, abdominal cramps, vomiting, diarrhea, and urinary urgency and incontinence.

Angina pectoris

- Acute anxiety may precede or follow an attack.
- Sharp, crushing substernal or anterior chest pain may radiate to the back, neck, arms, or jaw during an attack.
- Nitroglycerin or rest may relieve the pain and anxiety.

Asthma

- Acute anxiety occurs with dyspnea, wheezing, productive cough, accessory muscle use, hyperresonant lung fields, diminished breath sounds, coarse crackles, cyanosis, tachycardia, and diaphoresis.

Autonomic hyperreflexia

- Anxiety, severe headache, and dramatic hypertension may be early signs.
- Pallor and motor and sensory deficits occur below the level of the lesion.
- Flushing occurs above the level of the lesion.

Cardiogenic shock

- Acute anxiety is accompanied by cool, pale, clammy skin; tachycardia; weak, thready pulse; tachypnea; ventricular gallop; crackles; jugular vein distention; decreased urine output; hypotension; narrowing pulse pressure; and peripheral edema.

Chronic obstructive pulmonary disease

- Acute anxiety occurs with exertional dyspnea, cough, wheezing, crackles, hyperresonant lung fields, tachypnea, and accessory muscle use.
- Other signs include "barrel" chest, pursed-lip breathing, and finger clubbing (late in the disease).

Heart failure

- Acute anxiety is a symptom of inadequate oxygenation.
- Other signs and symptoms include restlessness, shortness of breath, tachypnea, decreased LOC, edema, crackles, ventricular gallop, hypotension, diaphoresis, and cyanosis.

Hyperthyroidism

- Acute anxiety may be an early sign.
- Classic signs and symptoms include heat intolerance, weight loss despite increased appetite, nervousness, tremor, palpitations, sweating, an enlarged thyroid gland, exophthalmos, and diarrhea.

Hypoglycemia

- Mild to moderate anxiety occurs.
- Other signs and symptoms include hunger, mild headache, palpitations, blurred vision, weakness, and diaphoresis.

Mitral valve prolapse

- Panic may occur.
- A hallmark sign of mitral valve prolapse is a midsystolic click, followed by an apical murmur.

■ Paroxysmal palpitations with sharp, stabbing, or aching precordial pain may also occur.

Mood disorder

■ Anxiety may be the chief complaint in the depressive or manic form.

■ In the depressive form, the patient may exhibit dysphoria; anger; insomnia or hypersomnia; decreased libido, energy, and concentration; appetite disturbance; multiple somatic complaints; and suicidal thoughts.

■ In the manic form, the patient may exhibit a reduced need for sleep, hyperactivity, increased energy, rapid or pressured speech and, in severe cases, paranoid ideas and other psychotic symptoms.

Myocardial infarction

■ A life-threatening disorder, acute anxiety occurs with persistent, crushing substernal pain that may radiate.

■ Accompanying signs and symptoms include shortness of breath, nausea, vomiting, diaphoresis, and cool, pale skin.

Obsessive-compulsive disorder

■ Chronic anxiety occurs along with thoughts or impulses to perform ritualistic acts.

■ Anxiety builds if the patient can't perform rituals and diminishes if he can.

■ The patient recognizes the acts as irrational, but he can't control them.

Pheochromocytoma

■ Acute, severe anxiety accompanies the main sign of persistent or paroxysmal hypertension.

■ Common signs and symptoms include tachycardia, diaphoresis, orthostatic hypotension, tachypnea, flushing, severe headache, palpitations, nausea, vomiting, epigastric pain, and paresthesia.

Phobias

■ Chronic anxiety occurs with persistent fear of an object, activity, or situation that results in a strong desire to avoid it.

■ The patient recognizes the fear as irrational, but he can't suppress it.

Postconcussion syndrome

■ Chronic anxiety or periodic attacks of acute anxiety may occur, especially in situations demanding attention, judgment, or comprehension.

■ Other symptoms include irritability, insomnia, dizziness, and mild headache.

Posttraumatic stress disorder

■ Chronic anxiety occurs with intrusive, vivid thoughts and memories of the traumatic event.

■ The event is relived in dreams and nightmares.

■ Related symptoms include insomnia, depression, and feelings of numbness and detachment.

Pulmonary edema

■ Acute anxiety occurs along with dyspnea, orthopnea, cough with frothy sputum, tachycardia, tachypnea, crackles, ventricular gallop, hypotension, thready pulse, and cool, clammy skin.

Pulmonary embolism

■ Hypoxia may result in acute anxiety and restlessness.

■ Other signs and symptoms include dyspnea, tachypnea, chest pain, tachycardia, blood-tinged sputum, and low-grade fever.

Somatoform disorder

■ Anxiety and multiple somatic complaints (that can't be explained) are severe enough to impair functioning.

Other causes

Drugs

- Many drugs cause anxiety, especially sympathomimetics and central nervous system stimulants.
- Antidepressants may cause paradoxical anxiety.

Nursing considerations

- Provide a calm, quiet atmosphere.
- Stay with the patient during an acute attack.
- Encourage the patient to express his feelings and concerns freely.
- Encourage anxiety-reducing measures, such as distraction, relaxation techniques, or biofeedback.
- The autonomic signs of anxiety tend to be more common and dramatic in children than in adults.
- Distractions from ritualistic activity may provoke anxiety or agitation in elderly patients.

Patient teaching

- Teach the patient about relaxation techniques.
- Encourage the patient's verbalization of anxiety.
- Help the patient to identify stressors.
- Help the patient better understand different coping mechanisms.
- Help the patient identify support systems, such as family and friends.

Aphasia

Aphasia, impaired expression or comprehension of written or spoken language, reflects disease or injury of the brain's language centers.

Depending on its severity, aphasia may slightly impede communication or may make it impossible. It can be classified as Broca's, Wernicke's, anomic, or global aphasia. Anomic aphasia eventually resolves in more than 50% of patients, but global aphasia is usually irreversible. (See *Identifying types of aphasia*.)

QUICK ACTION ***Quickly look for signs and symptoms of stroke or increased intracranial pressure (ICP), such as pupillary changes, a decreased level of consciousness (LOC), vomiting, seizures, bradycardia, widening pulse pressure, and irregular respirations. If you detect signs of increased ICP, administer mannitol (Osmitrol) I.V. to decrease cerebral edema. In addition, make sure that emergency resuscitation equipment is readily available to support respiratory and cardiac function if necessary. You may have to prepare the patient for emergency surgery.***

History

- Obtain a medical history, noting headaches, hypertension, seizure disorders, or drug use.
- Determine the patient's preaphasia ability to communicate and perform routine tasks.

Physical examination

- Perform a complete neurologic examination.
- Check for obvious signs of neurologic deficit.
- Take the patient's vital signs and assess his LOC.
- Assess the patient's pupillary response, eye movements, and motor function.

Causes

Medical causes

Alzheimer's disease

- Anomic aphasia may begin insidiously and then progress to severe global aphasia.
- Incontinence is a late symptom.
- Other signs and symptoms include behavioral changes, loss of memory,

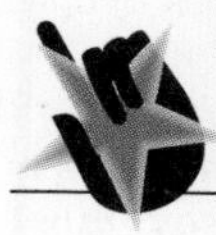

KNOW-HOW

Identifying types of aphasia

TYPE	LOCATION OF LESION	SIGNS AND SYMPTOMS
Anomic aphasia	Temporal-parietal area; may extend to angular gyrus, but sometimes poorly localized	The patient's understanding of written and spoken language is relatively unimpaired. His speech, although fluent, lacks meaningful content. Word-finding difficulty and circumlocution are characteristic. On rare occasions, the patient also displays paraphasias.
Broca's aphasia (expressive aphasia)	Broca's area; usually in third frontal convolution of the left hemisphere	The patient's understanding of written and spoken language is relatively spared, but speech lacks fluency, as evidenced by word-finding difficulty, use of jargon, paraphasias, limited vocabulary and simple sentence construction. He can't repeat words and phrases. If Wernicke's area is intact, he recognizes speech errors and shows frustration. He's commonly hemiparetic.
Global aphasia	Broca's and Wernicke's areas	The patient has profoundly impaired receptive and expressive ability. He can't repeat words or phrases and can't follow directions. His occasional speech is marked by paraphasias or jargon.
Wernicke's aphasia (receptive aphasia)	Wernicke's area; usually in posterior or superior temporal lobe	The patient has difficulty understanding written and spoken language. He can't repeat words or phrases and can't follow directions. His speech is fluent but may be rapid and rambling, with paraphasias. He has difficulty naming objects (anomia) and is unaware of speech errors.

poor judgment, restlessness, myoclonus, and muscle rigidity.

Brain abscess

- Any type of aphasia may occur.
- Aphasia may be accompanied by hemiparesis, ataxia, facial weakness, and signs of increased ICP.

Brain tumor

- Any type of aphasia may occur.
- As the tumor enlarges, behavioral changes, memory loss, motor weakness, seizures, auditory hallucinations, visual field deficits, and increased ICP may occur.

Creutzfeldt-Jakob disease

- Aphasia with a rapidly progressive dementia occurs.
- Other signs and symptoms may include myoclonic jerking, ataxia, vision disturbances, and paralysis.

Encephalitis

- Transient aphasia may occur.
- Early signs and symptoms include fever, headache, and vomiting.
- Other signs and symptoms include seizures, confusion, stupor or coma, hemiparesis, asymmetrical deep tendon reflexes, positive Babinski's reflex, ataxia, myoclonus, nystagmus, oculomotor palsies, and facial weakness.

Head trauma

- Sudden aphasia may occur.
- Aphasia may be transient or permanent, depending on the extent of brain damage.
- Other signs and symptoms include blurred or double vision, headache, pallor, diaphoresis, numbness and paresis, discharge containing cerebrospinal fluid from the ear or nose, altered respirations, tachycardia, behavioral changes, and increased ICP.

Seizure disorder

- Transient aphasia may occur if the seizures involve the language centers.

Stroke

- Wernicke's, Broca's, or global aphasia may occur.
- Other symptoms include decreased LOC, right-sided hemiparesis, homonymous hemianopsia, paresthesia, and loss of sensation.

Transient ischemic attack

- Sudden aphasia occurs, but resolves within 24 hours.
- Other symptoms include transient hemiparesis, hemianopsia, paresthesia, dizziness, and confusion.

Nursing considerations

- Tell the patient what has happened, where he is and why, and what the date is.
- Expect periods of depression as the patient recognizes his disability.
- Help the patient communicate by providing a relaxed environment with minimal distracting stimuli.
- Recognize that the term *childhood aphasia* is sometimes mistakenly applied to children who fail to develop normal language skills but who aren't considered mentally retarded or developmentally delayed. *Aphasia* refers solely to loss of previously developed communication skills.
- Brain damage associated with aphasia in children most commonly follows anoxia—the result of near drowning or airway obstruction.
- When assessing speech in an elderly patient, make sure that his dentures and hearing aid are in place.

Patient teaching

- Discuss alternate means of communication.
- Discuss risk reduction factors for stroke.

Apnea

Apnea, the cessation of spontaneous respiration, is occasionally temporary and self-limiting, as occurs during Cheyne-Stokes and Biot's respirations. More commonly, it's a life-threatening emergency that requires immediate intervention to prevent death.

Apnea usually results from one or more of six pathophysiologic mechanisms, each of which has numerous causes. Its most common causes include trauma, cardiac arrest, neurologic disease, aspiration of foreign objects, bronchospasm, and drug overdose. (See *Causes of apnea.*)

QUICK ACTION ***If you detect apnea, first establish and maintain a patent airway. Position the patient in a supine position and open his airway using the head-tilt, chin-lift technique.*** **(Caution: *If the patient has an obvious or suspected head or neck injury, use the jaw-thrust technique to prevent hyperextending the neck.) Next, quickly look, listen, and feel for spontaneous respiration; if it's absent, begin artificial ventilation until it occurs or until mechanical ventilation can be initiated.***

Because apnea may result from cardiac arrest (or may cause it), assess the patient's carotid pulse immediate-

Causes of apnea

Apnea may result from several causes, including airway obstruction, brain stem dysfunction, neuromuscular failure, parenchymatous lung disease, pleural pressure gradient disruption, and a decrease in pulmonary capillary perfusion. Each of these causes can result from many disorders, listed here.

Airway obstruction

- Asthma
- Bronchospasm
- Chronic bronchitis
- Chronic obstructive pulmonary disease
- Foreign body aspiration
- Hemothorax or pneumothorax
- Mucus plug
- Obstruction by tongue or tumor
- Obstructive sleep apnea
- Secretion retention
- Tracheal or bronchial rupture

Brain stem dysfunction

- Brain abscess
- Brain stem injury
- Brain tumor
- Central nervous system depressants
- Central sleep apnea
- Cerebral hemorrhage
- Cerebral infarction
- Encephalitis
- Head trauma
- Increased intracranial pressure
- Medullary or pontine hemorrhage or infarction
- Meningitis
- Transtentorial herniation

Neuromuscular failure

- Amyotrophic lateral sclerosis
- Botulism
- Diphtheria
- Guillain-Barré syndrome
- Myasthenia gravis
- Phrenic nerve paralysis
- Rupture of the diaphragm
- Spinal cord injury

Parenchymatous lung disease

- Acute respiratory distress syndrome
- Diffuse pneumonia
- Emphysema
- Near drowning
- Pulmonary edema
- Pulmonary fibrosis
- Secretion retention

Pleural pressure gradient disruption

- Flail chest
- Open chest wounds

Pulmonary capillary perfusion decrease

- Arrhythmias
- Cardiac arrest
- Myocardial infarction
- Pulmonary embolism
- Pulmonary hypertension
- Shock

ly after you have established a patent airway. If the patient is an infant or small child, assess the brachial pulse instead. If you can't palpate a pulse, begin cardiac compression.

History

- Investigate the underlying cause of apnea. Ask him (or, if he's unable to answer, anyone who witnessed the episode) about the onset of apnea and events immediately preceding it.

■ Take a patient history, especially noting reports of headache, chest pain, muscle weakness, sore throat, or dyspnea.
■ Ask about a history of respiratory, cardiac, or neurologic disease.
■ Ask about allergies and drug use.

Physical examination

■ Inspect the head, face, neck, and trunk for soft-tissue injury, hemorrhage, or skeletal deformity.
■ Don't overlook obvious clues, such as oral and nasal secretions (reflecting fluid-filled airways and alveoli) or facial soot and singed nasal hair (suggesting thermal injury to the tracheobronchial tree).
■ Auscultate over all lung lobes for adventitious breath sounds, particularly crackles and rhonchi, and percuss the lung fields for increased dullness or hyperresonance.
■ Auscultate the heart for murmurs, pericardial friction rub, and arrhythmias.
■ Check for cyanosis, pallor, jugular vein distention, and edema.
■ If appropriate, perform a neurologic assessment. Evaluate the patient's level of consciousness (LOC), orientation, and mental status; test cranial nerve and motor function, sensation, and reflexes in all extremities.

Causes

Medical causes

Airway obstruction

■ Occlusion or compression of the trachea, central airways, or smaller airways can cause sudden apnea by blocking the patient's airflow.
■ Acute respiratory failure may also occur.

Brain stem dysfunction

■ Primary or secondary brain stem dysfunction can cause apnea by destroying the brain stem's ability to initiate respirations.
■ Apnea may arise suddenly (as in trauma, hemorrhage, or infarction) or gradually (as in degenerative disease or tumor).
■ Apnea may be preceded by decreased LOC and various motor and sensory deficits.

Neuromuscular failure

■ Trauma or disease can disrupt the mechanics of respiration, causing sudden or gradual apnea.
■ Associated symptoms include diaphragmatic or intercostal muscle paralysis from injury, or respiratory weakness or paralysis from acute or degenerative disease.

Parenchymatous lung disease

■ An accumulation of fluid within the alveoli produces apnea by interfering with pulmonary gas exchange and producing acute respiratory failure.
■ Apnea may arise suddenly, as in near drowning and acute pulmonary edema, or gradually, as in emphysema.
■ Apnea may also be preceded by crackles and labored respirations with accessory muscle use.

Pleural pressure gradient disruption

■ Conversion of normal negative pleural air pressure to positive pressure by chest wall injuries (such as flail chest) causes lung collapse, producing respiratory distress and, if untreated, apnea.
■ Associated signs and symptoms include an asymmetrical chest wall and asymmetrical or paradoxical respirations.

Pulmonary capillary perfusion decrease

■ Apnea can stem from obstructed pulmonary circulation, most commonly due to heart failure or lack of circulatory patency.

■ It occurs suddenly in cardiac arrest, massive pulmonary embolism, and most cases of severe shock, and it occurs progressively in septic shock and pulmonary hypertension.
■ Other signs and symptoms include hypotension, tachycardia, and edema.

Sleep-related apneas
■ These repetitive apneas occur during sleep from airflow obstruction or brain stem dysfunction deficits.

Other causes
Drugs
■ Central nervous system (CNS) depressants may cause hypoventilation and apnea.
■ Benzodiazepines may cause respiratory depression and apnea when given I.V., along with other CNS depressants, to elderly or acutely ill patients.
■ Neuromuscular blockers—such as curariform drugs and anticholinesterases—may produce sudden apnea due to respiratory muscle paralysis.

Nursing considerations
■ Closely monitor the apneic patient's cardiac and respiratory status to prevent further apneic episodes.
■ Provide oxygen and ventilation, as necessary, and monitor arterial blood gas values and pulse oximetry effectiveness.
■ Premature neonates are especially susceptible to periodic apneic episodes because of CNS immaturity.
■ Other common causes of apnea in infants include sepsis, intraventricular and subarachnoid hemorrhage, seizures, bronchiolitis, and sudden infant death syndrome.
■ In toddlers and older children, the primary cause of apnea is acute airway obstruction from aspiration of foreign objects. Other causes include acute epiglottiditis, croup, asthma, and systemic disorders, such as muscular dystrophy and cystic fibrosis.
■ In elderly patients, increased sensitivity to analgesics, sedative-hypnotics, or a combination of these drugs may produce apnea, even with normal dosage ranges.

Patient teaching
■ Educate the patient about safety measures related to aspiration of medications.
■ Encourage cardiopulmonary resuscitation training for all adolescents and adults.

Ataxia

Classified as cerebellar or sensory, ataxia refers to incoordination and irregularity of voluntary, purposeful movements. Cerebellar ataxia results from disease of the cerebellum and its pathways to and from the cerebral cortex, brain stem, and spinal cord. It causes gait, trunk, limb, and possibly speech disorders. Sensory ataxia results from impaired position sense (proprioception) due to the interruption of afferent nerve fibers in the peripheral nerves, posterior roots, posterior columns of the spinal cord, or medial lemnisci or, occasionally, caused by a lesion in both parietal lobes. It causes gait disorders. (See *Identifying ataxia,* page 28.)

Ataxia occurs in acute and chronic forms. Acute ataxia may result from stroke, hemorrhage, or a large tumor in the posterior fossa. With this life-threatening condition, the cerebellum may herniate downward through the foramen magnum behind the cervical spinal cord or upward through the tentorium on the cerebral hemispheres. Herniation may also compress the brain stem. Acute ataxia may also result from drug toxicity or poisoning. Chronic ataxia can be progressive and, at times, can result from acute disease. It can also

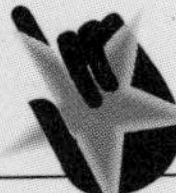

KNOW-HOW

Identifying ataxia

Ataxia may be observed in the patient's speech, in the movements of his trunk and limbs, or in his gait.

Cerebellar ataxia

With cerebellar ataxia, the patient may stagger or lurch in a zigzag fashion, turn with extreme difficulty, and lose his balance when his feet are together.

Gait ataxia

With gait ataxia, the patient's gait is widely spaced, unsteady, and irregular.

Limb ataxia

With limb ataxia, the patient loses the ability to gauge distance, speed, and power of movement, resulting in poorly controlled, variable, and inaccurate voluntary movements. He may move too quickly or too slowly, or his movements may break down into component parts, giving him the appearance of a puppet or robot. Other effects include a coarse, irregular tremor in purposeful movement (but not at rest) and reduced muscle tone.

Sensory ataxia

With sensory ataxia, the patient moves abruptly and stomps or taps his feet. This occurs because he throws his feet forward and outward, and then brings them down first on the heels and then on the toes. The patient also fixes his eyes on the ground, watching his steps. If he can't watch them, staggering worsens. When he stands with his feet together, he sways or loses his balance.

Speech ataxia

Speech ataxia is a form of dysarthria in which the patient typically speaks slowly and abnormally stresses certain words and syllables. Speech content is unaffected.

Truncal ataxia

Truncal ataxia is a disturbance in equilibrium in which the patient can't sit or stand without falling. Also, his head and trunk may bob and sway (titubation). If he can walk, his gait is reeling.

occur in metabolic and chronic degenerative neurologic disease.

QUICK ACTION ***If ataxic movements suddenly develop, examine the patient for signs of increased intracranial pressure and impending herniation. Determine his level of consciousness (LOC), and be alert for pupillary changes, motor weakness or paralysis, neck stiffness or pain, and vomiting. Check his vital signs, especially respirations; abnormal respiratory patterns may quickly lead to respiratory arrest. Elevate the head of the bed. Have emergency resuscitation equipment readily available. Prepare the patient for a computed tomography scan or surgery.***

History

- Ask about a history of multiple sclerosis, diabetes, central nervous system infection, neoplastic disease, or stroke.
- Inquire about a family history of ataxia.
- Ask about chronic alcohol abuse or prolonged exposure to industrial toxins.
- Find out if the ataxia developed suddenly or gradually.

Physical examination

- Perform Romberg's test to help distinguish between cerebellar and sensory ataxia.
- Check motor strength.

Causes

Medical causes

Cerebellar abscess

- Limb ataxia occurs on the same side as the lesion, with gait and truncal ataxia.
- The initial symptom is headache localized behind the ear or in the occipital region.
- Other signs and symptoms include oculomotor palsy, fever, vomiting, altered LOC, and coma.

Cerebellar hemorrhage

- In this life-threatening disorder, ataxia is usually acute but transient; it may affect the trunk, gait, or limbs.
- Initial signs and symptoms include repeated vomiting, occipital headache, vertigo, oculomotor palsy, dysphagia, and dysarthria.
- Late symptoms, such as decreased LOC or coma, signal impending herniation.

Creutzfeldt-Jakob disease

- Ataxia accompanies other neurologic signs, such as myoclonic jerking, aphasia, and rapidly progressing dementia.

Diabetic neuropathy

- Peripheral nerve damage may cause sensory ataxia.
- Other signs and symptoms include arm or leg pain, slight leg weakness, skin changes, bowel and bladder dysfunction, unsteady gait and, as neuropathy progresses, numbness in the feet.

Diphtheria

- In this life-threatening disorder, sensory ataxia may occur within 4 to 8 weeks of the onset of symptoms.
- Other symptoms include fever, paresthesia, and paralysis of the limbs and, sometimes, the respiratory muscles.

Hepatocerebral degeneration

- Residual neurologic defects, including mild cerebellar ataxia with a wide-based and unsteady gait, occur in those who survive hepatic coma.
- Other signs and symptoms include altered LOC, dysarthria, rhythmic arm tremors, and choreoathetosis of the face, neck, and shoulders.

Hyperthermia

- If the patient survives the coma and seizures characteristic of the acute phase, cerebellar ataxia can occur.
- Subsequent symptoms include spastic paralysis, dementia, and slowly resolving confusion.

Metastatic cancer

- If cancer metastasizes to the cerebellum, gait ataxia may occur along with headache, dizziness, muscle incoordination, nystagmus, decreased LOC, nausea, and vomiting.
- The patient may fall toward the side of the lesion.

Multiple sclerosis

- Cerebellar ataxia may occur.
- Spinal cord involvement may cause speech and sensory ataxia.
- Ataxia may subside or disappear during remissions.
- Other signs and symptoms include optic neuritis, optic atrophy, numbness and weakness, diplopia, dizziness, and bladder dysfunction.

Polyarteritis nodosa

- Sensory ataxia, abdominal and limb pain, hematuria, and elevated blood pressure may occur.

■ Other signs and symptoms include myalgia, headache, joint pain, and weakness.

Polyneuropathy
■ Ataxia, severe motor weakness, muscle atrophy, and sensory loss in the limbs occur.
■ Pain and skin changes may also occur.

Posterior fossa tumor
■ Gait, truncal, or limb ataxia is an early sign; ataxia may worsen as the tumor enlarges.
■ Other signs and symptoms include vomiting, headache, papilledema, vertigo, oculomotor palsy, decreased LOC, and motor and sensory impairment on the same side as the lesion.

Spinocerebellar ataxia
■ Fatigue occurs initially, followed by stiff-legged gait ataxia.
■ Eventually, limb ataxia, dysarthria, static tremor, nystagmus, cramps, paresthesia, and sensory deficits occur.

Stroke
■ Infarction in the medulla, pons, or cerebellum may lead to ataxia, which may remain as a residual symptom.
■ Worsening ataxia during the acute phase may indicate extension of stroke or severe swelling of the brain.
■ Accompanying signs and symptoms include motor weakness, sensory loss, vertigo, nausea, vomiting, oculomotor palsy, dysphagia and, possibly, altered LOC.

Wernicke's encephalopathy
■ Gait ataxia occurs.
■ With severe ataxia, the patient may not be able to stand or walk.
■ Other signs and symptoms include nystagmus, diplopia, oculomotor palsies, confusion, tachycardia, exertional dyspnea, and orthostatic hypotension.

Other causes

Drugs
■ Aminoglutethimide (Cytadren) may cause ataxia that disappears 4 to 6 weeks after the drug is stopped.
■ Toxic levels of anticonvulsants, anticholinergics, and tricyclic antidepressants may result in ataxia.

Poisoning
■ Chronic arsenic poisoning may cause sensory ataxia along with headache, seizures, altered LOC, motor deficits, and muscle aches.
■ Chronic mercury poisoning causes gait and limb ataxia, principally of the arms as well as dysarthria, mood changes, mental confusion, and tremors of the extremities, tongue, and lips.

Nursing considerations

■ If toxic drug levels are the cause, stop the drug.
■ Encourage physical therapy to improve function following a stroke.
■ If the patient has a brain tumor, prepare him for surgery, chemotherapy, or radiation therapy.

Patient teaching

■ Help the patient to identify rehabilitation goals.
■ Stress safety measures.
■ Discuss the use of assistive devices.
■ Refer the patient to counseling as needed.

B

Back pain

Back pain affects an estimated 80% of the population. In fact, it's the second leading reason—after the common cold—for lost time from work. Although this symptom may indicate a disorder of the vertebrae (spondylogenic), it may also result from a genitourinary, GI, cardiovascular, or neoplastic disorder, or from trauma or injury. Postural imbalance associated with pregnancy may also cause back pain.

The onset, location, and distribution of pain and its response to activity and rest provide important clues about the cause. Pain may be acute or chronic, constant or intermittent. It may remain localized in the back or radiate along the spine or down one or both legs. Pain may be worsened by activity—usually bending, stooping, lifting, or exercising—and alleviated by rest, or it may be unaffected by either.

Intrinsic back pain results from muscle spasm, nerve root irritation, fracture, or a combination of these mechanisms. It usually occurs in the lower back, or lumbosacral area. Back pain may also be referred from the abdomen or flank, possibly signaling a life-threatening perforated ulcer, acute pancreatitis, or dissecting abdominal aortic aneurysm.

QUICK ACTION ***If the patient reports acute, severe back pain, quickly check his vital signs, and then perform a rapid evaluation to rule out life-threatening causes. Ask him when the pain began. Can he relate it to any cause? For example, did the pain occur after eating? After falling on the ice? Have the patient describe the pain. Is it burning, stabbing, throbbing, or aching? Is it constant or intermittent? Does it radiate to the buttocks or legs? Does he have leg weakness? Does the pain seem to originate in the abdomen and radiate to the back? Has he had a pain like this before? What makes it better or worse? Is the pain affected by activity or rest? Is it worse in the morning or evening? Does it wake him up?***

Typically, visceral referred back pain is unaffected by activity and rest. In contrast, spondylogenic referred back pain worsens with activity and improves with rest. Pain of neoplastic origin is usually relieved by walking and worsens at night.

If the patient describes deep lumbar pain unaffected by activity, palpate for a pulsating epigastric mass. If this sign is present, suspect a dissecting abdominal aortic aneurysm. Withhold food and fluids in anticipation of emergency surgery. Prepare for I.V. fluid replacement and oxygen administration. Monitor the patient's vital signs and peripheral pulses closely.

If the patient describes severe epigastric pain that radiates through the abdomen to the back, assess him for absent bowel sounds and abdominal rigidity and tenderness. If these occur,

suspect a perforated ulcer or acute pancreatitis. Start an I.V. line for fluids and drugs, administer oxygen, and insert a nasogastric tube while withholding food.

History

- Obtain a medical, family, and drug history.
- Ask about unusual sensations in the legs.
- Ask about diet and alcohol use.

Physical examination

- Observe skin color, especially in the legs.
- Observe posture and body alignment.
- Palpate skin temperature and femoral, popliteal, posterior tibial, and pedal pulses.
- Ask the patient to bend forward, backward, and side to side while you palpate for paravertebral muscle spasms.
- Palpate the dorsolumbar spine for point tenderness.
- Ask the patient to walk—first on his heels and then on his toes.
- Evaluate Babinski's reflexes and the patellar and Achilles tendons.
- Evaluate the strength of the extensor hallucis longus by asking the patient to hold up his big toe against resistance.
- Measure leg length and hamstring and quadriceps muscles.
- Position the patient supine. Grasp his heel and slowly lift his leg. Note the exact location of the pain and the angle between the table and his leg when it occurs. Repeat this maneuver with the opposite leg.
- Note range of motion of the hip and knee.
- Palpate and percuss the flanks to elicit costovertebral angle (CVA) tenderness.

Causes

Medical causes

Abdominal aortic aneurysm, dissecting

- In this life-threatening disorder, lower back pain or dull abdominal pain may initially occur; however, upper abdominal pain is more common.
- A pulsating epigastric mass may be palpated; pulsating stops after rupture.
- Other signs and symptoms include mottled skin below the waist, absent femoral and pedal pulses, blood pressure lower in the legs than in the arms, abdominal rigidity, mild to moderate tenderness with guarding, and shock (if blood loss is significant).

Ankylosing spondylitis

- Sacroiliac pain radiates up the spine and is aggravated by pressure on the side of the pelvis.
- Pain is usually most severe in the morning or after a period of inactivity and isn't relieved by rest.
- Abnormal rigidity of the lumbar spine with forward flexion is common.
- Other signs and symptoms include local tenderness, fatigue, fever, anorexia, weight loss, and occasional iritis.

Intervertebral disk rupture

- Gradual or sudden lower back pain occurs with or without sciatica.
- Pain begins in the back and radiates to the buttocks and legs.
- Pain is worsened by activity, coughing, and sneezing, and is eased by rest.
- The patient walks slowly and rises from sitting to standing with extreme difficulty.
- Other signs and symptoms include paresthesia, paravertebral muscle spasm, and decreased reflexes on the affected side.

Lumbosacral sprain

- Aching, localized pain and tenderness are associated with muscle spasm caused by sideways motion.
- Flexion of the spine and movement intensify the pain; rest and lying down with the knees bent and the hips flexed relieves it.

Pancreatitis, acute

- In this life-threatening disorder, upper abdominal pain may radiate to the flanks and back.
- Bending forward, drawing the knees to the chest, or moving around may relieve pain.
- Early signs and symptoms include abdominal tenderness, nausea, vomiting, fever, pallor, tachycardia, hypoactive bowel sounds, rebound tenderness, and abdominal guarding and rigidity.
- Turner's sign (ecchymosis of the abdomen or flank) or Cullen's sign (bluish discoloration of skin around the umbilicus and in both flanks) signals hemorrhagic pancreatitis.

Perforated ulcer

- In this life-threatening disorder, sudden, prostrating epigastric pain may radiate throughout the abdomen and to the back.
- Other signs and symptoms include boardlike abdominal rigidity, tenderness with guarding, generalized rebound tenderness, absent bowel sounds, fever, tachycardia, hypotension, and grunting, shallow respirations.

Prostate cancer

- Chronic, aching back pain may be the only symptom, appearing in advanced stages.
- Other late signs and symptoms include hematuria, difficulty initiating a urine stream, dribbling, urine retention, unexplained cystitis, and a decrease in the urine stream.

Pyelonephritis, acute

- Progressive flank and lower abdominal pain accompanies back pain or tenderness (especially over the CVA).
- Other signs and symptoms include high fever and chills, nausea, vomiting, flank and abdominal tenderness, and urinary frequency and urgency.

Renal calculi

- Colicky pain travels from the CVA to the flank, suprapubic region, and external genitalia.
- If calculi travel down a ureter, the patient may feel excruciating pain.
- If calculi are in the renal pelvis and calyces, the patient may feel dull and constant flank pain.
- Other signs and symptoms include nausea, vomiting, urinary urgency, hematuria, and agitation.

Sacroiliac strain

- Sacroiliac pain may radiate to the buttock, hip, and lateral aspect of the thigh.
- Weight bearing on the affected side and abduction with resistance of the leg aggravates the pain.

Spinal stenosis

- Back pain occurs with or without sciatica.
- Pain may radiate to the toes and, if the patient doesn't rest, may progress to numbness or weakness.

Transverse process fractures and vertebral compression fractures

- In a transverse process fracture, severe, localized back pain occurs with muscle spasm and hematoma.
- In a vertebral compression fracture, pain may not occur for several weeks; then, back pain aggravated by weight bearing and local tenderness occurs.

Vertebral osteoporosis

- Chronic, aching back pain is aggravated by activity and relieved (somewhat) by rest.
- Vertebral collapse, causing a backache with pain that radiates around the trunk, is the most common characteristic.

Nursing considerations

- If the cause of back pain is life-threatening, monitor the patient closely.
- Look for increasing pain, altered neurovascular condition of the legs, loss of bowel or bladder control, altered vital signs, sweating, and cyanosis.
- Withhold food and fluids in case surgery is needed.
- Elevate the head of the bed and place a pillow under the patient's knees.
- Fit the patient for a corset or lumbosacral support.
- Apply heat or cold therapy, backboard, foam mattress, or pelvic traction.
- In children, back pain may stem from diskitis, neoplasms, idiopathic juvenile osteoporosis, and spondylolisthesis.

Patient teaching

- Provide information about the use of anti-inflammatory drugs and analgesics.
- Discuss lifestyle changes, such as losing weight or correcting posture.
- Teach relaxation techniques such as deep breathing.
- Instruct the patient on the correct use of a corset or lumbosacral support.
- Provide information about alternatives to drug therapy, such as biofeedback and transcutaneous electrical nerve stimulation.

Battle's sign

Battle's sign appears as ecchymosis over the mastoid process of the temporal bone. Commonly, it's the only outward sign of a basilar skull fracture. In fact, this type of fracture may go undetected even by skull X-rays. If left untreated, it can be fatal because of associated injury to the nearby cranial nerves and brain stem as well as to blood vessels and the meninges.

Appearing behind one or both ears, Battle's sign is easily overlooked or hidden by the patient's hair. During emergency care of a trauma victim, it may be overshadowed by more apparent or imminently life-threatening injuries.

Battle's sign is caused by a force that's strong enough to fracture the base of the skull. Such an impact damages supporting tissues of the mastoid area and leads to a seepage of blood from the fracture site to the mastoid. Battle's sign usually develops 24 to 36 hours after the fracture and may persist for several days to weeks.

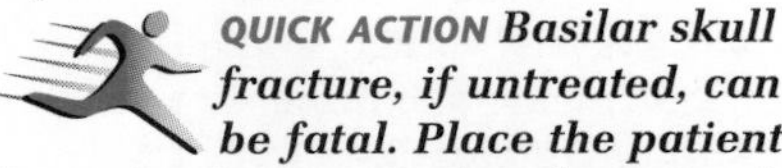

QUICK ACTION ***Basilar skull fracture, if untreated, can be fatal. Place the patient flat on his back in bed and monitor his neurologic status. If the patient has a large dural tear, prepare him for a craniotomy.***

History

- Ask about recent trauma, such as a severe blow to the head or a motor vehicle accident.

Physical examination

- Perform a complete neurologic examination, including mental status and speech, cranial nerve function, sensory and motor function, and reflexes.
- Assess the patient's level of consciousness (LOC).
- Check the patient's vital signs, and look for signs of increased intracranial pressure.
- Evaluate pupil size, response to light, and motor and verbal responses; relate data to the Glasgow Coma Scale.

- Note cerebrospinal fluid (CSF) leakage from the nose or ears.
- Test leakage with a glucose reagent strip to confirm that it's CSF. (If it's CSF, the strip will indicate the presence of glucose.)
- Look for the "halo" sign on bed linens or dressings.
- Perform a complete physical examination of all body systems.

Causes

Medical causes

Basilar skull fracture

- Battle's sign may be the only outward sign.
- Other signs and symptoms include periorbital ecchymosis ("raccoon" eyes), conjunctival hemorrhage, nystagmus, ocular deviation, epistaxis, anosmia, visible fracture lines on the external auditory canal, tinnitus, difficulty hearing, facial paralysis, vertigo, and a bulging tympanic membrane (from accumulation of CSF or blood).

Nursing considerations

- Keep the patient flat to decrease pressure on dural tears and to minimize CSF leakage.
- Monitor the patient's neurologic status.
- Avoid nasogastric intubation and nasopharyngeal suction, either of which may cause cerebral infection.
- Caution the patient against blowing his nose, which may worsen a dural tear.
- Prepare the patient for diagnostic tests, such as skull X-rays and computed tomography scan.
- Explain to the patient that basilar skull fracture and associated dural tears typically heal spontaneously within several days to weeks.
- Because a large dural tear may require a craniotomy to repair the tear with a graft patch, prepare the patient for surgery as indicated.
- Victims of abuse frequently sustain basilar skull fractures.
- If you suspect abuse, follow protocol for reporting the incident.

Patient teaching

- Explain what activities the patient should avoid, and emphasize the importance of bed rest.
- Explain to the patient or caregiver the signs and symptoms to look for and report, such as changes in mental status, LOC, or breathing.
- Tell the patient to take acetaminophen (Tylenol) for headaches.
- Explain what diagnostic tests the patient may need.
- Discuss the prospect of surgery with the patient, and respond to his questions and concerns.

Bladder distention

Bladder distention—abnormal enlargement of the bladder—results from an inability to excrete urine, which results in its accumulation. Distention can be caused by a mechanical or an anatomic obstruction, a neuromuscular disorder, or the use of certain drugs.

Distention usually develops gradually, but it occasionally has a sudden onset. Gradual distention usually remains asymptomatic until stretching of the bladder causes discomfort. Acute distention produces suprapubic fullness, pressure, and pain. If severe distention isn't corrected promptly by catheterization or massage, the bladder rises within the abdomen, its walls become thin, and renal function can be impaired.

Bladder distention is aggravated by the intake of caffeine, alcohol, large quantities of fluid, and diuretics.

QUICK ACTION ***If the patient has severe distention, insert an indwelling urinary catheter to help relieve discomfort and prevent bladder rupture. If more than***

700 ml is emptied from the bladder, compressed blood vessels dilate and may make the patient feel faint. Typically, the indwelling urinary catheter is clamped for 30 to 60 minutes to permit vessel compensation.

History

- Ask about voiding patterns and characteristics.
- Find out the time and amount of the patient's last voiding.
- Determine the amount of fluid consumed since last voiding.
- Obtain a medical history, including urinary tract obstruction or infections; sexually transmitted disease; neurologic, intestinal, or pelvic surgery; lower abdominal or urinary tract trauma; and systemic or neurologic disorders.
- Note drug history, including the use of over-the-counter drugs.

Physical examination

- Take the patient's vital signs.
- Percuss and palpate the bladder.
- Inspect the urethral meatus and measure its diameter.
- Note the appearance and amount of discharge.
- Test for perineal sensation and anal sphincter tone.
- Digitally examine the prostate gland (in men).

Causes

Medical causes

Benign prostatic hyperplasia

- Bladder distention develops gradually as the prostate enlarges.
- Initial signs and symptoms include urinary hesitancy, straining, and frequency; reduced force of the urine stream and the inability to stop the stream; nocturia; and postvoiding dribbling.
- Later signs and symptoms include prostate enlargement, perineal pain, constipation, hematuria, and sensations of suprapubic fullness and incomplete bladder emptying.

Multiple sclerosis

- Urine retention and bladder distention result from interrupted upper-motor-neuron control of the bladder.
- Other signs and symptoms include optic neuritis, paresthesia, impaired senses of position and vibration, diplopia, nystagmus, dizziness, abnormal reflexes, dysarthria, muscle weakness, emotional lability, Lhermitte's sign (transient, electric-like shocks that spread down the body when the head is dropped forward), Babinski's sign, and ataxia.

Prostatitis

- Bladder distention occurs rapidly along with perineal discomfort and suprapubic fullness.
- Other signs and symptoms include perineal pain; a tense, boggy, tender, and warm enlarged prostate; decreased libido; impotence; decreased force of the urine stream; dysuria; hematuria; urinary frequency and urgency; fatigue; malaise; myalgia; fever; chills; nausea; and vomiting.

Spinal neoplasms

- Upper-neuron control of the bladder is disrupted, causing neurogenic bladder and distention.
- Other signs and symptoms include a sense of pelvic fullness, continuous overflow dribbling, back pain that typically mimics sciatic pain, constipation, tender vertebral processes, sensory deficits, and muscle weakness, flaccidity, and atrophy.

Urethral calculi

- Urethral obstruction causes bladder distention and interrupted urine flow.

- Pain from the obstruction radiates to the penis or vulva and then to the perineum or rectum.
- A palpable calculus and urethral discharge may also be present.

Other causes

Catheterization

- Urine retention and bladder distention may occur from a kinked tube or an occluded lumen.

Drugs

- Anesthetics, anticholinergics, ganglionic blockers, opioids, parasympatholytics, and sedatives may cause urine retention and bladder distention.

Nursing considerations

- Monitor the patient's vital signs and the extent of bladder distention.
- Encourage the patient to change positions to alleviate discomfort.
- Give analgesics if needed.
- Prepare the patient for surgery as needed.
- Provide privacy for voiding and encourage a normal voiding position.
- Look for urine retention and bladder distention in an infant who fails to void normal amounts of urine.
- In boys, posterior urethral valves, meatal stenosis, phimosis, spinal cord anomalies, bladder diverticula, and other congenital defects may cause urinary obstruction and resultant bladder distention.
- Bladder distention is most common in elderly men with prostate disorders that cause urine retention.

Patient teaching

- Teach the patient to use Valsalva's maneuver or Credé's method to empty the bladder.
- Explain how to stimulate voiding.

Blood pressure, decreased

Low blood pressure is intravascular pressure that's inadequate to maintain the oxygen requirements of the body's tissues. Although commonly linked to shock, this sign may also result from a cardiovascular, respiratory, neurologic, or metabolic disorder. Hypoperfusion states especially affect the kidneys, brain, and heart, and may lead to renal failure, a change in the patient's level of consciousness (LOC), or myocardial ischemia. Low blood pressure may be drug-induced or may accompany diagnostic tests—most commonly those using contrast media. It may stem from stress or a change of position, such as rising abruptly from a supine or sitting position to a standing position (orthostatic hypotension).

Normal blood pressure varies considerably; what qualifies as low blood pressure for one person may be normal for another. Consequently, every blood pressure reading must be compared against the patient's baseline. Typically, a reading below 90/60 mm Hg, or a drop of 30 mm Hg from the baseline, is considered low blood pressure.

Low blood pressure can reflect an expanded intravascular space (as in severe infections, allergic reactions, or adrenal insufficiency), reduced intravascular volume (as in dehydration and hemorrhage), or decreased cardiac output (as in impaired cardiac muscle contractility). Because the body's pressure-regulating mechanisms are complex and interrelated, it's usually a combination of these factors that contributes to low blood pressure.

QUICK ACTION ***If the patient's systolic pressure is less than 80 mm Hg, or 30 mm Hg below his baseline, suspect shock.***

Quickly evaluate the patient for a decreased LOC. Check his apical pulse for tachycardia and his respirations for tachypnea. Inspect the patient for cool, clammy skin. Elevate the patient's legs above the level of his heart. If the bed can be adjusted, place him in Trendelenburg's position. Then, start an I.V. line using a large-bore needle to replace fluids and blood or to administer drugs. Prepare to administer oxygen with mechanical ventilation if necessary. Monitor the patient's intake and output and insert an indwelling urinary catheter to accurately measure urine output. The patient may need a central venous line or a pulmonary artery catheter to facilitate monitoring his fluid status. Prepare for cardiac monitoring to evaluate cardiac rhythm. Be ready to insert a nasogastric tube to prevent aspiration in the comatose patient.

Throughout emergency interventions, keep the patient's spinal column immobile until spinal cord trauma is ruled out.

History

- Ask the patient about symptoms, such as weakness, nausea, dizziness, and chest pain.

Physical examination

- Obtain the patient's vital signs.
- Inspect the skin for pallor, sweating, and clamminess.
- Palpate peripheral pulses.
- Auscultate for abnormal heart, breath, and bowel sounds and for abnormal heart and breath rates and rhythms.
- Look for signs of hemorrhage.
- Assess for abdominal rigidity and rebound tenderness and possible sources of infection.
- If the patient has episodes of dizziness when standing up suddenly, take blood pressure while he's lying down, sitting, and then standing. Compare readings. (See *Ensuring accurate blood pressure measurement.*)

Causes

Medical causes

Acute adrenal insufficiency

- Orthostatic hypotension is a characteristic sign.
- Other signs and symptoms include fatigue; weakness; nausea; vomiting; abdominal discomfort; weight loss; fever; tachycardia; pale, cool, clammy skin; restlessness; decreased urine output; tachypnea; hyperpigmentation of fingers, nails, scars, nipples, and body folds; and coma.

Anaphylactic shock

- Blood pressure falls dramatically and pulse pressure narrows.
- Initially, anxiety, restlessness, intense itching, pounding headache, and a feeling of doom occur.
- Later signs and symptoms include weakness, sweating, nasal congestion, coughing, difficulty breathing, nausea, abdominal cramps, involuntary defecation, seizures, flushing, change or loss of voice, urinary incontinence, and tachycardia.

Anthrax, inhalation

- Initial signs and symptoms are flu-like and include fever, chills, weakness, cough, and chest pain.
- The second stage develops abruptly with rapid deterioration marked by dyspnea, stridor, hypotension, and continuation of fever.

Cardiac arrhythmia

- Blood pressure fluctuates between normal and low.
- Dizziness, chest pain, difficulty breathing, light-headedness, weakness, fatigue, and palpitations occur.

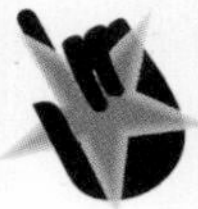

KNOW-HOW

Ensuring accurate blood pressure measurement

When taking the patient's blood pressure, begin by applying the cuff properly, as shown here.

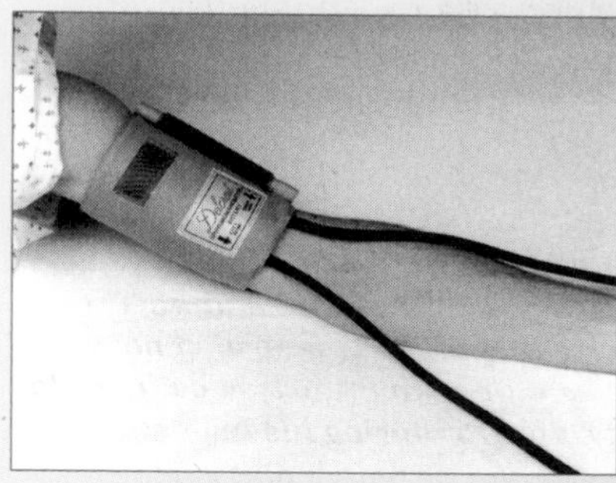

- For accuracy and consistency, position your patient with his upper arm at heart level and his palm turned up.
- Apply the cuff snugly, 1″ (2.5 cm) above the brachial pulse, as shown in the top photo.
- Position the manometer in line with your eye level.
- Palpate the brachial or radial pulse with your fingertips while inflating the cuff.
- Inflate the cuff to 30 mm Hg above the point where the pulse disappears.
- Place the bell of your stethoscope over the point where you felt the pulse, as shown in the bottom photo. Using the bell helps you hear Korotkoff sounds, which indicate pulse.
- Release the valve slowly and note the point at which Korotkoff sounds reappear. The start of the pulse sound indicates the systolic pressure.
- The sounds will become muffled and then disappear. The last Korotkoff sound you hear is the diastolic pressure.

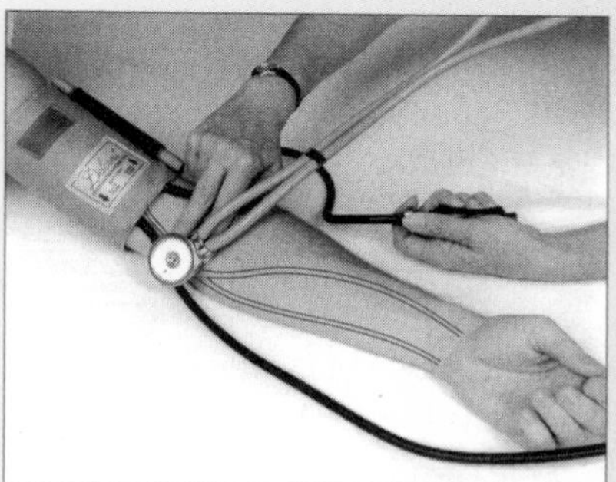

- Pulse rhythm is irregular, and heart rate is greater than 100 beats/minute or less than 60 beats/minute.

Cardiac tamponade

- Systolic pressure falls more than 10 mm Hg during inspiration (paradoxical pulse).
- Other signs and symptoms include restlessness, cyanosis, tachycardia, jugular vein distention, muffled heart sounds, dyspnea, and Kussmaul's sign.

Cardiogenic shock

- Systolic pressure falls to less than 80 mm Hg or 30 mm Hg below baseline.
- Signs and symptoms include tachycardia; narrowed pulse pressure; diminished Korotkoff sounds; peripheral cyanosis; restlessness and anxiety—which may progress to disorientation and confusion; and pale, cool, clammy skin.
- Angina, dyspnea, jugular vein distention, oliguria, ventricular gallop, tachypnea, or weak, rapid pulse may also occur.

Diabetic ketoacidosis

- Hypovolemia—triggered by osmotic diuresis in hyperglycemia—causes low blood pressure.
- Other signs and symptoms include polydipsia, polyuria, polyphagia, dehydration, weight loss, abdominal pain, nausea, vomiting, a fruity odor to the breath, Kussmaul's respirations, tachycardia, seizures, confusion, and stupor that may progress to coma.

Heart failure

- Blood pressure fluctuates between normal and low.
- Auscultation reveals ventricular gallop, tachycardia, crackles, and tachypnea.
- Dependent edema, jugular vein distention, and hepatomegaly may also occur.
- Other signs and symptoms include dyspnea of abrupt or gradual onset, exertional dyspnea, orthopnea, paroxysmal nocturnal dyspnea, fatigue, weight gain, pallor or cyanosis, sweating, and anxiety.

Hypovolemic shock

- Systolic pressure falls to less than 80 mm Hg or 30 mm Hg below baseline because of acute blood loss or dehydration.
- Other signs and symptoms include diminished Korotkoff sounds; narrowed pulse pressure; cyanosis of the extremities; pale, cool, clammy skin; rapid, weak, and irregular pulse; oliguria; confusion; disorientation; restlessness; and anxiety.

Hypoxemia

- Initially, blood pressure may be normal or slightly elevated.
- Blood pressure drops as hypoxemia becomes pronounced.
- Other signs and symptoms include tachycardia, tachypnea, dyspnea, confusion, and stupor that may progress to coma.

Myocardial infarction

- In this life-threatening disorder, blood pressure may be low or high.
- A precipitous drop in blood pressure may signal cardiogenic shock.
- Other signs and symptoms include chest pain that may radiate to the jaw, shoulder, arm, or epigastrium; dyspnea; anxiety; nausea or vomiting; sweating; and cool, pale, or cyanotic skin.

Neurogenic shock

- Low blood pressure and bradycardia occur.
- Other signs and symptoms include warm, dry skin and, possibly, motor weakness of the limbs or diaphragm, depending on the cause of shock.

Pulmonary embolism

- Low blood pressure with narrowed pulse pressure and diminished Korotkoff sounds occur.
- Early signs and symptoms include sharp chest pain, dyspnea, and cough.
- Other signs and symptoms include tachycardia, tachypnea, paradoxical pulse, jugular vein distention, and hemoptysis.

Septic shock

- Initially, fever and chills occur.
- Low blood pressure, tachycardia, and tachypnea may also develop early, but the skin remains warm.
- Blood pressure continues to decrease, accompanied by a narrowed pulse pressure.
- Other late signs and symptoms include pale skin, cyanotic extremities, apprehension, thirst, oliguria, and coma.

Vasovagal syncope

- Low blood pressure, pallor, cold sweats, nausea, palpitations or slowed heart rate, and weakness follow stressful, painful, or claustrophobic experiences.

Other causes

Diagnostic tests

- A gastric acid stimulation test, using histamine, and X-ray studies, using contrast media, may cause low blood pressure.

Drugs

- Alpha- and beta-adrenergic blockers, anxiolytics, calcium channel blockers, diuretics, general anesthetics, most I.V. antiarrhythmics, monoamine oxidase inhibitors, opioid analgesics, tranquilizers, and vasodilators can cause low blood pressure.

Nursing considerations

- Check the patient's vital signs frequently to determine if low blood pressure is constant or intermittent.
- If blood pressure remains extremely low, place an arterial catheter to allow close monitoring.
- Ensure bed rest.
- Assist ambulatory patients as needed.
- Don't leave a dizzy patient unattended when he's sitting or walking.
- Suspect trauma or shock as a possible cause of low blood pressure.
- Dehydration may also cause low blood pressure.
- Low blood pressure may occur as a result of taking several drugs that produce this adverse effect.
- Orthostatic hypotension may occur because of autonomic dysfunction.

Patient teaching

- Advise the patient with orthostatic hypotension to stand up slowly from a sitting position and, when getting out of bed, to first dangle his feet and rise slowly.
- For patients with vasovagal syncope, discuss how to avoid triggers.
- Discuss the need for a cane or walker.

Blood pressure, increased

Elevated blood pressure—an intermittent or sustained increase in blood pressure exceeding 140/90 mm Hg—strikes more men than women and twice as many blacks as whites. By itself, this common sign is easily ignored by the patient; after all, he can't see or feel it. However, be alert to the fact that its causes can be life-threatening.

Elevated blood pressure may develop suddenly or gradually. A sudden, severe rise in pressure (exceeding 180/110 mm Hg) may indicate life-threatening hypertensive crisis. Even a less dramatic rise may be equally significant if it indicates a dissecting aortic aneurysm, increased intracranial pressure, myocardial infarction, eclampsia, or thyrotoxicosis. (See *Responding to increased blood pressure,* pages 42 and 43.)

Usually associated with essential hypertension, elevated blood pressure may also result from a renal or endocrine disorder; a treatment that affects fluid status, such as dialysis; or a drug's adverse effect. Ingesting large amounts of certain foods—black licorice and cheddar cheese, for example—may also temporarily elevate blood pressure.

Sometimes, elevated blood pressure simply reflects inaccurate blood pressure measurement. Careful measurement alone doesn't ensure a clinically useful reading. To be useful, each blood pressure reading must be compared with the patient's baseline. Serial readings may be necessary to establish elevated blood pressure.

QUICK ACTION ***If blood pressure rises above 180/110 mm Hg, suspect hypertensive crisis and treat immediately.***

CASE CLIP

Responding to increased blood pressure

Ms. M. is a 57-year-old female who was admitted to the emergency department yesterday with a suspected transient ischemic attack (TIA). Her chief complaint on arrival was right-sided extremity weakness and facial droop. She also complained of a slight headache and mild dizziness. Her symptoms resolved within 2 hours of onset, but due to her past medical history, her practitioner admitted her for observation. The patient's history revealed poorly controlled hypertension, hypercholesterolemia, and atrial fibrillation. Both of Ms. M.'s parents had cardiac disease and her maternal aunt died of a massive stroke at age 61.

On admission, Ms. M.'s vital signs were:

- heart rate (HR): 94 beats/minute irregular
- respiratory rate (RR): 28 breaths/minute
- blood pressure (BP): 170/88 mm Hg
- oxygen saturation: 95% on room air.

The morning after Ms. M.'s admission to the stroke unit, the nursing assistant entered the room with the patient's breakfast tray. She noticed Ms. M. reaching with her left hand and trying to pull the tray closer without much success, so she asked if she would like help. Ms. M. attempted to answer, but the nursing assistant couldn't understand her. The nursing assistant asked the nurse to check on her.

The nurse found Ms. M. leaning toward her right side while still attempting to remain upright in bed. She asked if something was wrong, and when Ms. M. tried to reply, the nurse realized that Ms. M. appeared to have a new onset of expressive aphasia. Recalling that the admitting diagnosis was TIA, the nurse immediately checked Ms. M.'s BP and found it to be 200/94 mm Hg. In consideration of the marked hypertension and aphasia, the nurse activated the rapid response team (RRT). The RRT arrived within 3 minutes. An I.V. therapy nurse was also called to gain I.V. access.

The RRT found Ms. M. in semi-Fowler's position in bed. Vital signs were:

- HR: 110 beats/minute
- RR: 24 breaths/minute
- BP: elevated at 204/96 mm Hg
- oxygen saturation: 93% on room air.

Using the National Institute of Health Stroke Scale, the team discovered that Ms. M. demonstrated a marked right-sided facial droop along with her continued aphasia. They also noted that her right hand grasp was considerably weaker than her left. Assessment of her lower extremity strength showed that she was unable to exert any pressure with her left foot. She was able to communicate only by nodding or shaking her head. She affirmed that she had a slight headache and dizziness but denied any nausea, chest pain, shortness of breath, or change in level of consciousness.

The RRT ordered the following:

- Labetalol (Trandate) 10 mg I.V. push to lower Ms. M's blood pressure
- Labetalol 5 mg I.V. every 6 hours as needed for a systolic blood pressure of greater than 175 mm Hg
- Stat computed tomography scan of the head without contrast to rule out the presence of a hemorrhagic or embolic stroke
- Stat electrocardiography to determine ischemic or other changes
- Stat blood samples for electrolytes, complete blood count, prothrombin time, partial thromboplastin time, and glucose levels

Responding to increased blood pressure *(continued)*

- Stat portable chest X-ray, to rule out aspiration
- Echocardiogram
- Continuous cardiac monitoring
- Frequent vital sign assessments
- Strict bed rest
- Nothing by mouth
- I.V. fluid replacement at 50 ml/hour

Within ten minutes of receiving Labetalol 10 mg. I.V. push, Ms. M's blood pressure dropped to 170/90 mm Hg.

Since she responded well to the Labetalol, her physician decided to evaluate her eligibility for thrombolytic therapy to treat her stroke. One of the inclusion criteria to receive thrombolytic therapy is that the client's systolic blood pressure must be less than 185 and the diastolic pressure less than 110 mm Hg.

Maintain a patent airway in case the patient vomits, and use seizure precautions. Give an I.V. antihypertensive and a diuretic. Insert an indwelling urinary catheter to monitor urine output.

History

- Obtain a medical history, noting incidence of diabetes; cardiovascular, cerebrovascular, or renal disease; or a family history of high blood pressure.
- Ask the patient about the onset of high blood pressure.
- Note associated signs and symptoms, including headache, palpitations, blurred vision, sweating, wine-colored urine, and decreased urine output.
- Take a drug history, including past and present prescriptions, herbal preparations, and over-the-counter (OTC) drugs.
- If the patient is taking antihypertensives, determine compliance to the drug regimen.
- Explore psychosocial or environmental factors that affect blood pressure control.

Physical examination

- Perform a funduscopic (ophthalmoscopic) examination.
- Perform a cardiovascular assessment; check for carotid bruits and jugular vein distention.
- Assess skin color, temperature, and turgor.
- Palpate peripheral pulses.
- Auscultate for abnormal heart sounds, rate, or rhythm.
- Auscultate for abnormal breath sounds, rate, or rhythm.
- Auscultate for abdominal bruits.
- Palpate the abdomen for tenderness, masses, and liver or kidney enlargement.

Causes

Medical causes

Anemia

- Elevated systolic pressure may occur.
- Other signs and symptoms include pulsations in the capillary beds, bounding pulse, tachycardia, systolic ejection murmur, and pale mucous membranes.

Aortic aneurysm, dissecting

- Initially, a sudden rise in systolic pressure occurs, but diastolic pressure remains stable.
- Hypotension occurs as the body's ability to compensate fails.
- With an abdominal aneurysm, associated signs and symptoms include abdominal and back pain, weakness,

sweating, tachycardia, dyspnea, a pulsating abdominal mass, restlessness, confusion, and cool, clammy skin.

- With a thoracic aneurysm, associated signs and symptoms include a ripping or tearing sensation in the chest, which may radiate to the neck, shoulders, lower back, or abdomen; pallor; syncope; blindness; loss of consciousness; sweating; dyspnea; tachycardia; cyanosis; leg weakness; murmur; and absent radial and femoral pulses.

Atherosclerosis

- Systolic pressure rises, but diastolic pressure remains normal or slightly elevated.
- The patient may be asymptomatic.
- Other signs and symptoms may include a weak pulse, flushed skin, tachycardia, angina, and claudication.

Cushing's syndrome

- Blood pressure elevates and pulse pressure widens.
- Other findings include truncal obesity, "moon" face, and other cushingoid signs.

Hypertension

- Essential hypertension develops insidiously; blood pressure increases gradually.
- The patient may be asymptomatic.
- Malignant hypertension results when diastolic pressure abruptly rises above 120 mm Hg; systolic pressure may exceed 200 mm Hg.
- Pulmonary edema is a common sign.
- Other signs and symptoms include severe headache, confusion, blurred vision, tinnitus, epistaxis, muscle twitching, chest pain, nausea, and vomiting.

Increased intracranial pressure

- Respiratory rate increases initially, followed by increased systolic pressure and widened pulse pressure.
- Bradycardia is a late sign.
- Other signs and symptoms include headache, projectile vomiting, decreased level of consciousness, and fixed or dilated pupils.

Myocardial infarction

- Blood pressure may be high or low.
- Crushing chest pain may radiate to the jaw, shoulder, arm, or epigastrium.
- Other signs and symptoms include dyspnea, anxiety, nausea, vomiting, weakness, diaphoresis, atrial gallop, and murmurs.

Pheochromocytoma

- Paroxysmal or sustained elevated blood pressure occurs with possible orthostatic hypotension.
- Other findings include anxiety, diaphoresis, palpitations, tremors, pallor, nausea, weight loss, and headache.
- Hematuria, life-threatening retroperitoneal bleeding, proteinuria, and colicky abdominal pain may occur in advanced stages.

Renovascular stenosis

- Systolic and diastolic pressure rise abruptly.
- Other characteristic signs and symptoms include bruits over the upper abdomen or in the costovertebral angles, hematuria, and acute flank pain.

Thyrotoxicosis

- In this life-threatening disorder, elevated systolic pressure occurs.
- Other signs and symptoms include widened pulse pressure, tachycardia, bounding pulse, pulsations in the capillary nail beds, palpitations, weight loss, exophthalmos, enlarged thyroid gland, weakness, diarrhea, fever, nervousness, emotional instability, heat intolerance, exertional dyspnea, decreased or absent menses, and warm, moist skin.

Other causes

Drugs

- Central nervous system stimulants, corticosteroids, hormonal contraceptives, monoamine oxidase inhibitors, nonsteroidal anti-inflammatory drugs, sympathomimetics, and OTC cold remedies can increase blood pressure.
- Cocaine use may increase blood pressure.

Treatments

- Kidney dialysis or transplantation may cause a temporary elevation of blood pressure.

Nursing considerations

- Stress the need for follow-up diagnostic tests.
- In children, elevated blood pressure may result from such conditions as lead or mercury poisoning, chronic pyelonephritis, coarctation of the aorta, patent ductus arteriosus, glomerulonephritis, adrenogenital syndrome, or neuroblastoma.
- Atherosclerosis produces isolated systolic hypertension.

Patient teaching

- Emphasize the importance of weight loss and exercise.
- Explain the need for sodium restriction.
- Discuss stress management.
- Discuss ways of reducing other risk factors for coronary artery disease.
- Discuss the importance of regular blood pressure monitoring.
- Explain how to take prescribed antihypertensives correctly.
- Explain what adverse drug reactions the patient should report.
- Emphasize the importance of long-term follow-up care.

Bowel sounds, absent

Absent bowel sounds refers to an inability to hear any bowel sounds with a stethoscope in any quadrant after listening for at least 5 minutes in each quadrant. Bowel sounds cease when mechanical or vascular obstruction or neurogenic inhibition halts peristalsis. When peristalsis stops, gas from bowel contents and fluid secreted from the intestinal walls accumulate and distend the lumen, leading to life-threatening complications (such as perforation, peritonitis, and sepsis) or hypovolemic shock.

Simple mechanical obstruction, resulting from adhesions, hernia, or tumor, causes loss of fluids and electrolytes and induces dehydration. Vascular obstruction cuts off circulation to the intestinal walls, leading to ischemia, necrosis, and shock. Neurogenic inhibition, affecting innervation of the intestinal wall, may result from infection, bowel distention, or trauma. It may also follow mechanical or vascular obstruction or metabolic derangement such as hypokalemia.

Abrupt cessation of bowel sounds, when accompanied by abdominal pain, rigidity, and distention, signals a life-threatening crisis requiring immediate intervention. Absent bowel sounds following a period of hyperactive sounds are equally ominous and may indicate strangulation of a mechanically obstructed bowel. (See *Are bowel sounds really absent?* page 46.)

QUICK ACTION ***If you fail to detect bowel sounds and the patient reports sudden, severe abdominal pain and cramping or exhibits severe abdominal distention, prepare to insert a nasogastric (NG) or intestinal tube to suction lumen contents and decompress the bowel. Administer I.V. fluids and electrolytes to offset dehydration and im-***

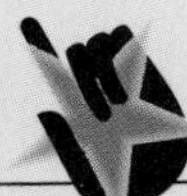

KNOW-HOW

Are bowel sounds really absent?

Before concluding that the patient has absent bowel sounds, ask yourself these questions.

Did you use the diaphragm of your stethoscope to auscultate for bowel sounds?
The diaphragm detects high-frequency sounds, such as bowel sounds, whereas the bell detects low-frequency sounds, such as a vascular bruit or venous hum.

Did you listen for at least 5 minutes in each quadrant for the presence of bowel sounds?
Normally, bowel sounds occur every 5 to 15 seconds, but the duration of a single sound may be less than 1 second.

Did you listen for bowel sounds in all quadrants?
Bowel sounds may be absent in one quadrant but present in another.

balances caused by the dysfunctioning bowel.

Because the patient may require surgery to relieve an obstruction, withhold oral intake. Take the patient's vital signs, and be alert for signs of shock, such as hypotension, tachycardia, and cool, clammy skin. Measure abdominal girth as a baseline for gauging subsequent changes. If the patient has emesis, be sure to check for occult blood.

History

- Ask about the onset and description of abdominal pain.
- Obtain a description of bowel movements and ask the patient if he has had diarrhea or has passed pencil-thin stools (a possible sign of a developing luminal obstruction).
- Obtain a medical and surgical history, including recent accidents, abdominal tumors, hernias, adhesions from past surgery, acute pancreatitis, diverticulitis, gynecologic infection, uremia, or spinal cord injury.

Physical examination

- Inspect abdominal contour.
- Observe for distention.
- Gently percuss and palpate the abdomen.
- Listen for dullness over fluid-filled areas and for tympany over pockets of gas.
- Palpate for abdominal rigidity and guarding.

Causes

Medical causes

Abdominal surgery

- Normally, bowel sounds are temporarily absent after abdominal surgery.

Complete mechanical intestinal obstruction

- In this potentially life-threatening condition, absent bowel sounds follow hyperactive sounds.
- Colicky abdominal pain, which may radiate, arises in the quadrant with the obstruction.
- Signs of shock, fever, rebound tenderness, and abdominal rigidity may occur in later stages.
- Other signs and symptoms include abdominal distention, bloating, constipation, nausea, and vomiting.

Mesenteric artery occlusion

- Bowel sounds disappear after a brief period of hyperactive sounds.
- Midepigastric or periumbilical pain occurs next, followed by abdominal distention, bruits, vomiting, constipation, and signs of shock.
- Abdominal rigidity may appear later.

Paralytic ileus

- Absent bowel sounds are a hallmark of this condition.
- If paralytic ileus follows acute abdominal infection, fever and abdominal pain may occur.
- Other signs and symptoms include abdominal distention, generalized discomfort, and constipation or passage of small, liquid stools.

Nursing considerations

- After NG or intestinal tube insertion, elevate the head of the bed at least 30 degrees.
- Turn the patient to facilitate passage of the tube through the GI tract.
- Ensure tube patency.
- Continue to give I.V. fluids and electrolytes, as prescribed.
- After mechanical obstruction and intra-abdominal sepsis have been ruled out, give drugs to control pain and stimulate peristalsis.
- In children, absent bowel sounds may result from Hirschsprung's disease or intussusception; these conditions may lead to life-threatening obstruction.
- If a bowel obstruction doesn't respond to decompression, early surgical intervention should be considered to avoid the risk of bowel infarct.

Patient teaching

- Explain diagnostic tests and therapeutic procedures that are needed.
- Explain which foods and fluids the patient should avoid.
- Explain the need for postoperative ambulation.

Bowel sounds, hyperactive

Sometimes audible without a stethoscope, hyperactive bowel sounds reflect increased intestinal motility (peristalsis). They're commonly characterized as rapid, rushing, gurgling waves of sounds.

Hyperactive bowel sounds may stem from life-threatening bowel obstruction or GI hemorrhage or from GI infection, inflammatory bowel disease (which usually follows a chronic course), food allergies, or stress.

QUICK ACTION ***After detecting hyperactive bowel sounds, quickly check the patient's vital signs and ask him about associated symptoms, such as abdominal pain, vomiting, and diarrhea. If he reports cramping, abdominal pain, or vomiting, continue to auscultate for bowel sounds. If bowel sounds stop abruptly, suspect complete bowel obstruction. Prepare to assist with GI suction and decompression, to give I.V. fluids and electrolytes, and possibly prepare the patient for surgery.***

If the patient has diarrhea, record its frequency, amount, color, and consistency. If you detect excessive watery diarrhea or bleeding, prepare to administer an antidiarrheal, I.V. fluids and electrolytes and, possibly, a blood transfusion.

History

- Obtain a medical and surgical history, including abdominal surgeries or previous inflammatory bowel disease.
- Ask the patient about recent exposure to gastroenteritis.
- Determine whether the patient has traveled recently.
- Ask about possible stress factors.
- Ask about allergies and recent food and fluid consumption.

Physical examination

- Take the patient's vital signs.
- Check for fever.
- After auscultation, gently inspect, percuss, and palpate the abdomen.

Causes

Medical causes

Crohn's disease

- Hyperactive bowel sounds arise insidiously.
- Muscle wasting, weight loss, and signs of dehydration may occur as the disease progresses.
- Other signs and symptoms include diarrhea, anorexia, low-grade fever, abdominal distention and tenderness, cramping abdominal pain that may be relieved by defecation, and a fixed mass in the right lower quadrant of the abdomen.

Gastroenteritis

- Hyperactive bowel sounds follow sudden nausea and vomiting.
- The patient has explosive diarrhea.
- Abdominal cramping or pain is common.
- Fever may occur, depending on the causative organism.

GI hemorrhage

- Hyperactive bowel sounds indicate upper GI bleeding.
- Decreased urine output, tachycardia, and hypotension accompany blood loss.
- Other signs and symptoms include hematemesis, coffee-ground vomitus, abdominal distention, bloody diarrhea, pain, and rectal passage of bright red clots and jellylike material or melena.

Malabsorption

- Lactose intolerance typically results in hyperactive bowel sounds.
- Other signs and symptoms include diarrhea and, possibly, nausea and vomiting, angioedema, and urticaria.

Mechanical intestinal obstruction

- In this potentially life-threatening disorder, hyperactive bowel sounds occur with cramping abdominal pain every few minutes.
- Bowel sounds may later become hypoactive and then disappear.
- Nausea and vomiting occur earlier and with greater severity in small-bowel obstruction than in large-bowel obstruction.
- Abdominal distention and constipation accompany hyperactive bowel sounds in complete obstruction, although the bowel farthest from the obstruction may continue to empty for up to 3 days.

Ulcerative colitis, acute

- Hyperactive bowel sounds arise abruptly.
- Bloody diarrhea occurs, with accompanying anorexia, abdominal pain, nausea and vomiting, fever, and tenesmus.
- Weight loss, arthralgia, and arthritis may also occur.

Nursing considerations

- If the patient has GI bleeding:
  - Insert an I.V. line for giving fluids and blood.
  - Restrict food and oral fluids.
  - Give drugs, such as vasopressin (Pitressin), to manage bleeding.
  - Insert a nasogastric tube to suction and monitor drainage.
- In children, hyperactive bowel sounds usually result from gastroenteritis, erratic eating habits, excessive ingestion of certain foods, or food allergy.

Patient teaching

- Explain dietary changes that are necessary or beneficial.
- Explain what physical activity the patient should avoid.
- Discuss stress reduction techniques.

Bradycardia

Bradycardia is a heart rate of less than 60 beats/minute. It occurs normally in young adults, trained athletes, and elderly people as well as during sleep. It's a normal response to vagal stimulation caused by coughing, vomiting, or straining during defecation. When bradycardia results from these causes, the heart rate rarely drops below 40 beats/minute. When it results from pathologic causes (such as cardiovascular disorders), the heart rate may be slower.

By itself, bradycardia is a nonspecific sign, but in conjunction with such symptoms as chest pain, dizziness, syncope, and shortness of breath, it can signal a life-threatening disorder. (See *Managing severe bradycardia.*)

History

- Ask about a family history of slow pulse rate.
- Obtain a medical history, including underlying metabolic disorders.
- Ask about current drugs and the patient's compliance.
- Find out if the patient is an athlete and his degree of physical activity.

Physical examination

- Monitor the patient's vital signs and oxygen saturation.

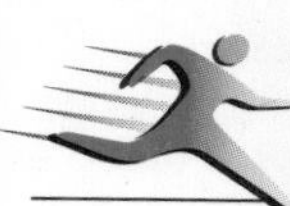

QUICK ACTION

Managing severe bradycardia

Bradycardia can signal a life-threatening disorder when accompanied by pain, shortness of breath, dizziness, syncope, or other symptoms. In addition, pay close attention if a patient with bradycardia has had prolonged exposure to cold or head or neck trauma. Take the patient's vital signs. Connect him to a cardiac monitor and insert an I.V. catheter. Depending on the cause of bradycardia, you'll need to initiate transcutaneous pacing and administer fluids, atropine, or thyroid medication. If indicated, insert an indwelling urinary catheter. Intubation or mechanical ventilation may be needed if the patient's respiratory rate falls.

Finding the cause

If appropriate, perform a focused evaluation to help locate the cause of bradycardia. For example, ask about pain. Viselike pressure or crushing or burning chest pain that radiates to the arms, back, or jaw may indicate an acute myocardial infarction (MI); a severe headache may be caused by increased intracranial pressure. Ask about nausea, vomiting, or shortness of breath—signs and symptoms associated with an acute MI and cardiomyopathy. Observe the patient for peripheral cyanosis, edema, or jugular vein distention, which may indicate cardiomyopathy. Look for a thyroidectomy scar because severe bradycardia may result from hypothyroidism caused by failure to take thyroid hormone replacements.

Providing supportive care

If the cause of bradycardia is evident, provide supportive care. For example, keep the hypothermic patient warm by applying blankets, and monitor his core temperature until it reaches 99° F (37.2° C); stabilize the head and neck of a trauma patient until cervical spinal injury is ruled out.

- Perform a complete cardiac assessment.
- After detecting bradycardia, look for related signs and symptoms to identify the cause.

Causes

Medical causes

Cardiac arrhythmia

- Bradycardia may be transient or sustained, benign, or life-threatening.
- Other signs and symptoms include hypotension, palpitations, dizziness, weakness, dyspnea, chest pain, decreased urine output, an altered level of consciousness (LOC), syncope, and fatigue.

Cardiomyopathy

- In this life-threatening disorder, transient or sustained bradycardia may occur.
- Other signs and symptoms include dizziness, syncope, edema, fatigue, jugular vein distention, orthopnea, dyspnea, and peripheral cyanosis.

Cervical spinal injury

- Bradycardia may be transient or sustained, depending on the severity of the injury.
- Other signs and symptoms include hypotension, decreased body temperature, slowed peristalsis, leg paralysis, and partial arm and respiratory muscle paralysis.

Hypothermia

- If the patient's core temperature drops below 86° F (30° C), he may not have a palpable pulse or audible heart sounds.
- Other signs and symptoms include shivering, peripheral cyanosis, muscle rigidity, bradypnea, and confusion leading to stupor.

Hypothyroidism

- Severe bradycardia is accompanied by fatigue, constipation, unexplained weight gain, and sensitivity to cold.
- Related signs and symptoms include cool, dry, thick skin; sparse, dry hair; facial swelling; periorbital edema; thick, brittle nails; and confusion leading to stupor.

Myocardial infarction

- Sinus bradycardia is common with this condition.
- Abnormal heart sounds may be heard on auscultation.
- Other signs and symptoms include an aching, burning, or viselike pressure in the chest, which may radiate to the jaw, shoulder, arm, back, or epigastric area; nausea and vomiting; cool, clammy, and pale or cyanotic skin; anxiety; and dyspnea.

Other causes

Diagnostic tests

- Cardiac catheterization and electrophysiologic studies can induce temporary bradycardia.

Drugs

- Protamine and some antiarrhythmics, beta-adrenergic blockers, cardiac glycosides, calcium channel blockers, sympatholytics, and topical miotics may cause transient bradycardia.
- Failure to take thyroid replacement medication may cause bradycardia.

Invasive treatments

- Cardiac surgery can result in edema or damage to the conduction tissue, causing bradycardia.
- Suctioning can induce hypoxia and vagal stimulation, causing bradycardia.

Nursing considerations

- Look for changes in cardiac rhythm, respiratory rate, and LOC.

- Prepare the patient for 24-hour Holter monitoring.
- Fetal bradycardia, characterized by a heart rate less than 120 beats/minute, may occur during prolonged labor or complications of delivery.
- Intermittent bradycardia commonly occurs in premature infants.
- Congenital heart defects, acute glomerulonephritis, and transient or complete heart block associated with cardiac catheterization or cardiac surgery can cause bradycardia in full-term infants and in children.
- Sinus node dysfunction is the most common bradyarrhythmia in elderly patients.
- Carefully scrutinize the patient's drug regimen.

Patient teaching

- Inform the patient about signs and symptoms he should report.
- Give instructions for pulse measurement, and explain the parameters for calling the practitioner and seeking emergency care.
- If the patient is getting a pacemaker, explain its use.

Bradypnea

Commonly preceding life-threatening apnea or respiratory arrest, bradypnea is a pattern of regular respirations with a rate of fewer than 10 breaths/minute. This sign results from neurologic and metabolic disorders or drug overdose, either of which depress the brain's respiratory control centers.

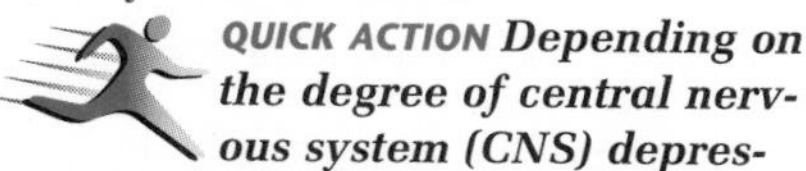

QUICK ACTION ***Depending on the degree of central nervous system (CNS) depression, the patient with severe bradypnea may require constant stimulation to breathe. If the patient seems excessively sleepy, try to arouse him by shaking and instructing him to breathe. Quickly take the patient's vital signs. Assess his neurologic status by checking pupil size and reactions and by evaluating his level of consciousness (LOC) and his ability to move his extremities.***

Place the patient on an apnea monitor and pulse oximeter, keep emergency airway equipment available, and be prepared to assist with endotracheal intubation and mechanical ventilation if spontaneous respirations cease. To prevent aspiration, position the patient on his side or keep his head elevated 30 degrees higher than the rest of his body, and clear his airway with suctioning if needed. Administer opioid antagonists, as ordered.

History

- Ask about a possible drug overdose; find out the names, doses, time frames, and routes of the drugs taken.
- Obtain a medical history.

Physical examination

- Assess the patient's vital signs.
- Perform a complete physical assessment, paying particular attention to the cardiopulmonary portion.

Causes

Medical causes

Diabetic ketoacidosis

- In patients with severe, uncontrolled diabetes, bradypnea occurs late.
- Other signs and symptoms include decreased LOC, fatigue, weakness, fruity breath odor, and oliguria.

Increased intracranial pressure

- Bradypnea is a late sign.
- Bradypnea is preceded by decreased LOC, deteriorating motor function, and fixed, dilated pupils.
- The triad of bradypnea, bradycardia, and hypertension is a classic sign of late medullary strangulation.

Respiratory failure

- Bradypnea occurs during end-stage respiratory failure.
- Restlessness, confusion, irritability, and decreased LOC may also occur.
- Other signs and symptoms include cyanosis, diminished breath sounds, tachycardia, and mildly increased blood pressure.

Other causes

Drugs

- Overdose with an opioid analgesic, sedative, barbiturate, phenothiazine, or another CNS depressant can cause bradypnea.
- Use of alcohol with these drugs can also cause bradypnea.

Nursing considerations

- Check respiratory status frequently, and give ventilatory support, if needed.
- Draw blood for arterial blood gas analysis, electrolyte studies, and drug screening.
- Give oxygen, being judicious in the patient with chronic carbon dioxide retention (such as chronic obstructive pulmonary disease) because excess oxygen therapy can decrease respiratory drive.
- Administer prescribed drugs, but avoid CNS depressants, which can worsen bradypnea.
- Review all drugs and dosages taken in the past 24 hours.
- Because respiratory rates are higher in children than in adults, bradypnea in children is defined according to age.
- Older patients have a higher risk of developing bradypnea from drug toxicity.

Patient teaching

- Explain the complications of opioid therapy such as bradypnea.
- Discuss the signs and symptoms of opioid toxicity.

Breath odor, fecal

Fecal breath odor typically accompanies fecal vomiting associated with a long-standing intestinal obstruction or gastrojejunocolic fistula. It represents an important late diagnostic clue to a potentially life-threatening GI disorder. That's because complete obstruction of any part of the bowel, if untreated, can cause death within hours from vascular collapse and shock.

When the obstructed or adynamic intestine attempts self-decompression by regurgitating its contents, vigorous peristaltic waves propel bowel contents backward into the stomach. When the stomach fills with intestinal fluid, further reverse peristalsis results in vomiting. The odor of feculent vomitus lingers in the mouth.

Fecal breath odor may also occur in patients with a nasogastric (NG) or intestinal tube. The odor is detectable only while the underlying disorder persists and subsides soon after its resolution.

QUICK ACTION ***Fecal breath odor signals a potentially life-threatening intestinal obstruction. Quickly evaluate the patient's condition. Monitor his vital signs, and be alert for signs of shock, such as hypotension, tachycardia, narrowed pulse pressure, and cool, clammy skin. Ask the patient if he's experiencing nausea or has vomited. Find out the frequency of vomiting as well as the color, odor, amount, and consistency of the vomitus. Place an emesis basin nearby to collect and accurately measure the vomitus.***

Anticipate possible surgery to relieve an obstruction or repair a fistula, and withhold all food and fluids. Be prepared to insert an NG or intestinal tube for GI tract decompression. Insert a peripheral I.V. line for vascular access, or assist with central line inser-

tion for large-bore access and central venous pressure monitoring. Obtain a blood sample and send it to the laboratory for complete blood count and electrolyte analysis because large fluid losses and shifts can produce electrolyte imbalances. Maintain adequate hydration and support circulatory status with additional fluids. Give a physiologic solution—such as lactated Ringer's, normal saline, or Plasmanate—to prevent metabolic acidosis from gastric losses and metabolic alkalosis from intestinal fluid losses.

History

- Ask about previous abdominal surgeries.
- Note the onset, duration, and location of abdominal pain.
- Find out about bowel habits, including time and description of last bowel movement.
- Ask about any loss of appetite.

Physical examination

- Auscultate for bowel sounds.
- Inspect the abdomen, noting its contour and surgical scars.
- Measure abdominal girth to provide a baseline.
- Percuss for tympany or dullness.
- Palpate for tenderness, distention, and rigidity.
- Perform rectal and pelvic examinations.

Causes

Medical causes

Distal small-bowel obstruction

- Fecal breath odor results from vomiting of fecal contents after vomiting of gastric contents and bilious contents.
- Other signs and symptoms include achiness, malaise, drowsiness, and polydipsia.
- Bowel changes (ranging from diarrhea to constipation) are accompanied by abdominal distention, persistent epigastric or periumbilical colicky pain, and hyperactive bowel sounds and borborygmi.
- Bowel sounds become hypoactive or absent as obstruction becomes complete.
- Fever, hypotension, tachycardia, and rebound tenderness may indicate strangulation or perforation.

Gastrojejunocolic fistula

- Fecal vomiting with resulting fecal breath odor may occur.
- Diarrhea with abdominal pain is the most common complaint.
- Other signs and symptoms include anorexia, weight loss, abdominal distention, and marked malabsorption.

Large-bowel obstruction

- Fecal vomiting with fecal breath odor occurs as a late sign.
- Colicky abdominal pain appears suddenly, followed by continuous hypogastric pain.
- Marked abdominal distention and tenderness occur.
- Constipation develops, but defecation may continue for up to 3 days.
- Leakage of stool is common with partial obstruction.

Nursing considerations

After an NG or intestinal tube has been inserted:

- Keep the head of the bed elevated at least 30 degrees.
- Turn the patient to facilitate passage of the intestinal tube through the GI tract.
- Don't tape the intestinal tube to the patient's face.
- Ensure tube patency by monitoring drainage and checking that suction devices function properly.
- Irrigate the tube as needed.
- Monitor GI drainage.

- At least once per day, send serum specimens to the laboratory for electrolyte analysis.

Patient teaching

- Explain to the patient the procedures and treatments he needs.
- Teach the patient the techniques of good oral hygiene.
- Explain to the patient the food and fluid restrictions that are needed.

Breath odor, fruity

Fruity breath odor results from respiratory elimination of excess acetone. This sign characteristically occurs with ketoacidosis—a potentially life-threatening condition that requires immediate treatment to prevent severe dehydration, irreversible coma, and death.

Ketoacidosis results from the excessive catabolism of fats for cellular energy in the absence of usable carbohydrates. This process begins when insulin levels are insufficient to transport glucose into the cells, as in diabetes mellitus, or when glucose is unavailable and hepatic glycogen stores are depleted, as in low-carbohydrate diets and malnutrition. Lacking glucose, the cells burn fat faster than enzymes can handle the ketones, the acidic end products. As a result, the ketones (acetone, beta-hydroxybutyric acid, and acetoacetic acid) accumulate in the blood and urine. To compensate for increased acidity, Kussmaul's respirations expel carbon dioxide with enough acetone to flavor the breath. Eventually, this compensatory mechanism fails, producing ketoacidosis.

QUICK ACTION ***When you detect fruity breath odor, check for Kussmaul's respirations and examine the patient's level of consciousness (LOC). Take his vital signs and check skin turgor. Be alert for fruity breath odor that accompanies rapid, deep respirations, stupor, and poor skin turgor. Try to obtain a brief history, noting especially diabetes mellitus, nutritional problems such as anorexia nervosa, and fad diets with little or no carbohydrates. Obtain venous blood samples for glucose, complete blood count, and electrolyte, acetone, and arterial blood gas (ABG) levels. Administer I.V. fluids and electrolytes to maintain hydration and electrolyte balance. For a patient with diabetic ketoacidosis (DKA), also give regular insulin to reduce blood glucose levels.***

If the patient is obtunded, you'll need to insert endotracheal and nasogastric (NG) tubes. Suction as needed. Insert an indwelling urinary catheter, and monitor intake and output. Insert central venous pressure and arterial lines to monitor the patient's fluid status and blood pressure. Place the patient on a cardiac monitor, monitor his vital signs and neurologic status, and draw blood as ordered to check glucose, electrolyte, acetone, and ABG levels.

History

- Ask about the onset and duration of odor.
- Find out about changes in breathing patterns.
- Review other signs and symptoms, including increased thirst, frequent urination, weight loss, fatigue, and abdominal pain.
- Ask the female patient if she has had candidal vaginitis or vaginal secretions with itching.
- If the patient has a history of diabetes mellitus, ask about stress, infections, and noncompliance to the treatment regimen.
- If anorexia nervosa is suspected, obtain a dietary and weight history.

Physical examination

- Take the patient's vital signs.
- Perform a physical examination.

Causes

Medical causes

Anorexia nervosa

- Severe weight loss may produce fruity breath odor.
- Nausea, constipation, and cold intolerance may be present.
- Dental enamel erosion and scars or calluses on the dorsum of the hand may indicate induced vomiting.

Ketoacidosis

- With alcoholic ketoacidosis, fruity breath odor occurs with vomiting, abdominal pain, abrupt onset of Kussmaul's respirations, signs of dehydration, minimal food intake over several days, and normal or slightly decreased blood glucose levels.
- With starvation ketoacidosis, fruity breath odor occurs with signs of cachexia and dehydration, decreased LOC, bradycardia, and a history of severely limited food intake.
- With DKA, fruity breath odor occurs as DKA develops over 1 or 2 days.
- Other signs and symptoms of DKA include polydipsia, polyuria, nocturia, weak and rapid pulse, hunger, weight loss, weakness, fatigue, nausea, vomiting, abdominal pain and, eventually, Kussmaul's respirations, orthostatic hypotension, dehydration, tachycardia, confusion, stupor, and coma.

Other causes

Drugs

- Drugs that cause metabolic acidosis, such as nitroprusside (Nitropress) and salicylates, can result in fruity breath odor.
- Low-carbohydrate diets may cause ketoacidosis and fruity breath odor.

Nursing considerations

- When the patient is more alert and his condition stabilizes, remove the NG tube and start him on an appropriate diet.
- Switch his insulin from I.V. to subcutaneous.
- In an infant or a child, fruity breath odor usually stems from uncontrolled diabetes mellitus.
- When evaluating the condition of an elderly patient with mouth odor, consider such factors as poor oral hygiene, increased dental caries, decreased salivary function, poor dietary intake, and use of multiple drugs.

Patient teaching

- Explain the signs of hyperglycemia.
- Emphasize the importance of wearing medical identification.
- Refer the patient to a psychologist or support group, as needed.

Brudzinski's sign

A positive Brudzinski's sign (flexion of the hips and knees in response to passive flexion of the neck) signals meningeal irritation. Passive flexion of the neck stretches the nerve roots, causing pain and involuntary flexion of the knees and hips.

Brudzinski's sign is a common and important early indicator of life-threatening meningitis and subarachnoid hemorrhage. It can be elicited in children as well as adults. For infants, however, there are more reliable indicators of meningeal irritation. Testing for Brudzinski's sign isn't part of the routine examination, unless meningeal irritation is suspected. (See *Testing for Brudzinski's sign,* page 56.)

QUICK ACTION ***Ask the patient about signs of increased intracranial pressure (ICP), such as headache, neck***

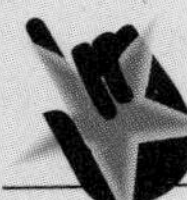

KNOW-HOW

Testing for Brudzinski's sign

Here's how to test for Brudzinski's sign when you suspect meningeal irritation:

With the patient in a supine position, place your hands behind her neck and lift her head toward her chest (as shown at right).

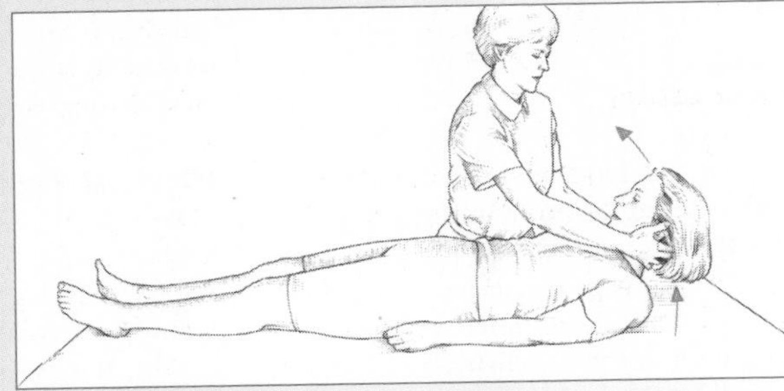

If your patient has meningeal irritation, she'll flex her hips and knees in response to the passive neck flexion (as shown at right).

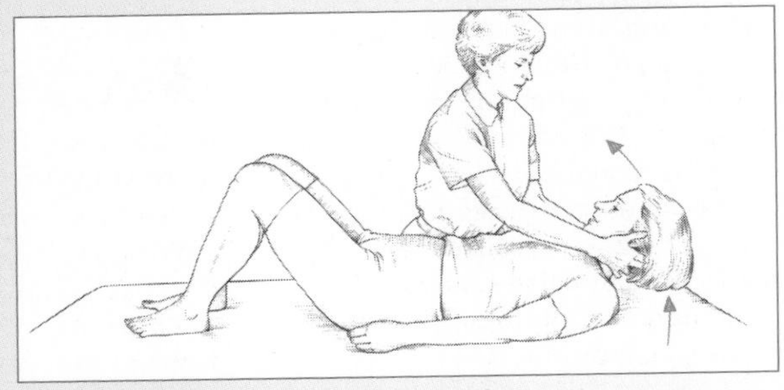

pain, nausea, and vision disturbances. Observe for altered level of consciousness (LOC), pupillary changes, bradycardia, widened pulse pressure, irregular respiratory patterns (such as Cheyne-Stokes or Kussmaul's respirations), vomiting, and moderate fever.

Keep artificial airways, intubation equipment, a handheld resuscitation bag, and suction equipment on hand in case the patient's condition suddenly deteriorates. Elevate the head of his bed 30 to 60 degrees to promote venous drainage. Administer an osmotic diuretic, such as mannitol (Osmitrol), to reduce cerebral edema.

Monitor ICP and be alert for ICP that continues to rise. You may have to provide mechanical ventilation and administer a barbiturate and additional doses of a diuretic. Cerebrospinal fluid may have to be drained.

History

- Ask about a history of hypertension, spinal arthritis, recent head trauma, open-head injury, dental work or abscessed teeth, endocarditis, or I.V. drug abuse.
- Ask about the sudden onset of headaches.

Physical examination

- Evaluate cranial nerve function, noting motor or sensory deficits.

■ Look for Kernig's sign (resistance to knee extension after flexion of the hip), which is a further indication of meningeal irritation.
■ Look for signs of central nervous system infection, such as fever and nuchal rigidity.

Causes

Medical causes

Meningitis

■ A positive Brudzinski's sign can usually be elicited 24 hours after the onset of this life-threatening disorder.
■ As ICP increases, arterial hypertension, bradycardia, widened pulse pressure, Cheyne-Stokes or Kussmaul's respirations, and coma may develop.
■ Other signs and symptoms include headache, a positive Kernig's sign, nuchal rigidity, irritability or restlessness, deep stupor or coma, vertigo, fever, chills, malaise, hyperalgesia, muscular hypotonia, opisthotonos, symmetrical deep tendon reflexes, papilledema, ocular and facial palsies, nausea, vomiting, photophobia, diplopia, and unequal, sluggish pupils.

Subarachnoid hemorrhage

■ In this life-threatening disorder, Brudzinski's sign may be elicited within minutes after initial bleeding.
■ Focal signs may occur, such as hemiparesis, vision disturbances, or aphasia.
■ As ICP increases, arterial hypertension, bradycardia, widened pulse pressure, Cheyne-Stokes or Kussmaul's respirations, and coma may develop.
■ Other signs and symptoms include sudden onset of severe headache, nuchal rigidity, altered LOC, dizziness, photophobia, cranial nerve palsies, nausea, vomiting, fever, and a positive Kernig's sign.

Nursing considerations

■ Provide constant ICP monitoring and perform frequent neurologic checks.
■ Monitor the patient's vital signs, fluid intake and urine output, and cardiorespiratory status.
■ Maintain low lights and minimal noise, and elevate the head of the bed to make the patient more comfortable.
■ In infants with meningeal irritation, bulging fontanels, a weak cry, fretfulness, vomiting, and poor feeding appear earlier than Brudzinski's sign.

Patient teaching

■ Teach the patient about diagnostic tests.
■ Discuss the signs and symptoms of meningitis and subdural hematoma.
■ Tell the patient and his family when to seek immediate medical attention.

Bruit

Commonly an indicator of life- or limb-threatening vascular disease, bruits are swishing sounds caused by turbulent blood flow. They're characterized by location, duration, intensity, pitch, and the time of onset in the cardiac cycle. Loud bruits produce intense vibration and a palpable thrill. A thrill doesn't provide a further clue to the causative disorder or to its severity.

Bruits are most significant when heard over the abdominal aorta; the renal, carotid, femoral, popliteal, or subclavian artery; or the thyroid gland. (See *Preventing false bruits,* page 58.) They're also significant when heard consistently despite changes in patient position, and when heard during diastole.

History

■ Obtain a medical history, noting past injuries, illnesses, surgeries, and family medical history.
■ Ask about alcohol use and diet.
■ Take a drug and social history.

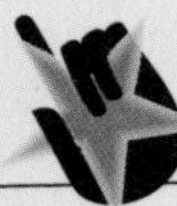

KNOW-HOW

Preventing false bruits

Auscultating bruits accurately requires practice and skill. These sounds typically stem from arterial luminal narrowing or arterial dilation, but they can also result from excessive pressure applied to the stethoscope's bell during auscultation. This pressure compresses the artery, creating turbulent blood flow and a false bruit.

To prevent false bruits, place the bell lightly on the patient's skin. Also, if you're auscultating for a popliteal bruit, help the patient to a supine position, place your hand behind his ankle, and lift his leg slightly before placing the bell behind the knee.

NORMAL BLOOD FLOW, NO BRUIT

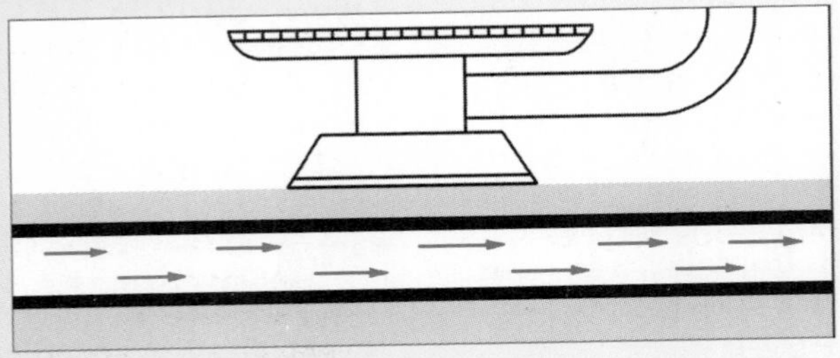

TURBULENT BLOOD FLOW AND RESULTANT BRUIT CAUSED BY ANEURYSM

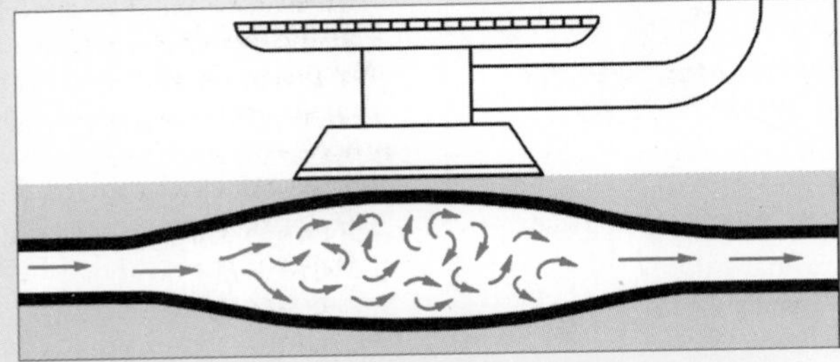

TURBULENT BLOOD FLOW AND FALSE BRUIT CAUSED BY COMPRESSION OF ARTERY

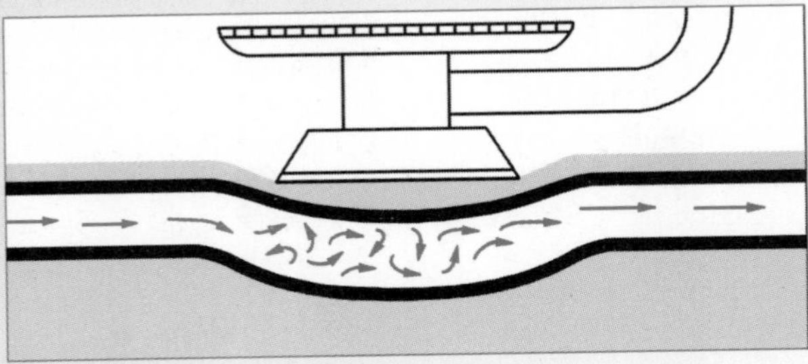

Physical examination

- Perform a cardiac assessment.

For bruits over abdominal aorta

- Check for a pulsating mass, Cullen's sign, or severe, tearing pain in the abdomen, flank, or lower back.
- Check peripheral pulses, comparing intensity in the upper versus lower extremities.
- Look for signs and symptoms of hypovolemic shock and dissection.

For bruits over thyroid gland

- Ask the patient about a history of hyperthyroidism.
- Watch for signs and symptoms of life-threatening thyroid storm.

For bruits over carotid artery

- Be alert for signs and symptoms of a transient ischemic attack (TIA).
- Evaluate frequently for changes in the patient's level of consciousness and muscle function.

For bruits over femoral, popliteal, or subclavian artery

- Watch for signs and symptoms of decreased or absent peripheral circulation.
- Ask the patient about a history of intermittent claudication.
- Frequently check distal pulses and skin color and temperature.
- Watch for pallor, coolness, or the sudden absence of a pulse.

Causes

Medical causes

Abdominal aortic aneurysm

- A systolic bruit over the aorta accompanies a pulsating periumbilical mass.
- Sharp, tearing pain in the abdomen, flank, or lower back signals imminent dissection.
- Other signs and symptoms include a rigid, tender abdomen, mottled skin, diminished peripheral pulses, and claudication.

Abdominal aortic atherosclerosis

- Loud systolic bruits in the epigastric and midabdominal areas are common findings.
- Other signs and symptoms may include leg weakness, numbness, paresthesia, or paralysis; leg pain; and decreased or absent femoral, popliteal, or pedal pulses.

Carotid artery stenosis

- Systolic bruits heard over one or both carotid arteries may be the only sign of this disorder.
- Dizziness, vertigo, headache, syncope, aphasia, dysarthria, sudden vision loss, hemiparesis, or hemiparalysis signals TIA and may indicate that a stroke is imminent.

Peripheral arteriovenous fistula

- A rough, continuous bruit with systolic accentuation may be heard over the fistula.
- A palpable thrill is also common.
- Other signs and symptoms depend on the location of the fistula, but may include claudication, absent pulses, and cool skin.

Peripheral vascular disease

- Bruits may be heard over the femoral artery and other arteries in the legs.
- Lower-leg ulcers that are difficult to heal may also occur.
- Other signs and symptoms include diminished or absent femoral, popliteal, or pedal pulses; intermittent claudication; numbness, weakness, pain, and cramping in the legs, feet, and hips; and cool, shiny skin and hair loss on the affected extremity.

Renal artery stenosis

- Systolic bruits are heard over the abdominal midline and flank on the affected side.
- Hypertension commonly accompanies stenosis.
- Other signs and symptoms include headache, palpitations, tachycardia, anxiety, dizziness, retinopathy, hematuria, and mental sluggishness.

Subclavian steal syndrome

- Systolic bruits may be heard over the subclavian artery.
- Other signs and symptoms include decreased blood pressure and claudication in the affected arm, hemiparesis, vision disturbances, vertigo, and dysarthria.

Thyrotoxicosis

- A systolic bruit is heard over the thyroid gland.
- Characteristic signs and symptoms include thyroid enlargement, fatigue, nervousness, tachycardia, heat intolerance, sweating, tremor, diarrhea, exophthalmos, and weight loss in spite of an increased appetite.

Nursing considerations

- Frequently check the patient's vital signs, and auscultate over affected arteries.
- Check for bruits that become louder or develop a diastolic component.
- Administer prescribed drugs, such as a vasodilator, anticoagulant, antihypertensive, or antiplatelet agent.
- In young children, bruits are common and usually of little significance.
- Auscultate for bruits in a child with port-wine spots or cavernous or diffuse hemangiomas.
- Elderly patients with atherosclerosis may have bruits over several arteries.
- Bruits from carotid artery stenosis are associated with stroke; therefore, close follow-up and prompt surgical referral are essential.

Patient teaching

- Tell the patient the signs and symptoms of stroke that he should report immediately.
- Discuss lifestyle changes, such as quitting smoking, exercising regularly, and eating a balanced, healthy diet.

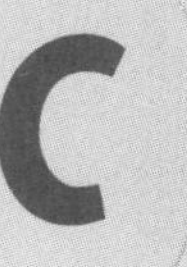

C

Carpopedal spasm

Carpopedal spasm is the violent, painful contraction of the muscles in the hands and feet. (See *Recognizing carpopedal spasm.*)

It's an important sign of tetany, a potentially life-threatening condition characterized by increased neuromuscular excitation and sustained muscle contraction, and is commonly associated with hypocalcemia.

Carpopedal spasm requires prompt evaluation and intervention. If the primary event isn't treated promptly, the patient can also develop laryngospasm, seizures, cardiac arrhythmias, and cardiac and respiratory arrest.

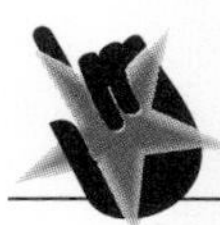

QUICK ACTION ***If you detect carpopedal spasm, quickly examine the patient for signs of respiratory distress (such as laryngospasm, stridor, loud crowing noises, and cyanosis) or cardiac arrhythmias, which indicate hypocalcemia. Obtain blood specimens for electrolyte analysis (especially calcium), and perform an electrocardiogram. Connect the patient to a cardiac monitor to watch for the appearance of arrhythmias. As ordered, administer an I.V. calcium preparation, and provide emergency respiratory and cardiac support. If a calcium infusion doesn't control seizures, give a sedative, such as chloral hydrate (Aquachloral) or phenobarbital (Luminal).***

History

- Ask about the onset and duration of spasms.
- Explore the extent of pain.
- Note related signs and symptoms of hypocalcemia.

KNOW-HOW

Recognizing carpopedal spasm

In the hand, carpopedal spasm involves adduction of the thumb over the palm, followed by flexion of the metacarpophalangeal joints, extension of the interphalangeal joints (fingers together), adduction of the hyperextended fingers, and flexion of the wrist and elbow joints. Similar effects occur in the joints of the feet.

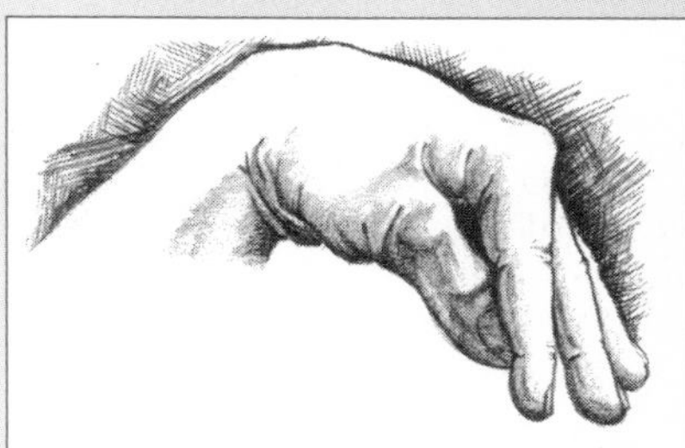

- Obtain the patient's immunization history, especially tetanus vaccine.
- Ask about previous neck surgery, calcium or magnesium deficiency, tetanus exposure, hypoparathyroidism, or recent puncture wounds.

Physical examination

- Perform a complete physical examination, including taking vital signs.
- Check for Chvostek's sign.
- Inspect the patient's skin and fingernails, noting dryness or scaling or ridged, brittle nails caused by hypocalcemia.
- Assess the patient's mental status and behavior.

Causes

Medical causes

Hypocalcemia

- Carpopedal spasm is an early sign.
- Signs and symptoms include paresthesia of the fingers, toes, and perioral area; muscle weakness, twitching, and cramping; hyperreflexia; chorea; fatigue; and palpitations.
- Positive Chvostek's and Trousseau's signs can be elicited.
- In chronic hypocalcemia, mental status changes; cramps; dry, scaly skin; brittle nails; and thin, patchy hair and eyebrows may occur.
- In severe hypocalcemia, laryngospasm, stridor, and seizures may appear.

Tetanus

- Muscle spasms and seizures develop.
- Other signs and symptoms include difficulty swallowing and low-grade fever.

Other causes

Surgery

- Surgery that impairs calcium absorption may cause hypocalcemia.

Treatments

- Multiple blood transfusions and parathyroidectomy may cause hypocalcemia.

Nursing considerations

- If hyperventilation occurs, help the patient slow his breathing.
- To reduce the patient's anxiety, provide a quiet, darkened environment.
- Monitor children with hypocalcemia caused by idiopathic hypoparathyroidism; carpopedal spasm may precede the onset of epileptiform seizures or generalized tetany.
- Ask the elderly patient about his immunization record and recent wounds.

Patient teaching

- Explain the importance of tetanus immunization and keeping an up-to-date immunization record and schedule.

Chest expansion, asymmetrical

Asymmetrical chest expansion is the uneven extension of portions of the chest wall during inspiration. During normal respiration, the thorax uniformly expands upward and outward and then contracts downward and inward. When this process is disrupted, breathing becomes uncoordinated, resulting in asymmetrical chest expansion.

Asymmetrical chest expansion may develop suddenly or gradually and may affect one or both sides of the chest wall. It may occur as delayed expiration (chest lag), as abnormal movement during inspiration (for example, intercostal retractions, paradoxical movement, or chest-abdomen asynchrony), or as a unilateral absence of movement. This sign usually results from pleural disorders, such as life-threatening hemothorax or

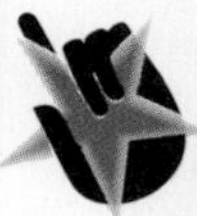

KNOW-HOW

Recognizing life-threatening causes of asymmetrical chest expansion

Asymmetrical chest expansion can result from several life-threatening disorders. Two common causes—bronchial obstruction and flail chest—produce distinctive chest wall movements that provide important clues about the underlying disorder.

With *bronchial obstruction,* only the unaffected portion of the chest wall expands during inspiration. Intercostal bulging during expiration may indicate that air is trapped in the chest.

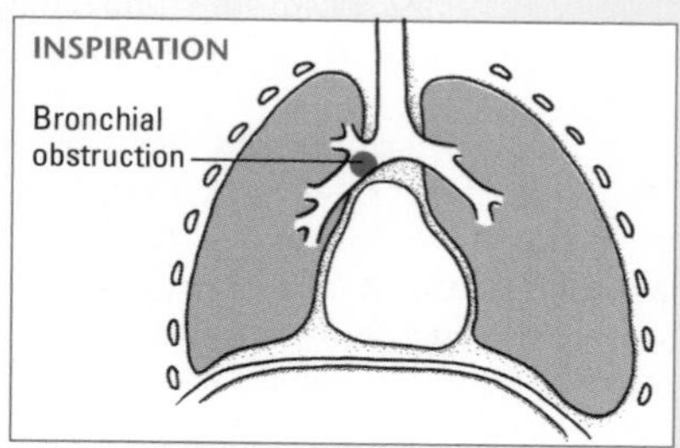

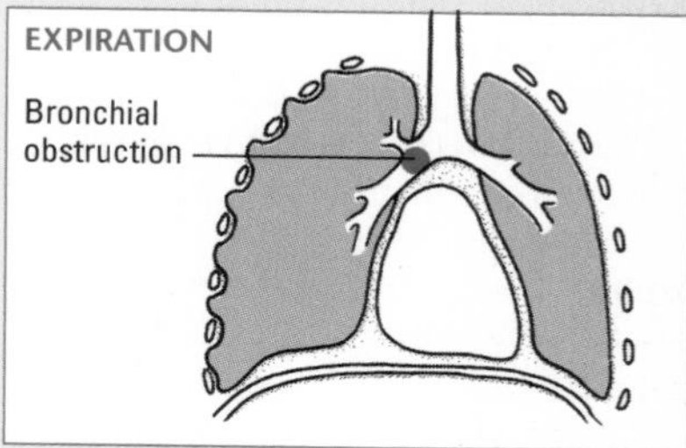

With *flail chest*—a disruption of the thorax due to multiple rib fracture—the unstable portion of the chest wall collapses inward at inspiration and balloons outward at expiration.

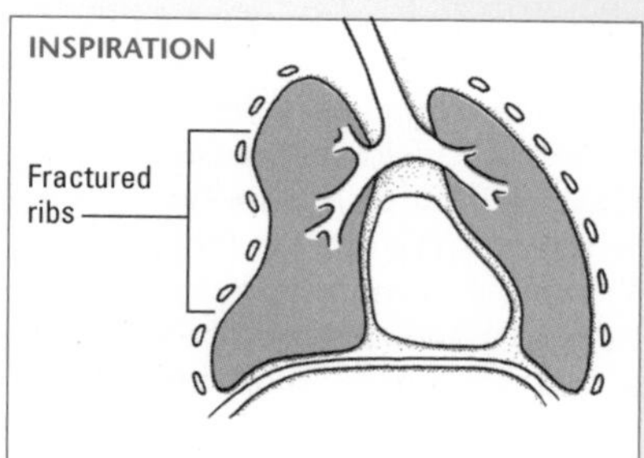

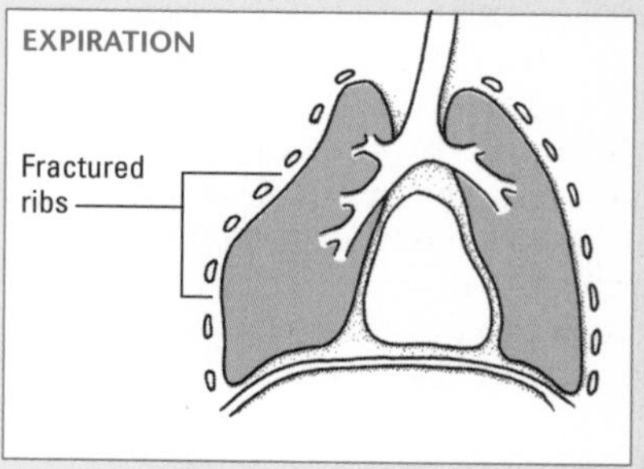

tension pneumothorax. (See *Recognizing life-threatening causes of asymmetrical chest expansion.*)

However, it can also result from a musculoskeletal or urologic disorder, airway obstruction, or trauma. Regardless of its underlying cause, asymmetrical chest expansion produces rapid and shallow or deep respirations that increase the work of breathing.

QUICK ACTION ***If you detect asymmetrical chest expansion, first consider flail chest, a life-threatening emergency characterized by paradoxical chest movement. Quickly take the patient's vital signs and look for signs of acute***

respiratory distress—rapid and shallow respirations, tachycardia, and cyanosis. Use tape or sandbags to temporarily splint the unstable flail segment.

Depending on the severity of respiratory distress, administer oxygen by nasal cannula, mask, or mechanical ventilator. Insert an I.V. line to allow fluid replacement and administration of pain medication. Draw a blood sample for arterial blood gas analysis, and connect the patient to a cardiac monitor.

Because any form of asymmetrical chest expansion can compromise the patient's respiratory status, don't leave the patient unattended, and be alert for signs of respiratory distress.

History

- Ask about the onset, duration, aggravating and alleviating factors, and extent of dyspnea or pain during breathing.
- Obtain a history of pulmonary or systemic illness, thoracic surgery, or blunt or penetrating chest trauma.
- Ask about occupational history.

Physical examination

- Palpate the trachea for midline positioning.
- Examine the posterior chest wall for tenderness or deformity.
- Evaluate the extent of asymmetrical chest expansion.
- Palpate for vocal or tactile fremitus on both sides of the chest. Note asymmetrical vibrations and areas of enhanced, diminished, or absent fremitus.
- Percuss and auscultate to detect air and fluid in the lungs and pleural spaces.
- Auscultate all lung fields for abnormal breath sounds.
- Examine the patient's anterior chest wall.

Causes

Medical causes

Bronchial obstruction

- In this life-threatening disorder, lack of chest movement indicates complete obstruction, while lagging chest signals partial obstruction.
- Intercostal bulging during expiration and hyperresonance on percussion suggest air trapped in the chest.
- Other signs and symptoms may include dyspnea, accessory muscle use, decreased or absent breath sounds, and suprasternal, substernal, or intercostal retractions.

Flail chest

- In this life-threatening disorder, the unstable portion of the chest wall collapses inward during inspiration and balloons outward during expiration.
- Ecchymoses and severe localized pain occur with traumatic injury to the chest wall.
- Rapid and shallow respirations, tachycardia, and cyanosis may also occur.

Hemothorax

- In this life-threatening disorder, bleeding into the pleural space causes the chest to lag during inspiration.
- Other signs and symptoms include signs of traumatic chest injury, stabbing pain at the injury site, anxiety, dullness on percussion, tachypnea, tachycardia, hypoxemia, and signs of shock.

Myasthenia gravis

- Progressive loss of ventilatory muscle function produces asynchrony of the chest and abdomen during inspiration.
- Shallow respirations and increased muscle weakness cause severe dyspnea, tachypnea, and possible apnea.

Pneumonia

- Inspiratory lagging chest or chest-abdomen asynchrony occurs.

■ Other signs and symptoms include fever, chills, tachycardia, fatigue, productive cough with rust-colored sputum, tachypnea, dyspnea, crackles, rhonchi, and chest pain that worsens with deep breathing.

Pneumothorax

■ In this life-threatening disorder, free air enters the pleural cavity, collapsing the lung and lagging the chest at end-inspiration.

■ Sudden, stabbing chest pain occurs that may radiate to the arms, face, back, or abdomen.

■ Other signs and symptoms include tachypnea, decreased tactile fremitus, tympany on percussion, decreased or absent breath sounds over the trapped air, tachycardia, restlessness, and anxiety.

■ In tension pneumothorax, the same findings occur as in pneumothorax but are more severe.

■ Other signs and symptoms of tension pneumothorax include cyanosis; hypotension; subcutaneous crepitation of the upper trunk, neck, and face; mediastinal and tracheal deviation from the affected side; and a crunching sound on auscultation over the precordium with each heartbeat.

Other causes

Treatments

■ Pneumonectomy and surgical removal of several ribs can cause asymmetrical chest expansion.

■ Mainstem bronchi intubation may also cause chest lag or the absence of chest movement.

Nursing considerations

■ Prepare the patient for pulmonary studies.

■ Auscultate breath sounds in the lung peripheries.

■ Give supplemental oxygen during acute events.

If the patient has a chest tube:

■ Maintain the water seal.

■ Check the system for air leaks.

■ Monitor drainage.

■ In children, asymmetrical chest expansion may develop with acute respiratory illnesses, congenital abnormalities, cerebral palsy, and life-threatening diaphragmatic hernia.

■ Asymmetrical chest expansion in the elderly patient may be more difficult to determine due to the structural deformities associated with aging.

Patient teaching

■ Explain to the patient or caregiver how to recognize early signs and symptoms of respiratory distress, and what to do if they occur.

■ Teach the patient coughing and deep-breathing exercises.

■ Teach the patient techniques that can help reduce his anxiety.

■ Teach the patient about all hospital procedures, tests, and interventions, such as chest tube insertion and oxygen administration.

Chest pain

Chest pain usually results from disorders that affect thoracic or abdominal organs—the heart, pleurae, lungs, esophagus, rib cage, gallbladder, pancreas, or stomach. An important indicator of several acute and life-threatening cardiopulmonary and GI disorders, chest pain can also result from a musculoskeletal or hematologic disorder, anxiety, and drug therapy.

Chest pain can arise suddenly or gradually, and initially, it may be difficult to discover its cause. The pain can radiate to the arms, neck, jaw, or back. It can be steady or intermittent, mild or acute. It can range in character from a sharp shooting sensation to a feeling of heaviness, fullness, or even indigestion. It can be provoked or aggravated by

QUICK ACTION

Managing severe chest pain

Sudden, severe chest pain may result from any one of several life-threatening disorders. Your evaluation and interventions will vary, depending on the pain's location and character. This flowchart will help you establish priorities for managing this emergency successfully.

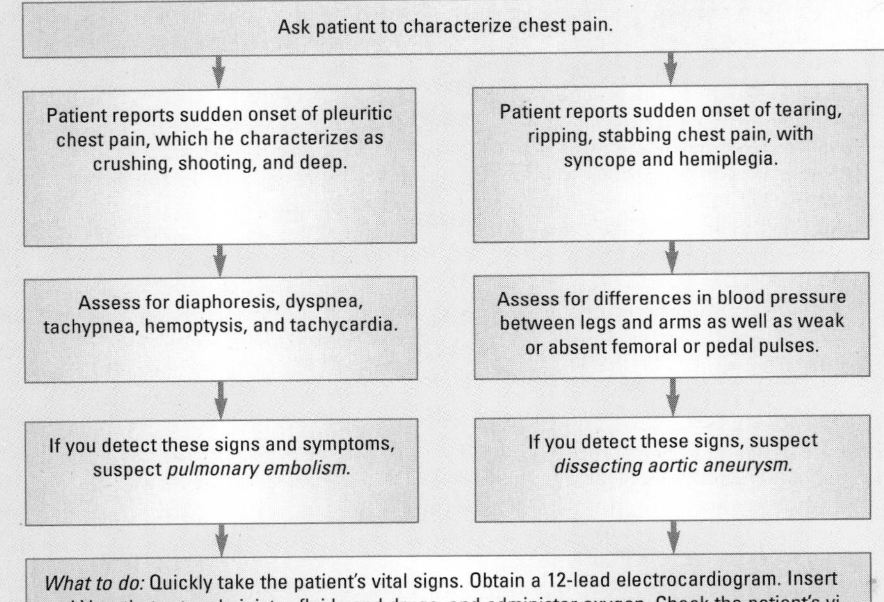

stress, anxiety, exertion, deep breathing, or eating certain foods.

Ask patient to characterize chest pain.
Patient reports sudden onset of pleuritic chest pain, which he characterizes as crushing, shooting, and deep.
Patient reports sudden onset of tearing, ripping, stabbing chest pain, with syncope and hemiplegia.
Assess for diaphoresis, dyspnea, tachypnea, hemoptysis, and tachycardia.
Assess for differences in blood pressure between legs and arms as well as weak or absent femoral or pedal pulses.
If you detect these signs and symptoms, suspect *pulmonary embolism.*
If you detect these signs, suspect *dissecting aortic aneurysm.*
What to do: Quickly take the patient's vital signs. Obtain a 12-lead electrocardiogram. Insert an I.V. catheter to administer fluids and drugs, and administer oxygen. Check the patient's vital signs frequently to detect changes from baseline. Begin cardiac monitoring to detect arrhythmias. As appropriate, prepare the patient for emergency surgery. Prepare the patient with a pulmonary embolism or myocardial infarction (MI) for possible thrombolytic therapy.

Sudden, severe chest pain requires prompt evaluation and treatment because it may signal a life-threatening disorder. (See *Managing severe chest pain.*)

History

- Ask about the onset and radiation of pain and its duration, quality, quantity, and what aggravates or alleviates it.
- Obtain a history of cardiac or pulmonary disease, chest trauma, GI disease, or sickle cell anemia.
- Obtain a drug history, including tobacco use.

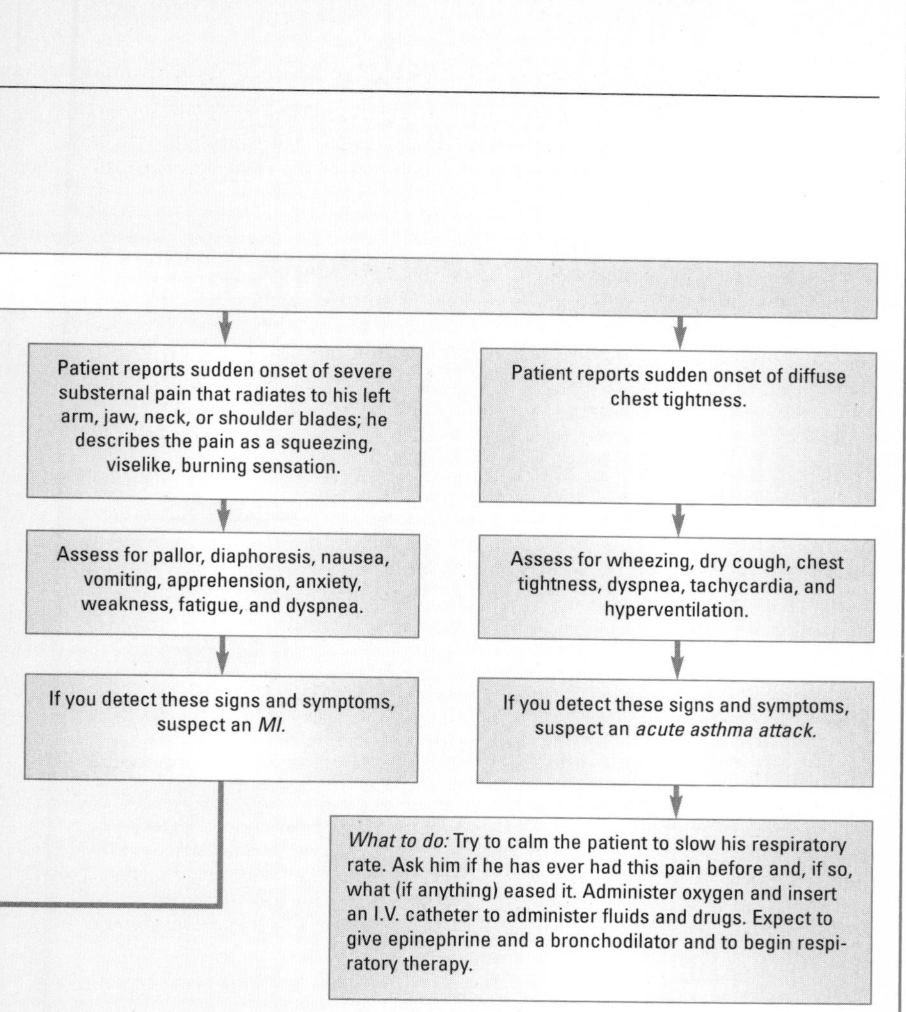

Patient reports sudden onset of severe substernal pain that radiates to his left arm, jaw, neck, or shoulder blades; he describes the pain as a squeezing, viselike, burning sensation.
Assess for pallor, diaphoresis, nausea, vomiting, apprehension, anxiety, weakness, fatigue, and dyspnea.
If you detect these signs and symptoms, suspect an *MI.*
Patient reports sudden onset of diffuse chest tightness.
Assess for wheezing, dry cough, chest tightness, dyspnea, tachycardia, and hyperventilation.
If you detect these signs and symptoms, suspect an *acute asthma attack.*
What to do: Try to calm the patient to slow his respiratory rate. Ask him if he has ever had this pain before and, if so, what (if anything) eased it. Administer oxygen and insert an I.V. catheter to administer fluids and drugs. Expect to give epinephrine and a bronchodilator and to begin respiratory therapy.

Physical examination

- Take the patient's vital signs; note tachypnea, fever, tachycardia, oxygen saturation, paradoxical pulse, and hypertension or hypotension.
- Look for jugular vein distention and peripheral edema.
- Observe the patient's breathing pattern; inspect the chest for asymmetrical expansion.
- Auscultate for pleural rub, crackles, rhonchi, wheezing, and diminished or absent breath sounds.
- Auscultate for murmurs, clicks, gallops, and pericardial rub.

■ Palpate for lifts, heaves, thrills, gallops, tactile fremitus, and abdominal masses or tenderness.

Causes

Medical causes

Angina pectoris

■ Chest discomfort may be described as pain or a sensation of indigestion or expansion.
■ Pain usually occurs in the retrosternal region behind the sternum and typically lasts 2 to 10 minutes.
■ Pain may radiate to the neck, jaw, and arms.
■ Emotional stress, exertion, or a heavy meal may provoke anginal pain.
■ Other signs and symptoms include dyspnea, nausea, vomiting, tachycardia, dizziness, diaphoresis, belching, and palpitations.
■ With Prinzmetal's angina, pain occurs at rest and with shortness of breath, nausea, vomiting, dizziness, and palpitations.

Anthrax, inhalation

■ Early signs and symptoms include low-grade fever, chills, cough, and chest pain.
■ Later signs and symptoms are characterized by abrupt development and rapid deterioration, including high fever, dyspnea, stridor, and hypotension, generally leading to death within 24 hours.

Anxiety

■ Intermittent, sharp, stabbing pain occurs behind the left breast.
■ Other signs and symptoms include precordial tenderness, palpitations, fatigue, headache, insomnia, breathlessness, nausea, vomiting, diarrhea, and tremors.

Aortic aneurysm, dissecting

■ In this life-threatening disorder, excruciating tearing, ripping, stabbing chest and neck pain begins suddenly and radiates to the upper and lower back and abdomen.
■ Other signs and symptoms include abdominal tenderness; tachycardia; murmurs; syncope; blindness; loss of consciousness; weakness or transient paralysis of the arms or legs; hypotension; asymmetrical brachial pulses; lower blood pressure in the legs than in the arms; pale, cool, diaphoretic, and mottled skin below the waist; weak or absent femoral or pedal pulses; a palpable abdominal mass; and systolic bruit.

Asthma

■ Diffuse and painful chest tightness, dry cough, and mild wheezing arise suddenly.
■ Signs may progress to a productive cough, audible wheezing, and severe dyspnea.
■ Associated respiratory signs and symptoms include rhonchi, crackles, prolonged expirations, intercostal and supraclavicular retractions on inspiration, accessory muscle use, flaring nostrils, and tachypnea.
■ Other signs and symptoms include anxiety, tachycardia, diaphoresis, flushing, and cyanosis.

Bronchitis

■ The acute form produces a burning chest pain or a sensation of substernal tightness.
■ Cough is initially dry but later productive.
■ Other signs and symptoms include low-grade fever, chills, sore throat, tachycardia, muscle and back pain, rhonchi, crackles, and wheezing.

Cardiomyopathy

■ Hypertrophic cardiomyopathy may cause angina-like chest pain, dyspnea, cough, dizziness, syncope, gallops, murmurs, and bradycardia associated with tachycardia.

- A medium-pitched systolic ejection murmur may be heard along the left sternal border and top of the heart.
- Palpation of peripheral pulses reveals a characteristic double impulse (*pulsus biferiens*).

Cholecystitis

- Epigastric or right upper quadrant pain occurs abruptly because of gallbladder inflammation.
- Pain may be sharp or intensely aching, steady or intermittent.
- Pain may radiate to the back or right shoulder.
- An abdominal mass, rigidity, distention, or tenderness may be palpable in the right upper abdomen.
- Other signs and symptoms include Murphy's sign, nausea, vomiting, fever, diaphoresis, and chills.

Costochondritis

- Pain and tenderness due to inflammation occur at the costochondral junctions, especially at the second costicartilage.
- Pain is elicited by palpating the inflamed joint, and worsens with movement.

Esophageal spasm

- Substernal chest pain mimics angina.
- Pain may last up to 1 hour and can radiate to the neck, jaw, arms, or back.
- Other signs and symptoms include dysphagia for solid foods, bradycardia, and nodal rhythm.

Hiatal hernia

- Heartburn and sternal ache or pressure occur and may radiate to the left shoulder and arm.
- Pain occurs after a meal and with bending or lying down.
- Other signs and symptoms include a bitter taste and pain while eating or drinking.

Interstitial lung disease

- Pleuritic chest pain, progressive dyspnea, "cellophane" crackles, nonproductive cough, fatigue, weight loss, decreased exercise tolerance, clubbing, and cyanosis occur.

Legionnaires' disease

- In this bacterial infection, pleuritic chest pain, malaise, headache, and general weakness develop early.
- Within 12 to 24 hours, a sudden high fever, chills, a nonproductive cough that eventually yields mucoid and then mucopurulent sputum and, possibly, hemoptysis occur.
- Other signs and symptoms include diarrhea, flushed skin, diaphoresis, prostration, anorexia, nausea, vomiting, diffuse myalgia, mild temporary amnesia, confusion, dyspnea, crackles, tachypnea, and tachycardia.

Mitral valve prolapse

- Sharp, stabbing precordial chest pain or precordial ache may occur.
- A midsystolic click is followed by a systolic murmur at the apex.
- Other signs and symptoms include cardiac awareness, migraine headache, dizziness, weakness, episodic severe fatigue, dyspnea, tachycardia, mood swings, and palpitations.

Myocardial infarction

- Crushing substernal pain occurs that isn't relieved by nitroglycerin.
- Pain lasts 15 minutes to hours, and may radiate to the left arm, jaw, neck, or shoulder blades.
- Other signs and symptoms include pallor, clammy skin, dyspnea, diaphoresis, nausea, vomiting, anxiety, restlessness, murmurs, crackles, hypotension or hypertension, a feeling of impending doom, and an atrial gallop.

Pancreatitis

- The acute form causes intense pain in the epigastric area.
- Pain radiates to the back and worsens in a supine position.
- Extreme restlessness, mottled skin, tachycardia, and cold, sweaty extremities may occur with severe pancreatitis.
- Massive hemorrhage, with resultant shock and coma, occurs with sudden, severe pancreatitis.
- Other signs and symptoms include nausea, vomiting, fever, abdominal tenderness and rigidity, diminished bowel sounds, and crackles at the lung bases.

Peptic ulcer

- Sharp and burning pain arises in the epigastric region hours after food intake, commonly during the night.
- Pain is relieved by food or antacids.
- Other signs and symptoms include nausea, vomiting, melena, and epigastric tenderness.

Pericarditis

- Sharp or cutting precordial or retrosternal pain is aggravated by deep breathing, coughing, and position changes.
- Pain radiates to the shoulder and neck.
- Other signs and symptoms include pericardial rub, fever, tachycardia, and dyspnea.

Pleurisy

- Sharp, usually one-sided pain in the lower aspects of the chest arises abruptly, reaching maximum intensity within a few hours.
- Deep breathing, coughing, or thoracic movement aggravates pain.
- Decreased breath sounds, inspiratory crackles, and a pleural rub may be heard on auscultation.
- Other signs and symptoms include dyspnea, shallow breathing, cyanosis, fever, and fatigue.

Pneumonia

- Pleuritic chest pain increases with deep inspiration.
- Shaking chills, fever, and a dry, hacking cough that later becomes productive occur.
- Other signs and symptoms include crackles, rhonchi, tachycardia, tachypnea, myalgia, fatigue, headache, dyspnea, abdominal pain, anorexia, cyanosis, decreased breath sounds, and diaphoresis.

Pneumothorax

- In this life-threatening disorder, sudden, severe, and sharp chest pain typically presents on one side and increases with chest movement.
- Dyspnea and cyanosis progressively worsen.
- Breath sounds are decreased or absent on the affected side, with hyperresonance or tympany, subcutaneous crepitation, and decreased vocal fremitus.
- Other signs and symptoms include asymmetrical chest expansion, accessory muscle use, nonproductive cough, tachypnea, tachycardia, anxiety, and restlessness.

Pulmonary embolism

- Sudden dyspnea occurs with intense angina-like or pleuritic pain that's aggravated by deep breathing and thoracic movement.
- Cyanosis and jugular vein distention occur with a large embolus.
- Other signs and symptoms include a choking sensation, tachycardia, tachypnea, cough, low-grade fever, restlessness, diaphoresis, crackles, pleural rub, diffuse wheezing, dullness on percussion, signs of respiratory collapse, paradoxical pulse, signs of cerebral ischemia, and signs of hypoxia.

Pulmonary hypertension, primary

- Angina-like pain develops late and typically occurs on exertion.

- Pain may radiate to the neck.
- Other signs and symptoms include exertional dyspnea, fatigue, syncope, weakness, cough, and hemoptysis.

Rib fracture

- Chest pain is usually sharp, severe, and aggravated by inspiration, coughing, or pressure on the affected area.
- Other signs and symptoms include dyspnea, cough, tenderness and slight edema at the fracture site, and shallow, splinted breathing.

Sickle cell crisis

- Pain may be vague at first and located in the back, hands, or feet.
- As pain worsens, it becomes generalized or localized to the abdomen or chest, causing severe pleuritic pain.
- Other signs and symptoms may include abdominal distention and rigidity, dyspnea, fever, and jaundice.

Tuberculosis

- Pleuritic chest pain and fine crackles occur after coughing.
- Other signs and symptoms include night sweats, anorexia, weight loss, fever, malaise, dyspnea, fatigue, mild to severe productive cough, hemoptysis, dullness on percussion, increased tactile fremitus, and amphoric breath sounds.

Other causes

Chinese restaurant syndrome

- A reaction to excessive ingestion of monosodium glutamate mimics the signs of an acute MI.

Drugs

- Abrupt withdrawal from a beta-adrenergic blocker can cause rebound angina in the patient with heart disease.

Nursing considerations

- Prepare the patient for cardiopulmonary studies.
- Perform a venipuncture to collect a serum specimen for cardiac enzyme and other studies.
- A child may complain of chest pain in an attempt to get attention or to avoid attending school.
- Because older patients have a higher risk of developing life-threatening conditions, carefully evaluate reports of chest pain.

Patient teaching

- Alert the patient or caregiver to signs and symptoms that require immediate medical attention.
- Explain the diagnostic tests the patient needs.
- Provide details to the patient about his prescribed drugs and how to take them.
- Teach the patient about the underlying diagnosis and ways to prevent chest pain in the future.

Cheyne-Stokes respirations

The most common pattern of periodic breathing, Cheyne-Stokes respirations are characterized by a waxing and waning period of hyperpnea that alternates with a shorter period of apnea. This pattern can occur normally in patients with heart or lung disease. It usually indicates increased intracranial pressure (ICP) from a deep cerebral or brain stem lesion, or a metabolic disturbance in the brain. (See *Respiratory pattern of Cheyne-Stokes,* page 72.)

Cheyne-Stokes respirations may indicate a major change in the patient's condition—usually deterioration. For example, in a patient who has had head trauma or brain surgery, Cheyne-Stokes respirations may signal increasing ICP. However, Cheyne-Stokes respirations can occur normally in a patient who lives at high altitudes.

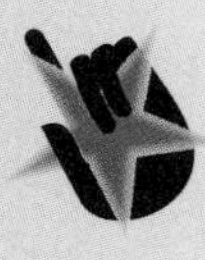

KNOW-HOW

Respiratory pattern of Cheyne-Stokes

When assessing a patient's respirations, determine the rate, rhythm, and depth. This schematic diagram shows the respiratory pattern of Cheyne-Stokes. Respirations gradually become faster and deeper than normal and then slow down. This pattern of respiration alternates with periods of apnea.

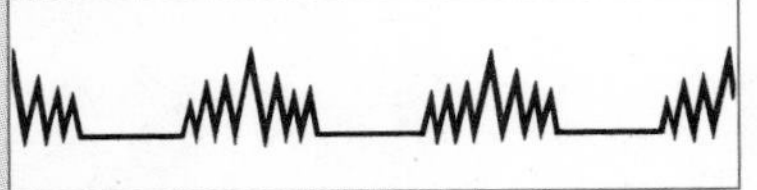

QUICK ACTION ***If you detect Cheyne-Stokes respirations in a patient with a history of head trauma, recent brain surgery, or another brain insult, quickly take his vital signs. Keep his head elevated 30 degrees, and perform a rapid neurologic examination to obtain baseline data. Reevaluate the patient's neurologic status frequently. If ICP continues to increase, you'll detect changes in the patient's level of consciousness (LOC), pupillary reactions, and ability to move his extremities. ICP monitoring is indicated.***

Time the periods of hyperpnea and apnea for 3 or 4 minutes to evaluate respirations and to obtain baseline data. Be alert for prolonged periods of apnea. Frequently check the patient's blood pressure; also check his skin color to detect signs of hypoxemia. Maintain airway patency and give oxygen as needed. If the patient's condition worsens, endotracheal intubation is necessary.

History

- Obtain a medical and surgical history.
- Ask about drug use.

Physical examination

- Perform a complete physical examination, focusing on the neurologic and cardiorespiratory systems.

Causes

Medical causes

Adams-Stokes syndrome

- Adams-Stokes attacks may precede Cheyne-Stokes respirations.
- A syncopal episode associated with atrioventricular block occurs.
- Other signs and symptoms include hypotension, heart rate of 20 to 50 beats/minute, confusion, shaking, and paleness.

Heart failure

- Cheyne-Stokes respirations may occur with exertional dyspnea and orthopnea in left-sided heart failure.
- Other signs and symptoms include fatigue, weakness, tachycardia, tachypnea, and crackles.

Hypertensive encephalopathy

- In this life-threatening disorder, severe hypertension precedes Cheyne-Stokes respirations.
- Other signs and symptoms include decreased LOC, vomiting, seizures, severe headache, vision disturbances, and transient paralysis.

Increased ICP

- Cheyne-Stokes respirations are the first irregular respiratory pattern to occur as ICP increases.
- Bradycardia and widened pulse pressure are late signs of increased ICP.

■ Accompanying signs and symptoms include decreased LOC, hypertension, headache, vomiting, impaired motor movement, and vision disturbances.

Renal failure

■ Cheyne-Stokes respirations occur with end-stage chronic renal failure.

■ Other signs and symptoms include bleeding gums, oral lesions, ammonia breath odor, and marked changes in every body system.

Other causes

Drugs

■ Large doses of an opioid, hypnotic, or barbiturate can precipitate Cheyne-Stokes respirations.

Nursing considerations

■ Don't mistake periods of hypoventilation or decreased tidal volume for complete apnea.

■ Cheyne-Stokes respirations rarely occur in children except during late heart failure.

■ Cheyne-Stokes respirations may occur normally in elderly people during sleep.

Patient teaching

■ Teach the patient and a responsible person to recognize the difference between sleep apnea and Cheyne-Stokes respirations.

■ Explain the causes and treatments of conditions leading to Cheyne-Stokes respirations.

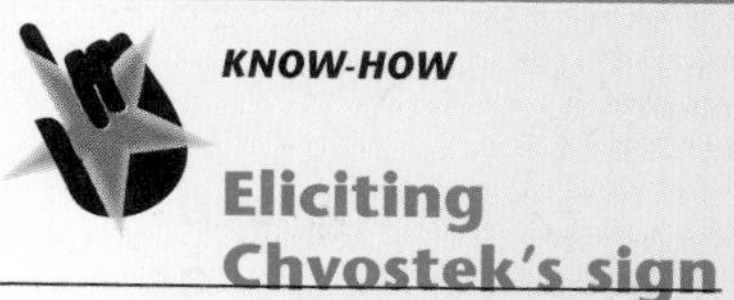

KNOW-HOW

Eliciting Chvostek's sign

Begin by telling the patient to relax his facial muscles. Then stand directly in front of him and tap the facial nerve either just anterior to the earlobe and below the zygomatic arch, or between the zygomatic arch and the corner of his mouth. A positive response varies from twitching of the lip at the corner of the mouth to spasm of all facial muscles, depending on the severity of hypocalcemia.

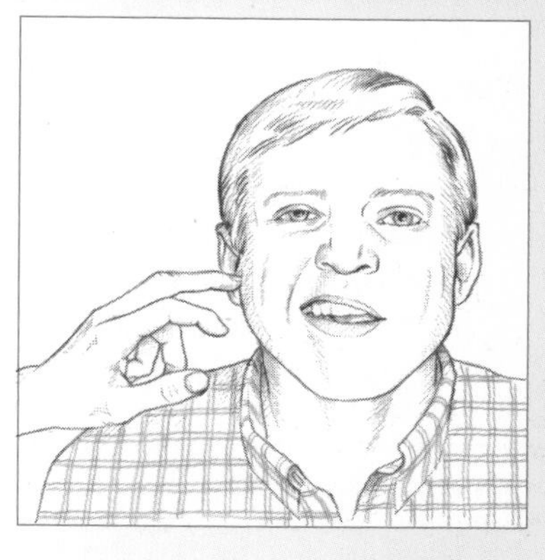

Chvostek's sign

Chvostek's sign is an abnormal spasm of the facial muscles that's elicited by lightly tapping the patient's facial nerve near his lower jaw. (See *Eliciting Chvostek's sign*.)

This sign usually suggests hypocalcemia, but can occur normally in about 25% of cases. Typically, it precedes other signs of hypocalcemia and persists until the onset of tetany. It can't be elicited during tetany because of strong muscle contractions.

Usually, eliciting Chvostek's sign is attempted only in patients with suspected hypocalcemic disorders. However, because the parathyroid gland regulates calcium balance, Chvostek's sign may also be tested in patients before neck surgery, to obtain a baseline.

QUICK ACTION ***Test for Trousseau's sign, a reliable indicator of hypocalcemia. Closely monitor the patient for signs of***

tetany, such as carpopedal spasms or circumoral and extremity paresthesia.

Be prepared to act quickly if a seizure occurs. Perform an electrocardiogram to check for changes associated with hypocalcemia that can predispose the patient to arrhythmias. Place the patient on a cardiac monitor.

History

- Obtain a medical history, including incidence of hypoparathyroidism, hypomagnesemia, or a malabsorption disorder.
- Ask about previous surgical removal of parathyroid glands.
- Determine whether mental changes have occurred.
- Question the patient about other symptoms, including tingling sensations around the mouth and in the fingertips and feet.

Physical examination

- Observe the patient's behavior.
- Watch for seizures, tetany, and facial spasms.
- Check for dry and scaling skin, brittle nails, and dry hair.
- Take the patient's vital signs because an irregular pulse and hypotension suggest hypocalcemia.
- Auscultate the lungs.
- Note signs of bronchospasm, laryngospasm, and airway obstruction.

Causes

Medical causes

Hypocalcemia

- The degree of muscle spasm elicited reflects the patient's calcium level.
- Initially, paresthesia in the fingers, toes, and circumoral area that progresses to muscle tension and carpopedal spasms occur.
- Muscle weakness, muscle twitching, hyperactive deep tendon reflexes, choreiform movements, muscle cramps, fatigue, and palpitations may be present.
- With chronic hypocalcemia, signs and symptoms include mental status changes; diplopia; difficulty swallowing; abdominal cramps; dry, scaly skin; brittle nails; and thin, patchy scalp hair and eyebrows.

Other causes

Treatments

- Massive blood transfusion can lower calcium levels.

Nursing considerations

- Collect blood samples for ongoing calcium studies.
- Administer oral or I.V. calcium supplements.
- Look for Chvostek's sign postoperatively.
- Because this sign may be observed in healthy infants, it isn't used to detect neonatal tetany.
- Consider malabsorption and poor nutritional status in the elderly patient with Chvostek's sign and hypocalcemia.

Patient teaching

- Explain which early signs and symptoms of hypocalcemia a patient should report immediately to the practitioner.
- Teach the patient about the underlying cause of hypocalcemia and how to prevent it.

Corneal reflex, absent

Tested bilaterally, a normal corneal reflex causes both eyes to blink each time either cornea is touched. (See *Eliciting the corneal reflex*.)

The site of the afferent fibers for this reflex is in the ophthalmic branch of the trigeminal nerve (cranial nerve [CN] V). The efferent fibers are located in the facial nerve (CN VII). Unilateral or bilateral absence of the corneal reflex may result from damage to these nerves.

History

■ Because an absent corneal reflex may signify such progressive neurologic disorders as Guillain-Barré syndrome, ask the patient about associated symptoms—facial pain, dysphagia, and limb weakness.

Physical examination

■ Test the corneal reflex bilaterally.
■ If you can't elicit the corneal reflex, look for other signs of trigeminal nerve dysfunction. To test the three sensory portions of the nerve, touch each side of the patient's face on the brow, cheek, and jaw with a cotton wisp, and ask him to compare the sensations.
■ If you suspect facial nerve involvement, note if the upper face (brow and eyes) and lower face (cheek, mouth, and chin) are weak bilaterally. Lower motor neuron facial weakness affects the face on the same side as the lesion, whereas upper motor neuron weakness affects the side opposite the lesion—predominantly the lower facial muscles.

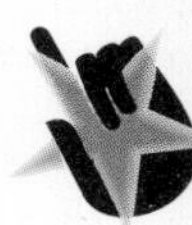

KNOW-HOW

Eliciting the corneal reflex

To elicit the corneal reflex, have the patient turn his eyes away from you to avoid involuntary blinking during the procedure. Then approach the patient from the opposite side, out of his line of vision, and brush the cornea lightly with a fine wisp of sterile cotton. Repeat the procedure on the other eye.

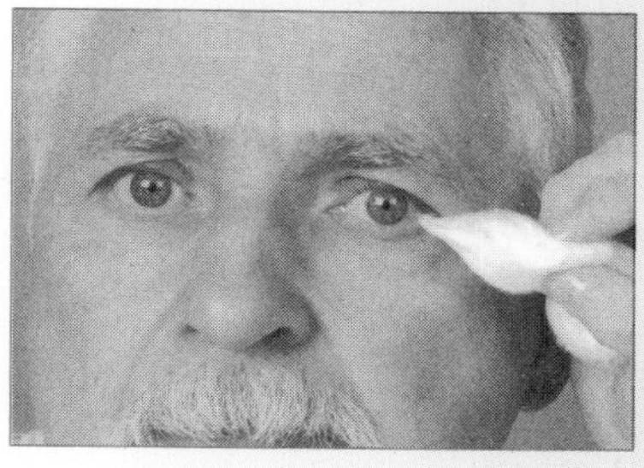

Causes

Medical causes

Acoustic neuroma

■ This condition affects the trigeminal nerve, causing a diminished or absent corneal reflex, tinnitus, and unilateral hearing impairment.
■ Facial palsy and anesthesia, palate weakness, and signs of cerebellar dysfunction (ataxia, nystagmus) may result if the tumor impinges on the adjacent cranial nerves, brain stem, and cerebellum.

Bell's palsy

■ This disorder is the most common cause of diminished or absent corneal reflex and paralysis of CN VII, probably due to a viral infection.
■ Other signs and symptoms include complete hemifacial weakness or paralysis; drooling on the affected side, which also sags and appears masklike; and constant tearing and inability of the eye on the affected side to close.

Brain stem infarction or injury

■ An absent corneal reflex can occur on the side opposite the lesion when infarction or injury affects CN V or VII or their connection in the central trigeminal tract.
■ With massive brain stem infarction or injury, the patient also displays respiratory changes, such as apneustic breathing or periods of apnea; bilateral pupillary dilation or constriction with decreased responsiveness to light; rising systolic blood pressure; widening pulse pressure; bradycardia; and coma.
■ Other signs and symptoms include decreased level of consciousness, dysphagia, dysarthria, contralateral limb

weakness, and early signs and symptoms of increased intracranial pressure, such as headache and vomiting.

Guillain-Barré syndrome

- With this polyneuropathic disorder, a diminished or absent corneal reflex accompanies ipsilateral loss of facial muscle control.
- Muscle weakness, the dominant neurologic sign, typically starts in the legs, and then extends to the arms and facial nerves within 72 hours.
- Other signs and symptoms include dysarthria, dysphagia, paresthesia, respiratory muscle paralysis, respiratory insufficiency, orthostatic hypotension, incontinence, diaphoresis, and tachycardia.

Nursing considerations

- When the corneal reflex is absent, take measures to protect the patient's affected eye from injury such as lubricating the eye with artificial tears to prevent drying.
- Cover the cornea with a shield and avoid excessive corneal reflex testing.
- Prepare the patient for cranial X-rays or computed tomography scanning.
- In children, brain stem lesions and injuries are usual causes of absent corneal reflexes; Guillain-Barré syndrome and trigeminal neuralgia are less common.
- Infants, especially those born prematurely, may have an absent corneal reflex due to anoxic damage to the brain stem.

Patient teaching

- Teach the patient and his family about the underlying diagnosis and prognosis.
- Teach the patient and his family about hospital procedures and testing.
- Provide the patient and his family with resources for home care and follow-up care.

Costovertebral angle tenderness

Costovertebral angle (CVA) tenderness indicates sudden distention of the renal capsule. It almost always accompanies unelicited, dull, constant flank pain in the CVA just lateral to the sacrospinalis muscle and below the 12th rib. This associated pain typically travels anteriorly in the subcostal region toward the umbilicus.

Percussing the CVA elicits tenderness, if present. (See *Eliciting CVA tenderness.*)

A patient who doesn't have this symptom will feel a thudding, jarring, or pressurelike sensation when tested, but no pain. A patient with a disorder that distends the renal capsule will experience intense pain as the renal capsule stretches and stimulates the afferent nerves, which emanate from the spinal cord at levels T11 through L2 and innervate the kidney.

History

- Find out about other signs and symptoms of renal or urologic dysfunction.
- Ask about voiding habits and the onset and description of any recent changes.
- Obtain a personal or family history of urinary tract infections, congenital anomalies, calculi, other obstructive nephropathies or uropathies, or renovascular disorders.

Physical examination

- Take the patient's vital signs.
- If the patient has hypertension and bradycardia, look for other autonomic effects of renal pain.
- Inspect, auscultate, and gently palpate the abdomen for clues to the underlying cause of CVA tenderness.

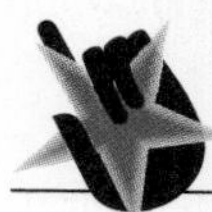

KNOW-HOW

Eliciting CVA tenderness

To elicit costovertebral angle (CVA) tenderness, have the patient sit upright facing away from you or have him in a prone position. Place the palm of your left hand over the left CVA, then strike the back of your left hand with the ulnar surface of your right fist (as shown at right). Repeat this percussion technique over the right CVA. A patient with CVA tenderness will experience intense pain.

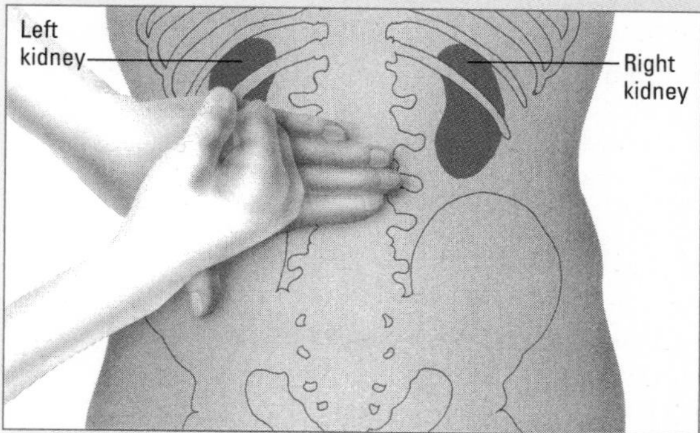

■ Look for abdominal distention, hypoactive bowel sounds, and palpable masses.

Causes

Medical causes

Calculi

■ CVA tenderness occurs with waves of waxing and waning flank pain that may radiate to the groin, testicles, suprapubic area, or labia, caused by calculi of the urinary tract system.

■ Other signs and symptoms include nausea, vomiting, severe abdominal pain, abdominal distention, and decreased bowel sounds.

Perirenal abscess

■ Exquisite CVA tenderness occurs with flank pain that may radiate to the groin or down the leg.

■ Other signs and symptoms include dysuria, persistent high fever, chills, erythema of the skin, and a palpable abdominal mass.

Pyelonephritis, acute

■ CVA tenderness occurs with persistent high fever, chills, flank pain, anorexia, nausea and vomiting, weakness, dysuria, hematuria, nocturia, urinary urgency and frequency, and tenesmus.

Renal artery occlusion

■ The patient experiences flank pain and CVA tenderness.

■ Other signs and symptoms include severe, continuous upper abdominal pain, nausea, vomiting, hematuria, decreased bowel sounds, and high fever.

Nursing considerations

■ Give prescribed drugs for pain.

■ Monitor the patient's vital signs and fluid intake and urine output.

■ Collect blood samples and urine specimens as ordered.

■ An infant won't exhibit CVA tenderness; instead, he'll display nonspecific signs and symptoms.

■ In older children, CVA tenderness has the same significance as in adults.

- Advanced age and cognitive impairment reduce an elderly patient's ability to perceive pain.

Patient teaching

- Explain any dietary restrictions the patient needs.
- Tell the patient to drink at least 2 qt (2 L) of fluids daily unless he's instructed otherwise.
- Explain which signs and symptoms of kidney infection he should report.
- Emphasize the importance of taking the full course of prescribed antibiotics.

Cough, nonproductive

A nonproductive cough is a noisy, forceful expulsion of air from the lungs that doesn't yield sputum or blood. It's one of the most common complaints of patients with respiratory disorders.

Coughing is a necessary protective mechanism that clears airway passages. However, a nonproductive cough is ineffective and can cause damage, such as airway collapse or rupture of alveoli or blebs. A nonproductive cough that later becomes productive is a classic sign of progressive respiratory disease.

The cough reflex generally occurs when mechanical, chemical, thermal, inflammatory, or psychogenic stimuli activate cough receptors.

However, external pressure—for example, from subdiaphragmatic irritation or a mediastinal tumor—can also induce it as well as voluntary expiration of air, which occasionally occurs as a nervous habit. Certain drugs, such as angiotensin-converting enzyme (ACE) inhibitors, may also cause a nonproductive cough.

A nonproductive cough may occur in paroxysms and can worsen by becoming more frequent. An acute cough has a sudden onset and may be self-limiting; a cough that persists beyond 1 month is considered chronic and commonly results from cigarette smoking.

History

- Ask about the onset, frequency, and description of coughing.
- Ask about aggravating factors.
- Obtain a smoking history.
- Find out the onset and location of associated pain.
- Obtain a history of surgery or trauma.
- Inquire about hypersensitivity to drugs, foods, pets, dust, or pollen.
- Find out which drugs the patient is taking.
- Ask about recent changes in appetite, weight, exercise tolerance, or energy level.
- Ask about recent exposure to irritating fumes, chemicals, or smoke.

Physical examination

- Observe the patient, and note behavior, cyanosis, clubbed fingers, or edema.
- Observe for use of accessory muscles, and note retractions.
- Take the patient's vital signs, checking the depth and rhythm of respirations; note if wheezing occurs with breathing.
- Inspect the neck for distended veins and a deviated trachea.
- Check the skin, noting whether it's cool or warm, dry or clammy.
- Check the mouth and nose for congestion, inflammation, drainage, and signs of infection.
- Examine the chest, looking for abnormal chest wall configuration and motion, such as accessory muscle use and retraction.
- Auscultate for wheezing, crackles, rhonchi, pleural rub, and decreased or absent breath sounds.
- Percuss for dullness, tympany, and flatness.

Causes

Medical causes

Airway occlusion

- Partial occlusion of the upper airway produces a sudden onset of dry, paroxysmal coughing.
- If choking on a foreign object, the patient may clutch his throat with his thumb and fingers extended.
- Other signs and symptoms include gagging, wheezing, hoarseness, stridor, tachycardia, and decreased breath sounds.

Anthrax, inhalation

- Initial signs and symptoms include low-grade fever, chills, weakness, cough, and chest pain.
- In the second stage, rapid deterioration is marked by fever, dyspnea, stridor, and hypotension, generally leading to death within 24 hours.

Aortic aneurysm, thoracic

- A brassy cough occurs with dyspnea, hoarseness, wheezing, and a substernal ache in the shoulders, lower back, or abdomen.
- Other signs and symptoms include facial or neck edema, jugular vein distention, dysphagia, prominent veins over the chest, stridor, paresthesia, and neuralgia.

Asthma

- Attacks start with a nonproductive cough and mild wheezing.
- As the attack progresses, severe dyspnea, audible wheezing, chest tightness, and a cough that produces thick mucus develop.
- Other signs and symptoms include anxiety, rhonchi, prolonged expiration, intercostal and supraclavicular retractions on inspiration, accessory muscle use, flaring nostrils, tachypnea, tachycardia, diaphoresis, and flushing or cyanosis.

Atelectasis

- As lung tissue deflates, it stimulates cough receptors, causing a nonproductive cough.
- The trachea may deviate toward the affected side.
- Other signs and symptoms include pleuritic chest pain, anxiety, cyanosis, diaphoresis, dullness on percussion, inspiratory lag, substernal or intercostal retractions, decreased vocal fremitus, dyspnea, tachypnea, and tachycardia.

Bronchitis, chronic

- A nonproductive, hacking cough later becomes productive.
- Clubbing may occur in stages.
- Other signs and symptoms include prolonged expiration, wheezing, dyspnea, accessory muscle use, barrel chest, cyanosis, tachypnea, crackles, and scattered rhonchi.

Bronchogenic carcinoma

- A chronic, nonproductive cough, dyspnea, and vague chest pain are early indicators.
- Other signs and symptoms include wheezing, hemoptysis, and stridor.

Common cold

- A nonproductive, hacking cough progresses to a mix of sneezing, headache, malaise, fatigue, rhinorrhea, myalgia, arthralgia, nasal congestion, and sore throat.

Esophagitis with reflux

- Regurgitation and aspiration produce a nonproductive nocturnal cough.
- Other signs and symptoms include chest pain that mimics angina pectoris, heartburn that worsens if the patient lies down soon after eating, and increased salivation, dysphagia, hematemesis, and melena.

Hodgkin's disease

- A crowing nonproductive cough may develop.
- Painless swelling of cervical lymph nodes or, occasionally, the axillary, mediastinal, or inguinal nodes, is an early sign.
- Pruritus is also an early sign.
- Other signs and symptoms include dyspnea, dysphagia, hepatosplenomegaly, edema, jaundice, nerve pain, and hyperpigmentation.

Hypersensitivity pneumonitis

- An acute, nonproductive cough, fever, dyspnea, and malaise occur 5 to 6 hours after exposure to an antigen.
- Chest tightness and extreme fatigue may also occur.

Interstitial lung disease

- A nonproductive cough and progressive dyspnea occur.
- Other signs and symptoms include cyanosis, clubbing, fine crackles, fatigue, chest pain, weight loss, and dyspnea on exertion.

Laryngeal tumor

- A mild nonproductive cough, minor throat discomfort, and hoarseness are early signs.
- Dysphagia, dyspnea, cervical lymphadenopathy, stridor, and earache occur later.

Legionnaires' disease

- A nonproductive cough progresses to a cough that may produce mucoid, mucopurulent, and bloody sputum.
- Prodromal signs and symptoms include malaise, headache, diarrhea, anorexia, diffuse myalgia, and generalized weakness.

Lung abscess

- A nonproductive cough, weakness, dyspnea, and pleuritic chest pain occur initially.
- Later, cough produces purulent, foul-smelling sputum.
- Other signs and symptoms include diaphoresis, fever, headache, malaise, fatigue, crackles, decreased breath sounds, anorexia, and weight loss.

Mediastinal tumor

- A nonproductive cough, dyspnea, and retrosternal pain occur.
- Snoring respirations with suprasternal retraction on inspiration, hoarseness, dysphagia, tracheal shift or tug, jugular vein distention, and facial or neck edema may develop.

Pleural effusion

- A nonproductive cough, dyspnea, pleuritic chest pain, and decreased chest motion are characteristic findings.
- Other signs and symptoms include pleural rub, tachycardia, tachypnea, egophony, flatness on percussion, decreased or absent breath sounds, and decreased tactile fremitus.

Pneumonia

- Bacterial pneumonia causes a nonproductive, hacking, painful cough that eventually becomes productive.
- Mycoplasmal pneumonia causes a nonproductive cough that may be paroxysmal, arising 2 to 3 days after the onset of malaise, headache, and sore throat.
- Viral pneumonia causes a nonproductive, hacking cough and the gradual onset of malaise, headache, and low-grade fever.
- Other signs and symptoms include shaking chills, headache, high fever, dyspnea, pleuritic chest pain, tachypnea, tachycardia, grunting respirations, nasal flaring, decreased breath sounds, fine crackles, rhonchi, and cyanosis.

Pneumothorax

- The patient with this life-threatening disorder exhibits dry cough and signs of respiratory distress as the lung is compressed due to free air in the pleural cavity.

- Other signs and symptoms include sudden, sharp chest pain that worsens with chest movement, subcutaneous crepitation, hyperresonance or tympany, decreased vocal fremitus, and decreased or absent breath sounds on the affected side.

Pulmonary edema

- Dry cough, exertional dyspnea, paroxysmal nocturnal dyspnea, orthopnea, tachycardia, tachypnea, dependent crackles, and ventricular gallop occur initially.
- Respirations become more rapid and labored, with diffuse crackles and coughing that produces frothy, bloody sputum as the condition worsens.

Pulmonary embolism

- In this life-threatening disorder, dry cough, dyspnea, and pleuritic or anginal chest pain may occur suddenly.
- More commonly, the cough produces blood-tinged sputum.
- Other signs and symptoms include tachycardia, low-grade fever, pleural rub, diffuse wheezing, dullness on percussion, and decreased breath sounds.

Sarcoidosis

- Sarcoidosis is a multisystem, granuloma-producing disorder that especially affects the lungs.
- A nonproductive cough is accompanied by dyspnea, substernal pain, and malaise.
- Other signs and symptoms include fatigue, arthralgia, myalgia, weight loss, tachypnea, crackles, lymphadenopathy, hepatosplenomegaly, skin lesions, vision impairment, difficulty swallowing, and arrhythmias.

Severe acute respiratory syndrome

- In this life-threatening disorder, severe acute respiratory syndrome begins with a fever; headache, malaise, dry nonproductive cough, and dyspnea also occur.

Sinusitis, chronic

- A chronic nonproductive cough may develop from postnasal drip.
- The nasal mucosa may appear inflamed; nasal congestion with profuse drainage and a musty breath odor may occur.

Tracheobronchitis, acute

- As secretions increase, a dry cough becomes productive.
- Chills, sore throat, slight fever, muscle and back pain, and substernal tightness generally precede the cough's onset.

Other causes

Diagnostic tests

- Pulmonary function tests and bronchoscopy may stimulate cough receptors, triggering coughing.

Drugs

- Certain medications, such as ACE inhibitors, may cause a cough.

Treatments

- Suctioning or deep endotracheal or tracheal tube placement can trigger a paroxysmal or hacking cough.
- Intermittent positive-pressure breathing or spirometry may cause a nonproductive cough.
- Inhalants, such as pentamidine (NebuPent), may stimulate coughing.

Nursing considerations

- A nonproductive, paroxysmal cough may induce life-threatening bronchospasm; the patient may need a bronchodilator.

- Unless the patient has chronic obstructive pulmonary disease, give an antitussive and a sedative to suppress the cough.
- Humidify the air in the patient's room.
- In children, the sudden onset of paroxysmal nonproductive coughing may indicate aspiration of a foreign body.
- Nonproductive coughing in children can also result from asthma, bacterial pneumonia, acute bronchiolitis, acute otitis media, measles, cystic fibrosis, airway hyperactivity, or a foreign body in the external auditory canal; it may also be psychogenic.
- In elderly patients, a nonproductive cough may indicate serious acute or chronic illness.

Patient teaching

- Explain how to use a humidifier.
- Teach the patient to avoid respiratory irritants; encourage the use of a respirator mask when he must be around respiratory irritants.
- Explain to the patient why nonproductive coughs should be suppressed and productive coughs should be encouraged.
- Explain the importance of adequate fluids and nutrition.
- If the patient smokes, stress the importance of smoking cessation, and refer him to appropriate resources, support groups, and information to help him quit.

Cough, productive

Productive coughing is the body's mechanism for clearing airway passages of accumulated secretions that normal mucociliary action doesn't remove. It's a sudden, forceful, noisy expulsion of air from the lungs that contains sputum, blood, or both. The sputum's color, consistency, and odor provide important clues about the patient's condition. A productive cough can occur as a single cough or as paroxysmal coughing. Although it's usually a reflexive response to stimulation of the airway mucosa, it can be voluntarily induced.

Usually due to a cardiovascular or respiratory disorder, productive coughing commonly results from an acute or chronic infection that causes inflammation, edema, and increased mucus production in the airways. However, this sign can also result from acquired immunodeficiency syndrome. Inhalation of antigenic or irritating substances or foreign bodies can also cause a productive cough. In fact, the most common cause of chronic productive coughing is cigarette smoking, which produces mucoid sputum ranging in color from clear to yellow to brown.

QUICK ACTION ***A patient with a productive cough can develop acute respiratory distress from thick or excessive secretions, bronchospasm, or fatigue, so examine him before you take his history. Take his vital signs, measure oxygen saturation, and check the rate, depth, and rhythm of respirations. Keep his airway patent, and be prepared to provide supplemental oxygen if he becomes restless or confused or if his respirations become shallow, irregular, rapid, or slow. Look for stridor, wheezing, choking, or gurgling. Be alert for nasal flaring and cyanosis.***

A productive cough may signal a severe, life-threatening disorder. For example, coughing due to pulmonary edema produces thin, frothy, pink sputum, and coughing due to an asthma attack produces thick, mucoid sputum. Help the patient clear excess mucus with tracheal suctioning if needed.

History

- Ask about the onset of coughing.
- Find out about the amount, color, odor, and consistency of the sputum.
- Note the time of day and what aggravates and alleviates coughing and sputum production.
- Ask the patient to describe the sound of the cough.
- Note the location and severity of pain.
- Ask about weight and appetite changes, smoking and alcohol use, asthma, allergies, and respiratory problems.
- Obtain a drug history.
- Review the patient's occupational history for exposure to chemicals or respiratory irritants.

Physical examination

- Examine the patient's mouth and nose for congestion, drainage, or inflammation.
- Note breath odor.
- Inspect the neck for distended veins, and palpate for tenderness and masses or enlarged lymph nodes.
- Observe the chest for accessory muscle use, retractions, and uneven chest expansion.
- Percuss the chest for dullness, tympany, or flatness.
- Auscultate for pleural rub and abnormal breath sounds.

Causes

Medical causes

Aspiration pneumonitis

- Sputum is pink, frothy, and possibly purulent.
- Other signs and symptoms include severe dyspnea, fever, tachypnea, fatigue, chest pain, halitosis, tachycardia, wheezing, and cyanosis.

Asthma, acute

- A life-threatening disorder, acute asthma may produce tenacious mucoid sputum and mucus plugs.
- As the attack progresses, severe dyspnea, audible wheezing, and chest tightness occur.
- Other signs and symptoms include apprehension, prolonged expirations, intercostal and supraclavicular retraction on inspiration, accessory muscle use, rhonchi, crackles, flaring nostrils, tachypnea, tachycardia, diaphoresis, and flushing or cyanosis.

Bronchiectasis

- Coughing produces copious, mucopurulent, layered sputum (top: frothy; middle: clear; bottom: dense, purulent particles).
- The odor of sputum is foul or sickeningly sweet.
- Other signs and symptoms include hemoptysis, persistent coarse crackles, wheezing, rhonchi, exertional dyspnea, weight loss, fatigue, malaise, weakness, fever, and late-stage clubbing.

Bronchitis, chronic

- Cough is nonproductive initially.
- Mucoid sputum becomes purulent.
- Cough usually occurs when the patient is recumbent or rising from sleep.
- Other signs and symptoms include prolonged expiration, accessory muscle use, barrel chest, tachypnea, cyanosis, wheezing, exertional dyspnea, scattered rhonchi, coarse crackles, and late-stage clubbing.

Chemical pneumonitis

- Cough produces purulent sputum.
- Other signs and symptoms include dyspnea; wheezing; orthopnea; malaise; crackles; mucus irritation of the conjunctivae, throat, and nose; laryngitis; and rhinitis.

Common cold

- Cough produces mucoid or mucopurulent sputum.
- Other signs and symptoms include dry hacking cough, sneezing, headache, malaise, fatigue, rhinorrhea, nasal congestion, sore throat, and myalgia.

Legionnaires' disease

- In this disease, caused by a bacterial infection, cough produces scant, mucoid, nonpurulent, and blood-streaked sputum.
- Early signs and symptoms include malaise, fatigue, weakness, anorexia, myalgia, and diarrhea.
- Within 12 to 48 hours, cough becomes dry, with accompanying sudden high fever and chills.
- Other signs and symptoms include pleuritic pain, headache, tachypnea, tachycardia, nausea, vomiting, dyspnea, crackles, and confusion.

Lung abscess, ruptured

- Cough produces purulent, foul-smelling, and blood-tinged sputum.
- Other signs and symptoms include diaphoresis, anorexia, clubbing, weight loss, weakness, fatigue, fever, chills, dyspnea, headache, malaise, pleuritic chest pain, and inspiratory crackles.

Lung cancer

- An early sign of the disease, chronic cough produces small amounts of purulent (or mucopurulent), blood-streaked sputum.
- With bronchoalveolar cancer, cough produces large amounts of frothy sputum.
- Other signs and symptoms include dyspnea, anorexia, fatigue, weight loss, chest pain, fever, diaphoresis, wheezing, and clubbing.

Pneumonia

- A dry cough becomes productive as the condition progresses.
- Other signs and symptoms develop suddenly and include shaking chills, high fever, myalgia, pleuritic chest pain, tachycardia, tachypnea, dyspnea, cyanosis, diaphoresis, decreased breath sounds, crackles, and rhonchi.

Pulmonary edema

- In this life-threatening disorder, early signs include exertional dyspnea, paroxysmal nocturnal dyspnea followed by orthopnea, and a nonproductive cough that eventually produces frothy, bloody sputum.
- Other signs and symptoms include fever, fatigue, tachycardia, tachypnea, crackles, and ventricular gallop.

Pulmonary embolism

- The first sign of this life-threatening disorder is usually severe dyspnea with angina or pleuritic chest pain.
- Cough may be nonproductive or may produce blood-tinged sputum.
- Severe anxiety, low-grade fever, tachycardia, tachypnea, and diaphoresis develop.
- Other symptoms include pleural rub, wheezing, crackles, chest dullness on percussion, decreased breath sounds, and signs of circulatory collapse.

Pulmonary emphysema

- Chronic cough produces scant, mucoid, translucent, grayish-white sputum, which can become mucopurulent.
- Other signs and symptoms include a thin appearance, weight loss, accessory muscle use, tachypnea, grunting expirations through pursed lips, diminished breath sounds, exertional dyspnea, rhonchi, barrel chest, anorexia, and late clubbing.

Pulmonary tuberculosis

- Cough may be mild to severe, with sputum that may be scant and mucoid or copious and purulent.
- Other signs and symptoms include hemoptysis, malaise, dyspnea, pleuritic chest pain, night sweats, fatigue, and weight loss.

Silicosis

- Silicosis occurs after inhalation of silica dust over a period of years, resulting in progressive fibrosis of the lungs.
- Cough with mucopurulent sputum is the first sign.
- Other signs and symptoms include exertional dyspnea, tachypnea, weight loss, fatigue, weakness, recurrent respiratory infections, and end-inspiratory crackles.

Tracheobronchitis

- After the onset of chills, sore throat, fever, muscle and back pain, and substernal tightness, cough becomes productive.
- Sputum is mucoid, mucopurulent, or purulent.
- Other signs and symptoms include rhonchi, wheezes, crackles, fever, and bronchospasm.

Other causes

Diagnostic tests

- Bronchoscopy and pulmonary function tests may cause productive coughing.

Drugs

- Expectorants increase productive coughing.

Respiratory therapy

- Incentive spirometry, intermittent positive-pressure breathing, and nebulizer therapy may cause productive coughing.

Nursing considerations

- Give a mucolytic and an expectorant, as prescribed, to increase productive coughing.
- Increase the patient's fluid intake to thin secretions.
- Give a bronchodilator, as prescribed, to relieve bronchospasm and open airways.
- If an infection is present, give antibiotics as prescribed.
- Humidify the air to relieve mucous membrane irritation and loosen secretions.
- Provide pulmonary physiotherapy to loosen secretions.
- Provide rest periods.
- Collect sputum specimens for culture and sensitivity testing.
- Be aware that a child with a productive cough can quickly develop airway occlusion and respiratory distress.
- Causes of a productive cough in children include asthma, bronchiectasis, bronchitis, acute bronchiolitis, cystic fibrosis, and pertussis.
- High humidity can induce bronchospasm in a hyperactive child or overhydration in an infant.
- An elderly patient with a productive cough may be suffering from a serious acute or chronic illness.

Patient teaching

- Refer the patient to resources to quit smoking.
- Teach the patient coughing and deep-breathing techniques.
- Teach the patient and caregiver to use chest percussion to loosen secretions.
- Explain the importance of adequate hydration and prescribed medications to thin secretions and improve expectoration.
- Explain infection control techniques.
- Explain how the patient can avoid respiratory irritants.

Crackles

A common finding in patients with certain cardiovascular and pulmonary disorders, crackles are nonmusical clicking or rattling noises heard during auscultation of breath sounds. They usually occur during inspiration and recur constantly from one respiratory cycle to the next. They can be unilateral or bilateral, moist or dry. They're characterized by their pitch, loudness, location, persistence, and occurrence during the respiratory cycle.

Crackles indicate abnormal movement of air through fluid-filled airways. They can be irregularly dispersed, as in pneumonia, or localized, as in bronchiectasis. (A few basilar crackles can be heard in normal lungs after prolonged shallow breathing. These normal crackles clear with a few deep breaths.) Usually, crackles indicate the degree of an underlying illness. When crackles result from a generalized disorder, they usually occur in the less distended and more dependent areas of the lungs (such as the lung bases) when the patient is standing. Crackles due to air passing through inflammatory exudate may not be audible if the involved portion of the lung isn't being ventilated because of shallow respirations. (See *How crackles occur.*)

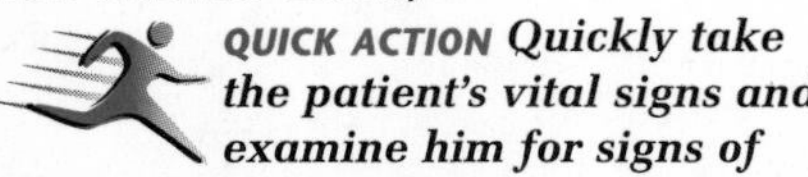

QUICK ACTION ***Quickly take the patient's vital signs and examine him for signs of respiratory distress or airway obstruction. Check the depth and rhythm of respirations. Is he struggling to breathe? Check for increased accessory muscle use and chest wall motion, retractions, stridor, or nasal flaring. Assess the patient for other signs and symptoms of fluid overload, such as jugular vein distention and edema. Provide supplemental oxygen and, if necessary, a diuretic. Endotracheal intubation may also be needed.***

History

- Ask about the onset, duration, and description of cough and pain.
- Note the sputum's consistency, amount, odor, and color.
- Obtain a medical history, including incidence of cancer, respiratory or cardiovascular problems, surgery, or trauma.
- Ask about smoking and alcohol use.
- Obtain a drug and occupational history.
- Inquire about recent weight loss, anorexia, nausea, vomiting, fatigue, weakness, vertigo, hoarseness, difficulty swallowing, and syncope.
- Determine exposure to respiratory irritants.

Physical examination

- Examine the nose and mouth for signs of infection.
- Note breath odor.
- Check the neck for masses, tenderness, lymphadenopathy, swelling, or venous distention.
- Inspect the chest for abnormal configuration or uneven expansion.
- Percuss the chest for dullness, tympany, or flatness.
- Auscultate the lungs for other abnormal, diminished, or absent breath sounds.
- Listen for abnormal heart sounds.
- Check the hands and feet for edema or clubbing.

Causes

Medical causes

Acute respiratory distress syndrome

- In this life-threatening disorder, diffuse, fine to coarse crackles are usually heard in the dependent portions of the lungs.
- Other signs and symptoms include cyanosis, nasal flaring, tachypnea, tachycardia, grunting respirations, rhonchi, dyspnea, anxiety, and decreased level of consciousness.

How crackles occur

Crackles occur when air passes through fluid-filled airways, causing collapsed alveoli to pop open as the airway pressure equalizes. They can also occur when membranes lining the chest cavity and lungs become inflamed. The illustrations below show a normal alveolus and two pathologic alveolar changes that cause crackles.

NORMAL ALVEOLUS

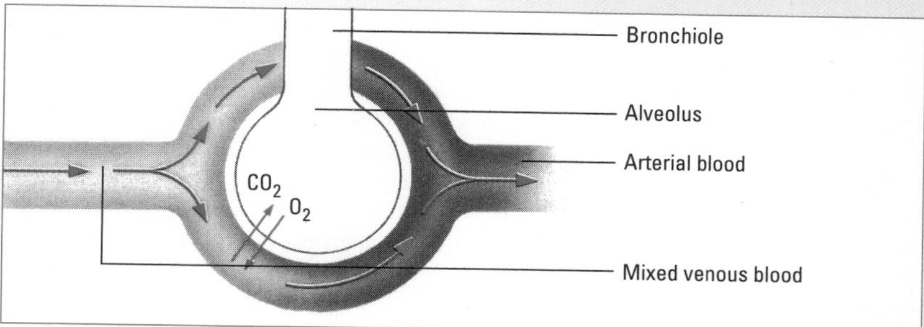

ALVEOLUS IN PULMONARY EDEMA

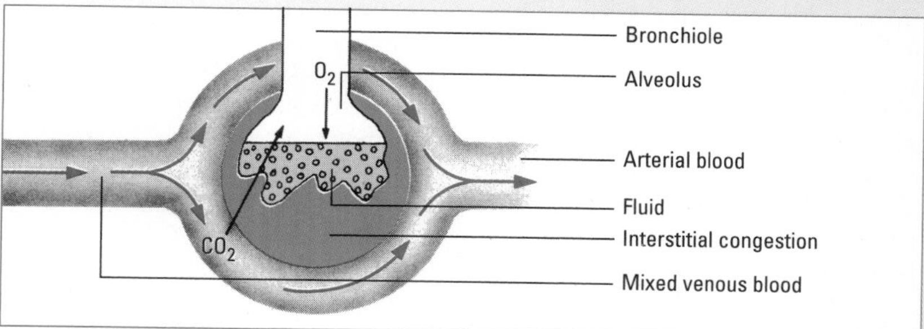

ALVEOLUS IN INFLAMMATION

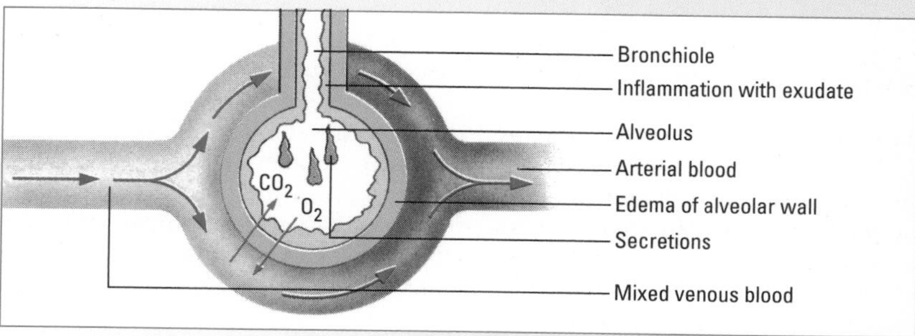

Asthma, acute

- Dry, whistling crackles occur.
- Dry cough and mild wheezing progress to severe dyspnea, audible wheezing, chest tightness, and a productive cough.
- Other signs and symptoms include anxiety, prolonged expirations, rhonchi, intercostal and supraclavicular retractions, accessory muscle use, flaring nostrils, tachypnea, tachycardia, diaphoresis, and flushing or cyanosis.

Bronchiectasis

- Persistent, coarse crackles are heard over the affected area of the lung.
- Chronic cough that produces copious amounts of mucopurulent sputum accompanies crackles.
- Other signs and symptoms include halitosis, wheezing, exertional dyspnea, rhonchi, weight loss, fatigue, malaise, weakness, recurrent fever, and late clubbing.

Bronchitis, chronic

- Coarse crackles are usually heard at the lung base.
- Other signs and symptoms include prolonged expirations, wheezing, rhonchi, exertional dyspnea, tachypnea, cyanosis, clubbing, and persistent, productive cough.

Chemical pneumonitis

- Diffuse, fine to coarse, moist crackles can be heard.
- Other signs and symptoms include a productive cough with purulent sputum, dyspnea, wheezing, orthopnea, fever, malaise, and mucous membrane irritation.

Interstitial fibrosis of the lungs

- Cellophane-like crackles can be heard over all lobes.
- As the disease progresses, other signs and symptoms include nonproductive cough, dyspnea, fatigue, weight loss, cyanosis, pleuritic chest pain, nasal flaring, and cyanosis.

Legionnaires' disease

- Diffuse, moist crackles can be heard in patients with this acute bronchopneumonia.
- Early signs and symptoms include malaise, fatigue, weakness, anorexia, myalgia, and diarrhea.
- Within 12 to 48 hours, a dry cough develops with accompanying sudden high fever and chills.
- Other signs and symptoms include pleuritic chest pain, headache, tachypnea, tachycardia, nausea, vomiting, dyspnea, confusion, flushing, diaphoresis, and prostration.

Lung abscess

- Fine to medium and moist inspiratory crackles occur.
- Other signs and symptoms include sweats, anorexia, weight loss, fever, fatigue, weakness, dyspnea, clubbing, pleuritic chest pain, pleural rub, and a cough that produces large amounts of foul-smelling, purulent, bloody sputum.

Pneumonia

- Bacterial pneumonia produces diffuse, fine crackles.
- Mycoplasmal pneumonia produces medium to fine crackles.
- Viral pneumonia causes gradually developing, diffuse crackles.
- Other signs and symptoms include sudden onset of shaking chills, high fever, tachypnea, pleuritic chest pain, cyanosis, grunting respirations, nasal flaring, decreased breath sounds, myalgia, headache, tachycardia, dyspnea, diaphoresis, rhonchi, and a dry cough that becomes productive.

Pulmonary edema

- One of the first signs of this life-threatening disorder are moist, bubbling crackles on inspiration.

■ Other signs and symptoms include exertional dyspnea; paroxysmal nocturnal dyspnea, then orthopnea; tachycardia; tachypnea; ventricular gallop; and a cough that's initially nonproductive, but later produces frothy, bloody sputum.

Pulmonary embolism

■ In this life-threatening disorder, fine to coarse crackles and severe dyspnea are early signs and may be accompanied by angina or pleuritic chest pain.
■ Cough may be nonproductive or produce blood-tinged sputum.
■ Acute anxiety, low-grade fever, tachycardia, tachypnea, and diaphoresis develop.
■ Other signs and symptoms include pleural rub, wheezing, chest dullness on percussion, decreased breath sounds, and signs of circulatory collapse.

Pulmonary tuberculosis

■ Fine crackles occur after coughing.
■ Sputum may be scant, mucoid or copious, and purulent.
■ Other signs and symptoms include hemoptysis, malaise, dyspnea, pleuritic chest pain, fatigue, night sweats, weakness, weight loss, and amphoric breath sounds.

Sarcoidosis

■ Sarcoidosis is a multisystem, granuloma-producing disorder that especially affects the lungs.
■ Fine, basilar, end-inspiratory crackles occur.
■ Other signs and symptoms include malaise, fatigue, weakness, weight loss, cough, dyspnea, and tachypnea.

Silicosis

■ End-inspiratory, fine crackles are heard at the lung bases, resulting from pulmonary fibrosis.
■ A productive cough with mucopurulent sputum is the first sign.
■ Other signs and symptoms include exertional dyspnea, tachypnea, weight loss, fatigue, weakness, and recurrent respiratory infections.

Tracheobronchitis

■ Moist or coarse crackles occur.
■ With severe disease, moderate fever and bronchospasm occur.
■ Other signs and symptoms include productive cough, chills, sore throat, slight fever, muscle and back pain, substernal tightness, rhonchi, and wheezes.

Nursing considerations

■ Raise the head of the bed to ease the patient's breathing.
■ Administer fluids and humidified air to liquefy secretions and relieve mucous membrane inflammation.
■ Administer oxygen.
■ If crackles result from cardiogenic pulmonary edema, give a diuretic, as prescribed.
■ Turn the patient every 1 to 2 hours, and encourage deep breathing.
■ Plan regular rest periods for the patient.
■ In children, pneumonias produce diffuse, sudden crackles; esophageal atresia and tracheoesophageal fistula can cause bubbling, moist crackles; pulmonary edema causes fine crackles; bronchiectasis produces moist crackles; cystic fibrosis produces widespread, fine to coarse inspiratory crackles in infants; and sickle cell anemia may produce crackles with pulmonary infection or infarction.
■ Crackles that clear after deep breathing may indicate mild basilar atelectasis.

Patient teaching

■ Teach the patient effective coughing techniques.
■ Teach the patient to avoid respiratory irritants.

- Stress the importance of quitting smoking, and refer the patient to appropriate resources to help him.
- Teach the patient energy conservation techniques, particularly with chronic disorders.

Crepitation, subcutaneous

When bubbles of air or other gases (such as carbon dioxide) are trapped in subcutaneous tissue, palpating or stroking the skin produces a crackling sound called *subcutaneous crepitation* or *subcutaneous emphysema*. The bubbles feel like small, unstable nodules and aren't painful, even though subcutaneous crepitation is commonly associated with painful disorders. Usually, the affected tissue is visibly edematous; this can lead to life-threatening airway occlusion if the edema affects the neck or upper chest.

The air or gas bubbles enter the tissues through open wounds from the action of anaerobic microorganisms or from traumatic or spontaneous rupture or perforation of pulmonary or GI organs.

QUICK ACTION ***For signs of respiratory distress, quickly test for Hamman's sign. Endotracheal intubation, an emergency tracheotomy, or chest tube insertion will be needed. Provide supplemental oxygen, and start an I.V. line to administer fluids and medications. Connect the patient to a cardiac monitor.***

History

- Ask if the patient is having difficulty breathing.
- Ask about the onset, location, and severity of any associated pain.
- Obtain a medical and surgical history, including recent thoracic surgery, diagnostic tests, and respiratory therapy, as well as trauma or chronic pulmonary disease.

Physical examination

- Palpate the affected skin to evaluate the location and extent of crepitus.
- Palpate frequently to determine if subcutaneous crepitation is increasing.
- Perform abbreviated cardiac, pulmonary, and GI assessments as the patient's condition allows.
- When the patient is stabilized, perform a complete physical examination.

Causes

Medical causes

Orbital fracture

- Subcutaneous crepitation of the eyelid and orbit develops when fracture allows air from the nasal sinus to escape into subcutaneous tissue.
- Periorbital ecchymosis is the most common sign.
- Other signs and symptoms include facial and eyelid edema, diplopia, a hyphema, impaired extraocular movements, and a dilated or unreactive pupil on the affected side.

Pneumothorax

- Subcutaneous crepitation occurs in the upper chest and neck in severe cases.
- One-sided chest pain increases on inspiration.
- Other signs and symptoms include dyspnea, anxiety, restlessness, tachypnea, cyanosis, tachycardia, accessory muscle use, asymmetrical chest expansion, decreased or absent breath sounds on the affected side, and a nonproductive cough.

Rupture of esophagus

- Subcutaneous crepitation may be palpable in the neck, chest wall, or supraclavicular fossa.
- With cervical esophagus rupture, signs and symptoms include excruciat-

ing pain in the neck or supraclavicular area, resistance to passive neck movement, local tenderness, soft-tissue swelling, dysphagia, odynophagia, and orthostatic vertigo.

- With life-threatening rupture of the intrathoracic esophagus, signs and symptoms include a positive Hamman's sign; severe retrosternal, epigastric, neck, or scapular pain; edema of the chest wall and neck; dyspnea; tachypnea; asymmetrical chest movement; nasal flaring; cyanosis; diaphoresis; tachycardia; hypotension; dysphagia; and fever.

Rupture of trachea or major bronchus

- In this life-threatening disorder, abrupt subcutaneous crepitation of the neck and anterior chest wall occurs.
- Other signs and symptoms include severe dyspnea with nasal flaring, tachycardia, accessory muscle use, hypotension, cyanosis, extreme anxiety, hemoptysis, and mediastinal emphysema with a positive Hamman's sign.

Other causes

Diagnostic tests

- Endoscopic tests can rupture or perforate respiratory or GI organs, producing subcutaneous crepitation.

Respiratory treatments

- Intermittent positive-pressure breathing and mechanical ventilation can rupture alveoli, producing subcutaneous crepitation.

Thoracic surgery

- If air escapes into the tissue in the area of the incision, subcutaneous crepitation can occur.

Nursing considerations

- Monitor the patient's vital signs frequently, especially respirations.
- Look for signs of respiratory distress and airway obstruction.
- Tell the patient that the affected tissues will eventually absorb the air or gas bubbles, decreasing subcutaneous crepitation.
- Provide reassurance to reduce anxiety.
- Children may develop subcutaneous crepitation in the neck from ingestion of corrosive substances that perforate the esophagus.

Patient teaching

- Explain diagnostic tests and procedures the patient needs.
- Explain the signs and symptoms of subcutaneous crepitation that should be reported.

Cyanosis

Cyanosis—a bluish or bluish black discoloration of the skin and mucous membranes—results from excessive concentration of unoxygenated hemoglobin in the blood. This common sign may develop abruptly or gradually. It's classified as central or peripheral, although the two types may coexist.

Central cyanosis reflects inadequate oxygenation of systemic arterial blood caused by right-to-left cardiac shunting, pulmonary disease, or hematologic disorders. It may occur anywhere on the skin and also on the mucous membranes of the mouth, lips, and conjunctiva.

Peripheral cyanosis reflects sluggish peripheral circulation caused by vasoconstriction, reduced cardiac output, or vascular occlusion. It may be widespread or may occur locally in one extremity; however, it doesn't affect mucous membranes. Typically, peripheral cyanosis appears on exposed areas, such as the fingers, nail beds, feet, nose, and ears. Although cyanosis is an important sign of cardiovascular and pulmonary disorders, it isn't always an accurate gauge of oxygenation. Several factors contribute to its development: hemoglobin concentration and oxygen saturation, cardiac output, and partial pressure of arterial oxygen (PaO_2). Cyanosis is usually undetectable until the oxygen saturation of hemoglobin falls below 80%. Severe cyanosis is quite obvious, whereas mild cyanosis is more difficult to detect, even in bright, natural light. In dark-skinned patients, cyanosis is most apparent in the mucous membranes and nail beds.

Transient, nonpathologic cyanosis may result from environmental factors. For example, peripheral cyanosis may result from cutaneous vasoconstriction following a brief exposure to cold air or water. Central cyanosis may result from reduced PaO_2 at high altitudes.

QUICK ACTION ***If the patient displays sudden, localized cyanosis and other signs of arterial occlusion, place the affected limb in a dependent position and protect it from injury. Don't, however, massage the limb. If you see central cyanosis stemming from a pulmonary disorder or shock, perform a rapid evaluation. Take immediate steps to maintain an airway, assist breathing, and monitor circulation.***

History

- Obtain a medical history, including cardiac, pulmonary, and hematologic disorders, and previous surgery.
- Evaluate the patient's mental status while obtaining his history.
- Ask about the onset, aggravating and alleviating factors, and characteristics of the cyanosis.
- Ask about other signs and symptoms.

Physical examination

- Take the patient's vital signs, measure oxygen saturation, and evaluate respiratory rate and rhythm.
- Check for nasal flaring and accessory muscle use.
- Inspect the skin, lips, and nail bed color and mucous membranes.
- Inspect for asymmetrical chest expansion or barrel chest.
- Inspect the abdomen for ascites.
- Palpate peripheral pulses, test capillary refill, and note edema.
- Percuss and palpate for liver enlargement and tenderness.
- Percuss the lungs for dullness or hyperresonance.
- Auscultate for decreased or adventitious breath sounds.
- Auscultate heart rate and rhythm.
- Auscultate the abdominal aorta and femoral arteries for bruits.

Causes

Medical causes

Arteriosclerotic occlusive disease, chronic

- Peripheral cyanosis occurs in the legs whenever they're in a dependent position.
- Leg ulcers and gangrene are late signs.
- Other signs and symptoms include intermittent claudication and burning pain at rest, paresthesia, pallor, muscle atrophy, weak leg pulses, and impotence.

Bronchiectasis

- Chronic central cyanosis develops.
- The classic sign is chronic productive cough with copious, foul-smelling, mucopurulent sputum, or hemoptysis.
- Other signs and symptoms include dyspnea, recurrent fever and chills, weight loss, malaise, clubbing, and signs of anemia.

Buerger's disease

- This is an occlusive inflammatory disorder of the leg and foot arteries.
- Exposure to cold initially causes the feet to become cold, cyanotic, and

numb; later, they redden, become hot, and tingle.

- Intermittent claudication of the instep is characteristic.
- Other signs and symptoms include weak, peripheral pulses and, in later stages, ulceration, muscle atrophy, and gangrene.

Chronic obstructive pulmonary disease

- Chronic central cyanosis occurs in advanced stages.
- Exertion aggravates cyanosis.
- Barrel chest and clubbing are late signs.
- Other signs and symptoms include exertional dyspnea, productive cough with thick sputum, anorexia, weight loss, pursed-lip breathing, tachypnea, accessory muscle use, and wheezing.

Heart failure

- Acute or chronic cyanosis may occur in a late phase.
- With left-sided heart failure, central cyanosis occurs with tachycardia, fatigue, dyspnea, cold intolerance, orthopnea, cough, ventricular or atrial gallop, and crackles.
- With right-sided heart failure, peripheral cyanosis occurs with fatigue, peripheral edema, ascites, jugular vein distention, and hepatomegaly.

Peripheral arterial occlusion, acute

- Acute cyanosis of the arm or leg occurs.
- Cyanosis is accompanied by sharp or aching pain that worsens with movement.
- Paresthesia, weakness, decreased or absent pulse, and pale, cool skin occur in the affected extremity.

Pneumonia

- Acute central cyanosis is usually preceded by fever, shaking chills, cough with purulent sputum, crackles, rhonchi, and pleuritic chest pain that's exacerbated by deep inspiration.
- Other signs and symptoms include tachycardia, dyspnea, tachypnea, diminished breath sounds, diaphoresis, myalgia, fatigue, headache, and anorexia.

Pneumothorax

- Acute central cyanosis is a cardinal sign.
- Signs and symptoms include rapid, shallow respirations; weak, rapid pulse; pallor; jugular vein distention; anxiety; and absence of breath sounds over the affected lobe.
- Sharp chest pain that's worsened by movement, deep breathing, and coughing; asymmetrical chest movement; and shortness of breath may also occur.

Polycythemia vera

- A ruddy complexion that can appear cyanotic is characteristic of this bone marrow disease.
- Other signs and symptoms include hepatosplenomegaly, headache, dizziness, fatigue, blurred vision, chest pain, intermittent claudication, and coagulation defects.

Pulmonary edema

- Acute central cyanosis occurs due to impaired gas exchange.
- Other signs and symptoms include dyspnea; orthopnea; frothy, blood-tinged sputum; tachycardia; tachypnea; crackles; ventricular gallop; cold, clammy skin; hypotension; weak, thready pulse; and confusion.

Pulmonary embolism

- Acute central cyanosis occurs when a large embolus obstructs pulmonary circulation.
- Other signs and symptoms include syncope, jugular vein distention, dyspnea, chest pain, tachycardia, paradoxical pulse, dry cough or productive

cough with blood-tinged sputum, fever, restlessness, and diaphoresis.

Raynaud's disease

- This is a vascular disorder characterized by episodes of vasospasm in the small peripheral arteries and arterioles.
- Exposure to cold or stress causes the fingers or hands to blanch, turn cold, then become cyanotic, and finally to redden with the return of a normal temperature.
- Numbness and tingling may also develop.

Shock

- Acute peripheral cyanosis develops in the hands and feet.
- Feet may be cold, clammy, and pale.
- Central cyanosis develops with progression of shock and organ system failures.
- Other signs and symptoms include lethargy, confusion, increased capillary refill, tachypnea, hyperpnea, hypotension, and a rapid, weak pulse.

Nursing considerations

- Provide supplemental oxygen to improve oxygenation.
- Deliver small doses of oxygen of 2 L/minute to patients with chronic obstructive pulmonary disease (COPD); use a low-flow oxygen rate for mild COPD exacerbations.
- For acute situations, a high-flow oxygen rate may be needed initially; in working with a patient who has COPD, remember to be attentive to his respiratory drive and adjust the amount of oxygen accordingly.
- Position the patient comfortably to ease breathing.
- Give a diuretic, bronchodilator, antibiotic, or cardiac drug, as prescribed.
- Provide rest periods to prevent dyspnea; encourage energy conservation.
- In children, central cyanosis may result from cystic fibrosis, asthma, airway obstruction, acute laryngotracheobronchitis, epiglottiditis, or congenital heart defects.
- Cyanosis around the mouth may precede generalized cyanosis.
- Acrocyanosis may occur in infants because of excessive crying or exposure to cold.
- Because of reduced tissue perfusion in elderly people, peripheral cyanosis can occur even with a slight decrease in cardiac output or systemic blood pressure.

Patient teaching

- Instruct the patient to seek medical attention if cyanosis occurs.
- Discuss the safe use of oxygen in the home.
- Teach the patient and his family about the medical diagnosis and treatment plan.
- Teach the importance of prescribed medications, how to administer them, and possible adverse effects.
- Discuss the importance of frequent rest periods.
- Discuss the importance of follow-up care.

D

Decerebrate posture

Decerebrate posture is characterized by adduction (internal rotation) and extension of the arms, with the wrists pronated and the fingers flexed. The legs are stiffly extended, with forced plantar flexion of the feet. In severe cases, the back is acutely arched (opisthotonos). This sign indicates upper brain stem damage, which may result from primary lesions, such as infarction, hemorrhage, or tumor; metabolic encephalopathy; a head injury; or brain stem compression associated with increased intracranial pressure (ICP).

Decerebrate posture may be elicited by noxious stimuli or may occur spontaneously. It may be unilateral or bilateral. With concurrent brain stem and cerebral damage, decerebrate posture may affect only the arms, with the legs remaining flaccid. Alternatively, decerebrate posture may affect one side of the body and decorticate posture the other. The two postures may also alternate as the patient's neurologic status fluctuates. Generally, the duration of each posturing episode correlates with the severity of brain stem damage.

QUICK ACTION ***Your first priority is to ensure a patent airway. Insert an artificial airway and take measures to prevent aspiration. (Don't disrupt spinal alignment if you suspect spinal cord injury.) Suction the patient as needed.***

Next, examine spontaneous respirations. Give supplemental oxygen, and ventilate the patient with a handheld resuscitation bag, if needed. Endotracheal intubation and mechanical ventilation may be indicated. Keep emergency resuscitation equipment handy. Monitor the patient's neurologic status, vital signs, and oxygen saturation.

History

- Determine when the patient's level of consciousness (LOC) began to deteriorate.
- Ask if the onset of decerebrate posture was abrupt or gradual and if other signs or symptoms occurred with it.
- Obtain a medical history, asking about diabetes, liver disease, cancer, blood clots, and aneurysm.
- Ask about recent trauma or accident.

Physical examination

- Take the patient's vital signs.
- Determine the patient's LOC using the Glasgow Coma Scale.
- Evaluate pupils for size, equality, and response to light.
- Test deep tendon reflexes (DTRs) and cranial nerve reflexes.
- Check for doll's eye sign.

Causes

Medical causes

Brain stem infarction

- Coma may occur with decerebrate posture.

■ Absence of doll's eye sign, positive Babinski's reflex, and flaccidity occur with deep coma.
■ Other signs and symptoms vary with the severity of infarct and may include cranial nerve palsies, cerebellar ataxia, and sensory loss.

Brain stem tumor
■ Decerebrate posture is a late sign that occurs with coma.
■ Earlier signs and symptoms include hemiparesis or quadriparesis, cranial nerve palsies, vertigo, dizziness, ataxia, and vomiting.

Cerebral lesion
■ Increased ICP may produce decerebrate posture, a late sign.
■ Other signs and symptoms include coma, abnormal pupil size and response to light, and the classic triad of increased ICP: bradycardia, increasing systolic blood pressure, and widening pulse pressure.

Hepatic encephalopathy
■ A late sign in this disorder, decerebrate posture occurs with coma resulting from increased ICP and ammonia toxicity.
■ Other signs and symptoms include fetor hepaticus, positive Babinski's reflex, and hyperactive DTRs.

Hypoglycemic encephalopathy
■ Decerebrate posture and coma may occur.
■ Low glucose levels are characteristic.
■ Muscle spasms, twitching, and seizures progress to flaccidity.
■ Other signs and symptoms include dilated pupils, slow respirations, and bradycardia.

Hypoxic encephalopathy
■ Decerebrate posture occurs.
■ Other signs and symptoms include coma, positive Babinski's reflex, absence of doll's eye sign, hypoactive DTRs, fixed pupils, and respiratory arrest.

Pontine hemorrhage
■ In this life-threatening disorder, decerebrate posture occurs rapidly along with coma.
■ Other signs and symptoms include paralysis, absence of doll's eye sign, positive Babinski's reflex, and small, reactive pupils.

Posterior fossa hemorrhage
■ Decerebrate posture occurs with vomiting, headache, vertigo, ataxia, stiff neck, drowsiness, papilledema, and cranial nerve palsies.
■ Eventually, coma and respiratory arrest may occur.

Other causes

Diagnostic tests
■ Removing spinal fluid during a lumbar puncture may cause the brain stem to compress, causing decerebrate posture and coma.

Nursing considerations

■ Monitor the patient's neurologic status and vital signs.
■ Look for symptoms of increased ICP and neurologic deterioration.
■ Children younger than age 2 may not display decerebrate posture because of nervous system immaturity.
■ In children, the most common cause of decerebrate posture is head injury.

Patient teaching

■ Explain that decerebrate posture is a reflex response.
■ Provide emotional support to the patient and his family.
■ Teach the patient and his family about the medical diagnosis, prognosis, and treatment plan.

Decorticate posture

A sign of corticospinal damage, decorticate posture is characterized by adduction of the arms and flexion of the elbows, with wrists and fingers flexed on the chest. The legs are extended and internally rotated, with plantar flexion of the feet. This posture may occur unilaterally or bilaterally. It usually results from stroke or head injury. It may be elicited by noxious stimuli or may occur spontaneously. The intensity of the required stimulus, the duration of the posture, and the frequency of spontaneous episodes vary with the severity and location of cerebral injury.

Although a serious sign, decorticate posture carries a more favorable prognosis than decerebrate posture. However, if the causative disorder extends lower in the brain stem, decorticate posture may progress to decerebrate posture. (See *Differentiating decerebrate from decorticate postures.*)

QUICK ACTION ***Obtain patient's vital signs and evaluate level of consciousness (LOC). If LOC is impaired, insert an oropharyngeal airway, and take measures to prevent aspiration. If spinal cord injury is suspected, don't disrupt alignment. Evaluate patient's respiratory rate, rhythm, and depth. Prepare***

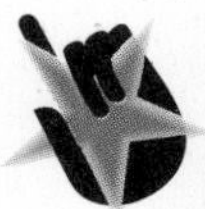

KNOW-HOW

Differentiating decerebrate from decorticate postures

Decerebrate posture results from damage to the upper brain stem. In this posture, the arms are adducted and extended, with the wrists pronated and the fingers flexed. The legs are stiffly extended, with plantar flexion of the feet.

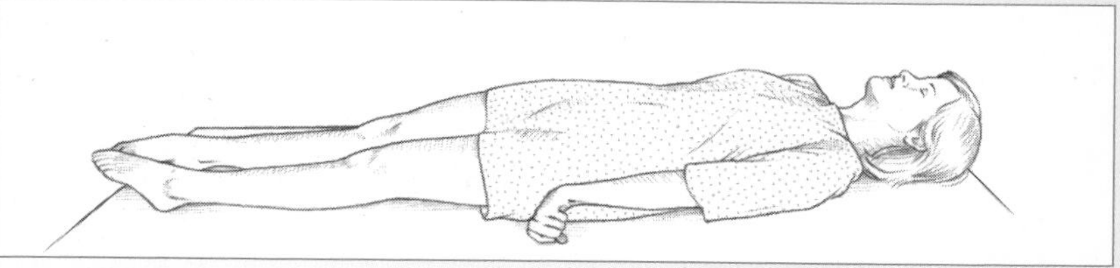

Decorticate posture results from damage to one or both corticospinal tracts. In this posture, the arms are adducted and flexed, with the wrists and fingers flexed on the chest. The legs are stiffly extended and internally rotated, with plantar flexion of the feet.

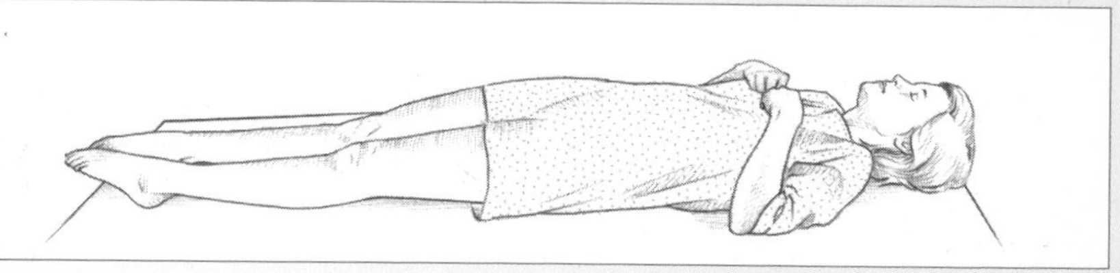

to assist respirations with a handheld resuscitation bag or with endotracheal intubation and mechanical ventilation, if necessary. Also, take seizure precautions.

History

- Check for symptoms, such as headache, dizziness, nausea, changes in vision, numbness or tingling, and behavioral changes. If a symptom is present, ask when it began.
- Obtain a medical history, asking about cerebrovascular disease, cancer, meningitis, encephalitis, upper respiratory tract infection, bleeding or clotting disorders, or recent trauma.

Physical examination

- Test motor and sensory functions.
- Evaluate pupil size, equality, and response to light.
- Test cranial nerve function and deep tendon reflexes.

Causes

Medical causes

Brain abscess

- Decorticate posture may occur along with aphasia, behavioral changes, altered vital signs, decreased LOC, hemiparesis, headache, dizziness, seizures, nausea, and vomiting.

Brain tumor

- Decorticate posture results from increased intracranial pressure (ICP).
- Other signs and symptoms include headache, behavioral changes, memory loss, diplopia, blurred vision or vision loss, seizures, ataxia, apraxia, aphasia, sensory loss, paresthesia, vomiting, papilledema, and signs of hormonal imbalance.

Head injury

- Decorticate posture may result, depending on the injury.
- Other signs and symptoms include headache, nausea, vomiting, dizziness, irritability, decreased LOC, aphasia, hemiparesis, seizures, and pupillary dilation.

Stroke

- A stroke involving the cerebral cortex produces decorticate posture on one side of the body.
- Other signs and symptoms include hemiplegia, dysarthria, dysphagia, sensory loss, apraxia, agnosia, aphasia, memory loss, decreased LOC, homonymous hemianopia, and blurred vision.

Nursing considerations

- Monitor the patient's neurologic status and vital signs frequently to detect signs of deterioration.
- Look for other signs of increased ICP.
- Decorticate posture is an unreliable sign before age 2 because of nervous system immaturity.
- In children, decorticate posture usually results from head injury.

Patient teaching

- Explain the signs and symptoms of decreased LOC and seizures.
- Discuss the patient's or caregiver's quality-of-life concerns.
- Provide referrals as appropriate.
- Explain to the caregiver how to keep the patient safe, especially during a seizure.

Deep tendon reflexes, hyperactive

A hyperactive deep tendon reflex (DTR) is an abnormally brisk muscle contraction that occurs in response to a sudden stretch induced by sharply tapping the muscle's tendon of insertion. This elicited sign may be graded as brisk or pathologically hyperactive. Hyperactive DTRs are commonly accompanied by clonus.

The corticospinal tract and other descending tracts govern the reflex arc—the relay cycle that produces any reflex response. A corticospinal lesion above the level of the reflex arc being tested may result in hyperactive DTRs. Abnormal neuromuscular transmission at the end of the reflex arc may also cause hyperactive DTRs.

Although hyperactive DTRs typically accompany other neurologic findings, they usually lack specific diagnostic value. By contrast, they're an early, cardinal sign of hypocalcemia.

History

- Obtain a medical history, including spinal cord injury, other trauma, or prolonged exposure to cold, wind, or water.
- Ask the female patient if she's pregnant.
- Determine the onset and progression of other signs and symptoms, including paresthesia, vomiting, and altered bladder habits.
- Obtain a drug history.
- Obtain immunization history, especially tetanus vaccine.

Physical examination

- Evaluate the patient's level of consciousness.
- Take the patient's vital signs.
- Test motor and sensory function in the limbs.
- Check for ataxia or tremors and for speech and visual deficits.
- Test for Chvostek's sign, Trousseau's sign, and carpopedal spasm.

Causes

Medical causes

Amyotrophic lateral sclerosis

- This motor neuron disease causes muscle atrophy.
- Generalized, hyperactive DTRs accompany weakness of the hands and forearms and spasticity of the legs.
- Atrophy of the neck and tongue muscles, fasciculations, weakness of the legs, and bulbar signs eventually develop.

Brain tumor

- Hyperactive DTRs occur on the side opposite the lesion.
- Other signs and symptoms include one-sided paresis or paralysis, visual field deficits, spasticity, and positive Babinski's reflex.

Hepatic encephalopathy

- Generalized hyperactive DTRs occur late in the comatose stage.
- Other signs and symptoms include positive Babinski's reflex, fetor hepaticus, and coma.

Hypocalcemia

- Onset of generalized hyperactive DTRs may be gradual or sudden.
- Other signs and symptoms include paresthesia, muscle twitching and cramping, positive Chvostek's and Trousseau's signs, carpopedal spasm, tetany, abdominal and muscle cramps, arrhythmias, and diarrhea.

Hypomagnesemia

- Onset of generalized hyperactive DTRs is gradual.
- Other signs and symptoms include muscle cramps, hypotension, tachycardia, paresthesia, ataxia, tetany, seizures, positive Chvostek's sign, confusion, and arrhythmias.

Hypothermia

- Mild hypothermia produces generalized hyperactive DTRs.
- Other signs and symptoms include shivering, fatigue, weakness, lethargy, slurred speech, ataxia, muscle stiffness, arrhythmias, diuresis, hypotension, and cold, pale skin.

Multiple sclerosis

- This progressive disease is caused by demyelination of the white matter of the brain and spinal cord.
- Hyperactive DTRs are preceded by weakness and paresthesia in the arms and legs.
- Ataxia, diplopia, vertigo, vomiting, and urine retention or incontinence occur later.
- Other signs and symptoms include clonus and positive Babinski's reflex.

Spinal cord lesion

- Incomplete lesions cause hyperactive DTRs below the lesion.
- In a traumatic lesion, hyperactive DTRs follow resolution of spinal shock.
- In a neoplastic lesion, hyperactive DTRs gradually replace normal DTRs.
- A lesion at or above T6 may produce autonomic hyperreflexia with diaphoresis and flushing above the lesion, headache, nasal congestion, nausea, hypertension, and bradycardia.
- Other signs and symptoms include paralysis and sensory loss below the level of the lesion, urine retention and overflow incontinence, and alternating constipation and diarrhea.

Stroke

- If the origin of the corticospinal tracts is affected, hyperactive DTRs on the side opposite the lesion suddenly occur.
- Other signs and symptoms include anesthesia, visual field deficits, spasticity, positive Babinski's reflex, and one-sided paresis or paralysis.

Tetanus

- Sudden onset of generalized hyperactive DTRs occurs.
- Other signs and symptoms include tachycardia, diaphoresis, low-grade fever, painful and involuntary muscle contractions, trismus (lockjaw), and *risus sardonicus* (a masklike grin).

Nursing considerations

- If motor weakness is present, perform range-of-motion exercises.
- Reposition the patient frequently, provide a special mattress, massage his back, and ensure adequate nutrition.
- Give a muscle relaxant and a sedative to relieve severe muscle contractions, as prescribed.
- Keep emergency resuscitation equipment on hand.
- Provide a quiet, calm atmosphere to reduce neuromuscular excitability.
- Assist with activities of daily living.
- Cerebral palsy typically causes hyperactive DTRs in children.
- Stage II Reye's syndrome causes generalized hyperactive DTRs; in stage V, DTRs are absent.
- Hyperreflexia may be normal in neonates.

Patient teaching

- Explain to the caregiver the procedures and treatments that the patient may need.
- Discuss safety measures that need to be taken.
- Provide emotional support.

Deep tendon reflexes, hypoactive

A hypoactive deep tendon reflex (DTR) is an abnormally diminished muscle contraction that occurs in response to a sudden stretch induced by sharply tapping the muscle's tendon of insertion. It may be graded as minimal (+) or absent (0). Symmetrically reduced (+) reflexes may be normal.

Normally, a DTR depends on an intact receptor, an intact sensory-motor nerve fiber, an intact neuromuscular-glandular junction, and a functional synapse in the spinal cord. Hypoactive DTRs may result from damage to the reflex arc involving the specific muscle, the peripheral nerve, the nerve roots, or the spinal cord at that level. Hypoactive DTRs are an important sign of many disorders, especially when they appear with other neurologic signs and symptoms.

History

- Obtain a medical history.
- Ask about other signs and symptoms.
- Take a family and drug history.

Physical examination

- Assess the patient's level of consciousness and speech.
- Test motor function in the limbs.
- Palpate for muscle atrophy or increased mass.
- Test sensory function, assessing for paresthesia.
- Observe gait and coordination.
- Check for Romberg's sign.
- Check for signs of vision and hearing loss.
- Take the patient's vital signs.
- Monitor for increased heart rate and blood pressure.
- Inspect the skin for pallor, dryness, flushing, and diaphoresis.
- Auscultate for hypoactive bowel sounds.
- Palpate for bladder distention.
- Document the muscles in which DTRs are lessened.

Causes

Medical causes

Botulism

- This life-threatening paralytic illness is caused by ingestion of contaminated food or, in rare cases, by a wound infection.
- Generalized hypoactive DTRs accompany progressive descending muscle weakness.
- Respiratory distress and severe constipation may also develop.
- Other signs and symptoms include blurred vision, double vision, anorexia, nausea, vomiting, vertigo, hearing loss, dysarthria, and dysphagia.

Cerebellar dysfunction

- Hypoactive DTRs occur with other findings, depending on the cause and location of the dysfunction.

Guillain-Barré syndrome

- This syndrome is an acute, rapidly progressing and potentially fatal form of polyneuritis.
- Hypoactive DTRs progress rapidly from hypotonia to areflexia.
- Muscle weakness begins in the legs and then extends to the arms and, possibly, to the trunk and neck, peaking in 10 to 14 days and then resolving.
- Weakness may progress to total paralysis.
- Other signs and symptoms include cranial nerve palsies, pain, paresthesia, and signs of autonomic dysfunction.

Peripheral neuropathy

- Progressive hypoactive DTRs occur.
- Other signs and symptoms include motor weakness, sensory loss, paresthesia, tremors, and possible autonomic dysfunction.

Polymyositis

- Hypoactive DTRs occur with accompanying muscle weakness, pain, stiffness, spasms and, possibly, increased size or atrophy.

Spinal cord lesions

- Transient hypoactive DTRs or areflexia occur below the lesion.
- Quadriplegia or paraplegia, flaccidity, loss of sensation, and pale, dry skin occur below the level of the lesion.
- Other signs and symptoms include urine retention with overflow incontinence, hypoactive bowel sounds, constipation, and genital reflex loss.

Other causes

Drugs

- Barbiturates and paralyzing drugs, such as pancuronium (Pavulon) and curare, may cause hypoactive DTRs.

Nursing considerations

- If the patient has sensory deficits, protect him from heat, cold, and pressure.
- Keep the skin clean and dry.
- Reposition the patient frequently.
- Encourage range-of-motion exercises.
- Provide a balanced diet with increased protein and fluids.
- Hypoactive DTRs commonly occur in children with muscular dystrophy, Friedreich's ataxia, syringomyelia, and spinal cord injury.
- Hypoactive DTRs accompany progressive muscular atrophy, which affects preschoolers and adolescents.
- Hypoactive DTRs occur because of a decrease in the number of nerve axons and demyelination of axons in elderly patients.

Patient teaching

- Teach skills that can help the patient be as independent as possible in his daily life.
- Discuss safety measures, including walking with assistance.

Diaphoresis

Diaphoresis is profuse sweating—at times, amounting to more than 1 L of sweat per hour. This sign represents an autonomic nervous system response to physical or psychogenic stress or to a fever or high environmental temperature. When caused by stress, diaphoresis may be generalized or limited to the palms, soles, and forehead. When caused by a fever or high environmental temperature, it's usually generalized.

Diaphoresis usually begins abruptly and may be accompanied by other autonomic system signs, such as tachycardia and increased blood pressure. (See *When diaphoresis spells crisis.*)

Night sweats may characterize intermittent fever because body temperature tends to return to normal between 2 a.m. and 4 a.m. before rising again. (Temperature is usually lowest around 6 a.m.) When caused by a high external temperature, diaphoresis is a normal response. Acclimatization usually requires several days of exposure to high temperatures; during this process, diaphoresis helps maintain normal body temperature. Diaphoresis also commonly occurs during menopause, preceded by a sensation of intense heat (a hot flash). Other causes include exercise or exertion that accelerates metabolism, creating internal heat, and mild to moderate anxiety that helps initiate the fight-or-flight response.

History

- Ask the patient to describe his chief complaint, and quickly rule out the possibility of a life-threatening cause.
- Note when diaphoresis occurs (day or night).
- Investigate other signs and symptoms.
- Find out about recent travel or exposure to high environmental temperatures or to pesticides.
- Ask about recent insect bites.
- Obtain a medical history, asking about partial gastrectomy or drug or alcohol abuse.
- Take a medication history.

Physical examination

- Inspect the trunk, extremities, palms, soles, and forehead to determine the extent of diaphoresis.
- Observe for flushing, abnormal skin texture or lesions, and an increased amount of coarse body hair.
- Note poor skin turgor and dry mucous membranes.

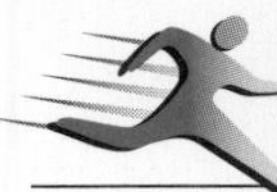

QUICK ACTION

When diaphoresis spells crisis

Diaphoresis is an early sign of certain life-threatening disorders. These guidelines will help you promptly detect such disorders and intervene to minimize harm to the patient.

Hypoglycemia

If you observe diaphoresis in a patient who complains of blurred vision, ask him about increased irritability and anxiety. Has the patient been unusually hungry lately? Does he have tremors? Take the patient's vital signs, noting hypotension and tachycardia. Then ask about a history of type 2 diabetes or antidiabetic therapy. If you suspect hypoglycemia, evaluate the patient's blood glucose level using a glucose reagent strip, or send a serum sample to the laboratory. Administer I.V. glucose 50% as ordered to return the patient's glucose level to normal. Monitor his vital signs and cardiac rhythm. Ensure a patent airway, and be prepared to assist with breathing and circulation, if necessary.

Heatstroke

If you observe profuse diaphoresis in a weak, tired, and apprehensive patient, suspect heatstroke, which can progress to circulatory collapse. Take his vital signs, noting a normal or subnormal temperature. Check for ashen gray skin and dilated pupils. Was the patient recently exposed to high temperatures and humidity? Was he wearing heavy clothing or performing strenuous physical activity at the time? Also, ask if he takes a diuretic, which interferes with normal sweating.

Then, take the patient to a cool room, remove his clothing, and use a fan to direct cool air over his body. Insert an I.V. line, and prepare for electrolyte and fluid replacement. Monitor the patient for signs of shock. Check his urine output carefully along with other sources of output (such as tubes, drains, and ostomies).

Autonomic hyperreflexia

If you observe diaphoresis in a patient with a spinal cord injury above T6 or T7, ask if he has a pounding headache, restlessness, blurred vision, or nasal congestion. Take the patient's vital signs, noting bradycardia or extremely elevated blood pressure. If you suspect autonomic hyperreflexia, quickly rule out its common complications. Examine the patient for eye pain associated with intraocular hemorrhage and for facial paralysis, slurred speech, or limb weakness associated with intracerebral hemorrhage.

Quickly reposition the patient to remove any pressure stimuli. Also, check for a distended bladder or fecal impaction. Remove any kinks from the urinary catheter if necessary, and administer a suppository or manually remove impacted feces. If you can't locate and relieve the causative stimulus, start an I.V. line. Prepare to administer hydralazine (Apresoline) for hypertension.

Myocardial infarction or heart failure

If the diaphoretic patient complains of chest pain and dyspnea or has arrhythmias or electrocardiogram changes, suspect a myocardial infarction or heart failure. Connect the patient to a cardiac monitor, ensure a patent airway, and administer supplemental oxygen. Start an I.V. line, and administer an analgesic. Be prepared to begin emergency resuscitation if cardiac or respiratory arrest occurs.

- Look for splinter hemorrhages and Plummer's nails.
- Evaluate the patient's mental status.
- Take the patient's vital signs.
- Observe for fasciculations and flaccid paralysis.
- Assess for seizures.
- Note the patient's facial expression and examine the eyes.
- Auscultate breath sounds.
- Palpate for lymphadenopathy and hepatosplenomegaly.

Causes

Medical causes

Acquired immunodeficiency syndrome

- Night sweats may occur early as a manifestation of the disease or from an opportunistic infection.
- Other signs and symptoms include fever, fatigue, lymphadenopathy, anorexia, weight loss, diarrhea, and a persistent cough.

Acromegaly

- Diaphoresis measures disease activity, which involves hypersecretion of growth hormone and increased metabolic rate.
- Other signs and symptoms include a hulking appearance; an enlarged supraorbital ridge and thickened ears and nose; warm, oily skin; enlarged hands, feet, and jaw; joint pain; weight gain; hoarseness; increased coarse body hair; elevated blood pressure; and visual field deficits or blindness.

Autonomic hyperreflexia

- Profuse diaphoresis above the level of injury, pounding headache, blurred vision, and dramatically elevated blood pressure occur after resolution of spinal shock in spinal cord injury above T6.
- Other signs and symptoms include flushing, restlessness, nausea, nasal congestion, and bradycardia.

Heart failure

- In left-sided heart failure, diaphoresis follows fatigue, dyspnea, orthopnea, and tachycardia.
- In right-sided heart failure, diaphoresis follows jugular vein distention and dry cough.
- Other signs and symptoms include tachypnea, cyanosis, edema, crackles, ventricular gallop, and anxiety.

Heat exhaustion

- Initially, profuse diaphoresis, fever, fatigue, weakness, and anxiety may occur.
- Later signs and symptoms include ashen gray appearance, dilated pupils, and normal or abnormally low temperature; the condition may progress to circulatory collapse and shock.

Hodgkin's disease

- An initial sign is usually a painless swelling of a cervical lymph node.
- Other signs and symptoms may include night sweats, fever, fatigue, pruritus, and weight loss.

Hypoglycemia

- Rapidly induced hypoglycemia may cause diaphoresis, irritability, tremors, hypotension, blurred vision, tachycardia, hunger, and loss of consciousness.
- Confusion, motor weakness, hemiplegia, seizures, or coma may also occur.

Infective endocarditis, subacute

- Generalized night sweats occur early.
- A sudden change in a murmur or a new murmur is a classic sign.
- Other signs and symptoms include intermittent low-grade fever, weakness, fatigue, petechiae, splinter hemorrhages, weight loss, anorexia, and arthralgia.

Liver abscess

- Diaphoresis, right upper quadrant pain, weight loss, fever, chills, nausea, vomiting, and anemia commonly occur.
- Other signs and symptoms include possible jaundice, chalk-colored stools, and dark urine.

Lung abscess

- Commonly, drenching night sweats occur.
- Cough produces copious purulent, foul-smelling, bloody sputum.
- Other signs and symptoms include fever with chills, pleuritic chest pain, dyspnea, weakness, anorexia, weight loss, headache, malaise, clubbing, tubular or amorphic breath sounds, and dullness on percussion.

Malaria

- Profuse diaphoresis marks the third stage of paroxysmal malaria, after chills (first stage) and high fever (second stage).
- Headache, arthralgia, and hepatosplenomegaly may occur.
- Severe malaria may progress to delirium, seizures, and coma.

Myocardial infarction

- Diaphoresis with acute, substernal, radiating chest pain occurs in this life-threatening condition.
- Anxiety, dyspnea, nausea, vomiting, tachycardia, blood pressure change, crackles, pallor, and clammy skin may also occur.

Pheochromocytoma

- This tumor of the adrenal medulla results in severe hypertension, increased metabolism, diaphoresis, and hyperglycemia.
- Other signs and symptoms include headache, palpitations, tachycardia, anxiety, tremors, paresthesia, abdominal pain, tachypnea, nausea, vomiting, and orthostatic hypotension.

Pneumonia

- Intermittent, generalized diaphoresis accompanies fever and chills.
- Other signs and symptoms include pleuritic pain, tachypnea, dyspnea, productive cough, headache, fatigue, myalgia, abdominal pain, anorexia, and cyanosis.

Tetanus

- Profuse sweating is accompanied by low-grade fever, tachycardia, and hyperactive deep tendon reflexes.
- Early restlessness, pain, and stiffness in the jaw, abdomen, and back progresses to spasms from lockjaw, risus sardonicus, dysphagia, and opisthotonos.

Thyrotoxicosis

- Diaphoresis with heat intolerance, weight loss despite increased appetite, tachycardia, palpitations, an enlarged thyroid gland, dyspnea, nervousness, diarrhea, tremors, Plummer's nails, and exophthalmos may occur.

Tuberculosis

- Night sweats may occur in patients with primary tuberculosis (TB) infection as well as low-grade fever, fatigue, weakness, anorexia, and weight loss.
- In the reactivation phase, mucopurulent productive cough, occasional hemoptysis, and chest pain may also be present.

Other causes

Alcohol and opioid withdrawal

- Generalized diaphoresis occurs with dilated pupils, tachycardia, tremors, and altered mental status.
- Other signs and symptoms include severe muscle cramps, paresthesia, tachypnea, altered blood pressure, nausea, vomiting, and seizures.

Drugs

- Aspirin or acetaminophen (Tylenol) poisoning cause diaphoresis.

■ Sympathomimetics, antipyretics, thyroid hormones, corticosteroids, and certain antipsychotics may cause diaphoresis.

Pesticide poisoning

■ Toxic effects of pesticide poisoning are diaphoresis, nausea, vomiting, diarrhea, blurred vision, miosis, and excessive lacrimation and salivation.

Nursing considerations

■ Sponge the patient's face and body.
■ Change wet clothes and sheets.
■ To prevent skin irritation, dust skin folds in the groin and axillae and under pendulous breasts with cornstarch.
■ Replace fluids and electrolytes.
■ Monitor fluid intake and urine output.
■ Encourage the patient to drink fluids high in electrolytes.
■ Keep the room temperature moderate.
■ Diaphoresis in children commonly results from environmental heat, overdressing, drug withdrawal from the mother's addiction, heart failure, thyrotoxicosis, and the effects of such drugs as antihistamines, ephedrine, haloperidol (Haldol), and thyroid hormone.
■ An elderly patient with TB may not have fever and night sweats, but instead may exhibit a change in activity or weight.
■ Elderly patients may not exhibit diaphoresis because of decreased sweating mechanisms, which increases their risk of developing heatstroke.

Patient teaching

■ Explain proper skin care.
■ Explain the causative disease process.
■ Discuss the importance of fluid replacement and how to make sure fluid intake is adequate.

Diarrhea

Usually a chief sign of an intestinal disorder, diarrhea is an increase in the volume of stools compared with the patient's normal bowel habits. It varies in severity and may be acute or chronic. Acute diarrhea may result from acute infection, stress, fecal impaction, or the effect of a drug. Chronic diarrhea may result from chronic infection, obstructive and inflammatory bowel disease, malabsorption syndrome, an endocrine disorder, or GI surgery. Periodic diarrhea may result from food intolerance or from ingestion of spicy or high-fiber foods or caffeine.

One or more pathophysiologic mechanisms may contribute to diarrhea. (See *What causes diarrhea,* pages 108 and 109.) The fluid and electrolyte imbalances it produces may precipitate life-threatening arrhythmias or hypovolemic shock.

QUICK ACTION ***If the patient's diarrhea is profuse, check for signs of shock—tachycardia, hypotension, and cool, pale, clammy skin. If you detect these signs, place the patient in the supine position and elevate his legs 20 degrees. Insert an I.V. line for fluid replacement. Monitor him for electrolyte imbalances, and look for an irregular pulse, muscle weakness, anorexia, and nausea and vomiting. Keep emergency resuscitation equipment handy.***

History

■ Check for other signs and symptoms, such as pain, cramps, difficulty breathing, weakness, and fatigue.
■ Find out about the patient's drug history.
■ Ask about recent GI surgery or radiation therapy.
■ Review the patient's diet and ask about food allergies.
■ Ask about possible stress factors.

Physical examination

- Check skin turgor and mucous membranes.
- Take blood pressure with the patient lying, sitting, and standing.
- Inspect the abdomen for distention, and palpate for tenderness.
- Percuss the abdomen for tympany.
- Auscultate bowel sounds.
- Take the patient's temperature and note any chills.
- Look for a rash.

Causes

Medical causes

Anthrax, GI

- Initial signs and symptoms include decreased appetite, nausea, vomiting, and fever.
- Later signs and symptoms include severe bloody diarrhea, abdominal pain, and hematemesis.

Clostridium difficile *infection*

- This infection commonly occurs after antibiotic treatment.
- Soft, unformed stools or watery diarrhea may be foul-smelling or bloody.
- Toxic megacolon, colon perforation, or peritonitis may develop in severe cases.
- Other signs and symptoms include abdominal pain, cramping and tenderness, fever, and a white blood cell count as high as 20,000/µl.

Crohn's disease

- This is an inflammation of the GI tract that extends through all layers of the intestinal wall.
- Diarrhea is accompanied by abdominal pain, with guarding and tenderness and nausea.
- Other signs and symptoms may include fever, chills, anorexia, weakness, and weight loss.

Escherichia coli *O157:H7*

- This strain of *E. coli* has been associated with animals and with eating undercooked meat.
- Watery or bloody diarrhea, nausea, vomiting, fever, and abdominal cramps occur.

Infections

- Acute viral, bacterial, and protozoan infections cause the sudden onset of watery diarrhea with abdominal pain, cramps, nausea, vomiting, and fever.
- Chronic tuberculosis and fungal and parasitic infections produce a less severe but more persistent diarrhea, along with epigastric distress, vomiting, weight loss, and passage of blood and mucus.

Intestinal obstruction

- Partial intestinal obstruction increases intestinal motility, resulting in diarrhea along with abdominal pain with tenderness and guarding, nausea and, possibly, distention.
- Other signs and symptoms include borborygmi, rushes on auscultation, and vomiting of fecal material.

Irritable bowel syndrome

- Diarrhea alternates with constipation or normal bowel function.
- Other signs and symptoms include abdominal pain, tenderness, and distention, dyspepsia, passage of mucus and pasty pencil-like stools, and nausea.

Ischemic bowel disease

- In this life-threatening disorder, bloody diarrhea occurs with abdominal pain.
- Other signs and symptoms include abdominal distention, nausea, vomiting and, if severe, shock.

Lactose intolerance

- Diarrhea occurs within hours of ingesting milk or milk products.

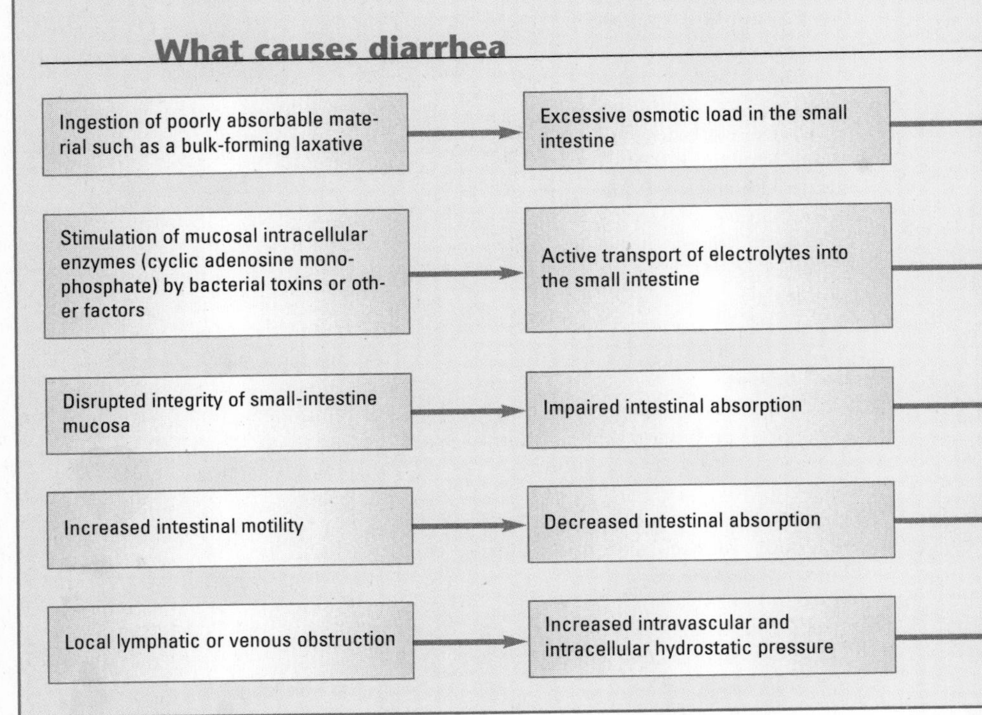

- Other signs and symptoms include cramps, abdominal pain, borborygmi, bloating, nausea, and flatus.

Large-bowel cancer

- Bloody diarrhea is seen with a partial obstruction.
- Other signs and symptoms include abdominal pain, anorexia, weight loss, weakness, fatigue, and exertional dyspnea.

Malabsorption syndrome

- Diarrhea occurs after meals along with steatorrhea, abdominal distention, and muscle cramps.
- Other signs and symptoms include anorexia, weight loss, bone pain, anemia, weakness, fatigue, bruising, and night blindness.

Pseudomembranous enterocolitis

- In this life-threatening disorder, copious watery, green, foul-smelling, bloody diarrhea rapidly precipitates signs of shock.
- Other signs and symptoms include colicky abdominal pain, distention, fever, and dehydration.

Rotavirus gastroenteritis

- Diarrhea occurs before fever, nausea, and vomiting.

Thyrotoxicosis

- Diarrhea accompanies diaphoresis, dyspnea, tachycardia, nervousness, tremors, palpitations, heat intolerance, weight loss despite increased appetite and, possibly, exophthalmos.

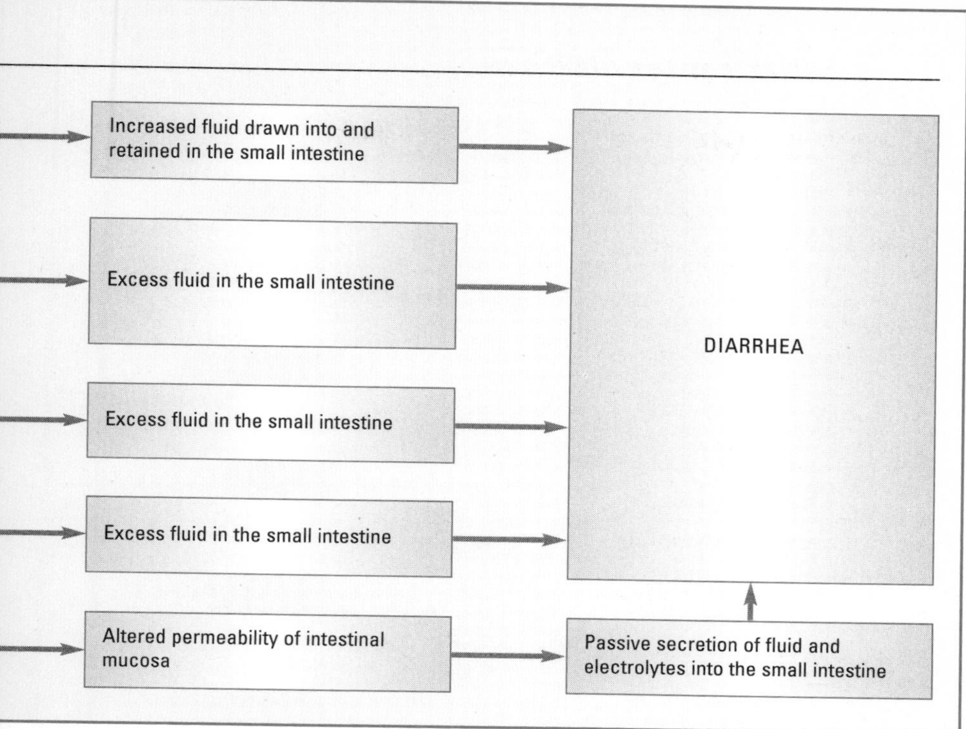

Ulcerative colitis

- Recurrent bloody diarrhea with pus or mucus is a characteristic sign.
- Weight loss, anemia, and weakness are late findings.
- Other signs and symptoms include tenesmus, hyperactive bowel sounds, cramping, lower abdominal pain, low-grade fever, anorexia, nausea, and vomiting.

Other causes

Drugs

- Many antibiotics, herbal remedies, and laxative abuse cause diarrhea.
- Other drugs that may cause diarrhea include antacids containing magnesium, colchicine, guanethidine (Ismelin), lactulose (Cephulac), dantrolene (Dantrium), ethacrynic acid (Edecrin), mefenamic acid (Ponstel), methotrexate, metyrosine (Demser) and, in high doses, cardiac glycosides and quinidine (Quinaglute).

Lead poisoning

- Diarrhea alternates with constipation.
- Other signs and symptoms include abdominal pain, anorexia, nausea, vomiting, a metallic taste, headache, dizziness, and a bluish gingival lead line.

Treatments

- Gastrectomy, gastroenterostomy, or pyloroplasty may produce diarrhea as part of dumping or postgastrectomy syndrome.
- High-dose radiation therapy may produce enteritis, leading to diarrhea.

Nursing considerations

- Administer an analgesic and an opioid as prescribed to decrease intestinal motility, unless the patient may have a stool infection.
- Clean the perineum thoroughly to prevent skin breakdown.
- Quantify the amount of liquid stools and monitor intake and output.
- Monitor electrolyte levels and hematocrit.
- Administer I.V. fluid replacements as prescribed.
- In children, diarrhea commonly results from infection.
- Chronic diarrhea may result from malabsorption syndrome, an anatomic defect, or allergies.
- In children, diarrhea can quickly cause life-threatening dehydration.
- In an elderly patient with new-onset segmental colitis, consider ischemia before assuming Crohn's disease.

Patient teaching

- Emphasize the importance of maintaining adequate hydration.
- Explain any foods or liquids the patient should avoid.
- Explain infection control techniques.
- Discuss stress-reduction techniques.
- Refer the patient for counseling as needed.
- Discuss the importance of medical follow-up with inflammatory bowel disease.

Dizziness

Dizziness is a sensation of imbalance or faintness, sometimes associated with giddiness, weakness, confusion, and blurred or double vision. Episodes are usually brief; they may be mild or severe with an abrupt or a gradual onset. Dizziness may be aggravated by standing up quickly and alleviated by lying down and by rest.

Dizziness typically results from inadequate blood flow and oxygen supply to the cerebrum and spinal cord. It may occur with anxiety, respiratory and cardiovascular disorders, and postconcussion syndrome. It's a key symptom in certain serious disorders, such as hypertension and vertebrobasilar artery insufficiency.

Dizziness is commonly confused with vertigo—a sensation of revolving in space or of surroundings revolving about oneself. However, unlike dizziness, vertigo is commonly accompanied by nausea, vomiting, nystagmus, a staggering gait, and tinnitus or hearing loss. Dizziness and vertigo may occur together, as in postconcussion syndrome.

QUICK ACTION ***If the patient complains of dizziness, first ensure his safety by assisting him back to bed and preventing falls. Then determine the severity and onset of the dizziness. Ask him to describe it. Is the dizziness associated with a headache or blurred vision? Next, take his blood pressure while he's lying down, sitting, and standing to check for orthostatic hypotension. Ask about a history of high blood pressure. Determine if he's at risk for hypoglycemia. Check his blood glucose level. Tell him to lie down, and recheck his vital signs every 15 minutes. Start an I.V. line, and prepare to administer medications as ordered.***

History

- Obtain a medical history, noting diabetes mellitus, head injury, anxiety disorders, and cardiovascular, pulmonary, and kidney disease.
- Take a drug history and determine whether the patient is taking antihypertensives.
- Determine the onset and characteristics of dizziness.
- Ask about emotional stress.

■ Ask about other signs and symptoms, such as palpitations, chest pain, diaphoresis, shortness of breath, and chronic cough.

Physical examination

■ Check the patient's neurologic status, including level of consciousness, motor and sensory functions, and reflexes.
■ Inspect for poor skin turgor and dry mucous membranes.
■ Auscultate heart rate and rhythm.
■ Inspect for barrel chest, clubbing, cyanosis, and accessory muscle use.
■ Auscultate breath and heart sounds.
■ Check for orthostatic hypotension.
■ Palpate for edema, capillary refill.

Causes

Medical causes

Anemia

■ Dizziness is aggravated by postural changes or exertion.
■ Other signs and symptoms include pallor, dyspnea, fatigue, tachycardia, and bounding pulse.

Cardiac arrhythmias

■ Dizziness lasts for several seconds or longer and may precede fainting.
■ Other signs and symptoms include palpitations; irregular, rapid, or thready pulse; hypotension; weakness; blurred vision; paresthesia; and confusion.

Carotid sinus hypersensitivity

■ Brief episodes of dizziness usually result in fainting.
■ An episode is preceded by stimulation of one or both carotid arteries.
■ Other signs and symptoms include sweating, nausea, and pallor.

Hypertension

■ Dizziness may precede fainting or may be relieved by rest.
■ Other signs and symptoms include headache, blurred vision, and retinal changes.

Hyperventilation syndrome

■ Dizziness lasts a few minutes.
■ With frequent hyperventilation, dizziness occurs between episodes.
■ Other signs and symptoms include apprehension, diaphoresis, pallor, dyspnea, chest tightness, palpitations, trembling, fatigue, and peripheral and circumoral paresthesia.

Hypoglycemia

■ Dizziness, headache, clouding of vision, restlessness, and mental status changes can result from fasting hypoglycemia.
■ Other signs and symptoms include irritability, trembling, hunger, cold sweats, and tachycardia.

Hypovolemia

■ Dizziness results from low circulating volume.
■ Other signs and symptoms include orthostatic hypotension, thirst, poor skin turgor, and flattened neck veins.

Orthostatic hypotension

■ Dizziness may terminate in fainting or disappear with rest after position change.
■ Other signs and symptoms include dim vision, spots before the eyes, pallor, diaphoresis, hypotension, tachycardia, and signs of dehydration.

Postconcussion syndrome

■ Dizziness, headache, emotional lability, alcohol intolerance, fatigue, anxiety and, possibly, vertigo occur 1 to 3 weeks after a head injury.
■ Dizziness or other symptoms are intensified by physical or mental stress.

Rift Valley fever

■ Typical signs and symptoms include dizziness, fever, myalgia, weakness, and back pain.

Transient ischemic attack

- Dizziness of varying severity, diplopia, blindness or visual field deficits, ptosis, tinnitus, hearing loss, paresis, and numbness occur.

Other causes

Drugs

- Antihistamines, antihypertensives, anxiolytics, central nervous system depressants, decongestants, opioids, and vasodilators commonly cause dizziness.
- Herbal remedies, such as St. John's wort, can produce dizziness.

Nursing considerations

- If the patient is dizzy, provide for his safety.
- Monitor the patient's vital signs, neurologic status, and intake and output.
- If you suspect a young patient of having dizziness, assess for vertigo, since that's a more common symptom in children.

Patient teaching

- Teach the patient how to control dizziness.
- Teach the patient safety measures for when dizziness happens in the future.
- Teach the patient about the underlying disease process and treatment.

Dysarthria

Dysarthria, poorly articulated speech, is characterized by slurring and labored, irregular rhythms. It may be accompanied by a nasal voice tone, caused by palate weakness. Whether it occurs abruptly or gradually, dysarthria is usually evident in ordinary conversation. It's confirmed by asking the patient to produce a few simple sounds and words, such as "ba," "sh," and "cat." However, dysarthria is occasionally confused with aphasia, the loss of the ability to produce or comprehend speech.

Dysarthria results from damage to the brain stem that affects cranial nerves IX, X, or XII. Degenerative neurologic disorders and cerebellar disorders commonly cause dysarthria. In fact, dysarthria is a chief sign of olivopontocerebellar degeneration. It may also result from ill-fitting dentures.

QUICK ACTION ***If the patient displays dysarthria, ask him about associated difficulty swallowing. Then determine his respiratory rate and depth. Measure his vital capacity with a Wright respirometer if available. Assess the patient's blood pressure and heart rate. Usually, tachycardia, slightly increased blood pressure, and shortness of breath are early signs of respiratory muscle weakness.***

Ensure a patent airway. Place the patient in Fowler's position and suction him, if necessary. Give oxygen, and keep emergency resuscitation equipment nearby. Anticipate endotracheal intubation and mechanical ventilation in progressive respiratory muscle weakness. Withhold oral fluids in the patient with associated dysphagia.

If dysarthria isn't accompanied by respiratory muscle weakness and dysphagia, continue to assess for other neurologic deficits. Compare muscle strength and tone in the limbs. Then evaluate tactile sensation. Ask the patient about numbness or tingling. Test deep tendon reflexes (DTRs), and note gait ataxia. Assess cerebellar function by observing rapid alternating movement, which should be smooth and coordinated. Next, test visual fields and ask about double vision. Check for signs of facial weakness such as ptosis. Finally, determine the patient's level of consciousness (LOC) and mental status.

History

- Ask about the onset and characteristics of dysarthria.
- Obtain a drug and alcohol history.
- Obtain a medical history, including the incidence of seizures.

Physical examination

- If the patient wears dentures, check them for proper fit.
- Have the patient produce a few simple sounds and words.
- Compare muscle strength and tone in the limbs on one side of the body with those on the other side.
- Assess the patient's tactile sense.
- Test DTRs, and note gait ataxia.
- Assess cerebellar function.
- Test visual fields and ask about double vision.
- Check for signs of facial weakness.
- Determine the patient's LOC and mental status.

Causes

Medical causes

Alcoholic cerebellar degeneration

- Chronic, progressive dysarthria occurs.
- Other signs and symptoms include ataxia, diplopia, ophthalmoplegia, hypotension, and altered mental status.

Amyotrophic lateral sclerosis

- Dysarthria occurs and worsens as the disease progresses.
- Other signs and symptoms include dysphagia; difficulty breathing; muscle atrophy and weakness, especially in the hands and feet; fasciculations; spasticity; hyperactive DTRs in the legs; and excessive drooling.

Basilar artery insufficiency

- Dysarthria accompanies diplopia, vertigo, facial numbness, ataxia, paresis, and visual field loss, lasting from minutes to hours.

Botulism

- This life-threatening paralytic illness is caused by ingestion of contaminated food or, in rare cases, a wound infection.
- Dysarthria, dysphagia, diplopia, and ptosis are characteristic signs.
- Initial signs and symptoms include dry mouth, sore throat, weakness, vomiting, and diarrhea.
- As the disorder progresses, descending weakness or paralysis of muscles in the extremities and trunk causes hyporeflexia and dyspnea.

Multiple sclerosis

- This progressive disease is caused by demyelination of the white matter of the brain and spinal cord.
- Dysarthria may occur with nystagmus, blurred or double vision, dysphagia, ataxia, and intention tremor.
- Other signs and symptoms include paresthesia, spasticity, hyperreflexia, muscle weakness or paralysis, constipation, emotional lability, and urinary frequency, urgency, and incontinence.

Myasthenia gravis

- This progressive disorder causes failure in the transmission of nerve impulses.
- Dysarthria, associated with a nasal voice, worsens during the day but may temporarily improve with short rest periods.
- Other signs and symptoms include dysphagia, drooling, facial weakness, diplopia, ptosis, dyspnea, and muscle weakness.

Olivopontocerebellar degeneration

- Dysarthria, a major sign of this genetic neurologic disease, accompanies cerebellar ataxia and spasticity.
- Other signs and symptoms include abnormal eye movement, sexual dysfunction, bowel and bladder problems, and difficulty swallowing.

Parkinson's disease

- Dysarthria and a monotone voice occur in this degenerative neurologic syndrome.
- Other signs and symptoms include muscle rigidity, bradykinesia, involuntary tremor usually beginning in the fingers, difficulty walking, muscle weakness, stooped posture, masklike facies, dysphagia, and drooling.

Stroke, brain stem

- Dysarthria that's most severe at the onset of a stroke occurs with dysphonia and dysphagia.
- Other signs and symptoms include facial weakness, diplopia, hemiparesis, spasticity, drooling, dyspnea, and decreased LOC.

Stroke, cerebral

- Weakness produces dysarthria that's most severe at the onset of the stroke.
- Other signs and symptoms include dysphagia, drooling, dysphonia, hemianopsia, aphasia, spasticity, and hyperreflexia.

Other causes

Drugs

- Large doses of anticonvulsants and barbiturates can cause dysarthria.

Manganese poisoning

- Progressive dysarthria is accompanied by weakness, fatigue, confusion, hallucinations, drooling, hand tremors, limb stiffness, spasticity, gross rhythmic movements of the trunk and head, and a propulsive gait.

Mercury poisoning

- Progressive dysarthria is accompanied by fatigue, depression, lethargy, irritability, confusion, ataxia, tremors, and changes in vision, hearing, and memory.

Nursing considerations

- Consult with a speech pathologist as needed.
- Give prescribed drugs and treatments as needed.
- Assess swallow and gag reflexes before feeding the patient.
- Give the patient time to express himself and encourage the use of gestures.
- Because dysarthria is difficult to detect in infants and young children, look for other neurologic deficits.

Patient teaching

- Encourage the patient to express his feelings by providing different ways in which he can communicate.
- Teach the patient about the underlying condition and treatment.

Dysphagia

Dysphagia—difficulty swallowing—is a common symptom that's usually easy to localize. It may be constant or intermittent. It's classified by the three phases of swallowing it affects: transfer (phase 1), transport (phase 2), or entrance (phase 3).

Dysphagia is the most common—and sometimes the *only*—symptom of esophageal disorders. However, it may also result from oropharyngeal, respiratory, neurologic, and collagen disorders or from the effects of toxins and treatments. Dysphagia increases the risk of choking and aspiration and may lead to malnutrition and dehydration.

QUICK ACTION ***If the patient suddenly complains of dysphagia and displays signs of respiratory distress, such as dyspnea and stridor, suspect an airway obstruction and quickly perform abdominal thrusts. Prepare to give oxygen by mask or nasal cannula, or to assist with endotracheal intubation.***

History

- Obtain a medical and surgical history.
- Ask about the onset and description of pain, if present.
- Determine aggravating and alleviating factors.
- Ask about recent vomiting, weight loss, anorexia, hoarseness, dyspnea, or cough.

Physical examination

- Evaluate swallowing and cough reflexes.
- If a sufficient swallow or cough reflex is present, check the gag reflex.
- Listen to the patient's speech for signs of muscle weakness.
- Check the mouth for dry mucous membranes and thick, sticky secretions.
- Observe for tongue and facial weakness and obstructions.
- Assess for disorientation.

Causes

Medical causes

Achalasia

- Gradually developing phase 3 dysphagia occurs and is precipitated or exacerbated by stress.
- Dysphagia is preceded by esophageal colic.
- Regurgitation of undigested food, especially at night, causes wheezing, coughing, choking, and halitosis.
- Other signs and symptoms include weight loss, cachexia, hematemesis, and heartburn.

Airway obstruction

- Phase 2 dysphagia occurs with gagging and dysphonia.
- When hemorrhage obstructs the trachea, dysphagia is sudden in onset but painless.
- When inflammation causes the obstruction, dysphagia is slow in onset and painful.
- Signs of respiratory distress occur with life-threatening upper airway obstruction.

Amyotrophic lateral sclerosis

- Dysphagia occurs with accompanying muscle weakness and atrophy, fasciculations, dysarthria, dyspnea, shallow respirations, tachypnea, slurred speech, hyperactive deep tendon reflexes (DTRs), and emotional lability.

Botulism

- Phase 1 dysphagia and dysuria usually begin within 36 hours of toxin ingestion.
- Blurred or double vision, dry mouth, sore throat, nausea, vomiting, and diarrhea occurs, with gradual symmetrical descending weakness or paralysis.

Bulbar paralysis

- Painful and progressive phase 1 dysphagia occurs with drooling, difficulty chewing, dysarthria, and nasal regurgitation.
- Other signs and symptoms include arm and leg spasticity, hyperreflexia, and emotional lability.

Esophageal cancer

- Painless dysphagia (phases 2 and 3) with weight loss are the earliest and most common findings.
- As the cancer advances, dysphagia becomes painful and is accompanied by steady chest pain, cough with hemoptysis, hoarseness, and sore throat.
- Other signs and symptoms include nausea, vomiting, fever, hiccups, hematemesis, melena, and halitosis.

Esophageal diverticulum

- Phase 3 dysphagia occurs when the enlarged diverticulum obstructs the esophagus.
- Other signs and symptoms include regurgitation, chronic cough, hoarseness, chest pain, and halitosis.

Esophageal obstruction by foreign body

- Sudden onset of phase 2 or 3 dysphagia occurs with gagging, coughing, and esophageal pain.
- If the obstruction compresses the trachea, dyspnea occurs.

Esophageal spasm

- Phase 2 dysphagia occurs along with substernal chest pain.
- Pain that radiates may be relieved by drinking water.
- Bradycardia may also occur.

Esophageal stricture

- Phase 3 dysphagia occurs, possibly with drooling, tachypnea, and gagging.
- With chemical ingestion, burns, ulcers, or erythema of the lips and mouth may develop.

Esophagitis

- Corrosive esophagitis, resulting from ingestion of alkalis or acids, causes severe phase 3 dysphagia with marked salivation, hematemesis, tachypnea, fever, and intense pain in the mouth and chest that's aggravated by swallowing.
- Candidal esophagitis causes phase 2 dysphagia, sore throat and, possibly, retrosternal pain on swallowing.
- Reflux esophagitis causes phase 3 dysphagia (late symptom) with heartburn; regurgitation; vomiting; a dry, nocturnal cough; and substernal chest pain.

Hypocalcemia

- Phase 1 dysphagia with numbness and tingling in the nose, ears, fingertips, toes, and around the mouth occurs.
- Other signs and symptoms include tetany with carpopedal spasms, muscle twitching, and laryngeal spasms.

Laryngeal cancer, extrinsic

- Phase 2 dysphagia and dyspnea develop late.
- Other signs and symptoms include muffled voice, stridor, pain, halitosis, weight loss, ipsilateral otalgia, chronic cough, and cachexia.

Lower esophageal ring

- Phase 3 dysphagia occurs with the feeling of a foreign body in the lower esophagus that may be relieved by drinking water or vomiting.

Myasthenia gravis

- This progressive disorder causes failure in nerve impulse transmission.
- Painless phase 1 dysphagia develops after ptosis and diplopia.
- Other signs and symptoms include masklike facies, nasal voice, nasal regurgitation, shallow respirations, dyspnea, and head bobbing.

Oral cavity tumor

- Painful phase 1 dysphagia occurs with hoarseness and ulcerating lesions.
- Other signs and symptoms include abnormal taste or bleeding in the mouth or dentures that no longer fit.

Pharyngitis, chronic

- Painful phase 2 dysphagia occurs with a dry, sore throat; cough; and thick mucus and sensation of fullness in the throat.

Progressive systemic sclerosis

- This diffuse connective tissue disease is also known as *scleroderma.*
- Preceded by Raynaud's phenomenon, mild dysphagia becomes so severe that only liquids can be swallowed.
- Heartburn, weight loss, abdominal distention, diarrhea, and malodorous and floating stools occur.
- Other signs and symptoms include joint pain and stiffness, masklike facies,

and thickening of the skin that becomes taut and shiny.

Tetanus

- Phase 1 dysphagia occurs about 1 week after the unimmunized patient receives a puncture wound.
- Other signs and symptoms include marked muscle hypotonicity, hyperactive DTRs, tachycardia, diaphoresis, drooling, trismus (lockjaw), risus sardonicus, opisthotonos, boardlike abdominal rigidity, seizures, and low-grade fever.

Other causes

Lead poisoning

- Painless, progressive dysphagia occurs.
- Other signs and symptoms include a lead line on the gums, metallic taste, papilledema, ocular palsy, footdrop or wristdrop, mental impairment, seizures, and signs of hemolytic anemia.

Procedures

- Recent tracheostomy or repeated or prolonged intubation may cause temporary dysphagia.

Radiation therapy

- Radiation therapy for oral cancer may cause scant salivation and temporary dysphagia.

Nursing considerations

- Stimulate salivation by talking about food, adding a lemon slice or dill pickle to the food tray, and providing mouth care.
- With decreased salivation, moisten food with liquid.
- Give an anticholinergic or antiemetic to control excess salivation, as prescribed.
- Consult with the dietitian to select foods with distinct temperatures, consistencies, and textures.
- Consult a therapist to assess the patient's aspiration risk and to begin exercises to aid swallowing.
- In feeding a child, coughing, choking, or regurgitation suggests dysphagia.
- Dysphagia in children results most commonly from esophageal obstruction by a foreign body or from corrosive esophagitis or congenital anomalies.
- In patients older than age 50, dysphagia is typically the first complaint in cases of head or neck cancer.

Patient teaching

- Discuss easy-to-swallow foods with the patient.
- Explain measures the patient can take to reduce the risk of choking and aspiration.
- Teach the patient about prescribed medications and possible adverse effects.
- Teach the patient about the underlying condition, diagnostic tests, and treatments.

Dyspnea

Typically a symptom of cardiopulmonary dysfunction, dyspnea is the sensation of difficult or uncomfortable breathing. It's usually reported as shortness of breath. Its severity varies greatly and is usually unrelated to the severity of the underlying cause. Dyspnea may arise suddenly or slowly, and may subside rapidly or persist for years.

Most people normally experience dyspnea when they exert themselves, and its severity depends on their physical condition. In a healthy person, dyspnea is quickly relieved by rest. Pathologic causes of dyspnea include pulmonary, cardiac, neuromuscular, and allergic disorders. It may also be caused by anxiety.

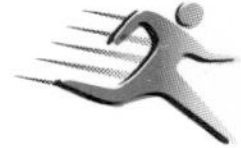

QUICK ACTION ***If a patient complains of shortness of breath, quickly look for***

signs of respiratory distress, such as tachypnea, cyanosis, restlessness, and accessory muscle use. Prepare to administer oxygen by nasal cannula, mask, or endotracheal tube. Ensure patent I.V. access, and begin cardiac monitoring and oxygen saturation monitoring to detect arrhythmias and low oxygen saturation, respectively. Expect to insert a chest tube for severe pneumothorax.

History

- Ask about the onset and progression of dyspnea.
- Determine aggravating and alleviating factors.
- Ask the patient if he has a cough.
- Obtain a history, including trauma, upper respiratory tract infection, deep vein phlebitis, orthopnea, paroxysmal nocturnal dyspnea, fatigue, smoking, or exposure to occupational hazards.
- Ask about current orthopnea, paroxysmal nocturnal dyspnea, or progressive fatigue.

Physical examination

- Look for pursed-lip exhalation, clubbing, peripheral edema, barrel chest, diaphoresis, jugular vein distention, and edema.
- Take the patient's vital signs.
- Auscultate for crackles, egophony, bronchophony, abnormal heart sounds or rhythms, and whispered pectoriloquy.
- Palpate the abdomen for hepatomegaly.

Causes

Medical causes

Acute respiratory distress syndrome

- A life-threatening condition, acute dyspnea is usually the first complaint.
- Progressive respiratory distress with restlessness, anxiety, decreased mental acuity, tachycardia, and crackles and rhonchi occur.
- Other signs and symptoms include cyanosis, tachypnea, motor dysfunction, intercostal and suprasternal retractions, and shock.

Amyotrophic lateral sclerosis

- Dyspnea is slow in onset, worsening over time.
- Other signs and symptoms include dysphagia, dysarthria, muscle weakness and atrophy, fasciculations, shallow respirations, tachypnea, and emotional lability.

Anemia

- Dyspnea is gradual in onset.
- Fatigue, weakness, syncope, tachycardia, tachypnea, restlessness, and anxiety occur.
- Other signs and symptoms include pallor, inability to concentrate, irritability, dysphagia, smooth tongue, and spoon-shaped and brittle nails.

Anthrax, inhalation

- In this life-threatening disorder, dyspnea occurs in the second stage, with fever, stridor, and hypotension.
- Other signs and symptoms include fever, chills, weakness, cough, and chest pain.

Asthma

- Dyspneic attacks occur with audible wheezing, dry cough, accessory muscle use, nasal flaring, intercostal and supraclavicular retractions, tachypnea, tachycardia, diaphoresis, prolonged expiration, flush or cyanosis, and anxiety.

Cor pulmonale

- Chronic dyspnea begins gradually with exertion and progressively worsens until it occurs even at rest.
- Other signs and symptoms include chronic productive cough, wheezing, tachypnea, jugular vein distention, edema, fatigue, weakness, and hepatomegaly.

Emphysema

- Progressive exertional dyspnea occurs.
- Other signs and symptoms include barrel chest, accessory muscle use, diminished breath sounds, anorexia, weight loss, malaise, peripheral cyanosis, tachypnea, pursed-lip breathing, prolonged expiration, a chronic and productive cough, and late clubbing.

Flail chest

- Sudden dyspnea is accompanied by paradoxical chest movement, severe chest pain, hypotension, tachypnea, tachycardia, and cyanosis.
- Bruising and decreased or absent breath sounds occur over the affected side.

Guillain-Barré syndrome

- Slowly worsening dyspnea occurs with fatigue and ascending muscle weakness and paralysis following a fever and upper respiratory tract infection.
- Other signs and symptoms include facial diplegia, dysphagia or dysarthria and, less commonly, weakness of the muscles supplied by cranial nerve XI.

Heart failure

- Dyspnea occurs gradually with orthopnea, tachypnea, tachycardia, palpitations, ventricular gallop, fatigue, dependent edema, jugular vein distention, paroxysmal nocturnal dyspnea, hepatosplenomegaly, cough, and weight gain.

Inhalation injury

- Dyspnea may be sudden or gradual (over several hours), with sooty or bloody sputum, persistent cough, and oropharyngeal edema.
- Other signs and symptoms include orofacial burns, singed nasal hairs, crackles, rhonchi, wheezing, and signs of respiratory distress.

Lung cancer

- Dyspnea develops slowly, progressively worsening over time.
- Other signs and symptoms include fever, hemoptysis, productive cough, wheezing, clubbing, pain, weight loss, anorexia, and pleural rub.

Myasthenia gravis

- This progressive disorder causes failure in nerve impulse transmission.
- Bouts of dyspnea occur with difficulty chewing and swallowing.
- With myasthenic crisis, acute respiratory distress with shallow respirations and tachypnea occur.

Myocardial infarction

- Dyspnea occurs suddenly with crushing substernal chest pain that may radiate to the back, neck, jaw, and arms.
- Other signs and symptoms include nausea, vomiting, diaphoresis, vertigo, tachycardia, anxiety, and pale, cool, clammy skin.

Pleural effusion

- Dyspnea develops slowly and progressively worsens over time.
- Initial signs and symptoms include pleural friction rub and pleuritic pain that worsens with cough and deep breathing.
- Other signs and symptoms include dry cough, dullness on percussion, tachycardia, tachypnea, weight loss, fever, and decreased breath sounds.

Pneumonia

- Dyspnea occurs suddenly with fever, shaking chills, pleuritic chest pain, and productive cough.
- Other signs and symptoms include fatigue, headache, myalgia, anorexia, abdominal pain, crackles, rhonchi, tachycardia, tachypnea, cyanosis, decreased breath sounds, and diaphoresis.

Pneumothorax

- Acute dyspnea occurs that's unrelated to the severity of pain.
- Sudden, stabbing chest pain radiates to the arms, face, back, or abdomen.
- Other signs and symptoms include anxiety, restlessness, dry cough, cyanosis, tachypnea, decreased or absent breath sounds on the affected side, splinting, and accessory muscle use.

Pulmonary edema

- Acute dyspnea is preceded by signs of heart failure.
- Other signs and symptoms include tachycardia, tachypnea, crackles, ventricular gallop, thready pulse, hypotension, diaphoresis, cyanosis, marked anxiety, and a cough that's dry or produces copious amounts of pink, frothy sputum.

Pulmonary embolism

- In this life-threatening disorder, acute dyspnea occurs usually with sudden pleuritic chest pain.
- Other signs and symptoms include tachycardia, low-grade fever, tachypnea, pleural rub, crackles, diffuse wheezing, dullness on percussion, nonproductive cough or productive cough with blood-tinged sputum, decreased breath sounds, diaphoresis, anxiety and, with a massive embolism, signs of shock.

Severe acute respiratory syndrome

- This life-threatening acute infectious disorder produces fever with headache, malaise, a dry, nonproductive cough, and dyspnea.

Shock

- In this life-threatening disorder, sudden dyspnea occurs, progressively worsening over time.
- Other signs and symptoms include severe hypotension, tachypnea, tachycardia, decreased peripheral pulses, decreased mental acuity, restlessness, anxiety, and cool, clammy skin.

Tuberculosis

- Dyspnea occurs with chest pain, crackles, and productive cough.
- Other signs and symptoms include night sweats, fever, anorexia, weight loss, palpitations on mild exertion, and dullness on percussion.

Nursing considerations

- Monitor the patient closely.
- Position the patient comfortably, usually in high-Fowler's or forward-leaning position.
- Administer oxygen if needed.
- Give a bronchodilator, an antiarrhythmic, a diuretic, and an analgesic, as prescribed.
- Suspect dyspnea in an infant who breathes costally, an older child who breathes abdominally, or any child who uses his neck or shoulder muscles to help him breathe.
- Acute epiglottiditis and laryngotracheobronchitis can cause severe dyspnea in a child.
- An older patient with dyspnea from chronic illness may not be aware of a significant change in his breathing pattern.

Patient teaching

- Teach the patient about the underlying condition, diagnostic tests, and treatment.
- Teach the patient about pursed-lip, diaphragmatic breathing and chest splinting.
- Instruct the patient to avoid chemical irritants, pollutants, and people with respiratory infections.
- Teach the patient with chronic dyspnea about oxygen use, if prescribed, and energy conservation.

Dysuria

Dysuria—painful or difficult urination—is commonly accompanied by urinary frequency, urgency, or hesitancy. This symptom usually reflects lower urinary tract infection—a common disorder, especially in women.

Dysuria results from lower urinary tract irritation or inflammation, which stimulates nerve endings in the bladder and urethra. The onset of pain provides clues to its cause. For example, pain just before voiding usually indicates bladder irritation or distention, whereas pain at the start of urination typically results from bladder outlet irritation. Pain at the end of voiding may signal bladder spasms; in women, it may indicate vaginal candidiasis.

History

- Obtain a description of the severity and location of the dysuria, and ask the patient what precipitates it and what alleviates or aggravates the pain.
- Ask about previous urinary or genital tract infections or if the patient has recently undergone an invasive procedure, such as cystoscopy or urethral dilatation.
- Ask about a history of intestinal disease, menstrual disorders, vaginal discharge or pruritus, or use of products that irritate the urinary tract—such as bubble bath salts, feminine deodorants, contraceptive gels, or perineal lotions.

Physical examination

- Inspect the urethral meatus for discharge, irritation, or other abnormalities.
- Percuss over the kidneys, costovertebral angle (CVA), and bladder.
- Palpate the kidneys and bladder. (See *Palpating the kidneys.*)
- A pelvic or rectal examination may be necessary.

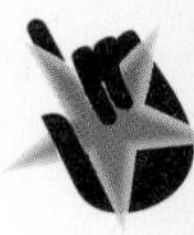

KNOW-HOW

Palpating the kidneys

To palpate the kidneys, first have the patient lie in a supine position. To palpate the right kidney, stand on his right side. Place your left hand under his back and your right hand on his abdomen.

Instruct him to inhale deeply, so his kidney moves downward. As he inhales, press up with your left hand and down with your right, as shown.

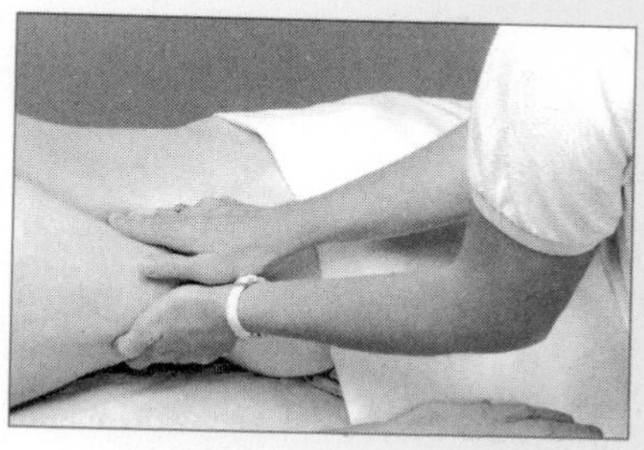

Causes

Medical causes

Appendicitis

- Dysuria may occur that persists throughout voiding and is accompanied by bladder tenderness.
- Other signs and symptoms include periumbilical abdominal pain that shifts to McBurney's point, anorexia, nausea, vomiting, constipation, slight fever, abdominal rigidity and rebound tenderness, and tachycardia.

Bladder cancer

- Dysuria occurs throughout voiding and is a late symptom.
- Other signs and symptoms include urinary frequency and urgency, nocturia, hematuria, and perineal, back, or flank pain.

Cystitis

- Dysuria throughout voiding is common in all types of cystitis, as are urinary frequency, nocturia, straining to void, and hematuria.
- Bacterial cystitis, the most common cause of dysuria in women, may also produce urinary urgency, perineal and lower back pain, suprapubic discomfort, fatigue and, possibly, low-grade fever.
- With chronic interstitial cystitis, dysuria is most acute at the end of voiding.
- With tubercular cystitis, symptoms may also include urinary urgency, flank pain, fatigue, and anorexia.
- With viral cystitis, severe dysuria occurs with gross hematuria, urinary urgency, and fever.

Diverticulitis

- Inflammation near the bladder may cause dysuria throughout voiding.
- Other signs and symptoms include urinary frequency and urgency, nocturia, hematuria, fever, abdominal pain and tenderness, perineal pain, constipation or diarrhea and, possibly, an abdominal mass.

Paraurethral gland inflammation

- Dysuria throughout voiding occurs with urinary frequency and urgency, a diminished urine stream, mild perineal pain and, occasionally, hematuria.

Prostatitis

- Acute prostatitis commonly causes dysuria throughout or toward the end of voiding as well as a diminished urine stream, urinary frequency and urgency, hematuria, suprapubic fullness, fever, chills, fatigue, myalgia, nausea, vomiting, and constipation.
- With chronic prostatitis, urethral narrowing causes dysuria throughout voiding.
- Other signs and symptoms include urinary frequency and urgency; a diminished urine stream; perineal, back, and buttock pain; urethral discharge; nocturia and, at times, hematospermia and ejaculatory pain.

Pyelonephritis, acute

- In this condition, more common in females, dysuria is present throughout voiding.
- Other signs and symptoms include persistent high fever with chills, CVA tenderness, unilateral or bilateral flank pain, weakness, urinary urgency and frequency, nocturia, straining on urination, hematuria, nausea, vomiting, and anorexia.

Reiter's syndrome

- In this condition, more common in males, dysuria occurs 1 to 2 weeks after sexual contact with an infected person.
- Initially, signs and symptoms include mucopurulent discharge, urinary urgency and frequency, meatal swelling and redness, suprapubic pain, anorexia, weight loss, and low-grade fever.
- Hematuria, conjunctivitis, arthritic symptoms, a papular rash, and oral and penile lesions may follow.

Urethritis

- In sexually active men, dysuria occurs throughout voiding and is accompanied by a reddened meatus and copious, yellow, purulent discharge (gonorrheal infection) or white or clear mucoid discharge (nongonorrheal infection).

Urinary obstruction

- Outflow obstruction by urethral strictures or calculi produces dysuria throughout voiding.
- With complete obstruction, bladder distention develops and dysuria precedes voiding.

- Other signs and symptoms include diminished urine stream, urinary frequency and urgency, and a sensation of fullness or bloating in the lower abdomen or groin.

Vaginitis

- Dysuria occurs throughout voiding along with urinary frequency and urgency, nocturia, hematuria, perineal pain, and vaginal discharge and odor.

Other causes

Chemical irritants

- Bubble bath, bath salts, feminine deodorants, and spermicides can cause dysuria.

Drugs

- Monoamine oxidase inhibitors and metyrosine (Demser) can cause dysuria.

Nursing considerations

- Monitor the patient's vital signs and intake and output.
- Give medications as prescribed.
- Obtain urine samples for testing as ordered.
- Be aware that elderly patients may underreport symptoms related to the urinary tract.

Patient teaching

- Explain the importance of increased fluid intake.
- Emphasize the importance of frequent urination.
- Teach the patient to perform proper perineal care.
- Discourage the use of bubble baths and vaginal deodorants.
- Discuss the importance of taking prescribed drugs as instructed.

E

Edema, generalized

A common sign in severely ill patients, generalized edema is the excessive accumulation of interstitial fluid throughout the body. Its severity varies widely; slight edema may be difficult to detect—especially if the patient is obese, whereas massive edema is immediately apparent.

Generalized edema is typically chronic and progressive. It may result from cardiac, renal, endocrine, or hepatic disorders as well as from severe burns, malnutrition, or the effects of certain drugs and treatments.

QUICK ACTION ***Quickly determine the location and severity of edema, including the degree of pitting. If the patient has severe edema, promptly take his vital signs and oxygen saturation, and check for jugular vein distention and cyanotic lips. Auscultate the lungs and heart. Be alert for signs of cardiac failure or pulmonary congestion, such as crackles, muffled heart sounds, or ventricular gallop. Unless the patient is hypotensive, place him in Fowler's position to promote lung expansion. Prepare to administer oxygen and an I.V. diuretic. Keep emergency resuscitation equipment nearby.***

History

- Note the onset, location, and description of edema.
- Ask about shortness of breath or pain.
- Obtain a medical history, including the incidence of previous burns and cardiac, renal, hepatic, endocrine, and GI disorders.
- Find out about recent weight gain and urine output changes.
- Ask the patient to describe his diet.
- Obtain a drug history.

Physical examination

- Compare the patient's arms and legs for symmetrical edema.
- Note ecchymoses and cyanosis.
- Assess the back, sacrum, and hips of a bedridden patient for dependent edema.
- Palpate peripheral pulses, noting coolness in the hands and feet.
- Perform complete cardiac and respiratory assessments.

Causes

Medical causes

Angioneurotic edema or angioedema

- Recurrent attacks of acute, painless, nonpitting edema involving the skin and mucous membranes may result from food or drug allergy, heredity, or emotional stress.
- Abdominal pain, nausea, vomiting, and diarrhea accompany visceral edema.
- Dyspnea and stridor accompany life-threatening laryngeal edema.

Burns

- Severe generalized edema may occur within 2 days of a major burn.
- Depending on the degree of edema, signs and symptoms of reduced or absent circulation and airway obstruction may occur.

Cirrhosis

- Edema is a late sign.
- Other signs and symptoms include abdominal pain, anorexia, nausea, vomiting, hepatomegaly, ascites, jaundice, pruritus, bleeding tendencies, musty breath, lethargy, mental changes, and asterixis.

Heart failure

- Severe, generalized pitting edema may follow leg edema.
- Edema may improve with exercise or elevation of limbs and is worst at the end of the day.
- Other classic, late signs and symptoms include hemoptysis, cyanosis, clubbing, crackles, marked hepatosplenomegaly, and ventricular gallop.

Myxedema

- Myxedema is a form of hypothyroidism characterized by generalized nonpitting edema with dry, flaky, inelastic, waxy, pale skin; puffy face; and upper eyelid droop.
- Other signs and symptoms include masklike facies, hair loss or coarsening, hoarseness, weight gain, fatigue, cold intolerance, bradycardia, constipation, abdominal distention, menorrhagia, impotence, and infertility.

Nephrotic syndrome

- Edema is initially localized around the eyes, and then becomes generalized and pitting.
- Anasarca develops in severe cases.
- Other signs and symptoms include ascites, anorexia, fatigue, malaise, depression, and pallor.

Pericardial effusion

- Generalized pitting edema may be most prominent in the arms and legs.
- Other signs and symptoms include chest pain, dyspnea, orthopnea, nonproductive cough, pericardial friction rub, jugular vein distention, dysphagia, and fever.

Renal failure

- Generalized pitting edema occurs as a late sign.
- With chronic renal failure, edema is less likely to become generalized; its severity depends on the degree of fluid overload.
- Other signs and symptoms include oliguria, anorexia, nausea, vomiting, drowsiness, confusion, hypertension, dyspnea, crackles, dizziness, and pallor.

Septic shock

- A late sign of this life-threatening disorder, generalized edema typically develops rapidly.
- Edema becomes pitting and moderately severe.
- Other signs and symptoms include cool skin, hypotension, oliguria, anxiety, and signs of respiratory failure.

Other causes

Drugs

- Drugs that cause sodium retention—such as antihypertensives, corticosteroids, androgenic and anabolic steroids, estrogens, and nonsteroidal anti-inflammatory drugs—may aggravate or cause generalized edema.

Treatments

- Enteral feedings and I.V. saline solution infusions may cause sodium and fluid overload, especially in patients with cardiac or renal disease.

Nursing considerations

- Position the patient with his limbs above heart level, to promote drainage.
- Periodically reposition the patient.
- If dyspnea develops, lower the patient's limbs, elevate the head of the bed, and administer oxygen.
- Prevent skin breakdown by placing a pressure mattress on the patient's bed.
- Restrict fluids and sodium, and administer a diuretic or I.V. albumin as prescribed.
- Monitor intake and output and daily weight.
- Monitor electrolyte levels.
- In children, renal failure typically causes generalized edema; kwashiorkor causes massive generalized edema.
- With an elderly patient, use caution when giving I.V. fluids or drugs that can raise sodium levels.

Patient teaching

- Explain signs and symptoms of edema that the patient should report.
- Discuss foods and fluids that the patient should avoid.

Epistaxis

A common sign, epistaxis (nosebleed) can be spontaneous or induced from the front or back of the nose. Most nosebleeds occur in the anterior-inferior nasal septum (Kiesselbach's plexus), but they may also occur at the point where the inferior turbinates meet the nasopharynx. Usually unilateral, they seem bilateral when blood runs from the bleeding side behind the nasal septum and out the other side. Epistaxis ranges from mild oozing to severe—possibly life-threatening—blood loss.

A rich supply of fragile blood vessels makes the nose particularly vulnerable to bleeding. Air moving through the nose can dry and irritate the mucous membranes, forming crusts that bleed when they're removed; dry mucous membranes are also more susceptible to infection, which can produce epistaxis as well. Additional causes include trauma; septal deviations; hematologic, coagulation, renal, and GI disorders; and certain drugs and treatments.

QUICK ACTION ***If the patient has severe epistaxis, quickly take his vital signs. Be alert for tachypnea, hypotension, and other signs of hypovolemic shock. Insert a large-gauge I.V. line for rapid fluid and blood replacement, and attempt to control bleeding by pinching the nares closed. (However, if you suspect a nasal fracture, don't pinch the nares. Instead, place gauze under the patient's nose to absorb the blood.)***

Have a hypovolemic patient lie down and turn his head to the side to prevent blood from draining down the back of his throat, which could cause aspiration or vomiting of swallowed blood. If the patient isn't hypovolemic, have him sit upright and tilt his head forward. Constantly check airway patency. If the patient's condition is unstable, begin cardiac monitoring and give supplemental oxygen by mask.

History

- Ask about recent trauma or surgery.
- Obtain a description of past nosebleeds.
- Take a medical history, including incidence of hypertension, bleeding or liver disorders, and other recent illnesses.
- Find out what drugs the patient is taking, especially anti-inflammatory drugs and anticoagulants.

Physical examination

- Inspect for other signs of bleeding, such as ecchymoses or petechiae.
- Look for trauma injuries.

Causes

Medical causes

Angiofibroma, juvenile

- Severe recurrent epistaxis and facial obstruction usually occurs in males.

Aplastic anemia

- Nosebleeds are accompanied by ecchymoses, retinal hemorrhages, menorrhagia, petechiae, and signs of GI bleeding.
- Other signs and symptoms may include fatigue, dyspnea, headache, tachycardia, and pallor.

Biliary obstruction

- Epistaxis occurs along with other bleeding tendencies.
- Other signs and symptoms include colicky right upper quadrant pain after eating fatty food, nausea, vomiting, fever, flatulence, and jaundice.

Cirrhosis

- Epistaxis and other bleeding tendencies are late signs.
- Other late findings include ascites, abdominal pain, shallow respirations, hepatomegaly or splenomegaly, and fever.
- Other signs and symptoms include muscle atrophy, pruritus, extremely dry skin, abnormal pigmentation, spider angiomas, jaundice, and central nervous system disturbances.

Coagulation disorders

- Signs and symptoms include epistaxis, ecchymoses, petechiae, menorrhagia, GI bleeding, and bleeding from the gums, mouth, and I.V. puncture sites.

Glomerulonephritis, chronic

- Nosebleeds occur with accompanying hypertension, proteinuria, hematuria, headache, edema, oliguria, hemoptysis, nausea, vomiting, pruritus, dyspnea, malaise, and fatigue.

Hepatitis

- Epistaxis occurs with accompanying jaundice, clay-colored stools, pruritus, hepatomegaly, abdominal pain, fever, fatigue, weakness, dark amber urine, anorexia, nausea, and vomiting.

Hypertension

- Severe hypertension can produce extreme epistaxis with accompanying dizziness, throbbing headache, anxiety, peripheral edema, nocturia, nausea, vomiting, drowsiness, and mental impairment.

Leukemia

- With acute leukemia, sudden epistaxis is accompanied by high fever and other types of abnormal bleeding tendencies, such as bleeding gums, ecchymoses, petechiae, easy bruising, and prolonged menses.
- Other signs and symptoms include chills, recurrent infections, low-grade fever, malaise, a systolic ejection murmur, and abdominal or bone pain.
- With chronic leukemia, epistaxis is a late sign that may be accompanied by other bleeding tendencies, extreme fatigue, weight loss, hepatosplenomegaly, bone tenderness, macular or nodular skin lesions, pallor, weakness, dyspnea, tachycardia, palpitations, and headache.

Maxillofacial injury

- Severe epistaxis may occur with accompanying facial pain, swelling, open-bite malocclusion or the inability to open the mouth, diplopia, conjunctival hemorrhage, lip edema, and buccal, mucosal, and soft palatal ecchymoses.

Nasal fracture

- One or both nostrils may bleed.
- Other signs and symptoms include nasal swelling, periorbital ecchymoses and edema, pain, nasal deformity, and crepitation of the nasal bones.

Polycythemia vera

- Spontaneous epistaxis is a common sign of this bone marrow disorder.
- Other signs and symptoms include bleeding gums; ecchymoses; ruddy cyanosis of the face, nose, ears, and lips; headache; dizziness; vision disturbances; hypertension; chest pain; splenomegaly; epigastric pain; pruritus; dyspnea; and congestion of the conjunctiva, retina, and oral mucous membranes.

Renal failure

- Epistaxis can occur with accompanying oliguria or anuria, weight loss, anorexia, abdominal pain, diarrhea, nausea, vomiting, tissue wasting, dry mucous membranes, uremic breath, Kussmaul's respirations, deteriorating mental condition, and tachycardia.

Sarcoidosis

- Oozing epistaxis may occur along with extensive nasal mucosal lesions, nonproductive cough, substernal pain, malaise, and weight loss.
- Other signs and symptoms include tachycardia, arrhythmias, parotid enlargement, cervical lymphadenopathy, skin lesions, hepatosplenomegaly, and arthritis in the ankles, knees, and wrists.

Sinusitis, acute

- Bloody or blood-tinged nasal discharge may become purulent and copious 48 hours after onset.
- Other signs and symptoms include nasal congestion, pain, and tenderness; malaise; headache; low-grade fever; and red, edematous nasal mucosa.

Skull fracture

- Epistaxis is direct or indirect, depending on the type of fracture.
- With a severe skull fracture, signs and symptoms include severe headache, decreased level of consciousness, hemiparesis, dizziness, seizures, projectile vomiting, and decreased pulse and respirations.
- With a basilar fracture, signs and symptoms include raccoon eyes; Battle's sign; bleeding from the pharynx, ears, and conjunctivae; and leakage of cerebrospinal fluid or brain tissue from the nose or ears.
- With a sphenoid fracture, blindness may also occur.
- With a temporal fracture, deafness in one ear or facial paralysis may also occur.

Systemic lupus erythematosus

- Oozing epistaxis occurs.
- Other signs and symptoms include butterfly rash, lymphadenopathy, joint pain and stiffness, anorexia, nausea, vomiting, myalgia, and weight loss.

Other causes

Chemical irritants

- Some chemicals, such as phosphorus, sulfuric acid, ammonia, printer's ink, and chromates, irritate the nasal mucosa, producing epistaxis.

Drugs

- Anticoagulants or anti-inflammatories can cause or worsen epistaxis.
- Frequent cocaine use may also cause epistaxis.

Vigorous nose blowing

- Vigorous nose blowing may rupture superficial blood vessels and cause epistaxis.

Nursing considerations

- Monitor for signs of hypovolemic shock.
- If external pressure doesn't control the bleeding, insert cotton saturated with a vasoconstrictor and local anesthetic into the nose as prescribed.
- If bleeding persists, insert anterior or posterior nasal packing.

- Administer humidified oxygen by face mask to a patient with posterior packing.
- Children are more likely to experience anterior nosebleeds.
- Causes of epistaxis in children include nose picking, allergic rhinitis, biliary atresia, cystic fibrosis, hereditary afibrinogenemia, nasal trauma from a foreign body, and rubeola.
- Elderly patients are more likely to have posterior nosebleeds.

Patient teaching

- Teach the patient or caregiver pinching pressure techniques.
- Discuss ways to prevent nosebleeds.

Erythema

Dilated or congested blood vessels that produce red skin, or erythema, is the most common sign of skin inflammation or irritation. It may be localized or generalized and may occur suddenly or gradually. Skin color can range from bright red in patients with acute conditions to pale violet or brown in those with chronic problems. Erythema must be differentiated from purpura, which causes redness from bleeding into the skin. When pressure is applied directly to the skin, erythema blanches momentarily, but purpura doesn't.

Erythema usually results from changes in the arteries, veins, and small vessels that lead to increased small-vessel perfusion. Drugs and neurogenic mechanisms can allow extra blood to enter the small vessels. Erythema can also result from trauma and tissue damage; changes in supporting tissues, which increase vessel visibility; and many rare disorders.

QUICK ACTION ***If the patient has sudden progressive erythema with a rapid pulse, dyspnea, hoarseness, and agitation, quickly take his vital signs. These may be indications of anaphylactic shock. Provide emergency respiratory support and give epinephrine.***

History

- Ask about the onset and duration of erythema.
- Obtain a medical history, including the incidence of recent fever, upper respiratory tract infection, skin disease, allergies, or asthma.
- Ask about pain or itching.
- Note recent falls or injury.
- Ask about exposure to anyone with a rash.
- Take a drug history, including recent immunizations.
- Review food intake and exposure to chemicals.

Physical examination

- Assess the extent, distribution, and intensity of erythema.
- Look for edema and other skin lesions.
- Examine the affected area for warmth.
- Gently palpate the affected area to check for tenderness or crepitus.

Causes

Medical causes

Allergic reactions

- A localized reaction produces erythema, hivelike eruptions, and edema.
- With life-threatening anaphylaxis, erythema is sudden and accompanied by flushing, facial edema, diaphoresis, weakness, bronchospasm with tachypnea and dyspnea, shock, and airway edema with hoarseness and stridor.

Burns

- With thermal burns, erythema and swelling appear first, possibly followed by blisters.
- Burns from ultraviolet rays cause delayed erythema and tenderness.

Cellulitis

- Erythema, tenderness, and edema occur with accompanying pain and warmth at the site of the infection.

Dermatitis

- With atopic dermatitis, erythema and intense pruritus precede the development of small papules that may redden, weep, scale, and lichenify.
- With contact dermatitis, erythema appears with vesicles, blisters, or ulcerations.
- With seborrheic dermatitis, erythema appears with dull-red or yellow lesions that are sharply marginated and may be ring-shaped and covered with greasy scales.

Erythema annulare centrifugum

- Small, pink, infiltrated papules appear on the trunk, buttocks, and inner thighs, slowly spreading at the margins and clearing in the center.
- Other signs and symptoms include itching, scaling, and tissue hardening.

Erythema marginatum rheumaticum

- Erythematous lesions caused by rheumatic fever are superficial, flat, and slightly hardened.
- Lesions shift, spread rapidly, and may last for hours or days.

Erythema multiforme

- This condition may result from allergies, pregnancy, or a drug sensitivity after infection, most commonly herpes simplex and *Mycoplasma.*
- In the minor form, burning or itching red-pink, iris-shaped, localized urticarial lesions occur on the flexor surfaces of extremities.
- Early signs and symptoms of the minor form include mild fever, cough, and sore throat.
- In the major form, blisters on the lips, tongue, and buccal mucosa and sore throat precede the development of widespread erythematous, symmetrical, bullous lesions.
- Early signs and symptoms of the major form include cough, vomiting, diarrhea, coryza, and epistaxis.
- Late signs and symptoms of the major form include fever, prostration, conjunctivitis, vulvitis, balanitis, and difficulty with oral intake because of oral lesions.

Erythema nodosum

- This condition may be caused by drug sensitivity, sarcoidosis, inflammatory bowel disease, or various infections.
- Tender erythematous nodules develop suddenly in crops on the shins, knees, and ankles.
- Other signs and symptoms include mild fever, chills, malaise, muscle and joint pain, and swollen feet and ankles.

Gout

- Tight, erythematous skin is seen over the inflamed, edematous joint.
- The metatarsophalangeal joint of the great toe usually becomes inflamed first, followed by the instep, ankle, heel, knee, or wrist joint.

Liver disease, chronic

- Local vasodilation and palmar erythema occur along with jaundice, pruritus, spider angiomas, xanthomas, and characteristic systemic signs.

Lupus erythematosus

- A characteristic erythematous butterfly rash develops.
- The rash may range from a blush with swelling to a scaly, sharply demarcated, macular rash with plaques that may spread to the forehead, chin, ears, chest, and other sun-exposed body parts.

■ With systemic lupus erythematosus, acute onset of erythema may accompany photosensitivity and mucous membrane ulcers.

Necrotizing fasciitis

■ Mild erythema begins at the site of the streptococcal infection.
■ The necrotizing process progresses rapidly, with the appearance of fluid-filled blisters and bullae.
■ After 7 to 10 days, dead skin begins to separate at the margins of the erythema, revealing extensive necrosis.
■ Other signs and symptoms include fever, hypovolemia and, in later stages, hypotension and respiratory insufficiency.

Psoriasis

■ Silvery white scales with a thickened erythematous base affect the elbows, knees, chest, scalp, and intergluteal folds.
■ Fingernails become thick and pitted.

Rheumatoid arthritis

■ During flare-ups, erythema, heat, swelling, pain, and stiffness occur at affected joints.
■ Early signs and symptoms include malaise, fatigue, myalgia, and morning stiffness.
■ As the disease progresses, other signs and symptoms include muscle atrophy, palmar erythema, edema, mottled skin, and structural deformities.

Rosacea

■ Scattered erythema develops across the center of the face, followed by superficial telangiectases, papules, pustules, and nodules.

Rubella

■ Flat solitary lesions form a blotchy pink erythematous rash that spreads rapidly to the trunk and extremities, clearing in 4 to 5 days.
■ Small red lesions may appear on the soft palate.
■ Other signs and symptoms include fever, headache, malaise, sore throat, a gritty eye sensation, lymphadenopathy, joint pain, and coryza.

Staphylococcal scalded-skin syndrome

■ Occurring mainly in infants and small children, erythema and widespread exfoliation of superficial epidermal layers occur.
■ Other signs and symptoms include low-grade fever and irritability.

Thrombophlebitis

■ Erythema may develop over the inflamed vein.
■ Fever, chills, and malaise may accompany severe, localized pain, warmth, and induration; distal edema; and a positive Homans' sign.

Other causes

Drugs

■ Many drugs commonly cause erythema. (See *Drugs associated with erythema,* page 132.)

Radiation therapy

■ Radiation therapy may produce dull erythema and edema within 24 hours.

Rare causes

■ A number of rare disorders, such as bullous pemphigoid and penphigus, cause erythema.

Nursing considerations

■ Monitor and replace fluids and electrolytes, as ordered.
■ Certain drugs may be withheld until the cause of erythema is identified.
■ Give an antibiotic and topical or systemic corticosteroid, as prescribed.

Drugs associated with erythema

Suspect drug-induced erythema in any patient who develops the sign within 1 week of starting a drug. Erythematous lesions can vary in size, shape, type, and amount, but they almost always appear suddenly and symmetrically on the trunk and inner arms. The following drugs can produce erythematous lesions:

allopurinol
anticoagulants
antimetabolites
barbiturates
cephalosporins
chlordiazepoxide
codeine
corticosteroids
co-trimoxazole
diazepam
erythromycin
gentamicin
gold
griseofulvin
hormonal contraceptives
indomethacin
iodide bromides
isoniazid
lithium
nitrofurantoin
penicillin
phenothiazines
phenytoin
quinidine
salicylates
sulfonamides
sulfonylureas
tetracyclines
thiazides

Some drugs—particularly barbiturates, hormonal contraceptives, salicylates, sulfonamides, and tetracycline—can cause a "fixed" drug eruption. In this type of reaction, lesions can appear on any body part and flake off after a few days, leaving a brownish purple pigmentation. Repeated drug administration causes the original lesions to recur and new ones to develop.

- To relieve itching skin, give soothing baths or apply open wet dressings containing starch, bran, or sodium bicarbonate.
- Give an antihistamine and an analgesic, as prescribed.
- Keep erythematous legs elevated above the heart level.
- For a burn patient with erythema, immerse the affected area in cold water, or apply a sheet soaked in cold water.
- Infections and other disorders can cause erythema in neonates and infants.
- Roseola, rubeola, scarlet fever, granuloma annulare, and cutis marmorata cause erythema in children.
- Well-defined purple macules or patches in the elderly, usually on the back of the hands and on the forearms, may result from blood leaking through fragile capillaries.

Patient teaching

- Teach the patient to recognize the signs and symptoms of flare-ups of disease.
- Stress the importance of using sunblock and avoiding sun exposure.
- Teach the patient methods to relieve itching.
- Teach the patient infection control techniques, as appropriate.

F

Facial pain

Facial pain may result from various neurologic, vascular, or infectious disorders. The most common cause of facial pain is trigeminal neuralgia (tic douloureux). In this disorder, intense, paroxysmal facial pain may occur along the pathway of a specific facial nerve or nerve branch, usually cranial nerve (CN) V (trigeminal nerve). Pain can also be referred to the face in disorders of the ear, nose, paranasal sinuses, teeth, neck, and jaw.

Atypical facial pain is a constant burning pain with limited distribution at onset. It usually spreads to the rest of the face and may involve the neck or back of the head as well. This type of facial pain is common in middle-aged women, especially those who are clinically depressed.

History

- Ask about the pain's onset, description, location, and duration.
- Determine what alleviates or aggravates the pain.
- Obtain a medical and dental history, noting the incidence of previous head trauma, dental disease, and infection.

Physical examination

- Inspect the ear for vesicles and changes in the tympanic membrane.
- Inspect the nose for deformity or asymmetry and characterize any secretions.
- Palpate the sinuses for tenderness and swelling.
- Evaluate oral hygiene.
- Ask about sensitivity to hot, cold, or sweet liquids or foods.
- Have the patient open and close his mouth as you palpate the temporomandibular joint.
- Assess CNs V and VII (facial nerve).

Causes

Medical causes

Angina pectoris

- Jaw pain may be described as burning, squeezing, or as feeling tight.
- Pain may radiate to the left arm, neck, and shoulder blade.

Dental caries

- Caries in the mandibular molars can produce ear, preauricular, and temporal pain.
- Caries in the maxillary teeth can produce maxillary, orbital, retro-orbital, and parietal pain.

Herpes zoster oticus

- Severe pain localizes around the ear, followed by the appearance of vesicles in the ear.
- Eye pain may occur with corneal and scleral damage and impaired vision.

Multiple sclerosis

- Facial pain may resemble that of trigeminal neuralgia.
- Pain is accompanied by jaw and facial weakness.

- Other signs and symptoms include visual blurring, diplopia, and nystagmus; sensory impairment; generalized muscle weakness and gait abnormalities; urinary disturbances; and emotional lability.

Postherpetic neuralgia

- Burning, itching, prickly pain occurs that worsens with contact or movement and persists along any of the three trigeminal nerve divisions.
- Mild hypoesthesia or paresthesia and vesicles affect the area before the onset of pain.

Sinusitis, acute

- Acute maxillary sinusitis produces pressure, fullness, or burning pain over the cheekbone, upper teeth, and around the eyes that worsens with bending over.
- Acute frontal sinusitis produces severe pain above or around the eyes that worsens when the patient is in a supine position.
- Acute ethmoid sinusitis produces pain at or around the inner corner of the eye.
- Acute sphenoid sinusitis produces persistent, deep-seated pain behind the eyes or nose or on the top of the head that increases with bending forward.

Sinusitis, chronic

- Chronic maxillary sinusitis produces a chronic toothache or a feeling of pressure below the eyes.
- Chronic frontal sinusitis produces persistent low-grade pain above the eyes.
- Chronic ethmoid sinusitis is characterized by nasal congestion and discharge and discomfort at medial corners of the eyes.
- Chronic sphenoid sinusitis produces a persistent low-grade, diffuse headache or retro-orbital discomfort.

Temporal arteritis

- Pain occurs behind one eye or in the scalp, jaw, tongue, or neck.
- A typical episode consists of a severe throbbing or boring temporal headache with redness, swelling, and nodulation of the temporal artery.

Temporomandibular joint syndrome

- An intermittent severe, dull ache or intense spasm, usually on one side, radiates to the cheek, temple, lower jaw, or ear.
- Other signs and symptoms include trismus (lockjaw), malocclusion, and clicking, crepitus, and tenderness of the joint.

Trigeminal neuralgia

- Paroxysms of intense pain shoot along the three branches of the trigeminal nerve.
- Pain may be triggered by touching the nose, cheek, or mouth; exposure to hot or cold; consuming hot or cold foods or beverages; or even smiling and talking.

Nursing considerations

- Administer pain medication, as prescribed.
- Apply direct heat or give a muscle relaxant, as prescribed.
- Provide a humidifier, vaporizer, or decongestant to relieve nasal or sinus congestion.
- Look for subtle signs of pain, such as facial rubbing, irritability, or poor eating habits in children.

Patient teaching

- Teach the patient about triggers to avoid.
- Explain which signs and symptoms to report.
- Teach the patient about prescribed medications, dosage, and possible adverse effects.

Fetor hepaticus

Fetor hepaticus—a distinctive musty, sweet breath odor—characterizes hepatic encephalopathy, a life-threatening complication of severe liver disease. The odor results from the damaged liver's inability to metabolize and detoxify mercaptans produced by the bacterial degradation of methionine, a sulfurous amino acid. These substances circulate in the blood, are expelled by the lungs, and affect the odor of the breath.

QUICK ACTION ***If you detect fetor hepaticus, quickly determine the patient's level of consciousness (LOC). If he's comatose, evaluate his respiratory status. Prepare to intubate and provide ventilatory support, if necessary. Start a peripheral I.V. line for fluid administration, begin cardiac monitoring, and insert an indwelling urinary catheter to monitor output. Obtain arterial and venous blood samples for analyzing blood gases, ammonia, and electrolytes.***

History

- Obtain a complete medical history, relying on the patient's family if necessary.
- Focus on any factors that may have precipitated liver disease or coma, such as a recent severe infection; overuse of sedatives, analgesics (especially acetaminophen [Tylenol]), alcohol, or diuretics; excessive protein intake; or recent blood transfusion, surgery, or GI bleeding.

Physical examination

- If the patient is conscious, closely observe him for signs of impending coma.
- Evaluate deep tendon reflexes, and test for asterixis and Babinski's reflex.
- Look for signs of GI bleeding and shock—common complications of end-stage liver failure, and watch for increased anxiety, restlessness, tachycardia, tachypnea, hypotension, oliguria, hematemesis, melena, or cool, moist, pale skin.
- Evaluate the degree of jaundice and abdominal distention, and palpate the liver to assess the degree of enlargement.

Causes

Medical causes

Hepatic encephalopathy

- Fetor hepaticus usually occurs in the final, comatose stage of this disorder, but it may occur earlier.
- Tremors progress to asterixis in the impending stage, which is also marked by lethargy, aberrant behavior, and apraxia.
- Hyperventilation and stupor mark the stuporous stage, during which the patient acts agitated when aroused.
- Seizures and coma indicate the final stage, along with decreased pulse and respiratory rates, positive Babinski's reflex, hyperactive reflexes, decerebrate posture, and opisthotonos.

Nursing considerations

- Administer neomycin (Neo-fradin) or lactulose (Cephulac) to suppress bacterial production of ammonia in the GI tract, give sorbitol solution to induce osmotic diarrhea, give potassium supplements to correct alkalosis, provide continuous gastric aspiration of blood, or maintain the patient on a low-protein diet.
- If these methods prove unsuccessful, hemodialysis or exchange transfusions may be performed.
- During treatment, closely monitor the patient's LOC, intake and output, and fluid and electrolyte balance.
- Place the patient in a supine position, with the head of the bed elevated 30 degrees. Administer oxygen if necessary.

■ Be prepared to draw blood samples for liver function tests, serum electrolyte levels, hepatitis panel, blood alcohol count, a complete blood cell count, typing and crossmatching, a clotting profile, and ammonia level.
■ Intubation, ventilation, or cardiopulmonary resuscitation may be necessary.
■ Along with fetor hepaticus, elderly patients with hepatic encephalopathy may exhibit disturbances of awareness and mentation, such as forgetfulness and confusion.

Patient teaching

■ Advise the patient to restrict his intake of dietary protein to as little as 40 g/day; recommend that he eat vegetable protein rather than animal protein.
■ Inform the patient that medications used to treat and prevent hepatic encephalopathy do so by causing diarrhea, so he shouldn't stop taking the drug when diarrhea occurs.
■ Teach the patient about all hospital procedures and the purpose of diagnostic tests and blood samples.

Fever

A fever is a common sign that can arise from many disorders. Because these disorders can affect virtually any body system, fever in the absence of other signs usually has little diagnostic significance. A persistent high fever, though, represents an emergency. (See *How fever develops*.)

A fever can be classified as low (oral reading of 99° to 100.4° F [37.2° to 38° C]), moderate (100.5° to 104° F [38.1° to 40° C]), or high (above 104° F). A fever greater than 106° F (41.1° C) causes unconsciousness and, if sustained, leads to permanent brain damage.

A fever may also be classified as remittent, intermittent, sustained, relapsing, or undulant. Remittent fever, the most common type, is characterized by daily temperature fluctuations above the normal range. Intermittent fever is marked by a daily temperature drop into the normal range and then a rise back to above normal. An intermittent fever that fluctuates widely, typically producing chills and sweating, is called *hectic,* or *septic,* fever. Sustained fever involves persistent temperature elevation with little fluctuation. Relapsing fever consists of alternating feverish and afebrile periods. Undulant fever refers to a gradual increase in temperature that stays high for a few days and then decreases gradually.

Further classification involves duration—either brief (less than 3 weeks) or prolonged. Prolonged fevers include fever of unknown origin, a classification used when careful examination fails to detect an underlying cause.

QUICK ACTION ***If you detect a fever higher than 106° F, take the patient's other vital signs and determine his level of consciousness (LOC). Administer an antipyretic and begin rapid cooling measures: Apply ice packs to the axillae and groin, give tepid sponge baths, or apply a hypothermia blanket. These methods may evoke a cooling response such as shivering, which increases metabolism and oxygen requirements and can lead to arrhythmias and rebound temperature. To prevent this, continually monitor the patient's rectal temperature using the thermistor probe of the hypothermia blanket. Avoid lowering the temperature more than 1° F every 15 minutes, or lower the temperature according to the physician's order.***

History

■ Ask about the onset of fever, temperature pattern, and highest reading.

How fever develops

Body temperature is regulated by the hypothalamic thermostat, which has a specific set point under normal conditions. Fever can result from a resetting of this set point or from an abnormality in the thermoregulatory system itself, as shown in this flowchart.

Disruption of hypothalamic thermostat by:
■ central nervous system disease
■ inherited malignant hyperthermia
Increased production of heat from:
■ strenuous exercise or other stress
■ chills (skeletal muscle response)
■ thyrotoxicosis
Decreased loss of heat from:
■ anhidrotic asthenia (heatstroke)
■ heart failure
■ skin conditions, such as ichthyosis and congenital absence of sweat glands
■ drugs that impair sweating
Failure of the body's temperature-regulating mechanisms
FEVER
Entrance of exogenous pyrogens, such as bacteria, viruses, or immune complexes, into the body
Production of endogenous pyrogens
Elevation of hypothalamic set point

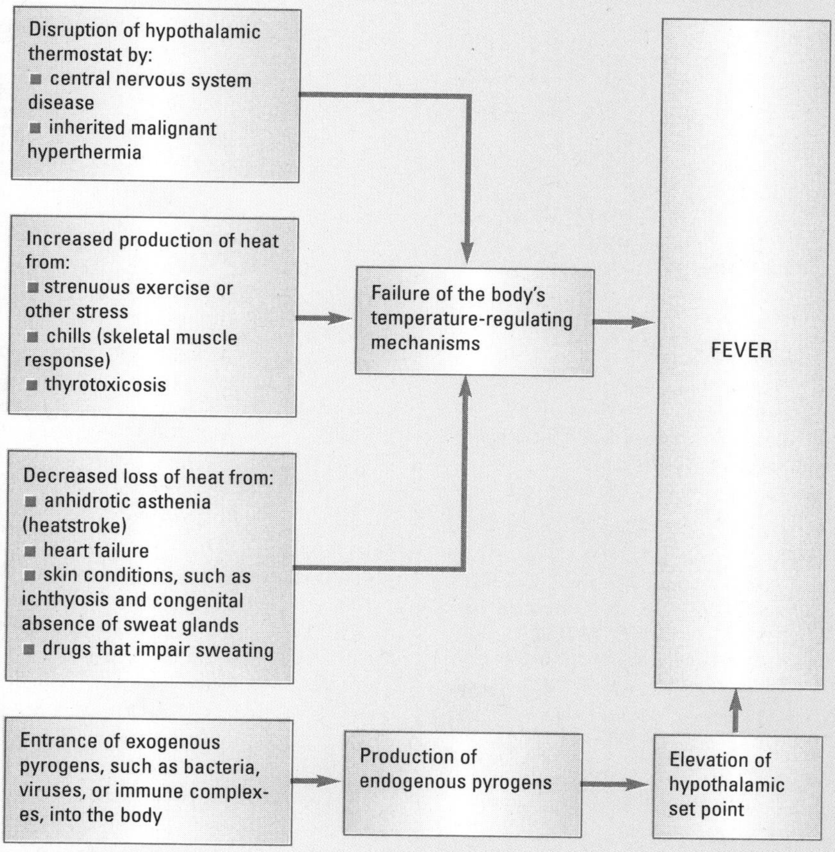

- Inquire about other symptoms, such as chills, fatigue, or pain.
- Obtain a medical history, including immunosuppressive treatments or disorders, infection, trauma, surgery, diagnostic testing, and use of anesthesia or other drugs.
- Ask about recent travel.

Physical examination

- Take the patient's vital signs.
- Let the history findings direct your physical examination, which may range from a brief evaluation of one body system to a comprehensive review of all systems. (See *Differential diagnosis: Fever,* pages 138 and 139.)

Differential diagnosis: Fever

History of present illness
Focused physical examination: All systems

↓

Common signs and symptoms
- Fatigue
- Malaise
- Anorexia

↓

Thermoregulatory dysfunction

Additional signs and symptoms
- Sudden onset of fever that rises rapidly and remains high
- Temperature that may rise to 107° F (41.7° C)
- Vomiting
- Anhidrosis
- Decreased level of consciousness (LOC)
- Hot, flushed skin
- Tachycardia
- Tachypnea
- Hypotension

Diagnosis: Patient history with additional signs or symptoms that would indicate source of thermoregulatory dysfunction (such as heatstroke, thyroid storm, neuroleptic malignant syndrome, malignant hyperthermia, lesions of the central nervous system)
Treatment: Cooling techniques to decrease temperature, treatment of cause, antipyretics
Follow-up: As needed (depending on cause of dysfunction)

Neoplasms

Additional signs and symptoms
- Prolonged fever of varying elevations
- Nocturnal diaphoresis
- Weight loss
- Lymphadenopathy
- Palpable mass

Diagnosis: Varies depending on additional signs and symptoms but usually includes imaging studies (computed tomography scan, magnetic resonance imaging)
Treatment: Varies based on type and location of neoplasm but may include medication (antipyretics, chemotherapy), radiation therapy and, possibly, surgery
Follow-up: Referral to oncologist

Causes

Medical causes

Anthrax, cutaneous

- Fever may occur with lymphadenopathy, malaise, and headache.
- A small, painless or pruritic, macular or papular lesion develops, changing to a vesicle in 1 to 2 days, and then into a painless ulcer with a characteristic black, necrotic center.

Anthrax, GI

- Fever, loss of appetite, nausea, and vomiting occur after eating contaminated food.

Infection and inflammatory disorders

Additional signs and symptoms
- Low or extremely high temperature that may be intermittent or sustained and may rise abruptly or insidiously
- Chills
- Diaphoresis
- Weakness
- Associated signs that may involve every system

Diagnosis: Varies depending on additional signs and symptoms
Treatment: Varies depending on source of fever but usually includes antipyretics
Follow-up: As needed (depending on source of infection)

Immune complex dysfunction

Additional signs and symptoms
- Low-grade fever that may be remittent, intermittent, or sustained
- Nocturnal diaphoresis

Diagnosis: Varies depending on additional signs and symptoms
Treatment: Varies depending on specific cause of fever but usually includes antipyretics
Follow-up: As needed (depending on cause of fever)

West Nile encephalitis

Additional signs and symptoms
- Mild to moderate fever
- Headache
- Myalgia
- Rash
- Swollen lymph glands
- Neck stiffness
- Decreased LOC
- Seizures

Diagnosis: History of recent mosquito bite, West Nile activity reported in locality, blood culture
Treatment: Supportive treatment, treatment of symptoms, medication (antipyretics, analgesics)
Follow-up: As needed (depending on severity of infection)

- Abdominal pain, severe bloody diarrhea, and hematemesis may also develop.

Anthrax, inhalation
- Initially, fever, chills, weakness, cough, and chest pain occur.
- Abrupt deterioration—marked by fever, dyspnea, stridor, and hypotension—occurs in the second stage, generally leading to death within 24 hours.

Escherichia coli *O157:H7*
- Fever, bloody diarrhea, nausea, vomiting, and abdominal cramps occur after eating contaminated food.

Immune complex dysfunction

- Fever usually remains low and may be remittent, intermittent, or sustained, relative to the underlying disease.
- Other signs and symptoms also depend on the underlying disease.

Infectious and inflammatory disorders

- Fever varies depending on the disorder and may be remittent, intermittent, sustained, or relapsing.
- Fever may occur abruptly or insidiously.
- Other signs and symptoms involve every body system.

Neoplasms

- Prolonged fever of varying elevations occurs.
- Other signs and symptoms include nocturnal diaphoresis, anorexia, fatigue, malaise, and weight loss.

Plague

- Bubonic form causes fever, chills, and swollen, inflamed, and tender lymph nodes near the bite from an infected rodent flea.
- Pneumonic form manifests as a sudden onset of chills, fever, headache, and myalgia.
- Other signs and symptoms of the pneumonic form include productive cough, chest pain, tachypnea, dyspnea, hemoptysis, increasing respiratory distress, and cardiopulmonary insufficiency.

Rhabdomyolysis

- This condition results in muscle breakdown and the release of myoglobin into the bloodstream.
- Signs and symptoms include fever, muscle weakness or pain, nausea, vomiting, malaise, and dark reddish-brown urine, leading to kidney damage and possible failure.

Severe acute respiratory syndrome

- Disease generally begins with fever greater than 100.4° F (38° C).
- Other symptoms include headache, malaise, a dry nonproductive cough, and dyspnea.

Smallpox

- Initial signs and symptoms include high fever, malaise, prostration, severe headache, backache, and abdominal pain.
- A maculopapular rash develops on the mucosa of the mouth, pharynx, face, and forearms and then spreads to the trunk and legs.
- Within 2 days, the rash becomes vesicular and later pustular; by day 8 or 9, crusts form that later separate, leaving a scar.

Thermoregulatory dysfunction

- Sudden onset of fever that rises rapidly and remains as high as 107° F (41.7° C) occurs in life-threatening disorders.
- Low or moderate fever appears in dehydrated patients.
- Prolonged high fever produces vomiting, anhidrosis, decreased LOC, and hot, flushed skin.

Typhus

- Initially in this rickettsial disease, headache, myalgia, arthralgia, and malaise occur.
- These signs and symptoms are followed by the abrupt onset of fever, chills, nausea, and vomiting.
- A maculopapular rash may be present in some cases.

West Nile encephalitis

- Fever, headache, body aches, skin rash, and swollen lymph nodes occur.
- Severe infection is marked by high fever, headache, neck stiffness, stupor, disorientation, coma, tremors, seizures, and paralysis.

Other causes

Diagnostic tests

- Immediate or delayed fever uncommonly follows radiographic tests that use contrast medium.

Drugs

- Fever can accompany chemotherapy.
- Drugs that impair sweating, such as anticholinergics, phenothiazines, and monoamine oxidase inhibitors, can result in fever.
- Hypersensitivity to antifungals, sulfonamides, penicillins, cephalosporins, tetracyclines, barbiturates, phenytoin (Dilantin), quinidine (Quinaglute), iodides, phenolphthalein, methyldopa (Aldoril), procainamide (Pronestyl), and some antitoxins can cause fever and rash.
- Muscle relaxants and inhaled anesthetics and muscle relaxants can trigger malignant hyperthermia.
- Toxic doses of salicylates, amphetamines, and tricyclic antidepressants can cause fever.

Nursing considerations

- Regularly monitor and record temperature.
- Increase fluid and nutritional intake.
- Maintain a stable room temperature.
- Provide frequent bedding and clothing changes for diaphoretic patients.
- Give antipyretics according to a regular dosage schedule to minimize chills and diaphoresis.
- For high fevers, initiate treatment with a hypothermia blanket.
- Common pediatric causes of fever include varicella, croup syndrome, dehydration, meningitis, mumps, otitis media, pertussis, roseola infantum, rubella, rubeola, tonsillitis, and adverse reactions to immunizations and antibiotics.
- Be aware that seizures commonly accompany extremely high fever in children.
- Elderly patients may have impaired thermoregulatory mechanisms, making temperature change a much less reliable measure of disease severity.

Patient teaching

- Instruct the patient about the proper way to take oral temperature measurements at home.
- Emphasize the importance of increased fluid intake (unless contraindicated).
- Discuss the use of antipyretics and antibiotics.
- Teach signs and symptoms that require immediate medical attention.

Flank pain

Pain in the flank, the area extending from the ribs to the ilium, is a leading indicator of renal and upper urinary tract disease or trauma. Depending on the cause, this symptom may vary from a dull ache to severe stabbing or throbbing pain, and may be unilateral or bilateral and constant or intermittent. It's aggravated by costovertebral angle (CVA) percussion and, in patients with renal or urinary tract obstruction, by increased fluid intake and ingestion of alcohol, caffeine, or diuretics. Unaffected by position changes, flank pain typically responds only to analgesics or to treatment of the underlying disorder.

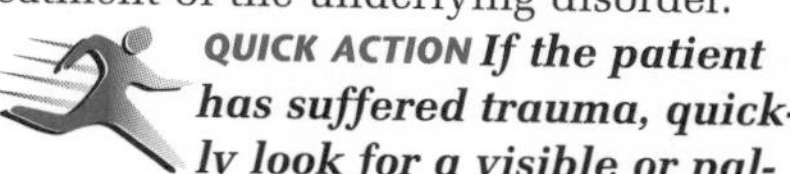

QUICK ACTION ***If the patient has suffered trauma, quickly look for a visible or palpable flank mass, associated injuries, CVA pain, hematuria, Turner's sign, and signs of shock, such as tachycardia and cool, clammy skin. If one or more is present, insert an I.V. line to allow fluid or drug infusion. Insert an indwelling urinary catheter to monitor urine output and evaluate hematuria. Obtain blood samples for typing and crossmatching, complete blood count, and electrolyte levels.***

History

- Ask about the onset, location, intensity, pattern, and duration of pain.
- Ask what alleviates or aggravates the pain.
- Explore precipitating events to pain.
- Ask about the patient's normal fluid intake and urine output and recent changes.
- Obtain a medical history, including the incidence of urinary tract infection (UTI), obstruction, renal disease, or recent streptococcal infection.

Physical examination

- Take the patient's vital signs.
- Palpate the flank area and percuss the CVA.
- Obtain a urine sample.

Causes

Medical causes

Bladder cancer

- Dull, constant flank pain radiates to the legs, back, and perineum.
- Initial signs include gross, painless, intermittent hematuria, usually with clots.
- Other signs and symptoms include urinary frequency and urgency, nocturia, dysuria, or pyuria; bladder distention; pain in the bladder, rectum, pelvis, back, or legs; diarrhea; vomiting; and sleep disturbances.

Calculi

- Intense colicky pain in one flank radiates from the CVA.
- Other signs and symptoms include intense nausea, vomiting, CVA tenderness, hematuria, hypoactive bowel sounds, and signs and symptoms of UTI.

Cystitis, bacterial

- Flank pain occurs along with perineal, lower back, and suprapubic pain.
- Other signs and symptoms include dysuria, nocturia, hematuria, urinary frequency and urgency, tenesmus, fatigue, and low-grade fever.

Glomerulonephritis, acute

- Constant and moderately intense flank pain occurs.
- Classic signs and symptoms include moderate facial and generalized edema, hematuria, oliguria or anuria, and fatigue.
- Other signs and symptoms include low-grade fever, malaise, nausea, vomiting, dyspnea, tachypnea, and crackles.

Obstructive uropathy

- With an acute obstruction, flank pain may be excruciating.
- With gradual obstruction, pain is typically a dull ache.
- A palpable abdominal mass, CVA tenderness, and bladder distention vary with the site and cause of the obstruction.
- Other signs and symptoms include nausea, vomiting, abdominal distention, anuria alternating with periods of oliguria and polyuria, and hypoactive bowel sounds.

Pancreatitis, acute

- Flank pain may develop as severe epigastric or left upper quadrant pain that radiates to the back.
- A severe attack causes extreme pain, nausea, persistent vomiting, abdominal tenderness and rigidity, hypoactive bowel sounds, restlessness, low-grade fever, tachycardia, hypotension, and positive Turner's and Cullen's signs.

Papillary necrosis, acute

- Intense flank pain occurs with renal colic, CVA tenderness, and abdominal pain and rigidity.
- Other signs and symptoms include oliguria or anuria, hematuria, and pyuria, with fever, chills, vomiting, and hypoactive bowel sounds.

Perirenal abscess

- Intense pain in one flank and CVA tenderness accompany dysuria, persistent high fever, and chills.

Polycystic kidney disease

- Dull, aching pain in both flanks is an early symptom.
- Pain may become severe and colicky if cysts rupture and clots migrate or cause obstruction.
- Early signs and symptoms include polyuria, increased blood pressure, and signs of UTI.
- Late signs and symptoms include hematuria and perineal, lower back, and suprapubic pain.

Pyelonephritis, acute

- Intense, constant flank pain develops.
- Typical signs and symptoms include dysuria, nocturia, hematuria, urgency, frequency, and tenesmus.
- Other common signs and symptoms include persistent high fever, chills, anorexia, weakness, fatigue, myalgia, abdominal pain, and CVA tenderness.

Renal cancer

- Classic signs and symptoms include pain in one flank that's dull and vague, gross hematuria, and a palpable flank mass.
- Signs of advanced disease include weight loss, leg edema, nausea, and vomiting.
- Other signs and symptoms include fever, increased blood pressure, and urine retention.

Renal infarction

- Constant, severe pain in one flank and tenderness typically accompany persistent, severe upper abdominal pain.
- Other signs and symptoms include CVA tenderness, anorexia, nausea, vomiting, fever, hypoactive bowel sounds, hematuria, and oliguria or anuria.

Renal trauma

- Variable flank pain is common.
- A visible or palpable flank mass and CVA or abdominal pain, which may be severe and radiate to the groin, may also develop.
- Other signs and symptoms include hematuria, oliguria, abdominal distention, Turner's sign, hypoactive bowel sounds, nausea, vomiting and, with severe injury, signs of shock.

Renal vein thrombosis

- Severe pain in one flank and lower back pain with CVA and epigastric tenderness are typical.
- Other signs and symptoms include fever, hematuria, and leg edema.

Nursing considerations

- Administer pain medication and evaluate effect.
- Continue to monitor the patient's vital signs.
- Maintain a precise record of intake and output.
- In children, transillumination of the abdomen and flanks may help assess bladder distention and identify masses.
- Common causes of flank pain in children include obstructive uropathy, acute poststreptococcal glomerulonephritis, infantile polycystic kidney disease, and nephroblastoma.

Patient teaching

- Explain the importance of increased fluid intake (unless contraindicated).
- Explain the patient's underlying condition, treatment plan, and signs and symptoms to report.
- Stress the importance of taking drugs as prescribed.
- Stress the importance of keeping follow-up appointments.

G

Gag reflex, abnormal

The gag reflex is a protective mechanism that prevents aspiration of food, fluid, and vomitus. Normally, it can be elicited by touching the posterior wall of the oropharynx with a tongue blade or by suctioning the throat. Prompt elevation of the palate, constriction of the pharyngeal musculature, and a sensation of gagging indicate a normal gag reflex. An abnormal gag reflex—either decreased or absent—interferes with the ability to swallow and, more important, increases susceptibility to life-threatening aspiration.

An impaired gag reflex can result from a lesion that affects its mediators—cranial nerve (CN) IX (glossopharyngeal) and X (vagus) or the pons or medulla. It can also occur during a coma, in muscle diseases such as severe myasthenia gravis, or as a temporary result of anesthesia.

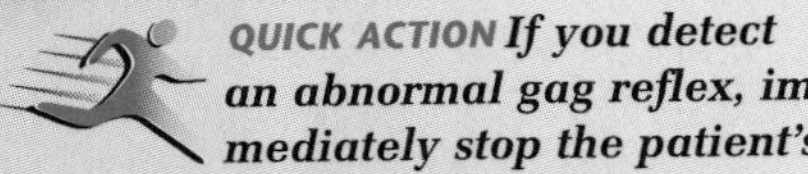

QUICK ACTION ***If you detect an abnormal gag reflex, immediately stop the patient's oral intake to prevent aspiration. Quickly evaluate his level of consciousness (LOC). If it's decreased, place him in a side-lying position to prevent aspiration; if not, place him in Fowler's position. Have suction equipment at hand.***

History

- Ask the patient (or a family member if the patient can't communicate) about the onset and duration of swallowing difficulties and if it's more difficult to swallow liquids than solids.
- If the patient also has trouble chewing, suspect more widespread neurologic involvement because chewing involves different cranial nerves.
- Explore the patient's medical history for vascular and degenerative disorders.

Physical examination

- Assess the patient's respiratory status for evidence of aspiration.
- Perform a neurologic examination.

Causes

Medical causes

Basilar artery occlusion

- This disorder may suddenly diminish or obliterate the gag reflex.
- Other signs and symptoms include diffuse sensory loss, dysarthria, facial weakness, extraocular muscle palsies, quadriplegia, and decreased LOC.

Brain stem glioma

- This lesion causes gradual loss of the gag reflex.
- Involvement of the corticospinal pathways causes spasticity and paresis of the arms and legs as well as gait disturbances.

■ Other signs and symptoms reflect bilateral brain stem involvement and include diplopia and facial weakness.

Bulbar palsy

■ Loss of the gag reflex reflects temporary or permanent paralysis of muscles supplied by CN IX and X.

■ Other signs and symptoms of this paralysis include jaw and facial muscle weakness, dysphagia, loss of sensation at the base of the tongue, increased salivation, fasciculations and, possibly, difficulty articulating and breathing.

Myasthenia gravis

■ In severe myasthenia, the motor limb of the gag reflex is reduced.

■ Weakness worsens with repetitive use and may also involve other muscles.

Wallenberg syndrome

■ Paresis of the palate and an impaired gag reflex usually develop within hours to days of stroke of the brain stem.

■ Other signs and symptoms may include analgesia and thermanesthesia, occurring ipsilaterally on the face and contralaterally on the body, as well as vertigo, nystagmus, ipsilateral ataxia of the arm and leg; signs of Horner syndrome (unilateral ptosis and miosis, hemifacial anhidrosis), and uncontrollable hiccups.

Other causes

Anesthesia

■ General and local (throat) anesthesia can produce temporary loss of the gag reflex.

Nursing considerations

■ Continually assess the patient's ability to swallow.

■ If his gag reflex is absent, provide tube feedings, as ordered; if it's diminished, try pureed foods.

■ Stay with the patient while he eats, and observe for choking.

■ Keep suction equipment handy in case of aspiration.

■ Maintain accurate intake and output records, and assess the patient's nutritional status daily.

■ Refer the patient to a speech therapist to determine his aspiration risk, and develop an exercise program to strengthen specific muscles.

■ In children, brain stem glioma is an important cause of an abnormal gag reflex.

Patient teaching

■ Advise the patient to eat small amounts slowly while sitting or in high Fowler's position.

■ Teach him techniques for safe swallowing and the types and textures of foods that reduce the risk of choking.

■ Teach the patient about scheduled diagnostic studies, such as swallow studies, computed tomography scan, magnetic resonance imaging, EEG, lumbar puncture, and arteriography.

■ Teach the patient about the underlying diagnosis.

Gait, bizarre

A bizarre gait has no obvious organic basis; rather, it's produced unconsciously by a person with a somatoform disorder (hysterical neurosis) or consciously by a malingerer. The gait has no consistent pattern. It may mimic an organic impairment, but characteristically has a more theatrical or bizarre quality with key elements missing, such as a spastic gait without hip circumduction, or leg "paralysis" with normal reflexes and motor strength. Its manifestations may include wild gyrations, exaggerated stepping, leg dragging, or mimicking unusual walks such as that of a tightrope walker.

History

- If you suspect that the patient's gait impairment has no organic cause, begin to investigate other possibilities.
- Ask when the gait first developed and whether it coincided with a stressful period or event, such as the death of a loved one or the loss of a job.
- Ask about associated symptoms, and explore reports of frequent unexplained illnesses and multiple physician visits.
- Subtly try to determine if the patient will gain anything from malingering—for instance, added attention or an insurance settlement.

Physical examination

- Test the patient's reflexes and sensorimotor function, noting abnormal response patterns.
- To quickly check reports of leg weakness or paralysis, perform a test for Hoover's sign: Place the patient in the supine position and stand at his feet. Cradle a heel in each of your palms, and rest your hands on the table. Ask the patient to raise the affected leg. In true motor weakness, the heel of the other leg will press downward; in hysteria, this movement will be absent.
- Observe the patient for normal movements when he's unaware of being watched.

Causes

Medical causes

Conversion disorder

- In this rare somatoform disorder, bizarre gait or paralysis may develop after severe stress and isn't accompanied by other symptoms.
- The patient typically shows indifference toward his impairment.

Malingering

- In this rare cause of bizarre gait, the patient may also complain of headache and chest and back pain.

Somatization disorder

- Bizarre gait is one of many possible somatic complaints.
- Other pseudoneurologic signs and symptoms include fainting, weakness, memory loss, dysphagia, visual problems (diplopia, vision loss, blurred vision), loss of voice, seizures, and bladder dysfunction.
- The patient may also report pain in the back, joints, and extremities (most commonly the legs) and complaints in almost any body system.
- The patient's reflexes and motor strength remain normal, but he may exhibit peculiar contractures and arm or leg rigidity.
- The patient may claim that he can't stand (astasia) or walk (abasia), remaining bedridden although still able to move his legs in bed.

Nursing considerations

- A full neurologic workup may be necessary to completely rule out an organic cause of the patient's abnormal gait.
- Remember, even though a bizarre gait has no organic cause, it's real to the patient (unless, of course, he's malingering).
- Avoid expressing judgment on the patient's actions or motives; you'll need to be supportive and reinforce positive progress.
- Because muscle atrophy and bone demineralization can develop in bedridden patients, encourage ambulation and resumption of normal activities.
- Consider a referral for psychiatric counseling, as appropriate.
- Bizarre gait is rare in patients younger than age 8. More common in prepubescence, it usually results from conversion disorder.

Patient teaching

- Instruct the patient in the use of assistive devices as necessary.
- Review the components of a safe environment, such as establishing a clear path to the bathroom and using proper footwear.

Gait, propulsive

Propulsive gait is characterized by a stooped, rigid posture—the patient's head and neck are bent forward; his flexed, stiffened arms are held away from the body; his fingers are extended; and his knees and hips are stiffly bent. During ambulation, this posture results in a forward shifting of the body's center of gravity and consequent impairment of balance, causing increasingly rapid, short, shuffling steps with involuntary acceleration (festination) and lack of control over forward motion (propulsion) or backward motion (retropulsion). (See *Identifying gait abnormalities,* pages 148 and 149.)

Propulsive gait is a cardinal sign of advanced Parkinson's disease; it results from progressive degeneration of the ganglia, which are primarily responsible for smooth-muscle movement. Because this sign develops gradually and its accompanying effects are usually wrongly attributed to aging, propulsive gait commonly goes unnoticed or unreported until severe disability results.

History

- Obtain a history of when the patient's gait impairment first developed and whether it has recently worsened. Because he may have difficulty remembering, include family members or friends when gathering information.
- Obtain a thorough drug history, including dosages. Ask about tranquilizers, especially phenothiazines.
- For the patient with Parkinson's disease, ask about levodopa (Larodopa) dosage because an overdose can cause acute worsening of signs and symptoms.
- Ask the patient if he has been acutely or routinely exposed to carbon monoxide or manganese.

Physical examination

- Begin the physical examination by testing the patient's reflexes and sensorimotor function, noting abnormal response patterns.

Causes

Medical causes

Parkinson's disease

- The characteristic and permanent propulsive gait associated with Parkinson's disease begins early as a shuffle; as the disease progresses, the gait slows.
- Besides the gait, akinesia also typically produces a monotone voice, drooling, masklike facies, stooped posture, and dysarthria, dysphagia, or both.
- Occasionally, it also causes an oculogyric crisis or blepharospasm.
- Other signs and symptoms include progressive muscle rigidity, which may be uniform (lead-pipe rigidity) or jerky (cogwheel rigidity), and an insidious tremor that begins in the fingers, increases during stress or anxiety, and decreases with purposeful movement and sleep.

Other causes

Carbon monoxide poisoning

- Propulsive gait commonly appears several weeks after acute carbon monoxide intoxication.
- Earlier signs and symptoms include muscle rigidity, choreoathetoid movements, generalized seizures, myoclonic jerks, masklike facies, and dementia.

Drugs

- Propulsive gait and other extrapyramidal effects can result from the use of phenothiazines, other antipsychotics (notably haloperidol [Haldol], thiothix-

Identifying gait abnormalities

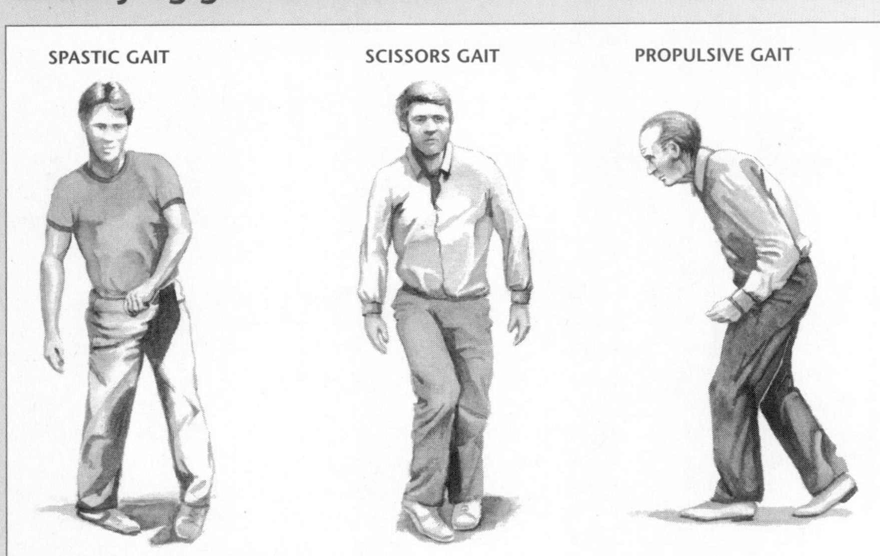

ene [Navane], and loxapine [Loxitane] and, infrequently, metoclopramide [Clopra] and metyrosine [Demser]).
- Such effects are usually temporary, disappearing within a few weeks after therapy is discontinued.

Manganese poisoning
- Chronic overexposure to manganese can cause an insidious, usually permanent, propulsive gait.
- Typical early signs and symptoms include fatigue, muscle weakness and rigidity, dystonia, resting tremor, choreoathetoid movements, masklike facies, and personality changes.
- Those at risk for manganese poisoning are welders, railroad workers, miners, steelworkers, and workers who handle pesticides.

Nursing considerations
- The patient may have problems performing activities of daily living; therefore, assist him as appropriate, while at the same time encouraging his independence, self-reliance, and confidence.
- Encourage the patient to maintain ambulation; for safety reasons, remember to stay with him while he's walking, especially if he's on unfamiliar or uneven ground.
- Refer the patient to a physical therapist for exercise therapy and gait retraining.
- Propulsive gait, usually with severe tremors, typically occurs in juvenile parkinsonism, a rare form of parkinsonism.

Patient teaching
- Teach the patient and his family about the underlying diagnosis and prevention, if appropriate.

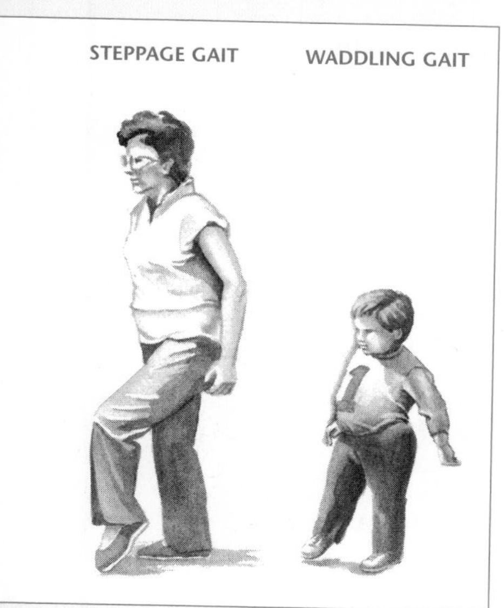

■ Advise the patient and his family to allow plenty of time for activities, especially walking, to avoid falling.
■ Teach them about safety measures.
■ Teach the patient about prescribed medication administration, dosage, and possible adverse effects.

Gait, scissors

Resulting from bilateral spastic paresis (diplegia), scissors gait affects both legs and has little or no effect on the arms. The patient's legs flex slightly at the hips and knees, so he looks as if he's crouching. With each step, his thighs adduct and his knees hit or cross in a scissorslike movement. His steps are short, regular, and laborious, as if he were wading through waist-deep water. His feet may be plantar flexed and turned inward, with a shortened Achilles tendon; as a result, he walks on his toes or on the balls of his feet and may scrape his toes on the ground.

History

■ Ask the patient (or a family member if the patient can't answer) about the onset and duration of the gait and whether it has progressively worsened or remained constant.
■ Ask about a history of trauma, including birth trauma, and neurologic disorders.

Physical examination

■ Thoroughly evaluate motor and sensory function and deep tendon reflexes (DTRs) in the legs.

Causes

Medical causes

Cerebral palsy

■ In the spastic form of this central nervous system disorder, patients walk on their toes with a scissors gait.
■ Other signs and symptoms include hyperactive DTRs, increased stretch reflexes, rapid alternating muscle contraction and relaxation, muscle weakness, underdevelopment of affected limbs, and a tendency toward contractures.

Cervical spondylosis with myelopathy

■ Scissors gait develops in the late stages of this degenerative disease and steadily worsens.
■ Related findings mimic those of a herniated disk: severe low back pain, which may radiate to the buttocks, legs, and feet; muscle spasms; sensorimotor loss; and muscle weakness and atrophy.

Hepatic failure

■ Scissors gait may appear several months before the onset of hepatic failure due to altered glycogen metabolism.
■ Other signs and symptoms may include asterixis, generalized seizures, jaundice, purpura, dementia, and fetor hepaticus.

Multiple sclerosis

- Progressive scissors gait usually develops gradually, with infrequent remissions.
- Characteristic muscle weakness, usually in the legs, ranges from minor fatigability to paraparesis with urinary urgency and constipation.
- Other signs and symptoms include facial pain, vision disturbances, paresthesia, incoordination, and loss of proprioception and vibration sensation in the ankle and toes.

Pernicious anemia

- Scissors gait sometimes occurs as a late sign in neurologic complications of untreated pernicious anemia.
- Besides this disorder's classic triad of symptoms—weakness, sore tongue, and numbness and tingling in the extremities—the patient may exhibit pale lips, gums, and tongue; faintly jaundiced sclerae and pale to bright yellow skin; impaired proprioception; incoordination; and vision disturbances (diplopia, blurring).

Spinal cord trauma

- Scissors gait may develop during recovery from partial spinal cord compression, particularly with an injury below C6.
- Other signs and symptoms may include sensory loss or paresthesia, muscle weakness or paralysis distal to the injury, and bladder and bowel dysfunction.

Spinal cord tumor

- Scissors gait can develop gradually from a thoracic or lumbar tumor.
- Other signs and symptoms reflect the location of the tumor, and may include radicular, subscapular, shoulder, groin, leg, or flank pain; muscle spasms or fasciculations; muscle atrophy; sensory deficits, such as paresthesia and a girdle sensation of the abdomen and chest; hyperactive DTRs; bilateral Babinski's reflex; spastic neurogenic bladder; and sexual dysfunction.

Stroke

- Scissors gait occasionally develops during the late recovery stage of bilateral occlusion of the anterior cerebral artery.
- Other signs and symptoms may include leg muscle paraparesis and atrophy, incoordination, numbness, urinary incontinence, confusion, and personality changes.

Syphilitic meningomyelitis

- Scissors gait appears late in this inflammatory disorder and may improve with treatment.
- Other signs and symptoms include sensory ataxia, changes in proprioception and vibration sensation, optic atrophy, and dementia.

Syringomyelia

- Scissors gait usually occurs late in this spinal cord disorder along with analgesia and thermanesthesia, muscle atrophy and weakness, and Charcot's joint.
- Skin in the affected areas is typically dry, scaly, and grooved.
- Other signs and symptoms may include loss of fingernails, fingers, or toes; Dupuytren's contracture of the palms; scoliosis; and clubfoot.

Nursing considerations

- Because of the sensory loss associated with scissors gait, provide meticulous skin care to prevent skin breakdown and pressure ulcer formation.
- Promote daily active and passive range-of-motion exercises.
- Refer the patient to a physical therapist, if appropriate, for gait retraining and for possible application of in-shoe splints or leg braces to maintain proper

foot alignment for standing and walking.

Patient teaching

- Give the patient and his family complete skin care instructions to prevent skin breakdown.
- If appropriate, provide bladder and bowel retraining.
- Reinforce the proper use of splints or braces, if appropriate.
- Teach the patient and his family about the underlying diagnosis.
- Explain the prescribed medication: how to give it, the dosage, and possible adverse effects.

Gait, spastic

Spastic gait—sometimes referred to as *paretic* or *weak* gait—is a stiff, foot-dragging walk caused by unilateral leg muscle hypertonicity. This gait indicates focal damage to the corticospinal tract. The affected leg becomes rigid, with a marked decrease in flexion at the hip and knee and possibly plantar flexion and equinovarus deformity of the foot. Because the patient's leg doesn't swing normally at the hip or knee, his foot tends to drag or shuffle, scraping his toes on the ground. To compensate, the pelvis of the affected side tilts upward in an attempt to lift the toes, causing the patient's leg to abduct and circumduct. Also, arm swing is hindered on the same side as the affected leg.

Spastic gait usually develops after a period of flaccidity (hypotonicity) in the affected leg. Whatever the cause, the gait is usually permanent after it develops.

History

- Obtain a history of when the patient first noticed the gait impairment and whether it developed suddenly or gradually.
- Ask if it waxes and wanes or if it has worsened progressively. Ask if fatigue, hot weather, or warm baths or showers worsen the gait. Such worsening typically occurs in multiple sclerosis (MS).
- Focus your medical history questions on neurologic disorders, recent head trauma, and degenerative diseases.

Physical examination

- Test and compare strength, range of motion, and sensory function in all limbs.
- Observe and palpate for muscle flaccidity or atrophy.

Causes

Medical causes

Brain abscess

- In this disorder, spastic gait generally develops slowly after a period of muscle flaccidity and fever.
- Early signs and symptoms reflect increased intracranial pressure (ICP) and include headache, nausea, vomiting, and focal or generalized seizures.
- Later, site-specific signs and symptoms may include hemiparesis, tremors, vision disturbances, nystagmus, and pupillary inequality.
- The patient's level of consciousness may range from drowsiness to stupor.

Brain tumor

- Depending on the site and type of tumor, spastic gait usually develops gradually and worsens over time.
- Other possible characteristics include signs of increased ICP, papilledema, sensory loss on the affected side, dysarthria, ocular palsies, aphasia, and personality changes.

Head trauma

- Spastic gait typically follows the acute stage of head trauma.
- The patient may also experience focal or generalized seizures, personality changes, headache, and focal neurologic

signs, such as aphasia and visual field deficits.

Multiple sclerosis

- Spastic gait begins insidiously and follows a cycle of worsening and remission characteristic of this neurologic disorder.
- Like other signs and symptoms of MS, the gait commonly worsens in warm weather or after a warm bath or shower.
- Characteristic weakness, usually affecting the legs, ranges from minor fatigability to paraparesis with urinary urgency and constipation.
- Other signs and symptoms include vision disturbances, facial pain, paresthesia, incoordination, and loss of proprioception and vibration sensation in the ankle and toes.

Stroke

- Spastic gait usually appears after a period of muscle weakness and hypotonicity on the affected side.
- Other signs and symptoms may include unilateral muscle atrophy, sensory loss, and footdrop; aphasia; dysarthria; dysphagia; visual field deficits; diplopia; and ocular palsies.

Nursing considerations

- Because leg muscle contractures are commonly associated with spastic gait, promote daily exercise and range of motion—both active and passive.
- The patient may have poor balance and a tendency to fall to the paralyzed side, so stay with him while he's walking.
- Provide a cane or walker if indicated.
- Refer the patient to a physical therapist, if appropriate, for gait retraining and possible application of in-shoe splints or leg braces to maintain proper foot alignment for standing and walking.
- In children, causes of spastic gait include sickle cell crisis, cerebral palsy, porencephalic cysts, and arteriovenous malformation that cause hemorrhage or ischemia.

Patient teaching

- Teach the patient how to use a cane or walker, if appropriate.
- Teach the patient and his family safety measures to reduce the risk of falling.
- Teach the patient about the underlying diagnosis and treatment options.

Gait, steppage

Steppage gait typically results from footdrop caused by weakness or paralysis of pretibial and peroneal muscles. Usually, this results from lower motor neuron lesions. Footdrop causes the foot to hang with the toes pointing down, causing the toes to scrape the ground during walking. To compensate, the hip rotates outward and the hip and knee flex in an exaggerated fashion to lift the advancing leg off the ground. The foot is thrown forward and the toes hit the ground first, producing an audible slap. The rhythm of the gait is usually regular, with even steps and normal upper body posture and arm swing. Steppage gait can be unilateral or bilateral and permanent or transient, depending on the site and type of neural damage.

History

- Begin by asking the patient about the onset of the gait and any recent changes in its character.
- Ask about a family history of gait disturbance; traumatic injury to the buttocks, hips, legs, or knees; or chronic disorders that may be associated with polyneuropathy, such as diabetes mellitus, polyarteritis nodosa, and alcoholism.

Physical examination

- Observe whether the patient crosses his legs while sitting because this may put pressure on the peroneal nerve.
- Inspect and palpate the patient's calves and feet for muscle atrophy and wasting.
- Using a pin, test for sensory deficits along the entire length of both legs.

Causes

Medical causes

Guillain-Barré syndrome

- Typically occurring after recovery from the acute stage of this neurologic disorder, steppage gait can be mild or severe and unilateral or bilateral; it's invariably permanent.
- Muscle weakness usually begins in the legs, extends to the arms and face within 72 hours, and can progress to total motor paralysis and respiratory failure.
- Other signs and symptoms include footdrop, transient paresthesia, hypernasality, dysphagia, diaphoresis, tachycardia, orthostatic hypotension, and incontinence.

Herniated lumbar disk

- Unilateral steppage gait and footdrop commonly occur with late-stage weakness and atrophy of the leg muscles.
- The most pronounced symptom of a herniated lumbar disk is severe low back pain, which may radiate to the buttocks, legs, and feet, usually unilaterally.
- Sciatic pain follows, commonly accompanied by muscle spasms and sensorimotor loss. Paresthesia and fasciculations may also occur.

Multiple sclerosis

- Steppage gait and footdrop follow a characteristic cycle of periodic worsening and remission in this neurologic disorder.
- Muscle weakness, usually affecting the legs, can range from minor fatigability to paraparesis with urinary urgency and constipation.
- Other signs and symptoms include facial pain, vision disturbances, paresthesia, incoordination, and sensory loss in the ankle and toes.

Peroneal muscle atrophy

- Bilateral steppage gait and footdrop begin insidiously in this disorder.
- Other early signs and symptoms include paresthesia, aching, cramping, coldness, swelling, and cyanosis in the feet and legs. Foot, peroneal, and ankle dorsiflexor muscles are affected first.
- As the disorder progresses, all leg muscles become weak and atrophic, with hypoactive or absent deep tendon reflexes (DTRs). Later, atrophy and sensory loss spread to the hands and arms.

Peroneal nerve trauma

- Temporary ipsilateral steppage gait occurs suddenly but resolves with the release of peroneal nerve pressure.
- Steppage gait is associated with footdrop, muscle weakness, and sensory loss over the lateral surface of the calf and foot.

Poliomyelitis

- Steppage gait, usually permanent and unilateral, commonly develops after the acute stage of poliomyelitis.
- Fever typically occurs first, accompanied by such signs and symptoms as asymmetrical muscle weakness, coarse fasciculations, paresthesia, hypoactive or absent DTRs, and permanent muscle paralysis and atrophy.
- Dysphagia, urine retention, and respiratory difficulty may also occur.

Polyneuropathy

- Diabetic polyneuropathy is a rare cause of bilateral steppage gait, which appears as a late but permanent effect.

- This sign is preceded by burning pain in the feet and is accompanied by leg weakness, sensory loss, and skin ulcers.
- In polyarteritis nodosa with polyneuropathy, unilateral or bilateral steppage gait is a late finding.
- Other signs and symptoms include vague leg pain, abdominal pain, hematuria, fever, and increased blood pressure.
- In alcoholic polyneuropathy, steppage gait appears 2 to 3 months after the onset of vitamin B deficiency. The gait may be bilateral, and it resolves with treatment of the deficiency. Early signs and symptoms include paresthesia in the feet, leg muscle weakness and, possibly, sensory ataxia.

Spinal cord trauma

- In an ambulatory patient, spinal cord trauma may cause steppage gait.
- Paresthesia, sensory loss, asymmetrical or absent DTRs, and muscle weakness or paralysis may occur distal to the injury.
- Fecal and urinary incontinence may also occur.
- Other signs and symptoms vary with the severity of the injury and may include unilateral or bilateral footdrop, neck and back pain, and vertebral tenderness and deformity.

Nursing considerations

- The patient with steppage gait may tire rapidly when walking because of the extra effort he must expend to lift his feet off the ground. Help the patient recognize his exercise limits, and encourage him to get adequate rest.
- Refer the patient to a physical therapist, if appropriate, for gait retraining and possible application of in-shoe splints or leg braces to maintain correct foot alignment.
- Help the patient ambulate.

Patient teaching

- Teach the patient about safety measures he can take at home to prevent falls.
- Teach the patient about the underlying diagnosis and treatment options.

Gait, waddling

Waddling gait, a distinctive ducklike walk, is an important sign of muscular dystrophy, spinal muscle atrophy or, in rare cases, congenital hip displacement. It may be present when a child begins to walk or may appear only later in life. The gait results from deterioration of the pelvic girdle muscles—primarily the gluteus medius, hip flexors, and hip extensors. Weakness in these muscles hinders stabilization of the weight-bearing hip during walking, causing the opposite hip to drop and the trunk to lean toward that side in an attempt to maintain balance.

Typically, the legs assume a wide stance and the trunk is thrown back to further improve stability, exaggerating lordosis and abdominal protrusion. In severe cases, leg and foot muscle contractures may cause equinovarus deformity of the foot, combined with circumduction or bowing of the legs.

History

- Ask the patient (or a family member if the patient is a young child) when the gait first appeared and if it has recently worsened.
- To determine the extent of pelvic girdle and leg muscle weakness, ask if the patient falls frequently or has difficulty climbing stairs, rising from a chair, or walking. Also find out if he was late in learning to walk or holding his head upright.
- Obtain a family history, focusing on problems of muscle weakness and gait and on congenital motor disorders.

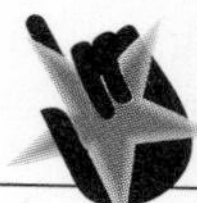

KNOW-HOW

Identifying Gowers' sign

To check for Gowers' sign, place the patient in the supine position and ask him to rise. A positive Gowers' sign—an inability to lift the trunk without using the hands and arms to brace and push—indicates pelvic muscle weakness, as occurs in muscular dystrophy and spinal muscle atrophy.

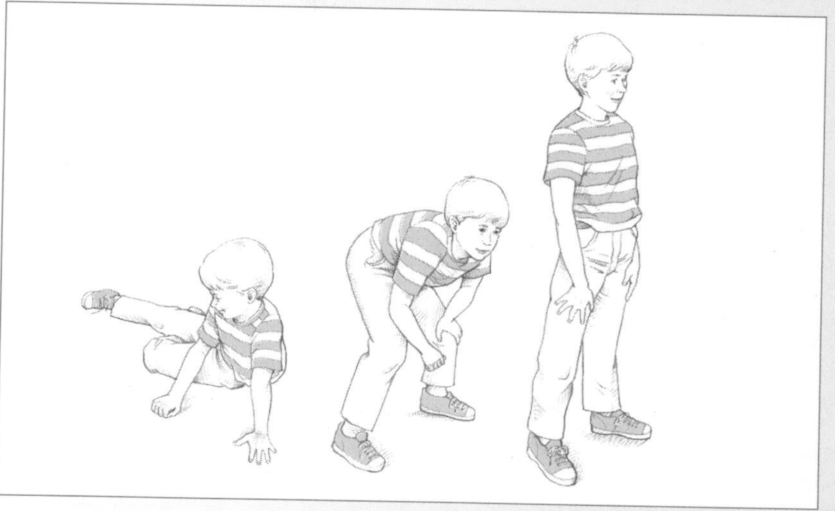

Physical examination

- Inspect and palpate leg muscles, especially in the calves, for size and tone.
- Check for a positive Gowers' sign, which indicates pelvic muscle weakness. (See *Identifying Gowers' sign*.)
- Assess motor strength and function in the shoulders, arms, and hands, looking for weakness or asymmetrical movements.

Causes

Medical causes

Developmental dysplasia of the hip

- Bilateral hip dislocation produces a waddling gait with lordosis and pain.

Muscular dystrophy

- In *Duchenne's muscular dystrophy*, waddling gait becomes clinically evident by ages 3 to 5. The gait worsens as the disease progresses, until the child loses the ability to walk and needs a wheelchair, usually between ages 10 and 12.
  - Early signs are usually subtle and include a delay in learning to walk, frequent falls, gait or posture abnormalities, and intermittent calf pain.
  - Common later signs and symptoms include lordosis with abdominal protrusion, a positive Gowers' sign, and equinovarus foot position.
  - As the disease progresses, its signs and symptoms become more prominent;

they commonly include rapid muscle wasting beginning in the legs and spreading to the arms (although calf and upper arm muscles may become hypertrophied, firm, and rubbery), muscle contractures, limited dorsiflexion of the feet and extension of the knees and elbows, obesity and, possibly, mild mental retardation.
– If kyphoscoliosis develops, it may lead to respiratory dysfunction and, eventually, death from cardiac or respiratory failure.

- In *Becker's muscular dystrophy,* waddling gait typically becomes apparent in late adolescence, slowly worsens during the third decade, and culminates in total loss of ambulation. Muscle weakness first appears in the pelvic and upper arm muscles. Progressive wasting with selected muscle hypertrophy produces lordosis with abdominal protrusion, poor balance, a positive Gowers' sign and, possibly, mental retardation.
- In *facioscapulohumeral muscular dystrophy,* which usually occurs late in childhood or during adolescence, waddling gait appears after muscle wasting has spread downward from the face and shoulder girdle to the pelvic girdle and legs.
  – Early signs and symptoms include progressive weakness and atrophy of facial, shoulder, and arm muscles; slight lordosis; and pelvic instability.

Spinal muscle atrophy

- In *Kugelberg-Welander syndrome,* waddling gait occurs early (usually after age 2) and typically progresses slowly, culminating in total loss of ambulation up to 20 years later.
  – Other signs and symptoms may include muscle atrophy in the legs and pelvis, progressing to the shoulders; a positive Gowers' sign; ophthalmoplegia; and tongue fasciculations.
- In *Werdnig-Hoffmann disease,* waddling gait typically begins when the child learns to walk. Reflexes may be absent. The gait progressively worsens, culminating in complete loss of ambulation by adolescence.
  – Other signs and symptoms include lordosis with abdominal protrusion and muscle weakness in the hips and thighs.

Nursing considerations

- Provide daily passive and active muscle-stretching exercises to both arms and legs.
- Encourage the patient to walk at least 3 hours each day (with leg braces if necessary) to maintain muscle strength, reduce contractures, and delay further gait deterioration.
- Stay with the patient when he's walking to provide support, especially if he's on unfamiliar or uneven ground.
- Provide a balanced diet to maintain energy levels and prevent obesity.
- Because of the grim prognosis associated with muscular dystrophy and spinal muscle atrophy, provide emotional support for the patient and his family.

Patient teaching

- Caution the patient against long, unbroken periods of bed rest, which accelerate muscle deterioration.
- Refer him to a local chapter of the Muscular Dystrophy Association.
- Recommend that parents seek genetic testing and counseling if they're considering having another child.

Gallop, atrial (S_4)

An atrial or presystolic gallop is an extra heart sound (known as S_4) that's heard or typically palpated immediately before the first heart sound (S_1), late in diastole. This low-pitched sound is heard best with the bell of the stethoscope pressed lightly against the cardiac apex. Some clinicians say that an S_4 has

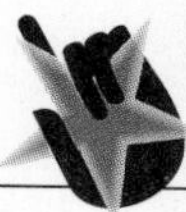

KNOW-HOW

Locating heart sounds

When auscultating heart sounds, remember that certain sounds are heard best in specific areas. Use the auscultatory points shown below to locate heart sounds quickly and accurately. Then expand your auscultation to nearby areas. Note that the numbers indicate pertinent intercostal spaces.

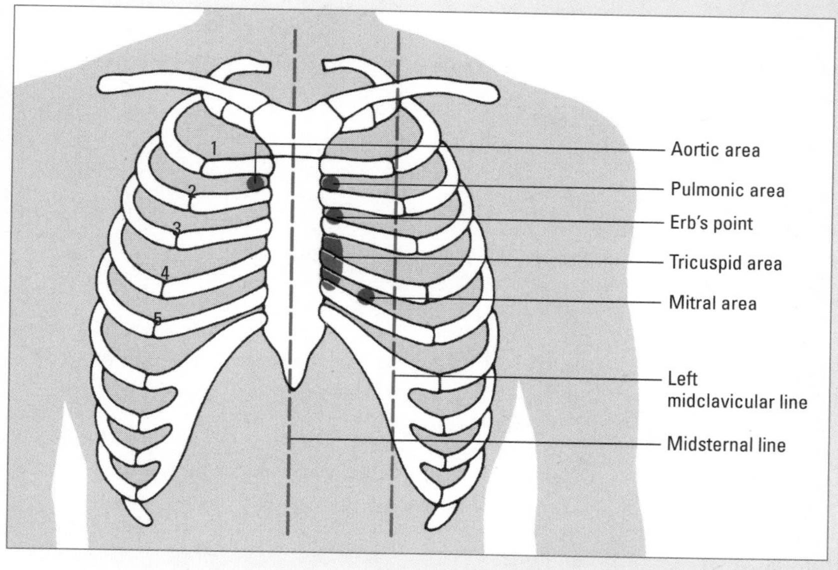

the cadence of the "Ten" in Tennessee (Ten = S_4; nes = S_1; see = S_2).

This gallop typically results from hypertension, conduction defects, valvular disorders, or other problems such as ischemia. Occasionally, it helps differentiate angina from other causes of chest pain. It results from abnormal forceful atrial contraction, caused by augmented ventricular filling or by decreased left ventricular compliance. An atrial gallop usually originates from left atrial contraction, is heard at the apex, and doesn't vary with inspiration. A left-sided S_4 can occur in hypertensive heart disease, coronary artery disease, aortic stenosis, and cardiomyopathy. It may also originate from right atrial contraction. A right-sided S_4 indicates pulmonary hypertension and pulmonary stenosis. In that case, it's heard best at the lower left sternal border and intensifies with inspiration.

An atrial gallop seldom occurs in normal hearts; however, it may occur in elderly people and in athletes with physiologic hypertrophy of the left ventricle.

QUICK ACTION ***Suspect myocardial ischemia if you auscultate an atrial gallop in a patient with chest pain. (See* **Locating heart sounds.** *Also see* **Interpreting heart sounds,** *pages 158 and 159.)***

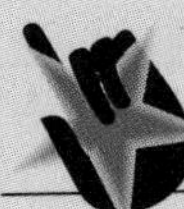

KNOW-HOW

Interpreting heart sounds

Detecting subtle variations in heart sounds requires concentration and practice. When you can recognize normal heart sounds, the abnormal heart sounds become more obvious.

HEART SOUND AND CAUSE | **TIMING AND CADENCE**

First heart sound (S_1)

Vibrations associated with mitral and tricuspid valve closure

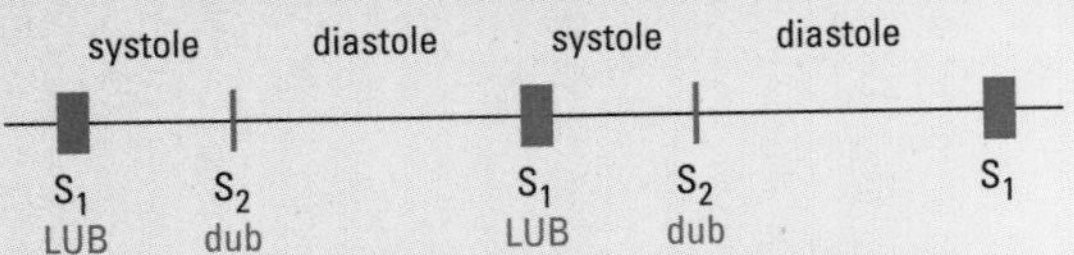

Second heart sound (S2)

Vibrations associated with aortic and pulmonic valve closure

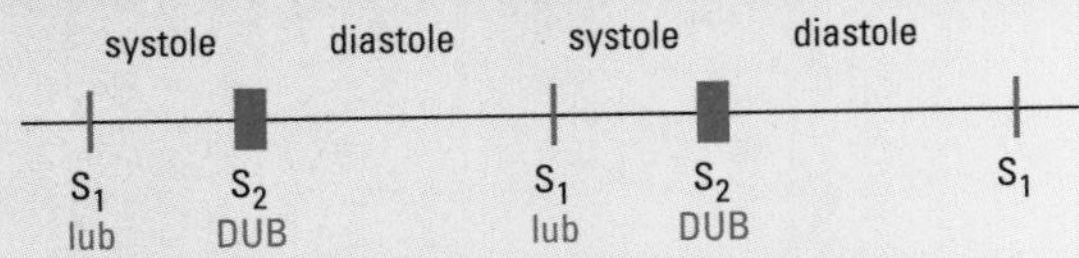

Ventricular gallop (S_3)

Vibrations produced by rapid blood flow into the ventricles

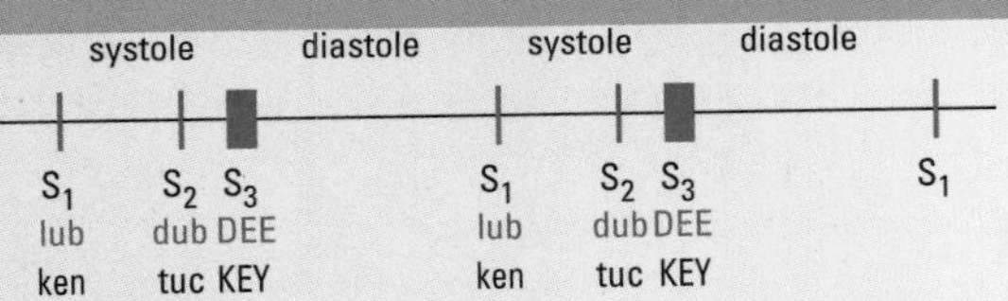

Atrial gallop (S_4)

Vibrations produced by an increased resistance to sudden, forceful ejection of atrial blood

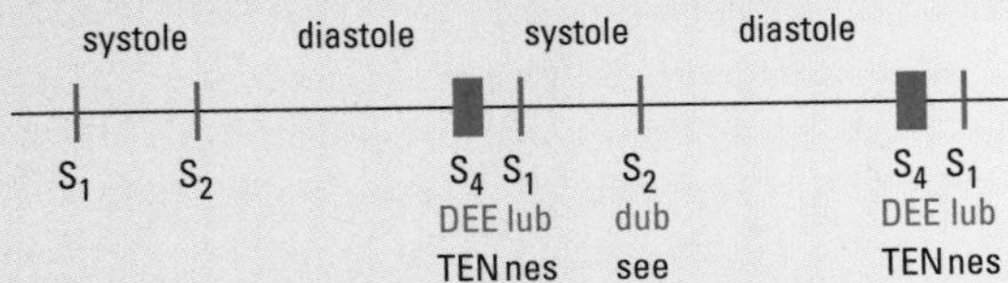

Summation gallop

Vibrations produced in mid-diastole by a simultaneous S_3 and S_4, usually caused by tachycardia

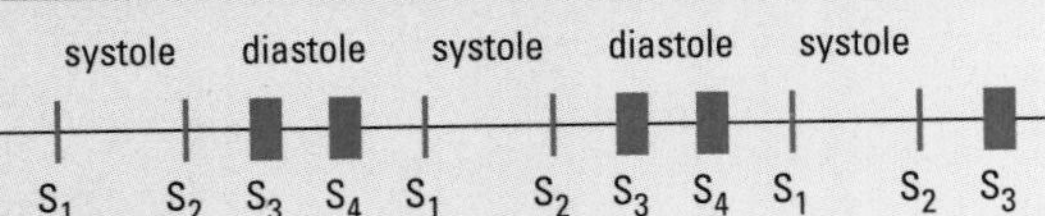

AUSCULTATION TIPS

Best heard with the diaphragm of the stethoscope at the apex (mitral area)

Best heard with the diaphragm of the stethoscope in the second or third right and left parasternal intercostal spaces with the patient sitting or in a supine position

Best heard through the bell of the stethoscope at the apex with the patient in the left lateral position; may be visible and palpable during early diastole at the midclavicular line between the fourth and fifth intercostal spaces

Best heard through the bell of the stethoscope at the apex with the patient in the left semilateral position; may be visible in late diastole at the midclavicular line between the fourth and fifth intercostal spaces; may also be palpable in the midclavicular area with the patient in the left lateral decubitus position

Best heard through the bell of the stethoscope at the apex with the patient in the left lateral position; may be louder than S_1 or S_2; may be visible and palpable during diastole

Take the patient's vital signs and quickly assess for signs of heart failure, such as dyspnea, crackles, and jugular vein distention. If you detect these signs, connect the patient to a cardiac monitor and obtain an electrocardiogram. Administer an antianginal and oxygen. If the patient has dyspnea, elevate the head of the bed. Then auscultate for abnormal breath sounds. If you detect coarse crackles, ensure patent I.V. access and give oxygen and diuretics as needed. If the patient has bradycardia, he may require atropine and a pacemaker.

History

- Obtain a medical history, including incidence of hypertension, angina, cardiomyopathy, or valvular stenosis.
- Ask about the frequency and severity of anginal attacks.

Physical examination

- Take the patient's vital signs.
- Perform a complete cardiopulmonary examination.

Causes

Medical causes

Anemia

- An atrial gallop may accompany compensatory increased cardiac output.
- Other signs and symptoms may include fatigue, pallor, dyspnea, tachycardia, a bounding pulse, crackles, and a systolic bruit over the carotid arteries.

Angina

- An intermittent atrial gallop typically occurs during an attack.
- The gallop may be accompanied by paradoxical S_2 or a new murmur.
- Other signs and symptoms include chest tightness, pressure, aching, or burning that radiates to the neck, jaw, left shoulder, and arm; dyspnea; tachycardia; increased blood pressure; di-

aphoresis; dizziness; nausea; and vomiting.

Aortic insufficiency, acute

- Atrial gallop is accompanied by a soft, short diastolic murmur along the left sternal border.
- S_2 may be soft or absent and a soft, short midsystolic murmur may be heard over the second right intercostal space.
- Other signs and symptoms include tachycardia, dyspnea, jugular vein distention, crackles, cool extremities, and angina.

Aortic stenosis

- Atrial gallop occurs with severe valvular obstruction.
- Auscultation reveals a harsh, crescendo-decrescendo (louder-then-softer), systolic-ejection murmur.
- Angina and syncope are principal symptoms.
- Other signs and symptoms include crackles, palpitations, fatigue, and diminished carotid pulses.

Atrioventricular block

- First-degree atrioventricular (AV) block may cause an atrial gallop accompanied by a faint S_1, but the patient remains asymptomatic.
- Second-degree AV block produces an atrial gallop.
- Third-degree AV block produces an atrial gallop that varies in intensity with S_1.
- Other signs and symptoms include hypotension, light-headedness, dizziness, angina, and syncope.

Cardiomyopathy

- Atrial gallop is accompanied with such signs and symptoms as dyspnea, orthopnea, crackles, fatigue, syncope, chest pain, palpitations, edema, jugular vein distention, S_3, and tachycardia-bradycardia syndrome.

Hypertension

- Atrial gallop is an early symptom.
- Other signs and symptoms include headache, weakness, epistaxis, tinnitus, dizziness, and fatigue.

Mitral insufficiency

- Atrial gallop occurs with an S_3.
- Other signs and symptoms include a harsh holosystolic murmur, fatigue, dyspnea, tachypnea, orthopnea, tachycardia, crackles, and jugular vein distention.

Myocardial infarction

- Atrial gallop signifies a life-threatening myocardial infarction and may persist after the infarction heals.
- Crushing substernal chest pain may radiate to the back, neck, jaw, shoulder, and left arm.
- Other signs and symptoms include dyspnea, restlessness, anxiety, a feeling of impending doom, diaphoresis, pallor, clammy skin, nausea, vomiting, and increased or decreased blood pressure.

Pulmonary embolism

- A life-threatening disorder, right-sided atrial gallop is heard along the lower left sternal border with a loud pulmonic closure sound.
- Other signs and symptoms include tachycardia, tachypnea, fever, chest pain, diaphoresis, syncope, cyanosis, and a nonproductive or productive cough with blood-tinged sputum.

Thyrotoxicosis

- Atrial gallop occurs with an S_3.
- Other signs and symptoms include tachycardia, bounding pulse, widened pulse pressure, palpitations, weight loss despite increased appetite, diarrhea, tremors, an enlarged thyroid gland, dyspnea, nervousness, difficulty concentrating, heat intolerance, exophthalmos, weakness, fatigue, and muscle atrophy.

Nursing considerations

- Monitor the patient for signs and symptoms of heart failure.
- Give drugs and oxygen, as prescribed.

Patient teaching

- Discuss with the patient ways to reduce his cardiac risk.
- Teach the patient the correct way to measure his pulse rate.
- Emphasize conditions that require medical attention.
- Stress the importance of follow-up appointments.

Gallop, ventricular (S_3)

A ventricular gallop is a heart sound (known as S_3) associated with rapid ventricular filling in early diastole. Usually palpable, this low-frequency sound occurs about 0.15 second after the second heart sound (S_2). It may originate in either the left or right ventricle. A right-sided gallop usually sounds louder on inspiration and is heard best along the lower left sternal border or over the xiphoid region. A left-sided gallop usually sounds louder on expiration and is heard best at the apex.

Ventricular gallops are easily overlooked because they're usually faint. Fortunately, certain techniques make their detection more likely. These include auscultating in a quiet environment; examining the patient in the supine, left lateral, and semi-Fowler's positions; and having the patient cough or raise his legs to augment the sound.

A physiologic ventricular gallop normally occurs in children and adults younger than age 40; however, most people lose this third heart sound by age 40. This gallop may also occur during the third trimester of pregnancy. Abnormal S_3 (in adults older than age 40) can be a sign of decreased myocardial contractility, myocardial failure, and volume overload of the ventricle, as in mitral and tricuspid valve insufficiency. Although the physiologic S_3 has the same timing as the pathologic S_3, its intensity increases and decreases with respiration. It's also heard more faintly if the patient is sitting or standing.

A pathologic ventricular gallop may be one of the earliest signs of ventricular failure. It may result from one of two mechanisms: rapid deceleration of blood entering a stiff, noncompliant ventricle or rapid acceleration of blood associated with increased flow into the ventricle. A gallop that persists despite therapy indicates a poor prognosis.

Patients with cardiomyopathy or heart failure may develop a ventricular and an atrial gallop—a condition known as a *summation gallop*.

History

- Ask about the location, frequency, and duration of chest pain, if present, and what aggravates and alleviates it.
- Ask about palpitations, dizziness, syncope, difficulty breathing, or cough.
- Obtain a medical history, including the incidence of cardiac disorders.
- Obtain a drug history.

Physical examination

- Auscultate for murmurs or abnormalities in S_1 and S_2.
- Listen for pulmonary crackles.
- Assess peripheral pulses.
- Palpate the liver.
- Check for jugular vein distention and peripheral edema.

Causes

Medical causes

Aortic insufficiency

- In acute cases, ventricular and atrial gallops may occur with a soft, short diastolic murmur.

- Other signs and symptoms include tachycardia, dyspnea, jugular vein distention, and crackles.
- In chronic cases, a ventricular gallop and a high-pitched, blowing, decrescendo diastolic murmur occur.
- Other signs and symptoms include tachycardia, palpitations, angina, fatigue, dyspnea, orthopnea, and crackles.

Cardiomyopathy

- Ventricular gallop is a common symptom.
- When associated with fluctuating pulse and altered S_1 and S_2, it signals advanced heart disease.
- Other signs and symptoms include fatigue, dyspnea, orthopnea, chest pain, palpitations, syncope, crackles, peripheral edema, jugular vein distention, and an atrial gallop.

Heart failure

- Ventricular gallop is a classic symptom.
- Sinus tachycardia occurs with left-sided heart failure.
- Other signs and symptoms of left-sided heart failure include fatigue, exertional dyspnea, paroxysmal nocturnal dyspnea, orthopnea, and a dry cough.
- Jugular vein distention occurs with right-sided heart failure.
- Other late signs and symptoms of right-sided heart failure include tachypnea, chest tightness, palpitations, anorexia, nausea, dependent edema, weight gain, slowed mental response, hepatomegaly, and pallor.

Mitral insufficiency

- In acute cases, ventricular gallop may be accompanied by an early or holosystolic decrescendo murmur at the apex, an atrial gallop, and a widely split S_2.
- Other signs and symptoms of acute valvular disease include tachycardia, tachypnea, orthopnea, dyspnea, crackles, jugular vein distention, peripheral edema, hepatomegaly, and fatigue.
- In chronic cases, ventricular gallop is progressively severe and accompanied by fatigue, exertional dyspnea, and palpitations.

Thyrotoxicosis

- Ventricular and atrial gallops may occur.
- Other signs and symptoms include an enlarged thyroid gland, weight loss despite increased appetite, heat intolerance, diaphoresis, nervousness, tremors, tachycardia, palpitations, diarrhea, and dyspnea.

Nursing considerations

- Assess for tachycardia, dyspnea, crackles, and jugular vein distention.
- To prevent pulmonary edema, give oxygen, diuretics, and other drugs, such as digoxin (Lanoxin) and angiotensin-converting enzyme inhibitors, as prescribed.
- Ventricular gallop is normally heard in children, but may accompany congenital abnormalities associated with heart failure or result from sickle cell anemia.

Patient teaching

- Explain dietary and fluid restrictions the patient needs.
- Stress the importance of scheduled rest periods.
- Explain signs and symptoms of fluid overload that the patient should report.
- Teach the patient how to measure and monitor his weight daily.
- Teach the patient about the underlying condition and treatment options,

H

Headache

The most common neurologic symptom, headaches may be localized or generalized, producing mild to severe pain. About 90% of headaches are benign and can be described as vascular, muscle-contraction, or a combination of both. Occasionally, however, headaches indicate a severe neurologic disorder associated with intracranial inflammation, increased intracranial pressure (ICP), or meningeal irritation. They may also result from an ocular or a sinus disorder, tests, drugs, or other treatments.

Other causes of headache include fever, eyestrain, dehydration, and systemic febrile illnesses and stress. Headaches may occur in certain metabolic disturbances—such as hypoxemia, hypercapnia, hyperglycemia, and hypoglycemia—but they aren't a diagnostic or prominent symptom. Some individuals get headaches after seizures or from coughing, sneezing, heavy lifting, or stooping.

History

- Ask about the characteristics and location of the headache.
- Find out about precipitating or alleviating factors.
- Obtain a drug and alcohol history.
- Find out about recent head trauma, nausea, vomiting, photophobia, or vision changes.
- Ask about associated drowsiness, confusion, dizziness, or seizures.

Physical examination

- Evaluate the patient's level of consciousness (LOC).
- Take the patient's vital signs.
- Be alert for signs of increased ICP.
- Check pupil size and response to light.
- Note any neck stiffness.

Causes

Medical causes

Anthrax, cutaneous

- A maculopapular lesion develops into a vesicle and finally a painless ulcer.
- Other signs and symptoms include headache, lymphadenopathy, fever, and malaise.

Arteriovenous malformations

- Vascular malformations usually result from developmental defects of the cerebral veins and arteries.
- Although many are present from birth, they manifest in adulthood with a triad of symptoms, including headache, hemorrhage, and seizures.

Brain abscess

- Headache is localized to the abscess site and intensifies over a few days.
- Straining aggravates headache.
- Other signs and symptoms include nausea, vomiting, focal or generalized seizures, changes in LOC and, depending on the location of the abscess, aphasia, impaired visual acuity, hemiparesis,

ataxia, tremors, and personality changes.

Brain tumor

- Headache is localized near the tumor site but becomes generalized as the tumor grows.
- Pain is usually intermittent, deep-seated, dull, and most intense in the morning; aggravating factors include coughing, stooping, Valsalva's maneuver, and changes in head position; alleviating factors include sitting and rest.
- Other signs and symptoms include personality changes, altered LOC, motor and sensory dysfunction, and signs of increased ICP.

Cerebral aneurysm, ruptured

- A life-threatening condition, headache is sudden and excruciating and usually peaks within minutes of the rupture.
- Loss of consciousness may be immediate or a variably altered LOC may occur.
- Depending on the location and severity of the bleeding, other signs and symptoms may include nausea, vomiting, nuchal rigidity, blurred vision, and hemiparesis.

Encephalitis

- A severe, generalized headache is characteristic.
- Within 48 hours, the patient's LOC typically deteriorates.
- Other signs and symptoms include fever, nuchal rigidity, irritability, seizures, nausea, vomiting, photophobia, cranial nerve palsies, and focal neurologic deficits.

Epidural hemorrhage, acute

- A progressively severe headache occurs with nausea, vomiting, bladder distention, confusion, and a rapid decrease in LOC.
- Other signs and symptoms include unilateral seizures, hemiparesis, hemiplegia, high fever, decreased pulse rate and bounding pulse, widened pulse pressure, increased blood pressure, positive Babinski's reflex, and decerebrate posture.

Glaucoma, acute angle-closure

- Excruciating headache as well as acute eye pain, blurred vision, halo vision, nausea, and vomiting may occur in this ophthalmic emergency.
- Other signs and symptoms include conjunctival injection, a cloudy cornea, and a moderately dilated, fixed pupil.

Hypertension

- Upon awakening, a slightly throbbing occipital headache may occur; severity decreases during the day (if diastolic pressure remains greater than 120 mm Hg, the headache is constant).
- Other signs and symptoms include atrial gallop, restlessness, confusion, nausea, vomiting, blurred vision, seizures, and altered LOC.

Influenza

- A severe generalized or frontal headache usually begins suddenly.
- Other signs and symptoms include stabbing retro-orbital pain, weakness, myalgia, fever, chills, coughing, rhinorrhea, and hoarseness.

Intracerebral hemorrhage

- A severe generalized headache may develop.
- Signs and symptoms vary with the size and location of the hemorrhage and may include altered LOC, hemiplegia, hemiparesis, abnormal pupil size and response, aphasia, dizziness, nausea, vomiting, seizures, decreased sensation, irregular respirations, positive Babinski's reflex, decorticate or decerebrate posture, and increased blood pressure.

Meningitis

■ The onset of a severe, constant, generalized headache is sudden and worsens with movement.

■ Other signs and symptoms include altered LOC, seizures, fever, chills, nuchal rigidity, ocular palsies, facial weakness, hearing loss, positive Kernig's and Brudzinski's signs, hyperreflexia, opisthotonos, and signs of increased ICP.

Plague

■ The pneumonic form results in the sudden onset of headache, chills, fever, myalgia, productive cough, chest pain, tachypnea, dyspnea, hemoptysis, respiratory distress, and cardiopulmonary insufficiency.

Postconcussional syndrome

■ A generalized or localized headache may develop 1 to 30 days after head trauma and last for 2 to 3 weeks.

■ Pain may be aching, pounding, pressing, stabbing, or throbbing.

■ Other signs and symptoms include giddiness or dizziness, blurred vision, fatigue, insomnia, inability to concentrate, noise and alcohol intolerance, fever, chills, malaise, chest pain, nausea, vomiting, and diarrhea.

Sinusitis, acute

■ A dull periorbital headache is usually aggravated by bending over or touching the face and is relieved by sinus drainage.

■ Other signs and symptoms may include fever, sinus tenderness, nasal turbinate edema, sore throat, malaise, cough, and nasal discharge.

Smallpox

■ Initial signs and symptoms include severe headache, backache, abdominal pain, high fever, malaise, prostration, and a maculopapular rash on the mucosa of the mouth, pharynx, face, and forearms, gradually developing on the trunk and legs.

■ The rash becomes vesicular, then pustular, and finally forms a crust and scab, leaving a pitted scar.

Subarachnoid hemorrhage

■ A sudden, violent headache occurs along with nuchal rigidity, nausea and vomiting, seizures, dizziness, ipsilateral pupil dilation, and altered LOC that may progress to coma.

■ Other signs and symptoms include positive Kernig's and Brudzinski's signs, photophobia, blurred vision, fever, hemiparesis, hemiplegia, sensory disturbances, aphasia, and signs of increased ICP.

Subdural hematoma

■ Headache develops and LOC decreases.

■ In acute cases, early signs and symptoms include drowsiness, confusion, and agitation that may progress to coma; late signs include signs of increased ICP and focal neurologic deficits.

■ In chronic cases, pounding headache fluctuates in severity and is located over the hematoma.

■ Giddiness, personality changes, confusion, seizures, and progressively worsening LOC may develop weeks or months after the trauma.

Temporal arteritis

■ A throbbing unilateral headache in the temporal or frontotemporal region may be accompanied by vision loss, hearing loss, confusion, and fever.

■ The temporal arteries are tender, swollen, nodular and, possibly, erythematous.

Other causes

Diagnostic tests

- Lumbar puncture or a myelogram may produce a throbbing frontal headache that worsens on standing.

Drugs

- Indomethacin (Indocin), vasodilators, and drugs with a vasodilating effect may produce headaches.
- Withdrawal from vasopressors may also result in headaches.

Traction

- Cervical traction with pins commonly causes a headache, which may be generalized or localized to pin insertion sites.

Nursing considerations

- Monitor the patient's vital signs and LOC.
- Watch for a change in the headache's severity or location.
- Administer an analgesic, darken the room, and minimize stimuli to ease the headache.
- In children older than age 3, headache is the most common symptom of a brain tumor.
- Suspect a headache if a young child is banging or holding his head.

Patient teaching

- Discuss the underlying disorder, diagnostic testing, and treatment options.
- Explain the signs of reduced LOC and seizures that the patient or his caregivers should report.
- Explain ways to maintain a safe, quiet environment and reduce environmental stress.
- Discuss the use of analgesics.

Hearing loss

Affecting nearly 16 million U.S. residents, hearing loss may be temporary or permanent and partial or complete. This common symptom may involve reception of low-, middle-, or high-frequency tones. If the hearing loss doesn't affect speech frequencies, the patient may be unaware of it.

Normally, sound waves enter the external auditory canal, and then travel to the middle ear's tympanic membrane and ossicles (incus, malleus, and stapes) and into the inner ear's cochlea. The cochlear division of cranial nerve (CN) VIII (auditory nerve) carries the sound impulse to the brain. This type of sound transmission, called *air conduction,* is normally better than bone conduction—sound transmission through bone to the inner ear.

Hearing loss can be classified as conductive, sensorineural, mixed, or functional. Conductive hearing loss results from external- or middle-ear disorders that block sound transmission. This type of hearing loss usually responds to medical or surgical intervention (or in some cases, both). Sensorineural hearing loss results from disorders of the inner ear or of CN VIII. Mixed hearing loss combines aspects of conductive and sensorineural hearing loss. Functional hearing loss results from psychological factors rather than identifiable organic damage.

Hearing loss may also result from trauma, infection, allergy, tumors, certain systemic and hereditary disorders, and the effects of ototoxic drugs and treatments. In most cases, however, it results from presbycusis, a type of sensorineural hearing loss that usually affects people older than age 50. Other physiologic causes of hearing loss include cerumen (earwax) impaction; barotitis media (unequal pressure on the eardrum) associated with descent in an airplane or elevator, diving, or close proximity to an explosion; and chronic exposure to noise over 90 dB, which can occur on the job, with certain hobbies, or from listening to live or recorded music.

History

- Ask for a description of the hearing loss.
- Obtain a medical history, including the incidence of chronic ear infections, ear surgery, ear or head trauma, and recent upper respiratory tract infection.
- Obtain a drug history.
- Ask for a description of the occupational environment.
- Ask about other signs and symptoms, such as pain; discharge; ringing, buzzing, hissing, or other noises; and dizziness.

Physical examination

- Inspect the external ear for inflammation, boils, foreign bodies, and discharge.
- Apply pressure to the tragus and mastoid to elicit tenderness.
- During otoscopic examination, note a color change, perforation, bulging, or retraction of the tympanic membrane.
- Evaluate hearing acuity.
- Perform Weber's and the Rinne tests. (See *Differentiating conductive from sensorineural hearing loss,* page 168.)

Causes

Medical causes

Acoustic neuroma

- Unilateral, progressive, sensorineural hearing loss occurs; tinnitus, vertigo, and facial paralysis may also develop.

Adenoid hypertrophy

- Gradual conductive hearing loss occurs.
- Other signs and symptoms include ear discharge, mouth breathing, and a sensation of ear fullness.

Allergies

- Conductive hearing loss may result.
- Other signs and symptoms include ear pain or a feeling of fullness, nasal congestion, and conjunctivitis.

Cholesteatoma

- Gradual hearing loss may be accompanied by vertigo and facial paralysis.
- Other signs and symptoms include eardrum perforation, pearly white balls in the ear canal, and discharge.

External ear canal tumor, malignant

- Progressive conductive hearing loss occurs with deep, boring ear pain, purulent discharge, and facial paralysis.

Head trauma

- Conductive or sensorineural hearing loss is sudden in onset.
- Headache and bleeding from the ear also occur.
- Neurologic findings depend on the type of trauma that occurred.

Hypothyroidism

- Reversible sensorineural hearing loss may occur.
- Other signs and symptoms include bradycardia, weight gain despite anorexia, mental dullness, cold intolerance, facial edema, brittle hair, and dry, pale, cool and doughy skin.

Ménière's disease

- Intermittent, unilateral sensorineural hearing loss that involves only low tones progresses to constant hearing loss that involves other tones.
- Other signs and symptoms include intermittent severe vertigo, nausea, vomiting, a sensation of fullness in the ear, a roaring or hollow-seashell tinnitus, diaphoresis, and nystagmus.

Osteoma

- Sudden or intermittent conductive hearing loss occurs.
- Other signs and symptoms include bony projections in the ear canal.

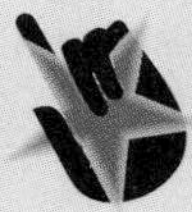

KNOW-HOW

Differentiating conductive from sensorineural hearing loss

Weber's and the Rinne tests can help determine whether the patient's hearing loss is conductive or sensorineural. Weber's test evaluates bone conduction; the Rinne test, bone and air conduction. Using a 512-Hz tuning fork, perform these preliminary tests as described here.

Weber's test

Place the base of a vibrating tuning fork firmly against the midline of the patient's skull at the forehead. Ask her if she hears the tone equally well in both ears. If she does, Weber's test is graded *midline*—a normal finding. In an abnormal Weber's test (graded *right* or *left*), sound is louder in one ear, suggesting a conductive hearing loss in that ear, or a sensorineural loss in the opposite ear.

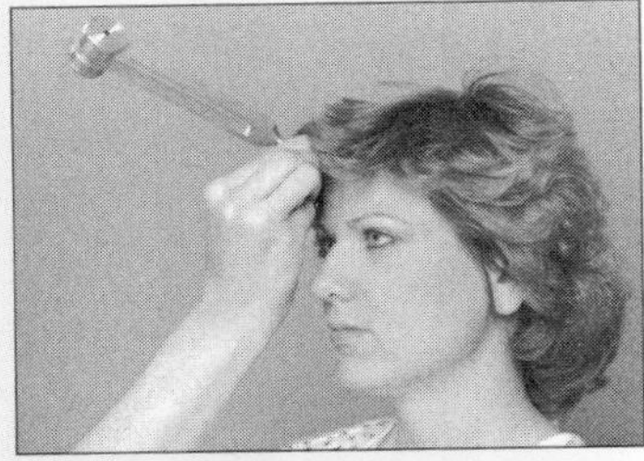

Rinne test

Hold the base of a vibrating tuning fork against the patient's mastoid process to test bone conduction. Then quickly move the vibrating fork in front of her ear canal to test air conduction. Ask her to tell you which location has the louder or longer sound. Repeat the procedure for the other ear. In a positive Rinne test, air conduction lasts longer or sounds louder than bone conduction—a normal finding. In a negative test, the opposite is true: Bone conduction lasts longer or sounds louder than air conduction.

After performing both tests, correlate the results with other assessment data.

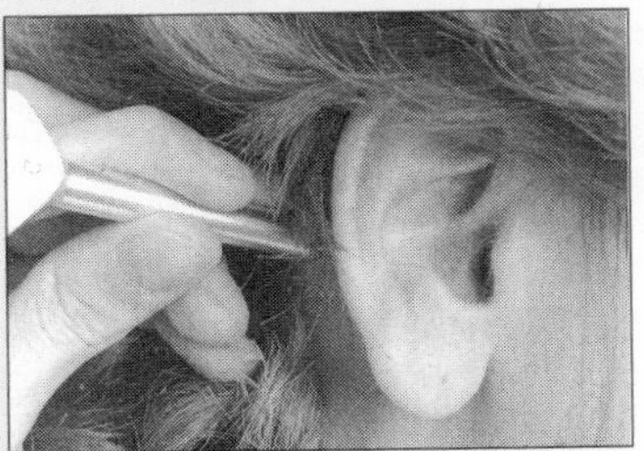

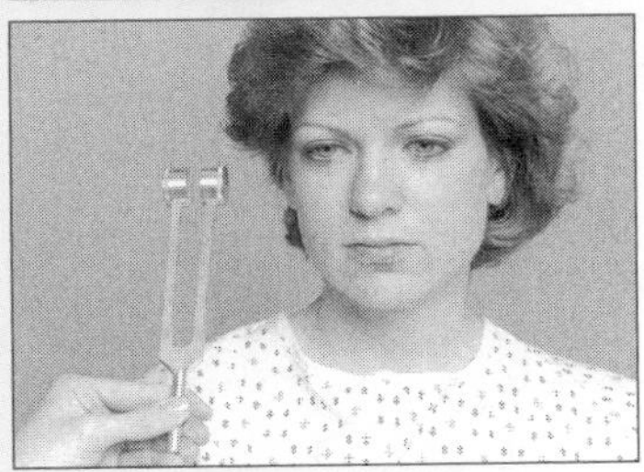

Implications of results

Conductive hearing loss produces:
- abnormal Weber's test result
- negative Rinne test result
- improved hearing in noisy areas
- normal ability to discriminate sounds
- difficulty hearing when chewing
- a quiet speaking voice.

Sensorineural hearing loss produces:
- positive Rinne test
- poor hearing in noisy areas
- difficulty hearing high-frequency sounds
- complaints that others mumble or shout
- tinnitus.

Otitis externa

■ Conductive hearing loss is a characteristic symptom.

■ The acute form produces pain, headache on the affected side, low-grade fever, lymphadenopathy, itching, and a foul-smelling sticky yellow discharge.

■ The malignant form involves visible debris in the ear canal, pruritus, tinnitus, and severe ear pain.

Otitis media

■ In the acute and chronic forms, hearing loss develops gradually.

■ Other signs and symptoms of the acute form include upper respiratory tract infection with sore throat, cough, nasal discharge, headache, dizziness, a sensation of fullness in the ear, intermittent or constant ear pain, fever, nausea, and vomiting.

■ Other signs and symptoms of the chronic form include a perforated tympanic membrane, purulent ear drainage, earache, nausea, and vertigo.

■ In the serous form, a stuffy feeling in the ear occurs with pain that worsens at night.

Otosclerosis

■ Unilateral conductive hearing loss usually begins in the early 20s and may gradually progress to bilateral mixed loss.

■ Tinnitus and the ability to hear better in a noisy environment may occur.

Skull fracture

■ Sudden, unilateral, sensorineural hearing loss may occur if the auditory nerve is damaged.

■ Other signs and symptoms include ringing tinnitus, blood behind the tympanic membrane, and scalp wounds.

Temporal arteritis

■ Unilateral, sensorineural hearing loss may occur along with throbbing unilateral facial pain, pain behind the eye, temporal or frontotemporal headache and, occasionally, vision loss.

■ Other signs and symptoms include malaise, anorexia, weight loss, weakness, low-grade fever, myalgia, and a nodular, swollen artery.

Tympanic membrane perforation

■ Abrupt hearing loss occurs with ear pain, tinnitus, vertigo, and a feeling of fullness in the ear.

Other causes

Drugs

■ Chloroquine (Aralen HCL), cisplatin (Platinol AQ), vancomycin (Vancocin), and aminoglycosides (especially neomycin [Neo-fradin], kanamycin [Kantrex], and amikacin [Amikin]) may cause irreversible hearing loss.

■ Loop diuretics, quinine (Quinamm), quinidine (Quinaglute), and high doses of erythromycin (Ilosone) or salicylates may cause reversible hearing loss.

Radiation therapy

■ Radiation of the middle ear, thyroid, face, skull, or nasopharynx may cause eustachian tube dysfunction, resulting in hearing loss.

Surgery

■ Myringotomy, myringoplasty, simple or radical mastoidectomy, or fenestrations may cause scarring that result in hearing loss.

Nursing considerations

■ When talking to the patient, face him and speak slowly and clearly.

■ Provide an alternate means of communication if necessary.

Patient teaching

■ Explain interventions to the patient, such as a hearing aid or cochlear implant, to improve his hearing.

- Explain the importance of ear protection and avoidance of loud noise.
- Stress the importance of following instructions for taking prescribed antibiotics.
- Teach the patient about the underlying diagnosis and treatment options.

Hematemesis

Hematemesis, the vomiting of blood, usually indicates GI bleeding above the ligament of Treitz, which suspends the duodenum at its junction with the jejunum. Bright red or blood-streaked vomitus indicates fresh or recent bleeding. Dark red, brown, or black vomitus (the color and consistency of coffee grounds) indicates that blood has been retained in the stomach and partially digested.

Although hematemesis usually results from a GI disorder, it may stem from a coagulation disorder or a treatment that irritates the GI tract. Esophageal varices may also cause hematemesis. Swallowed blood from epistaxis or oropharyngeal erosion may also cause bloody vomitus. Hematemesis may be precipitated by straining, emotional stress, and the use of an anti-inflammatory, anticoagulant, or alcohol. In a patient with esophageal varices, hematemesis may be a result of trauma from swallowing hard or partially chewed food.

Hematemesis is always an important sign, but its severity depends on the amount, source, and rapidity of the bleeding. Massive hematemesis (vomiting 500 to 1,000 ml of blood) may be life-threatening.

QUICK ACTION ***If the patient has massive hematemesis, check his vital signs. If you detect signs of shock—such as tachypnea, hypotension, and tachycardia—place the patient in a supine position, and elevate his feet 20 to 30 degrees. Start a large-bore I.V. line for emergency fluid replacement. Also, send a blood sample for typing and crossmatching, hemoglobin level, and hematocrit, and administer oxygen. Emergency endoscopy may be necessary to locate, and possibly treat, the source of bleeding. Prepare to insert a nasogastric (NG) tube for suction or iced lavage. A Sengstaken-Blakemore tube may be used to compress esophageal varices.***

History

- Ask about the onset, amount, color, and consistency of vomitus.
- Ask for a description of stools.
- Inquire about associated nausea, flatulence, diarrhea, or weakness.
- Obtain a medical history, including the incidence of ulcers or liver or coagulation disorders.
- Find out about alcohol use.
- Obtain a drug history, including aspirin and nonsteroidal anti-inflammatory drugs (NSAIDs).

Physical examination

- Check for orthostatic hypotension.
- Obtain other vital signs.
- Inspect the mucous membranes, nasopharynx, and skin for signs of bleeding.
- Palpate the abdomen for tenderness, pain, or masses.
- Note lymphadenopathy.

Causes

Medical causes

Anthrax, GI

- Initial findings include loss of appetite, nausea, vomiting, and fever.
- Signs and symptoms may progress to hematemesis, abdominal pain, and severe bloody diarrhea.

Coagulation disorders

- GI bleeding and moderate to severe hematemesis may occur.

■ Other signs and symptoms vary with the specific coagulation disorder and may include epistaxis and ecchymoses.

Esophageal cancer

■ Hematemesis is a late sign and occurs with steady chest pain that radiates to the back.

■ Other signs and symptoms include substernal fullness, severe dysphagia, nausea, vomiting with nocturnal regurgitation and aspiration, hemoptysis, fever, hiccups, sore throat, melena, and halitosis.

Esophageal rupture

■ Severity of hematemesis depends on the cause of the rupture.

■ Severe retrosternal, epigastric, neck, or scapular pain accompanied by chest and neck edema may occur.

■ Other signs and symptoms include subcutaneous crepitation in the chest wall, supraclavicular fossa, and neck and signs of respiratory distress.

Esophageal varices, ruptured

■ A life-threatening condition, coffee-ground or massive, bright red vomitus may occur.

■ Other signs and symptoms include signs of shock, abdominal distention, and melena or painless hematochezia, ranging from slight oozing to massive rectal hemorrhage.

Gastric cancer

■ Painless, bright red or dark brown vomitus is a late sign; additional late findings include fatigue, weakness, weight loss, feelings of fullness, melena, altered bowel habits, and signs of malnutrition.

■ Other signs and symptoms include upper-abdominal discomfort, anorexia, mild nausea, and chronic dyspepsia unrelieved by antacids and made worse by eating.

Gastritis, acute

■ Hematemesis and melena are the most common signs.

■ Other signs and symptoms include mild epigastric discomfort, nausea, fever, malaise and, with massive blood loss, signs of shock.

GI leiomyoma

■ Hematemesis occurs, possibly with dysphagia and weight loss.

Mallory-Weiss syndrome

■ Hematemesis and melena may occur because of a mucosal tear at the junction of the esophagus and the stomach, preceded by severe vomiting, retching, or straining.

■ Signs of shock may accompany severe bleeding.

Peptic ulcer

■ Hematemesis, possibly life-threatening, may occur.

■ Other signs and symptoms include melena or hematochezia, chills, fever, and signs of shock.

Other causes

Esophageal injury by caustic substances

■ Hematemesis occurs with epigastric and anterior or retrosternal chest pain that's intensified by swallowing.

Treatments

■ Nose or throat surgery, and traumatic NG or endotracheal intubation may cause hematemesis.

Nursing considerations

■ Monitor the patient's vital signs, and watch for signs of shock.

■ Check stools for occult blood; monitor NG tube drainage for blood.

■ Keep accurate intake and output records.

■ Place the patient on bed rest in low or semi-Fowler's position.

- Keep suctioning equipment nearby and use as needed.
- Provide frequent oral hygiene.
- Give a histamine-2 blocker and antacids, as prescribed; vasopressin (Pitressin) may be required for variceal hemorrhage.
- Prepare the patient for endoscopic evaluation, as needed.
- In infants, hemorrhagic disease and esophageal erosion may cause hematemesis.
- Chronic obstructive pulmonary disease, chronic liver or renal failure, and chronic NSAID use predispose elderly people to hemorrhage caused by coexisting ulcerative disorders.

Patient teaching

- Discuss the underlying condition and treatment options.
- Explain foods or fluids the patient should avoid, as appropriate.
- Stress the importance of avoiding alcohol, if applicable.
- Teach the patient and family about all hospital procedures and testing as well as prescribed medications and what drugs to avoid.

Hematochezia

The passage of bloody stools, also known as *hematochezia,* usually indicates—and may be the first sign of—GI bleeding below the ligament of Treitz. However, this sign—usually preceded by hematemesis—may also accompany rapid hemorrhage of 1 L or more from the upper GI tract.

Hematochezia ranges from formed, blood-streaked stools to liquid, bloody stools that may be bright red, dark mahogany, or maroon. This sign usually develops abruptly and is accompanied by abdominal pain.

Although hematochezia is commonly associated with GI disorders, it may also result from a coagulation disorder, exposure to toxins, or certain diagnostic tests. Always a significant sign, hematochezia may precipitate life-threatening hypovolemia.

QUICK ACTION ***If the patient has severe hematochezia, check his vital signs. If you detect signs of shock, such as hypotension and tachycardia, place the patient in a supine position and elevate his feet 20 to 30 degrees. Prepare to administer oxygen, and start a large-bore I.V. line for emergency fluid replacement. Next, obtain a blood sample for typing and crossmatching, hemoglobin level, and hematocrit. Insert a nasogastric tube. Iced lavage may be indicated to control bleeding. Endoscopy may be necessary to detect the source of bleeding.***

History

- Ask about the onset, amount, color, and consistency of stools.
- Find out about associated signs and symptoms.
- Obtain a medical history, including the incidence of GI and coagulation disorders.
- Determine the use of GI irritants, such as alcohol, aspirin, and nonsteroidal anti-inflammatory drugs.

Physical examination

- Check for orthostatic hypotension.
- Examine the skin for petechiae or spider angiomas.
- Palpate the abdomen for tenderness, pain, or masses.
- Note lymphadenopathy.
- Perform a digital rectal examination to detect rectal masses or hemorrhoids.

Causes

Medical causes

Anal fissure

- Slight hematochezia occurs; blood may streak the stools or appear on toilet tissue.

- Severe rectal pain occurs, leading to a reluctance to defecate and eventual constipation.

Angiodysplastic lesions

- Most common in elderly patients, angiodysplastic lesions cause chronic, bright red rectal bleeding.
- Occasionally, this condition may result in life-threatening blood loss and signs of shock.

Anorectal fistula

- Blood, pus, mucus, and occasionally stools may drain from an anorectal fistula.
- Other signs and symptoms include rectal pain and pruritus.

Coagulation disorders

- GI bleeding marked by moderate to severe hematochezia may occur.
- Other signs and symptoms vary with the specific coagulation disorder but may include epistaxis and purpura.

Colitis

- Ischemic colitis commonly causes slight or massive hematochezia; severe, cramping lower abdominal pain; abdominal distention and tenderness; absent bowel sounds; and hypotension.
- Severe ischemic colitis may cause hypovolemic shock and peritonitis.
- Ulcerative colitis typically causes hematochezia that may also contain mucus.
- Other signs and symptoms of ulcerative colitis include abdominal cramps, fever, tenesmus, anorexia, nausea, vomiting, hyperactive bowel sounds, tachycardia and, later, weight loss and weakness.

Colon cancer

- Bright red rectal bleeding occurs with or without pain.
- With a left colon tumor, early signs of obstruction occur; later, obstipation, diarrhea or ribbon-shaped stools, and pain relieved by passage of stools or flatus occurs.
- With a right colon tumor, melena, abdominal aching, pressure, and dull cramps occur; later, weakness, fatigue, diarrhea, anorexia, weight loss, anemia, vomiting, an abdominal mass, and signs of obstruction develop.

Colorectal polyps

- Intermittent hematochezia occurs.

Diverticulitis

- Mild to moderate rectal bleeding occurs after the patient feels the urge to defecate.
- Other signs and symptoms include left lower quadrant pain that's relieved by defecation, alternating episodes of constipation and diarrhea, anorexia, nausea, vomiting, rebound tenderness, and a distended, tympanic abdomen.

Esophageal varices, ruptured

- In this life-threatening condition, hematochezia ranges from slight rectal oozing to grossly bloody stools.
- Other signs and symptoms include hematemesis, melena, and signs of shock.

Food poisoning, staphylococcal

- Bloody diarrhea may occur 1 to 6 hours after ingesting food toxins.
- Other signs and symptoms include nausea, vomiting, prostration, and severe, cramping abdominal pain.

Hemorrhoids

- Hematochezia may accompany external hemorrhoids, causing painful defecation, possibly leading to constipation.
- Internal hemorrhoids usually produce chronic bleeding with bowel movements, leading to signs of anemia.

Peptic ulcer
- Hematochezia, hematemesis, or melena may occur.
- Other signs and symptoms include pain relieved by food or antacids, chills, fever, nausea, vomiting, and signs of dehydration and shock.

Small-intestine cancer
- Slight hematochezia or blood-streaked stools occur.
- Other signs and symptoms include colicky pan, postprandial vomiting, weight loss, anorexia, and fever.

Ulcerative proctitis
- The patient has an intense urge to defecate, but passes only bright red blood, pus, or mucus.
- Constipation and tenesmus (a painful spasm of the anal sphincter) may develop.

Other causes

Diagnostic tests
- Certain procedures, especially colonoscopy, polypectomy, and proctosigmoidoscopy may cause rectal bleeding.

Heavy metal poisoning
- Heavy metal poisoning may cause bloody diarrhea accompanied by cramping abdominal pain, nausea, vomiting, tachycardia, hypotension, seizures, paresthesia, depressed or absent deep tendon reflexes, and an altered level of consciousness.

Nursing considerations
- Place the patient on bed rest.
- Check the patient's vital signs frequently, watching for signs of shock.
- Monitor intake and output hourly.
- Administer blood products as ordered.
- Visually examine stools and test them for occult blood.
- If necessary, send a stool sample to the laboratory to check for parasites.

Patient teaching
- Discuss the underlying condition, diagnostic tests, and treatment options.
- Explain the signs and symptoms the patient should report.
- Teach the patient about ostomy self-care.
- Discuss proper bowel elimination habits.
- Explain dietary recommendations and restrictions.

Hematuria

A cardinal sign of renal and urinary tract disorders, hematuria is the abnormal presence of blood in urine. Strictly defined, it means three or more red blood cells (RBCs) per high-power microscopic field in urine. Microscopic hematuria is confirmed by an occult blood test, whereas macroscopic hematuria is immediately visible. However, macroscopic hematuria must be distinguished from pseudohematuria. Macroscopic hematuria may be continuous or intermittent, is commonly accompanied by pain, and may be aggravated by prolonged standing or walking.

Hematuria may be classified by the stage of urination it predominantly affects. Bleeding at the start of urination—initial hematuria—usually indicates urethral disease. Bleeding at the end of urination—terminal hematuria—usually indicates disease of the bladder neck, posterior urethra, or prostate. Bleeding throughout urination—total hematuria—usually indicates disease above the bladder neck.

Hematuria may result from one of two mechanisms: rupture or perforation of vessels in the renal system or urinary tract, or impaired glomerular filtration, which allows RBCs to seep into the urine. The color of the bloody urine provides a clue to the source of bleeding. Generally, dark or brownish blood indicates renal or upper urinary tract bleeding, whereas bright red blood indicates lower urinary tract bleeding.

Although hematuria usually results from renal and urinary tract disorders, it may also result from certain GI, prostate, vaginal, or coagulation disorders or from the effects of certain drugs. Invasive therapy and diagnostic tests that involve manipulative instrumentation of the renal and urologic systems may also cause hematuria. Nonpathologic hematuria may result from fever and hypercatabolic states. Transient hematuria may follow strenuous exercise.

History

- Ask about the onset, description, and severity.
- Find out about associated pain or burning.
- Obtain a medical history, including the incidence of renal, urinary, prostatic, or coagulation disorders and recent abdominal or flank trauma.
- Find out about recent strenuous exercise.
- Take a drug history, noting the use of anticoagulants or aspirin.

Physical examination

- Percuss and palpate the abdomen and flanks.
- Percuss the costovertebral angle (CVA) to elicit tenderness.
- Check the urinary meatus for bleeding or other abnormalities.
- Obtain a urine specimen for testing.
- Perform a vaginal or digital rectal examination.

Causes

Medical causes

Bladder cancer

- Gross hematuria occurs with pain in the bladder, rectum, pelvis, flank, back, or leg.
- Other signs and symptoms include nocturia, dysuria, urinary frequency and urgency, vomiting, diarrhea, and insomnia.

Bladder trauma

- Hematuria occurs with lower abdominal pain.
- Other signs and symptoms include anuria despite a strong urge to void; swelling of the scrotum, buttocks, or perineum; and signs of shock.

Calculi

- Bladder calculi causes gross hematuria, pain that's referred to the lower back or penile or vulvar area, and bladder distention.
- Renal calculi causes microscopic or gross hematuria; colicky pain (cardinal sign) that travels from the CVA to the flank, suprapubic region, and external genitalia when a calculus is passed; nausea; vomiting; restlessness; fever; chills; and abdominal distention.

Coagulation disorders

- Macroscopic hematuria is the first sign of hemorrhage.
- Other signs and symptoms include epistaxis, purpura, and signs of GI bleeding.

Cystitis

- Bacterial cystitis usually produces macroscopic hematuria with urinary urgency and frequency, dysuria, perineal and lumbar pain, suprapubic discomfort, and nocturia.
- Chronic interstitial cystitis occasionally causes grossly bloody hematuria

with urinary frequency, dysuria, nocturia, and tenesmus.
- Tubercular cystitis produces microscopic and macroscopic hematuria.
- Viral cystitis usually produces hematuria, urinary urgency and frequency, dysuria, nocturia, tenesmus, and fever.

Diverticulitis
- When the bladder is involved, diverticulitis usually causes microscopic hematuria, urinary frequency and urgency, dysuria, and nocturia.
- Other signs and symptoms include left lower quadrant pain, abdominal tenderness, constipation or diarrhea, a palpable abdominal mass, mild nausea, flatulence, and low-grade fever.

Glomerulonephritis
- The acute form causes gross hematuria that tapers off to microscopic hematuria and RBC casts.
- Other acute signs and symptoms include oliguria or anuria, proteinuria, mild fever, fatigue, flank and abdominal pain, edema, increased blood pressure, nausea, vomiting, and crackles.
- The chronic form causes hematuria that's accompanied by proteinuria, generalized edema, and increased blood pressure.

Nephritis, interstitial
- Microscopic hematuria is typical, but some patients may develop gross hematuria.
- Other signs and symptoms include fever, a maculopapular rash, and oliguria or anuria.

Nephropathy, obstructive
- Microscopic or macroscopic hematuria occurs with colicky flank and abdominal pain, CVA tenderness, and anuria or oliguria that alternates with polyuria.

Polycystic kidney disease
- Microscopic or gross hematuria occurs.
- Increased blood pressure, polyuria, dull flank pain, and signs of urinary tract infection also occur.
- Late signs and symptoms include a swollen, tender abdomen and lumbar pain that's aggravated by exertion and relieved by lying down.

Prostatic hyperplasia, benign
- Macroscopic hematuria occurs with significant obstruction.
- Early signs and symptoms include a diminished urinary stream, tenesmus, and a feeling of incomplete voiding.
- Late signs and symptoms include urinary hesitancy, frequency, and incontinence; nocturia; perineal pain; an enlarged prostate on rectal palpation; and constipation.

Prostatitis
- Macroscopic hematuria occurs at the end of urination.
- Urinary frequency and urgency and dysuria occur, followed by visible bladder distention.
- The acute form causes fatigue, malaise, myalgia, arthralgia, fever, chills, nausea, vomiting, perineal and lower back pain, decreased libido, and a tender, swollen, firm prostate on palpation.
- The chronic form causes persistent urethral discharge, dull perineal pain, ejaculatory pain, and decreased libido.

Pyelonephritis, acute
- Microscopic or macroscopic hematuria progresses to grossly bloody hematuria.
- After the infection resolves, microscopic hematuria may persist for a few months.
- Other signs and symptoms include persistent high fever, flank pain, CVA tenderness, shaking chills, weakness,

nausea, vomiting, anorexia, fatigue, dysuria, urinary frequency and urgency, nocturia, and tenesmus.

Renal cancer

- Grossly bloody hematuria; dull, aching flank pain; and a smooth, firm, palpable flank mass are the classic triad of signs and symptoms.
- Colicky pain also occurs accompanied by the passage of clots, CVA tenderness, fever, and increased blood pressure.
- In advanced disease, weight loss, nausea, vomiting, and leg edema with varicoceles occurs.

Renal infarction

- Gross hematuria occurs.
- Constant, severe flank and upper abdominal pain occurs with CVA tenderness, anorexia, nausea, and vomiting.
- Other signs and symptoms include oliguria or anuria, proteinuria, hypoactive bowel sounds, fever, and increased blood pressure.

Renal papillary necrosis, acute

- Grossly bloody hematuria occurs.
- Other signs and symptoms include intense flank pain, CVA tenderness, abdominal rigidity and colicky pain, oliguria or anuria, pyuria, fever, chills, hypertension, arthralgia, vomiting, and hypoactive bowel sounds.

Renal trauma

- Microscopic or gross hematuria occurs.
- Other signs and symptoms include flank pain, a palpable flank mass, oliguria, hematoma or ecchymoses over the upper abdomen or flank, nausea, vomiting, hypoactive bowel sounds and, in severe trauma, signs of shock.

Renal tuberculosis

- Gross hematuria is commonly the first sign.
- Other signs and symptoms include urinary frequency, dysuria, pyuria, tenesmus, colicky abdominal pain, lumbar pain, and proteinuria.

Renal vein thrombosis

- Grossly bloody hematuria occurs.
- With abrupt venous obstruction, severe flank and lumbar pain and epigastric and CVA tenderness occurs.
- Other signs and symptoms include fever, pallor, proteinuria, peripheral edema, and oliguria or anuria if the obstruction is bilateral.

Sickle cell anemia

- Gross hematuria occurs.
- Other signs and symptoms include pallor, dehydration, chronic fatigue, tachycardia, heart murmurs, polyarthralgia, leg ulcers, dyspnea, chest pain, impaired growth and development, hepatomegaly, and jaundice.

Systemic lupus erythematosus

- Gross hematuria occurs along with proteinuria if the kidneys are involved.
- Other signs and symptoms include joint pain and stiffness, butterfly rash, photosensitivity, Raynaud's phenomenon, seizures, psychoses, recurrent fever, lymphadenopathy, oral or nasopharyngeal ulcers, anorexia, and weight loss.

Other causes

Diagnostic tests

- Renal biopsy and biopsy or manipulative instrumentation of the urinary tract may result in hematuria.

Drugs

- Drugs that may cause hematuria include anticoagulants, aspirin toxicity, analgesics, cyclophosphamide (Cytoxan), metyrosine (Demser), penicillin, rifampin (Rifadin), and thiabendazole (Mintezol).

Treatments

- Any therapy that involves manipulative instrumentation of the urinary tract, such as transurethral prostatectomy, may cause microscopic hematuria.
- Following a kidney transplant, a patient may experience hematuria with or without clots.

Nursing considerations

- Check the patient's vital signs frequently.
- Monitor intake and output, including the amount and pattern of hematuria.
- If the patient has an indwelling urinary catheter in place, ensure its patency; irrigate if necessary.
- Administer analgesics as indicated.

Patient teaching

- Discuss the underlying condition, diagnostic testing, and treatment options.
- Instruct the patient in the three-glass technique for collecting serial urine specimens.
- Emphasize increasing fluid intake.
- Tell the patient the signs and symptoms to report.

Hemoptysis

Frightening to the patient and commonly ominous, hemoptysis is the expectoration of blood or bloody sputum from the lungs or tracheobronchial tree. It's sometimes confused with bleeding from the mouth, throat, nasopharynx, or GI tract. (See *Identifying hemoptysis.*) Expectoration of 200 ml of blood in a single episode suggests severe bleeding, whereas expectoration of 400 ml in 3 hours or more than 600 ml in 16 hours signals a life-threatening crisis.

Hemoptysis usually results from chronic bronchitis, lung cancer, or bronchiectasis. However, it may also result from inflammatory, infectious, cardiovascular, or coagulation disorders and, rarely, from a ruptured aortic aneurysm. In up to 15% of patients, the cause is unknown. The most common causes of *massive hemoptysis* are lung cancer, bronchiectasis, active tuberculosis (TB), and cavitary pulmonary disease from necrotic infections or TB.

Several pathophysiologic processes can cause hemoptysis. It can result from hemorrhage and diapedesis of red blood cells from the pulmonary microvasculature into the alveoli; necrosis of lung tissue that causes rupture of blood vessels into alveolar spaces; rupture of aortic aneurysm into the tracheobronchial tree; rupture of distended endobronchial blood vessels from pulmonary hypertension; rupture of pulmonary arteriovenous fistula; or an ulceration and erosion of the bronchial epithelium.

QUICK ACTION ***If the patient coughs up copious amounts of blood, endotracheal intubation may be required. Suction frequently to remove blood. Lavage may be necessary to loosen tenacious secretions or clots. Massive hemoptysis can cause airway obstruction and asphyxiation. Insert an I.V. line to allow fluid replacement, drug administration, and blood transfusions, if needed. An emergency bronchoscopy should be performed to identify the bleeding site. Monitor the patient's blood pressure and pulse to detect hypotension and tachycardia, and draw an arterial blood sample for laboratory analysis to monitor respiratory status.***

History

- Ask about the onset and extent of hemoptysis.
- Obtain a medical history of cardiac, pulmonary, or bleeding disorders, recent infection, and exposure to TB.
- Ask about the date and results of the last tuberculin tine test.

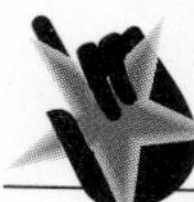

KNOW-HOW

Identifying hemoptysis

These guidelines will help you distinguish hemoptysis from epistaxis, hematemesis, and brown, red, or pink sputum.

Hemoptysis

Typically frothy because it's mixed with air, hemoptysis is commonly bright red with an alkaline pH (tested with nitrazine paper). It's strongly suggested by the presence of respiratory signs and symptoms, including a cough, a tickling sensation in the throat, and blood produced from repeated coughing episodes. (You can rule out epistaxis because the patient's nasal passages and posterior pharynx are usually clear.)

Hematemesis

The usual site of hematemesis is the GI tract; the patient vomits or regurgitates coffee-ground material that contains food particles, tests positive for occult blood, and has an acid pH. However, he may vomit bright red blood or swallowed blood from the oral cavity and nasopharynx. After an episode of hematemesis, the patient may have stools with traces of blood and may also complain of dyspepsia.

Brown, red, or pink sputum

Brown, red, or pink sputum can result from oxidation of inhaled bronchodilators. Sputum that looks like old blood may result from rupture of an amebic abscess into the bronchus. Red or brown sputum may occur in a patient with pneumonia caused by the enterobacterium *Serratia marcescens.*

- Obtain a drug history, including the use of anticoagulants.
- Obtain a smoking history.

Physical examination

- Take the patient's vital signs.
- Examine the nose, mouth, and pharynx for sources of bleeding.
- Inspect the chest; look for abnormal movement during breathing and accessory muscle use.
- Observe the respiratory rate, depth, and rhythm.
- Examine the skin for lesions.
- Palpate the chest for diaphragm level and for tenderness, respiratory excursion, fremitus, and abnormal pulsations.
- Percuss the chest for flatness, dullness, resonance, hyperresonance, and tympany.
- Auscultate for breath sounds.
- Auscultate for heart murmurs, bruits, and pleural rubs.
- Obtain a sputum sample, and examine it for quantity, amount of blood, color, odor, and consistency.

Causes

Medical causes

Bronchial adenoma

- Recurring hemoptysis occurs along with a chronic cough and local wheezing.
- Recurrent infection, dyspnea, and wheezing may also occur.

Bronchiectasis

- Hemoptysis appearance varies from blood-tinged sputum to frank blood, depending on the extent of bronchial blood vessel erosion.

- Other signs and symptoms include chronic cough, coarse crackles, late clubbing, fever, weight loss, fatigue, weakness, malaise, dyspnea on exertion, and copious, foul-smelling, and purulent sputum.

Bronchitis, chronic

- A productive cough leads to the production of blood-streaked sputum.
- Other signs and symptoms include dyspnea, prolonged expirations, wheezing, scattered rhonchi, accessory muscle use, barrel chest, tachypnea, and late clubbing.

Coagulation disorders

- Hemoptysis occurs with multisystem hemorrhaging and purpuric lesions.

Laryngeal cancer

- Hemoptysis occurs, but hoarseness is the usual early sign.
- Other signs and symptoms include dysphagia, dyspnea, stridor, cervical lymphadenopathy, and neck pain.

Lung abscess

- Blood-streaked sputum occurs.
- Other signs and symptoms include fever, chills, diaphoresis, anorexia, dyspnea, pleuritic or dull chest pain, clubbing, and a cough with purulent, foul-smelling sputum.

Lung cancer

- Recurring hemoptysis is an early sign.
- Other signs and symptoms include productive cough, dyspnea, fever, anorexia, weight loss, wheezing, and chest pain (a late sign).

Plague

- The pneumonic form can produce hemoptysis, productive cough, chest pain, tachypnea, dyspnea, increasing respiratory distress, and cardiopulmonary insufficiency.
- Other signs and symptoms include the sudden onset of chills, fever, headache, and myalgia.

Pneumonia

- *Klebsiella* pneumonia produces dark brown or red tenacious sputum that the patient has difficulty expelling from his mouth. It's abrupt in onset with accompanying chills, fever, dyspnea, productive cough, severe pleuritic chest pain, cyanosis, tachycardia, decreased breath sounds, and crackles.
- Pneumococcal pneumonia causes pinkish or rust-colored mucoid sputum; its onset is marked by sudden shaking chills, a rapidly rising temperature, tachycardia, and tachypnea.
- Other signs and symptoms include rapid, shallow, grunting respirations with splinting; accessory muscle use; malaise; weakness; myalgia; and prostration.

Pulmonary contusion

- Cough and hemoptysis occur after blunt chest trauma.
- Other signs and symptoms include dyspnea, tachypnea, chest pain, tachycardia, hypotension, crackles, decreased or absent breath sounds over the affected area and, possibly, severe respiratory distress.

Pulmonary edema

- A life-threatening condition, frothy, blood-tinged pink sputum accompanies severe dyspnea, orthopnea, gasping, anxiety, cyanosis, diffuse crackles, ventricular gallop, and cold, clammy skin.

■ Other signs and symptoms include tachycardia, lethargy, arrhythmias, tachypnea, hypotension, and a thready pulse.

Pulmonary embolism with infarction
■ A life-threatening disorder, hemoptysis is a common sign.
■ Initial symptoms typically include dyspnea and anginal or pleuritic chest pain.

Pulmonary hypertension, primary
■ Hemoptysis, exertional dyspnea, and fatigue are common but generally develop late in the disease process.
■ Other signs and symptoms include arrhythmias, syncope, cough, hoarseness, and angina-like pain that occur with exertion and may radiate to the neck.

Pulmonary tuberculosis
■ Hemoptysis is a common sign.
■ Other signs and symptoms include chronic productive cough, fine crackles after coughing, dyspnea, dullness to percussion, increased tactile fremitus, amphoric breath sounds, night sweats, malaise, fatigue, fever, anorexia, weight loss, and pleuritic chest pain.

Silicosis
■ A productive cough with mucopurulent sputum becomes blood-streaked; occasionally, massive hemoptysis may occur.
■ Other signs and symptoms include exertional dyspnea, tachypnea, weight loss, fatigue, weakness, and fine, end-inspiratory crackles.

Systemic lupus erythematosus
■ Pleuritis and pneumonitis may cause hemoptysis.
■ Other signs and symptoms include butterfly rash, nondeforming joint pain and stiffness, photosensitivity, Raynaud's phenomenon, convulsions or psychoses, anorexia with weight loss, and lymphadenopathy.

Tracheal trauma
■ Torn tracheal mucosa may cause hemoptysis, hoarseness, dysphagia, neck pain, airway occlusion, and respiratory distress.

Other causes

Diagnostic tests
■ Lung or airway injury from bronchoscopy, laryngoscopy, mediastinoscopy, or lung biopsy may cause bleeding and hemoptysis.

Treatments
■ Traumatic or prolonged intubation may produce hemoptysis.
■ Surgery to the lungs, throat, or upper airways may cause hemoptysis.

Nursing considerations
■ To protect the nonbleeding lung, place the patient in the lateral decubitus position, with the suspected bleeding lung facing down.
■ Monitor the patient's respiratory status, vital signs, and blood test results closely.
■ In children, hemoptysis may stem from Goodpasture's syndrome or cystic fibrosis.
■ If the patient is receiving anticoagulants, determine any changes that need to be made in diet or medications because these factors may affect clotting.

Patient teaching
■ Explain the importance of reporting recurrent episodes.
■ Give the patient instructions for providing sputum samples.
■ Teach the patient and his family about all hospital procedures and tests.
■ Teach the patient about the cause of hemoptysis.

Hepatomegaly

Hepatomegaly, an enlarged liver, indicates potentially reversible primary or secondary liver disease. This sign may stem from diverse pathophysiologic mechanisms, including dilated hepatic sinusoids (in heart failure), persistently high venous pressure leading to liver congestion (in chronic constrictive pericarditis), dysfunction and engorgement of hepatocytes (in hepatitis), fatty infiltration of parenchymal cells causing fibrous tissue (in cirrhosis), distention of liver cells with glycogen (in diabetes), and infiltration of amyloid (in amyloidosis).

Hepatomegaly may be confirmed by palpation, percussion, or radiologic tests. It may be mistaken for displacement of the liver by the diaphragm, in a respiratory disorder; by an abdominal tumor; by a spinal deformity, such as kyphosis; by the gallbladder; or by fecal material or a tumor in the colon.

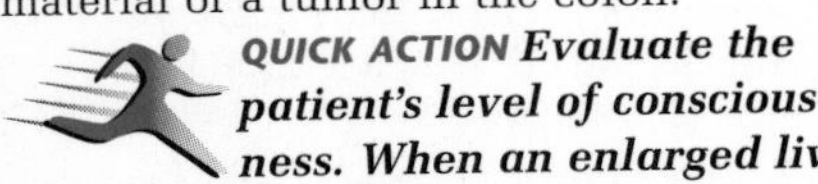

QUICK ACTION ***Evaluate the patient's level of consciousness. When an enlarged liver loses its ability to detoxify waste products, metabolic substances toxic to brain cells accumulate. As a result, watch for personality changes, irritability, agitation, memory loss, inability to concentrate, poor mentation, and—in a severely ill patient—coma.***

History

- Ask about alcohol use.
- Determine exposure to hepatitis.
- Obtain a drug history.
- Ask about the location and description of any associated abdominal pain.

Physical examination

- Inspect the skin and sclerae for jaundice, dilated veins, scars from previous surgery, and spider angiomas.
- Inspect the contour of the abdomen and measure abdominal girth.
- Percuss the liver. (See *Percussing the liver for size and position.*)
- During deep inspiration, palpate the liver's edge.
- Take the patient's vital signs.
- Assess the patient's nutritional status.
- Evaluate the patient's level of consciousness (LOC).

Causes

Medical causes

Cirrhosis

- In the late stage of this disease, the liver becomes enlarged, nodular, and hard.
- Other late signs and symptoms affect all body systems and include jaundice, ascites, hypoxia, encephalopathy, bleeding disorders, and portal hypertension.

Diabetes mellitus

- Hepatomegaly and right upper quadrant tenderness along with polydipsia, polyphagia, and polyuria may occur in overweight patients with poorly controlled diabetes.

Heart failure

- Hepatomegaly occurs along with jugular vein distention, cyanosis, nocturia, dependent edema of the legs and sacrum, steady weight gain, confusion and, possibly, nausea, vomiting, abdominal discomfort, and anorexia.
- Massive right-sided heart failure may cause anasarca, oliguria, severe weakness, and anxiety.
- If left-sided heart failure precedes right-sided heart failure, signs and symptoms include dyspnea, orthopnea, paroxysmal nocturnal dyspnea, tachypnea, arrhythmias, tachycardia, and fatigue.

Hepatic abscess

- Hepatomegaly may accompany fever (primary sign), nausea, vomiting, chills, weakness, diarrhea, anorexia, an elevated right hemidiaphragm, and right upper quadrant pain and tenderness.

Hepatitis

- Hepatomegaly occurs in the icteric phase and continues during the recovery phase.
- Early signs and symptoms include nausea, vomiting, fatigue, malaise, photophobia, sore throat, cough, and headache.
- Other signs and symptoms of the icteric phase include liver tenderness, slight weight loss, dark urine, clay-colored stools, jaundice, pruritus, right upper quadrant pain, and splenomegaly.

Leukemia and lymphomas

- Moderate to massive hepatomegaly, splenomegaly, and abdominal discomfort are common.
- Other signs and symptoms include malaise, low-grade fever, fatigue, weakness, tachycardia, weight loss, bleeding disorders, and anorexia.

Liver cancer

- Primary liver tumors cause irregular, nodular, firm hepatomegaly, with pain or tenderness in the right upper quadrant and a friction rub or bruit over the liver.
- Metastatic liver tumors cause hepatomegaly, but accompanying signs and symptoms reflect the primary cancer.
- Other signs and symptoms include weight loss, anorexia, cachexia, nausea, vomiting, peripheral edema, ascites, jaundice, and a palpable right upper quadrant mass.

Mononucleosis, infectious

- Hepatomegaly may occur.
- Prodromal symptoms include headache, malaise, and extreme fatigue.
- After 3 to 5 days, signs and symptoms include sore throat, cervical lymphadenopathy, temperature fluctuations,

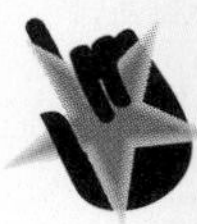

KNOW-HOW

Percussing the liver for size and position

With the patient in a supine position, begin at the right iliac crest to percuss up the right midclavicular line, as shown below. The percussion note becomes dull when you reach the liver's inferior border—usually at the costal margin, but sometimes at a lower point in the patient with liver disease. Mark this point and then percuss down from the right clavicle, again along the right midclavicular line. The liver's superior border usually lies between the fifth and seventh intercostal spaces. Mark the superior border.

The distance between the two marked points represents the approximate span of the liver's right lobe, which normally ranges from 2¼″ to 4¾″ (6 to 12 cm).

Next, assess the liver's left lobe similarly, percussing along the sternal midline. Again, mark the points where you hear dull percussion notes. Also, measure the span of the left lobe, which normally ranges from 1½″ to 3⅛″ (4 to 8 cm). Record your findings for use as a baseline.

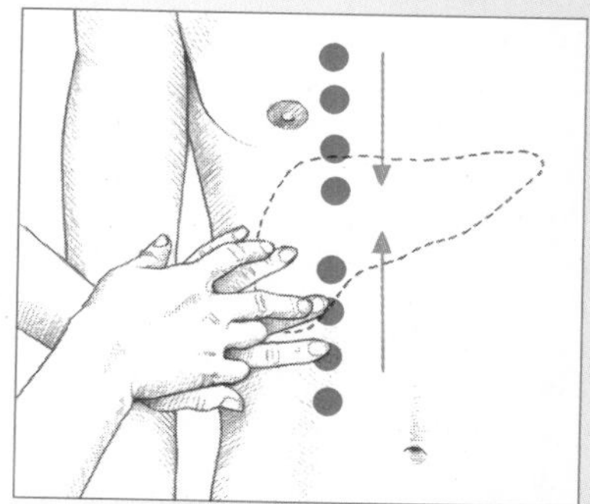

stomatitis, palatal petechiae, periorbital edema, splenomegaly, exudative tonsillitis, pharyngitis, and a maculopapular rash.

Obesity

- Hepatomegaly may occur along with respiratory difficulties, cardiovascular disease, diabetes, renal disease, gallbladder disease, and psychological difficulties.

Pancreatic cancer

- Hepatomegaly accompanies anorexia, weight loss, abdominal or back pain, and jaundice.
- Other signs and symptoms include nausea, vomiting, fever, fatigue, weakness, pruritus, and skin lesions.

Pericarditis

- In chronic constrictive pericarditis, there's marked congestive hepatomegaly.
- Other signs and symptoms include jugular vein distention, peripheral edema, ascites, fatigue, and decreased muscle mass.

Nursing considerations

- Provide bed rest, relief from stress, and adequate nutrition.
- Monitor and restrict dietary protein as needed.
- Give hepatotoxic drugs or drugs metabolized by the liver in very small doses, if at all.

Patient teaching

- Explain the treatment plan for the underlying disorder and diagnostic tests.
- Stress the avoidance of alcohol and people with infections.
- Emphasize personal hygiene.
- Discuss the importance of pacing activities and rest periods.

Hyperpnea

Hyperpnea indicates increased respiratory effort for a sustained period. It may take the form of a normal rate (at least 12 breaths/minute) with increased depth (a tidal volume greater than 7.5 ml/kg), an increased rate (more than 20 breaths/minute) with normal depth, or an increased rate and depth. This sign differs from sighing (intermittent deep inspirations) and may be associated with tachypnea (increased respiratory frequency).

The typical patient with hyperpnea breathes at a normal or increased rate and inhales deeply, displaying marked chest expansion. He may complain of shortness of breath if a respiratory disorder is causing hypoxemia. However, he may not be aware of his breathing if a metabolic, psychiatric, or neurologic disorder is causing involuntary hyperpnea. (See *Managing hyperpnea*.) Other causes of hyperpnea include profuse diarrhea or dehydration, loss of pancreatic juice or bile from GI drainage, and ureterosigmoidostomy. All these conditions and procedures cause a loss of bicarbonate ions, resulting in metabolic acidosis. Of course, hyperpnea may also accompany strenuous exercise, and voluntary hyperpnea can promote relaxation in the patient experiencing stress or pain—for example, a woman in labor.

Hyperventilation, a consequence of hyperpnea, is characterized by alkalosis (arterial pH above 7.45 and partial pressure of arterial carbon dioxide below 35 mm Hg). In central neurogenic hyperventilation, brain stem dysfunction (such as results from a severe cranial injury) increases the rate and depth of respirations. In acute intermittent hyperventilation, the respiratory pattern may be a response to hypoxemia, anxiety, fear, pain, or excitement. Hyperpnea may also be a compensatory mechanism

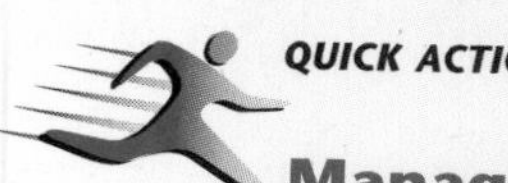

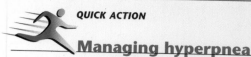

QUICK ACTION

Managing hyperpnea

Carefully examine the patient with hyperpnea for related signs of life-threatening conditions, such as increased intracranial pressure (ICP), metabolic acidosis, and diabetic ketoacidosis (DKA).

Increased ICP

If you observe hyperpnea in a patient who has signs of head trauma from a recent accident and has lost consciousness, act quickly to prevent further brain stem injury and irreversible deterioration. Take the patient's vital signs, noting bradycardia, increased systolic blood pressure, and a widening pulse pressure (signs of increased ICP).

Examine the patient's pupillary reaction. Elevate the head of the bed 30 degrees (unless you suspect spinal cord injury), and insert an artificial airway. Connect the patient to a cardiac monitor, and continuously observe his respiratory pattern. Insert an I.V. catheter and begin fluids at a slow infusion rate and prepare to administer an osmotic diuretic, such as mannitol (Osmitrol), to decrease cerebral edema. Catheterize the patient to measure urine output, administer supplemental oxygen, and keep emergency resuscitation equipment close by. Obtain an arterial blood gas analysis to help guide treatments.

Metabolic acidosis

If the patient with hyperpnea doesn't have a head injury, his increased respiratory rate probably indicates metabolic acidosis. If the patient's level of consciousness is decreased, check his history to help you determine the cause of his metabolic acidosis, and intervene appropriately. Suspect shock if the patient has cold, clammy skin. Palpate for a rapid, thready pulse and take his blood pressure, noting hypotension. Elevate the patient's legs 30 degrees, apply pressure dressings to any obvious hemorrhage, insert several large-bore I.V. catheters, and prepare to administer fluids, vasopressors, and blood products.

A patient with hyperpnea who has a history of alcohol abuse, is vomiting profusely, has diarrhea or profuse abdominal drainage, has ingested an overdose of aspirin, or is cachectic and has a history of starvation may also have metabolic acidosis. Inspect his skin for dryness and poor turgor, indicating dehydration. Take his vital signs, looking for a low-grade fever and hypotension. Insert an I.V. catheter for fluid administration. Obtain blood specimens for electrolyte studies, and prepare to administer sodium bicarbonate, as ordered.

Diabetic ketoacidosis

If the patient has a history of diabetes mellitus, is vomiting, and has a fruity breath odor (acetone breath), suspect DKA. Catheterize him to monitor urine output. Infuse an I.V. saline solution. Perform a fingerstick to estimate blood glucose level with a reagent strip. Obtain a urine specimen to test for glucose and acetone, and obtain a blood specimen for glucose and ketone tests. Also administer fluids, insulin, potassium, and sodium bicarbonate I.V., as ordered.

to metabolic acidosis. Under these conditions, it's known as *Kussmaul's respirations.*

History

- Ask about recent illnesses or infections.
- Find out about the ingestion of aspirin or other drugs, or the inhalation of drugs or chemicals.
- Obtain a medical history, including the incidence of diabetes mellitus, renal disease, or pulmonary conditions.
- Ask about associated signs and symptoms, such as thirst, hunger, nausea, vomiting, severe diarrhea, or upper respiratory tract infection.

Physical examination

- Assess the patient's level of consciousness (LOC).
- Observe for clues to abnormal breathing pattern.
- Examine for cyanosis, restlessness, and anxiety.
- Observe for intercostal and abdominal retractions, accessory muscle use, and diaphoresis.
- Inspect for draining wounds or signs of infection.
- Take the patient's vital signs, including oxygen saturation.
- Auscultate the heart and lungs.
- Assess for dehydration.

Causes

Medical causes

Head injury

- Hyperpnea occurs along with signs of increased intracranial pressure; loss of consciousness; soft-tissue injury or bony deformity of the face, head, or neck; facial edema; cloudy or bloody drainage from the mouth, nose, or ears; raccoon eyes; Battle's sign; an absent doll's eye sign; and motor and sensory disturbances.

Hyperventilation syndrome

- Acute anxiety triggers episodic hyperpnea.
- Other signs and symptoms include agitation, vertigo, syncope, pallor, circumoral and peripheral cyanosis, muscle twitching, carpopedal spasm, weakness, and arrhythmias.

Hypoxemia

- Many pulmonary disorders that cause hypoxemia may cause hyperpnea and episodes of hyperventilation with chest pain, dizziness, and paresthesia.
- Other signs and symptoms include dyspnea, cough, crackles, rhonchi, wheezing, and decreased breath sounds.

Ketoacidosis

- In alcoholic ketoacidosis, Kussmaul's respirations begin abruptly and are accompanied by vomiting for several days, fruity breath odor, dehydration, abdominal pain and distention, and absent bowel sounds.
- In diabetic ketoacidosis (DKA), a potentially life-threatening disorder, Kussmaul's respirations occur with polydipsia, polyphagia, and polyuria.
- Other signs and symptoms of DKA include fruity breath odor, orthostatic hypotension, weakness, decreased LOC, nausea, vomiting, anorexia, abdominal pain, and a rapid, thready pulse.
- In starvation ketoacidosis, also a life-threatening disorder, Kussmaul's respirations occur gradually and may be accompanied by cachexia, dehydration, decreased LOC, bradycardia, and a history of severely limited food intake.

Renal failure

- Life-threatening acidosis and Kussmaul's respirations can occur.
- Other signs and symptoms include oliguria or anuria, uremic fetor, severe pruritus, uremic frost, purpura, ecchymoses, nausea, vomiting, weakness,

burning in the legs and feet, diarrhea or constipation, altered LOC, seizures, and yellow, dry, scaly skin.

Sepsis

- Severe infection may cause acidosis, resulting in Kussmaul's respirations.
- Other signs and symptoms include tachycardia, fever or a low temperature, chills, headache, lethargy, profuse diaphoresis, anorexia, cough, change in mental status, and signs of infection.

Shock

- This life-threatening condition may be characterized by Kussmaul's respirations, hypotension, tachycardia, narrowed pulse pressure, weak pulse, dyspnea, oliguria, anxiety, restlessness, stupor that can progress to coma, and cool, clammy skin.
- Other signs and symptoms include external or internal bleeding, in hypovolemic shock; chest pain, arrhythmias, and signs of heart failure, in cardiogenic shock; high fever and chills, in septic shock; or stridor, in anaphylactic shock.

Other causes

Drugs

- Toxic levels of salicylates, ammonium chloride, acetazolamide (Dazamide), and other carbonic anhydrase inhibitors can cause Kussmaul's respirations.
- Ingestion of methanol and ethylene glycol can also cause Kussmaul's respirations.

Nursing considerations

- Monitor the patient's vital signs, including oxygen saturation.
- Observe for increasing respiratory distress or an irregular respiratory pattern.
- Start an I.V. line for administration of fluids, blood transfusions, and vasopressors, as ordered.
- Prepare to give ventilatory support.

Patient teaching

- Discuss the underlying condition, diagnostic tests, and treatment options.
- Teach the diabetic patient how to monitor his blood glucose level, and stress the importance of compliance with diabetes therapy.
- Explain fluids and foods the patient should avoid.
- Discuss pulmonary hygiene.
- Teach the patient ways to avoid respiratory infections.
- Emphasize the importance of alcohol cessation and provide information about groups or other resources that can help, as appropriate.

Hyperthermia

Hyperthermia, also known as *heat syndrome,* refers to a core body temperature elevated above normal. It results when environmental and internal factors increase heat production or decrease heat loss beyond the body's ability to compensate. Hyperthermia affects males and females equally; however, incidence increases among elderly patients and neonates during excessively hot days. Risk factors for hyperthermia include obesity, salt and water depletion, alcohol use, poor physical condition, age, and socioeconomic status.

A temperature between 99° and 102° F (37.2° and 38.9° C) is considered mild hyperthermia; a temperature between 102° and 105° F (38.9° and 40.6° C) is considered moderate hyperthermia. A temperature of 105° F or above is considered critical hyperthermia and represents an emergency—particularly if the temperature rises rapidly or stays elevated for a prolonged period.

QUICK ACTION ***For critical hyperthermia, immediate action should include providing supplemental oxygen and preparing the patient for endotracheal***

intubation and mechanical ventilation, if necessary. The goal is to reduce the patient's temperature, but not too rapidly; rapid reduction can lead to vasoconstriction, which can lead to shivering. Administer diazepam (Valium) or chlorpromazine (Thorazine) to control shivering. Shivering must be treated because it increases metabolic demands and oxygen consumption. Continuous cardiac monitoring should be instituted, and the patient should be monitored for arrhythmias. Prepare the patient for pulmonary artery catheter insertion to monitor the body's core temperature. Closely observe the patient's vital signs and level of consciousness (LOC). Administer fluids and replace electrolytes as ordered. Remove the patient's clothing and apply cool water to the skin, and then fan the patient with cool air.

In mild hyperthermia, provide a cool, calm environment and allow the patient to rest. Encourage the oral intake and administration of I.V. fluids. Replace electrolytes as necessary.

History

- Ask the patient about the onset and duration of the fever.
- Ask the patient to describe the pattern of the fever.
- Find out if the patient has a history of endocrine dysfunction or malignant hyperthermia.
- Ask the patient about drug history.
- Find out about the medical and surgical history, including recent trauma, burns, or blood transfusions.
- Ask about the patient's work environment and water consumption while working.

Physical examination

- Perform a complete physical examination.
- Monitor the patient's vital signs and the cardiac rate, rhythm, and intensity.
- Note the rate and depth of the patient's breathing and any changes from normal respiratory patterns.
- Inspect skin color and temperature; check skin turgor and monitor for diaphoresis.
- Check for signs of trauma or needle marks on the arms or legs.
- Inspect for shivering of the body or flushing of the face.
- Assess the patient's mental status and be alert for signs of malaise, fatigue, restlessness, or anxiety.
- Auscultate lung fields and the abdomen.

Causes

Medical causes

Infection and inflammatory disorders

- Depending on the specific disorder, the temperature elevation may be insidious or abrupt.
- It can be a prodromal symptom and is commonly accompanied by chills, goose bumps, generalized symptoms of fatigue, headache, weakness, anorexia, malaise and, possibly, pain.
- Other signs and symptoms depend on the disease and can involve any body system.

Malignant hyperthermia

- Rapid temperature increases occur at a rate of about 2° F (1.1° C) every 15 minutes to as high as 109.4° F (43° C). Usually the rise is preceded by skeletal rigidity, cardiac arrhythmias, tachycardia, and tachypnea.

Neuroleptic malignant syndrome

- This syndrome is marked by an explosive onset of hyperthermia.
- Other accompanying signs and symptoms include muscle rigidity, altered LOC, cardiac arrhythmias, tachycardia, wide fluctuations in blood pressure, postural instability, dyspnea, and tachypnea.

Thermoregulatory dysfunction

- The patient's temperature rises suddenly and rapidly, then stays at 105° F to 107° F (40.6° C to 41.7° C).
- Signs and symptoms include hot flushed skin, decreased LOC, tachycardia, and hypotension.
- Other signs and symptoms include mottled cyanosis, if the patient has malignant hyperthermia; diarrhea, if he's experiencing thyroid storm; and signs of increased intracranial pressure, if the problem is central nervous system trauma or hemorrhage.

Other causes

Drugs

- Hyperthermia can result from the use of tricyclic antidepressants and drugs that impair sweating, such as anticholinergics, phenothiazines, and monoamine oxidase inhibitors.

Impaired heat dissipation

- This condition occurs with severe dehydration in which sweat production decreases to conserve further fluid loss, which impairs heat loss by evaporation.
- Impaired heat dissipation also occurs when the environmental temperature is high, and the body can't rid itself of heat as fast as it's being received.

Nursing considerations

Treat mild to moderate hyperthermia by doing the following:

- Provide a cool, restful environment.
- Replace oral or I.V. fluid and electrolyte losses.

If the patient experiences heatstroke:

- Apply cool water to the skin and fan the patient.
- Apply a hyperthermia blanket or ice packs to the groin or axilla.
- Expect treatment to continue until the patient's body temperature drops to 102.2° F (39° C).
- Continuously monitor the patient's vital signs, especially the core body temperature.
- Monitor hemodynamic parameters, fluid and electrolyte balance, and laboratory and diagnostic tests.

Patient teaching

- Caution the patient to reduce activity, especially outdoor activity, in hot, humid weather.
- Advise him to wear light-colored, lightweight, loose-fitting clothing as well as a hat and sunglasses during hot weather.
- Instruct the patient to drink sufficient fluids—especially water—in hot weather and after vigorous physical activity.
- Warn him to avoid caffeine and alcohol in hot weather.
- Advise the patient to use air conditioning or to open windows and use a fan to help circulate air indoors.

Hypotension, orthostatic

In orthostatic hypotension, the patient's blood pressure drops 15 to 20 mm Hg or more—with or without an increase in the heart rate of at least 20 beats/minute—when he rises from a supine to a sitting or standing position. (Blood pressure should be measured 5 minutes after the patient has changed his position.) This common sign indicates failure of compensatory vasomotor responses to adjust to position changes. It's typically associated with lightheadedness, syncope, or blurred vision and may occur in a hypotensive, normotensive, or hypertensive patient. Although commonly a nonpathologic sign in an elderly person, orthostatic hypotension may result from prolonged bed rest, fluid and electrolyte imbalance, endocrine or systemic disorders, and the effects of drugs.

To detect orthostatic hypotension, take and compare blood pressure readings with the patient supine, sitting, and then standing.

QUICK ACTION ***If you detect orthostatic hypotension, quickly check for tachycardia, an altered level of consciousness (LOC), and pale, clammy skin. If these signs are present, suspect hypovolemic shock. Insert a large-bore I.V. catheter for fluid or blood replacement. Take the patient's vital signs every 15 minutes, and monitor his intake and output. Encourage bed rest until the patient's condition is stable.***

History

- Ask about dizziness, weakness, or fainting when standing.
- Inquire about fatigue, orthopnea, nausea, headache, abdominal or chest discomfort, and GI bleeding.
- Obtain a drug history.

Physical examination

- Obtain the patient's vital signs, and weigh him.
- Check skin turgor.
- Palpate peripheral pulses.
- Auscultate the heart and lungs.
- Test muscle strength and observe gait for unsteadiness.
- Obtain blood samples for laboratory studies.

Causes

Medical causes

Adrenal insufficiency

- Orthostatic hypotension may be accompanied by fatigue, muscle weakness, poor coordination, anorexia, nausea, vomiting, fasting hypoglycemia, weight loss, irritability, abdominal pain, hyperpigmentation, and a weak, irregular pulse.
- Other signs and symptoms include diarrhea, constipation, decreased libido, amenorrhea, syncope, and enhanced taste, smell, and hearing.

Amyloidosis

- Orthostatic hypotension is common.
- Other signs and symptoms include angina, tachycardia, dyspnea, orthopnea, fatigue, and cough.

Diabetic autonomic neuropathy

- Orthostatic hypotension is accompanied by syncope, dysphagia, constipation or diarrhea, painless bladder distention with overflow incontinence, impotence, and retrograde ejaculation.

Hyperaldosteronism

- Orthostatic hypotension with sustained elevated blood pressure occurs.
- Other signs and symptoms include muscle weakness, intermittent flaccid paralysis, fatigue, headache, paresthesia, vision disturbances, nocturia, polydipsia, personality changes and, possibly, tetany.

Hyponatremia

- Orthostatic hypotension occurs with headache, profound thirst, nausea, vomiting, muscle twitching and weakness, fatigue, oliguria or anuria, tachycardia, abdominal cramps, irritability, seizures, decreased LOC, and cold, clammy skin.
- If severe, cyanosis, thready pulse and, eventually, vasomotor collapse occurs.

Hypovolemia

- Orthostatic hypotension occurs with apathy, fatigue, muscle weakness, anorexia, nausea, and profound thirst.
- Other signs and symptoms include dizziness, oliguria, sunken eyeballs, poor skin turgor, and dry mucous membranes.

Other causes

Drugs

- Antihypertensives, diuretics in large doses, levodopa (Larodopa), monoamine oxidase inhibitors, morphine, nitrates, phenothiazines, spinal anesthesia, and tricyclic antidepressants may cause orthostatic hypotension.

Treatments

- Orthostatic hypotension is common with prolonged bed rest.
- Sympathectomy may cause orthostatic hypotension by disrupting normal vasoconstrictive mechanisms.

Nursing considerations

- Elevate the head of the bed, and help the patient to a sitting position with his feet dangling over the side of the bed; if tolerated, have him sit in a chair briefly.
- Monitor intake and output and weigh the patient daily.
- Evaluate the need for assistive devices.
- Help the patient with walking.

Patient teaching

- Discuss the underlying condition, diagnostic tests, and treatment options.
- Explain the importance of avoiding volume depletion.
- Explain how to change position gradually.
- Teach the patient preambulation exercises to do before getting out of bed.

Hypothermia

Hypothermia refers to a core body temperature below 95° F (35° C) and affects chemical changes in the body. It may be classified as mild—89.6° to 95° F (32° to 35° C), moderate—86° to 89.6° F (30° to 32° C), or severe, which may be fatal—77° to 86° F (25° to 30° C). Risk factors that contribute to serious cold injury, especially hypothermia, include the lack of insulating body fat, wet or inadequate clothing, drug abuse, cardiac disease, smoking, fatigue, malnutrition and depletion of calorie reserves, and excessive alcohol intake. The incidence of hypothermia is highest in children and elderly people.

Hypothermia commonly results from cold-water near drowning and prolonged exposure to cold temperatures. It can also occur in normal temperatures if disease or debility alters the patient's homeostasis. The administration of large amounts of cold blood or blood products can also cause hypothermia. A process such as hemodialysis, which circulates the blood outside of the body and then returns it to the body, will result in hypothermia.

***QUICK ACTION** Initiate cardiopulmonary resuscitation (CPR), if necessary. Hypothermia helps protect the brain from anoxia, which normally accompanies prolonged cardiopulmonary arrest. Therefore, even if the patient has been unresponsive for a long time, CPR may resuscitate him, especially after cold-water near drowning. Institute continuous cardiac monitoring and administer supplemental oxygen. Prepare the patient for intubation and mechanical ventilation, if necessary. Prepare the patient for placement of a pulmonary artery catheter to monitor core body temperature. Monitor the patient's vital signs closely. Continue warming the patient until the core body temperature is within 1° to 2° F (0.6° to 1.1° C) of the desired body temperature. If the patient has been hypothermic for longer than 45 minutes, administer additional fluids, as ordered, to compensate for the expansion of the vascular space that occurs during vasodilation in warming.*

If oxygen therapy is needed, be sure to use warm, humidified oxygen to prevent additional cooling.

History

- Obtain the patient's history for clues to the causative factor. Was he exposed to cold and, if so, what temperature and for what length of time?
- Ask whether he has recently undergone hemodialysis therapy, had major surgery, or recently received a blood transfusion where the blood was still cold.
- Find out about a history of thyroid, adrenal, liver, or cerebrovascular diseases.
- Ask about ingestion of such substances as alcohol or barbiturates.

Physical examination

- Assess the patient's level of consciousness; a patient with mild hypothermia will have amnesia, a patient with moderate hypothermia is unresponsive, and the patient with severe hypothermia will be comatose.
- Assess for shivering, slurred speech, and peripheral cyanosis.
- Assess the patient's neurologic status and presence or absence of deep tendon reflexes.
- Assess the muscle rigidity that can produce a rigor mortis-like state.

Causes

Medical causes

Prolonged exposure to extremely low temperatures

- The patient has severe hypothermia, accompanied by lethargy or coma, depressed respiratory rate and depth, bradycardia, and muscle stiffness.

Other causes

Disorders

- Hypothermia may be a result of a certain disorder, but may require immediate intervention.
- Endocrine disorders, such as hypothyroidism, hypoadrenalism, hypopituitarism, diabetes mellitus, cirrhosis, stroke, and renal failure, also affect the body's ability to regulate temperature.

Drugs

- Alcohol ingestion and an overdose of barbiturates can induce mild to moderate hypothermia as a result of vasodilation, lowered metabolism, and central nervous system effects.

Nursing considerations

- Specific rewarming techniques include passive rewarming (the patient rewarms on his own), active rewarming (using heating blankets, warm-water immersion, heated objects such as water bottles, and radiant heat), and active core warming (using heated I.V. fluids, genitourinary tract irrigation, extracorporeal warming, and lavage).
- Administration of oxygen, endotracheal intubation, controlled ventilation, I.V. fluids, and treatment of metabolic acidosis depend upon test results and careful patient monitoring.
- Stay alert for signs and symptoms of hyperkalemia.

Patient teaching

- Advise the patient, especially if he's elderly, to maintain proper insulation in the home and keep the indoor temperature set to 70° F (21.1° C) or higher.
- Caution the patient to wear warm clothing and use warm bedding.
- Advise the patient of the importance of adequate nutrition, rest, and exercise.
- Advise the patient to wear loose-fitting clothing in layers, cover his feet and head, wear wind- and water-resistant outer garments, and avoid alcohol intake when out in the cold, especially for prolonged periods.

I

Insomnia

Insomnia is the inability to fall asleep, remain asleep, or feel refreshed by sleep. Acute and transient during periods of stress, insomnia may become chronic, causing constant fatigue, extreme anxiety as bedtime approaches, and psychiatric disorders. This common complaint is experienced occasionally by about 25% of U.S. residents and chronically by another 10%.

Physiologic causes of insomnia include jet lag, arguing, and lack of exercise. Pathophysiologic causes range from medical and psychiatric disorders to pain, adverse effects of a drug, and idiopathic factors. Complaints of insomnia are subjective and require close investigation; for example, the patient may mistakenly attribute his fatigue from an organic cause, such as anemia, to insomnia.

History

- Obtain a sleep history.
- Determine when the onset of insomnia occurred.
- Obtain a drug history, noting the use of central nervous system (CNS) stimulants and over-the-counter medications.
- Ask about the use of caffeine and caffeinated beverages.
- Obtain a medical history of chronic or acute conditions, including painful or pruritic conditions.
- Ask about alcohol use.
- Determine the patient's emotional status and stress factors.
- Obtain a psychosocial history, noting factors such as frequent travel, exercise, and personal or job-related problems.

Physical examination

- Perform a complete physical examination.
- Pay close attention to findings that suggest a neurologic, cardiac, respiratory, or endocrine disorder.

Causes

Medical causes

Alcohol withdrawal syndrome

- Insomnia may persist for up to 2 years.
- Other early effects include excessive diaphoresis, tachycardia, hypertension, tremors, restlessness, irritability, headache, nausea, flushing, and nightmares.
- Progression to alcohol withdrawal delirium as soon as 48 hours after cessation produces confusion, disorientation, paranoia, delusions, hallucinations, and seizures.

Depression

- Chronic insomnia occurs with difficulty falling asleep, waking and being unable to fall back to sleep, or waking early in the morning.
- The patient also experiences loss of interest in his usual activities, feelings of worthlessness and guilt, fatigue, difficulty concentrating, indecisiveness, and recurrent thoughts of death.
- Other signs and symptoms include dysphoria, decreased appetite with weight loss or increased appetite with

weight gain, and psychomotor agitation or retardation.

Generalized anxiety disorder

- Chronic insomnia occurs with fatigue, restlessness, diaphoresis, dyspepsia, high resting pulse and respiratory rates, and signs of apprehension.

Nocturnal myoclonus

- Involuntary and fleeting muscle jerks of the legs occur every 5 to 90 seconds, disturbing sleep.
- The patient reports poor sleep and daytime somnolence.
- The condition can occur in patients with diabetes or restless leg syndrome.

Pain

- Conditions that cause pain can also cause insomnia.
- Behavioral responses include altered body position, moaning, grimacing, withdrawal, crying, restlessness, muscle twitching, and immobility.
- With mild or moderate pain, signs and symptoms include pallor, elevated blood pressure, dilated pupils, skeletal muscle tension, dyspnea, tachycardia, and diaphoresis.
- With severe and deep pain, signs and symptoms include pallor, decreased blood pressure, bradycardia, nausea, vomiting, weakness, dizziness, and loss of consciousness.

Restless leg syndrome

- Uncomfortable sensations in the leg cause uncontrollable urges to move the limb; movement brings relief, and sleep is usually disrupted, causing insomnia.

Sleep apnea syndrome

- Sleep is disturbed by apneic periods that end with a series of gasps and eventual wakefulness.
- With central sleep apnea, respiratory movement ceases for the apneic period.
- With obstructive sleep apnea, upper airway obstruction blocks incoming air, but breathing movements continue.
- Other signs and symptoms include morning headache, daytime fatigue, hypertension, ankle edema, and personality changes.

Thyrotoxicosis

- Difficulty falling asleep and then sleeping for only a brief period is a characteristic symptom.
- Other signs and symptoms include dyspnea, tachycardia, palpitations, atrial or ventricular gallop, weight loss despite increased appetite, diarrhea, tremors, nervousness, diaphoresis, hypersensitivity to heat, an enlarged thyroid gland, and exophthalmos.

Other causes

Drugs

- Use of, abuse of, or withdrawal from sedatives or hypnotics may produce insomnia.
- CNS stimulants may also produce insomnia.

Nursing considerations

- Prepare the patient for tests to evaluate his insomnia.
- Institute measures to help relieve insomnia.
- Caffeine intake should be avoided, especially 2 to 4 hours before bedtime.

Patient teaching

- Teach the patient techniques to increase comfort and relaxation.
- Advise him to wake up at the same time each day, go to bed at the same time each night, and exercise regularly—but not close to bedtime.
- Discuss the appropriate use of tranquilizers or sedatives.
- Refer the patient for counseling or to a sleep disorder clinic as needed.

Intermittent claudication

Most common in the legs, intermittent claudication is cramping limb pain brought on by exercise and relieved by 1 to 2 minutes of rest. This pain may be acute or chronic; when acute, it may signal acute arterial occlusion. Intermittent claudication is most common in men ages 50 to 60 with a history of diabetes mellitus, hyperlipidemia, hypertension, or tobacco use. Without treatment, it may progress to pain at rest. With chronic arterial occlusion, limb loss is uncommon because collateral circulation usually develops.

With occlusive artery disease, intermittent claudication results from an inadequate blood supply. Pain in the calf (the most common area) or foot indicates disease of the femoral or popliteal arteries. Pain in the buttocks and upper thigh indicates disease of the aortoiliac arteries. During exercise, pain typically results from the release of lactic acid due to anaerobic metabolism in the ischemic segment, secondary to obstruction. When exercise stops, the lactic acid clears and the pain subsides.

Intermittent claudication may also have a neurologic cause: narrowing of the vertebral column at the level of the cauda equina. This condition creates pressure on the nerve roots to the lower extremities. Walking stimulates circulation to the cauda equina, causing increased pressure on those nerves and resultant pain.

Physical findings include pallor on elevation, rubor on dependency (especially the toes and soles), loss of hair on the toes, and diminished arterial pulses.

QUICK ACTION ***If the patient has sudden intermittent claudication with severe or aching leg pain at rest, check the leg's temperature and color and palpate femoral, popliteal, posterior tibial, and dorsalis pedis pulses. Ask about numbness and tingling. Suspect acute arterial occlusion if pulses are absent; if the leg feels cold and looks pale, cyanotic, or mottled; and if paresthesia and pain are present. Mark the area of pallor, cyanosis, or mottling, and reassess it frequently, noting an increase in the area.***

Don't elevate the leg. Protect it, allowing nothing to press on it. Prepare the patient for preoperative blood tests, urinalysis, electrocardiography, chest X-rays, lower-extremity Doppler studies, and angiography. Insert an I.V. catheter, and administer an anticoagulant and analgesics, as ordered.

History

- Ask the patient how far he can walk before pain occurs, how long it takes for pain to subside, and recent changes in the pattern and characteristics of the pain.
- Explore risk factors, such as smoking, diabetes, hypertension, and hyperlipidemia.
- Ask about associated signs and symptoms, such as paresthesia in the affected limb and visible changes in the color of the fingers.

Physical examination

- Palpate lower extremity pulses; note character, strength, and bilateral equality.
- Note color and temperature differences between the legs and compare with the arms.
- Auscultate for bruits over major arteries.
- Elevate the affected leg for 2 minutes and assess color changes; note how long it takes for color to return when legs are dependent.
- Examine the feet, toes, and fingers for ulceration.
- Inspect the hands and lower legs for small, tender nodules and erythema along blood vessels.

- If the patient has arm pain, inspect the arms for a change in color (to white) on elevation.
- Palpate and compare upper extremity pulses.

Causes

Medical causes

Aortic arteriosclerotic occlusive disease

- Intermittent claudication occurs in the buttock, hip, thigh, and calf, along with absent or diminished femoral pulses.
- Other signs and symptoms include bruits over the femoral and iliac arteries, pallor and coolness of the affected limb on elevation, and profound limb weakness.

Arterial occlusion, acute

- Intense intermittent claudication occurs.
- The limb is cool, pale, and cyanotic with absent pulses below the occlusion.
- Other signs and symptoms include paresthesia, paresis, increased capillary refill time, and a sensation of cold in the affected limb.

Arteriosclerosis obliterans

- Intermittent claudication appears in the calf along with diminished or absent popliteal and pedal pulses, coolness in the affected limb, pallor on elevation, and profound limb weakness with continuing exercise.
- Other signs and symptoms include numbness, paresthesia and, in more severe disease, pain in the toes or foot while at rest, ulceration, and gangrene.

Buerger's disease

- Intermittent claudication of the instep is typical in this inflammatory vascular disorder.
- Early signs include migratory superficial nodules and erythema along extremity blood vessels and migratory venous phlebitis.
- With exposure to cold, the feet initially become cold, cyanotic, and numb; later, they redden, become hot, and tingle.
- Other signs and symptoms include impaired peripheral pulses, paresthesia of the hands and feet, and migratory superficial thrombophlebitis.

Leriche syndrome

- Arterial occlusion causes intermittent claudication of the hip, thigh, buttocks, and calf and also causes impotence in men.
- Other signs and symptoms include bruits, global atrophy, absent or diminished pulses, gangrene of the toes, and legs that become cool and pale with elevation.

Neurogenic claudication

- Pain from intermittent claudication requires a longer rest time than pain from vascular claudication.
- Other signs and symptoms include paresthesia, weakness and clumsiness when walking, and hypoactive deep tendon reflexes after walking.

Nursing considerations

- Encourage the patient to exercise.
- Advise the patient to avoid prolonged sitting or standing as well as crossing his legs at the knees.

Patient teaching

- Discuss with the patient the risk factors, diagnostic tests, and treatment options, including medications, for intermittent claudication.
- Stress the importance of inspecting his legs and feet for ulcers.
- Explain ways the patient can protect his extremities from injury and elements.
- Teach the patient the signs and symptoms he should report.
- Teach the patient exercises to improve circulation in his legs.

J

Jaundice

A yellow discoloration of the skin, mucous membranes, or sclera of the eyes, jaundice indicates excessive levels of conjugated or unconjugated bilirubin in the blood. In fair-skinned patients, it's most noticeable on the face, trunk, and sclera; in dark-skinned patients, on the hard palate, sclera, and conjunctiva.

Jaundice is most apparent in natural sunlight. In fact, it may be undetectable in artificial or poor light. It's commonly accompanied by pruritus (because bile pigment damages sensory nerves), dark urine, and clay-colored stools.

Jaundice may result from any of three pathophysiologic processes. It may be the only warning sign of certain disorders such as pancreatic cancer.

History

- Ask about the onset of jaundice.
- Inquire about associated pruritus, clay-colored stools, dark urine, fatigue, fever, chills, GI signs or symptoms, and cardiopulmonary symptoms.
- Obtain a medical history, including incidence of cancer; liver, pancreatic, or gallbladder disease; hepatitis; or gallstones.
- Ask about drug and alcohol use.
- Find out about recent weight loss.

Physical examination

- Perform the physical examination in a room with natural light.
- Rule out hypercarotenemia, which is more prominent on the palms and soles and doesn't affect the sclera.
- Inspect the skin for texture, dryness, hyperpigmentation, spider angiomas, petechiae, and xanthomas.
- Note clubbed fingers and gynecomastia.
- Palpate the abdomen for tenderness, pain, and swelling.
- Palpate and percuss the liver and spleen for enlargement.
- Test for ascites.
- Auscultate for arrhythmias, murmurs, or gallops.
- Palpate lymph nodes for swelling.
- Obtain baseline data on mental status.

Causes

Medical causes

Carcinoma

- Cancer of the hepatopancreatic ampulla produces fluctuating jaundice, occult bleeding, mild abdominal pain, recurrent fever, weight loss, pruritus, back pain, and chills.
- Hepatic cancer produces jaundice, right upper quadrant discomfort and tenderness, nausea, weight loss, slight fever, ascites, edema, and an irregular, nodular, firm, enlarged liver.
- With pancreatic cancer, progressive jaundice may be the only sign. However, other signs and symptoms that may occur are weight loss, back or abdominal pain, anorexia, nausea, vomiting, fever, steatorrhea, fatigue, weakness, diarrhea, pruritus, and skin lesions.

Cholangitis

- Jaundice along with right upper quadrant pain and high fever with chills make up Charcot's triad.
- Other signs and symptoms include pruritus and clay-colored stools.

Cholecystitis

- Nonobstructive jaundice occurs.
- Biliary colic typically peaks abruptly, persisting for 2 to 4 hours, and then localizes to the right upper quadrant and becomes constant.
- Other signs and symptoms include nausea, vomiting, fever, profuse diaphoresis, chills, tenderness on palpation, a positive Murphy's sign, and abdominal distention and rigidity.

Cholelithiasis

- Jaundice and biliary colic are common.
- Pain is severe and steady in the right upper quadrant or epigastrium, radiates to the right scapula or shoulder, and intensifies over several hours.
- Other signs and symptoms include nausea, vomiting, tachycardia, restlessness and, if the common bile duct is occluded, fever, chills, jaundice, clay-colored stools, and abdominal tenderness.

Cholestasis

- Prolonged attacks of jaundice (sometimes spaced several years apart) are accompanied by pruritus.
- Other signs and symptoms include fatigue, nausea, weight loss, anorexia, pale stools, and right upper quadrant pain.

Cirrhosis

- With Laënnec's cirrhosis, mild to moderate jaundice occurs with pruritus; common early signs and symptoms include ascites, weakness, leg edema, nausea, vomiting, diarrhea or constipation, anorexia, massive hematemesis, weight loss, and right upper quadrant pain.
- With primary biliary cirrhosis, fluctuating jaundice may appear years after the onset of other signs and symptoms, such as pruritus that worsens at bedtime (commonly the first sign), weakness, fatigue, weight loss, and vague abdominal pain.

Glucose-6-phosphate dehydrogenase deficiency

- Jaundice occurs along with pallor, dyspnea, tachycardia, malaise, and hepatosplenomegaly in this congenital abnormality.

Heart failure

- Jaundice occurs with severe right-sided heart failure due to liver dysfunction.
- Other signs and symptoms include jugular vein distention, cyanosis, dependent edema, weight gain, weakness, confusion, hepatomegaly, nausea, vomiting, abdominal discomfort, anorexia, and ascites (a late sign).

Hemolytic anemia, acquired

- Prominent jaundice appears with dyspnea, fatigue, pallor, tachycardia, and palpitations.
- With rapid hemolysis, chills, fever, irritability, headache, and abdominal pain may occur, and signs of shock may appear.

Hepatitis

- Jaundice occurs late and is preceded by dark urine and clay-colored stools.
- Signs and symptoms during the icteric phase include weight loss, anorexia, right upper quadrant pain and tenderness, and an enlarged liver.
- Other signs and symptoms include fatigue, nausea, vomiting, malaise, arthralgia, myalgia, headache, anorexia, photophobia, pharyngitis, cough, diar-

rhea or constipation, and low-grade fever.

Pancreatitis, acute

- Jaundice may occur.
- The primary symptom is usually severe epigastric pain that may radiate to the back and is relieved by lying with the knees flexed on the chest or sitting up and leaning forward.
- Other signs and symptoms include nausea, persistent vomiting, Turner's or Cullen's sign, fever, and abdominal distention, rigidity, and tenderness.

Sickle cell anemia

- Jaundice occurs with impaired growth and development, increased susceptibility to infection, thrombotic complications, leg ulcers, swollen and painful joints, fever, chills, bone aches, and chest pain.

Other causes

Drugs

- Jaundice may occur with drugs that cause hepatic injury, such as acetaminophen (Tylenol), isoniazid (Nydrazid), hormonal contraceptives, sulfonamides, mercaptopurine (Purinethol), erythromycin estolate (Ilosone), niacin, troleandomycin (TAO), androgenic steroids, 3-hydroxy-3-methylglutaryl coenzyme A reductase inhibitors, phenothiazines, ethanol, methyldopa (Aldoril), rifampin (Rifadin), phenytoin (Dilantin), and I.V. tetracyclines.

Treatments

- Upper abdominal surgery may result in jaundice because of organ manipulation leading to edema and obstructed bile flow.
- Surgical shunts used to reduce portal hypertension may also produce jaundice.
- Prolonged surgery resulting in shock, blood loss, or blood transfusion can cause jaundice.

Nursing considerations

- To decrease pruritus:
  - Frequently bathe the patient.
  - Apply an antipruritic lotion such as calamine.
  - Administer diphenhydramine (Benadryl) or hydroxyzine (Atarax, Vistaril).

Patient teaching

- Discuss the underlying condition, diagnostic tests, and treatment options.
- Teach the patient appropriate dietary changes he can make.
- Discuss ways to reduce pruritus.

Jaw pain

Jaw pain may arise from either of the two bones that hold the teeth in the jaw—the maxilla (upper jaw) and the mandible (lower jaw). Jaw pain also includes pain in the temporomandibular joint (TMJ), where the mandible meets the temporal bone.

Jaw pain may develop gradually or abruptly and may range from barely noticeable to excruciating, depending on its cause. It usually results from disorders of the teeth, soft tissue, or glands of the mouth or throat or from local trauma or infection. Systemic causes include musculoskeletal, neurologic, cardiovascular, endocrine, immunologic, metabolic, and infectious disorders. Life-threatening disorders, such as a myocardial infarction (MI) and tetany, also produce jaw pain as well as certain drugs (especially phenothiazines) and dental or surgical procedures.

Jaw pain is seldom a primary indicator of any one disorder; however, some causes are medical emergencies.

QUICK ACTION ***Ask the patient when the jaw pain began. Did it arise suddenly or gradually? Is it more severe or frequent now than when it first occurred? Sudden, severe jaw pain, especially***

when associated with chest pain, shortness of breath, or arm pain, requires prompt evaluation because it may indicate a life-threatening MI.

Perform an electrocardiogram and obtain blood samples for cardiac enzyme levels. Administer oxygen, morphine sulfate, and a vasodilator as indicated.

History

- Determine the onset, character, intensity, and frequency of jaw pain.
- Ask whether the jaw pain radiates to other areas.
- Ask about recent trauma, surgery, or procedures.
- Inquire about associated signs and symptoms, such as joint or chest pain, dyspnea, palpitations, fatigue, headache, malaise, anorexia, weight loss, intermittent claudication, diplopia, and hearing loss.
- Ask about aggravating or alleviating factors.

Physical examination

- Inspect the painful area for redness; palpate for edema or warmth.
- Look for facial asymmetry.
- Check the TMJs, noting crepitus and ability to open the mouth.
- Palpate the parotid area for pain and swelling.
- Inspect and palpate the oral cavity for lesions, elevation of the tongue, or masses.

Causes

Medical causes

Angina pectoris

- Jaw and left arm pain may radiate from the substernal area.
- It may be triggered by exertion, emotional stress, or ingestion of a heavy meal and subsides with rest or administration of nitroglycerin.
- Other signs and symptoms include shortness of breath, nausea, vomiting, tachycardia, dizziness, diaphoresis, and palpitations.

Arthritis

- Osteoarthritis causes aching jaw pain that increases with activity and may be accompanied by crepitus, enlarged joints with restricted range of motion (ROM), and stiffness on awakening that improves with activity.
- Rheumatoid arthritis causes symmetrical pain in all joints, including the jaw.
- Other signs and symptoms of rheumatoid arthritis include tender, swollen joints with limited ROM that are stiff after inactivity; myalgia; fatigue; weight loss; malaise; anorexia; lymphadenopathy; mild fever; painless, movable nodules on the elbows, knees, and knuckles; joint deformities and crepitus; and multiple systemic complications.

Head and neck cancer

- Jaw pain has an insidious onset.
- Other signs and symptoms include a history of leukoplakia ulcers on the mucous membranes; palpable masses in the jaw, mouth, and neck; dysphagia; bloody discharge; drooling; lymphadenopathy; and trismus.

Hypocalcemic tetany

- Painful muscle contractions of the jaw and mouth occur with paresthesia and carpopedal spasms.
- Other signs and symptoms include weakness, fatigue, palpitations, hyperreflexia, positive Chvostek's and Trousseau's signs, muscle twitching, choreiform movements, muscle cramps and, with severe hypocalcemia, laryngospasm with stridor, cyanosis, seizures, and arrhythmias.

Ludwig's angina

- Severe jaw pain in the mandibular area occurs with tongue elevation, sub-

lingual edema, fever, and drooling caused by cellulitis.
■ Progressive disease produces dysphagia, dysphonia, stridor, and dyspnea.

Myocardial infarction
■ In this life-threatening disorder, crushing substernal pain may radiate to the lower jaw, left arm, neck, back, or shoulder blades.
■ Other signs and symptoms include pallor, clammy skin, dyspnea, excessive diaphoresis, nausea, vomiting, anxiety, restlessness, a feeling of impending doom, low-grade fever, decreased or increased blood pressure, arrhythmias, an atrial gallop, new murmurs, and crackles.

Osteomyelitis
■ Aching jaw pain may occur along with warmth, swelling, tenderness, erythema, and restricted jaw movement.
■ Tachycardia, sudden fever, nausea, and malaise may occur with acute osteomyelitis.

Sinusitis
■ Maxillary sinusitis produces intense boring pain in the maxilla and cheek that may radiate to the eye along with a feeling of fullness, increased pain on percussion of the first and second molars and, in those with nasal obstruction, the loss of the sense of smell.
■ Sphenoid sinusitis produces chronic pain at the mandibular ramus and vertex of the head and in the temporal area.
■ Other signs and symptoms of both types of sinusitis include fever, halitosis, headache, malaise, cough, sore throat, and fever.

Suppurative parotitis
■ Onset of jaw pain, high fever, and chills is abrupt.
■ Other signs and symptoms include erythema and edema of the overlying skin; a tender, swollen gland; and pus at the second molar.

Temporal arteritis
■ Sharp jaw pain occurs after chewing or talking.
■ Other signs and symptoms include low-grade fever; generalized muscle pain; malaise; fatigue; anorexia; weight loss; throbbing, unilateral headache in the frontotemporal regions; swollen, nodular, tender and, possibly, pulseless temporal arteries; and erythema of the overlying skin.

Temporomandibular joint disorders
■ Jaw pain at the TMJ; spasm and pain of the masticating muscle; clicking, popping, or crepitus of the TMJ; and restricted jaw movement may occur.
■ Other signs and symptoms include localized pain that may radiate to other head and neck areas, teeth clenching, bruxism, ear pain, headache, deviation of the jaw to the affected side upon opening the mouth, and jaw subluxation or dislocation, especially after yawning.

Trauma
■ Jaw pain may occur with swelling and decreased jaw mobility.
■ Other signs and symptoms include hypotension, tachycardia, lacerations, ecchymoses, hematomas, blurred vision, and rhinorrhea or otorrhea.

Trigeminal neuralgia
■ Paroxysmal attacks of intense unilateral jaw pain (stopping at the facial midline) or rapid-fire shooting sensations in one division of the trigeminal nerve (usually the mandibular or maxillary division) occur.
■ Pain is felt mainly over the lips and chin and in the teeth, mouth and nose areas may be hypersensitive, and

corneal reflexes are diminished or absent (if the ophthalmic branch is involved).

Other causes

Drugs

- Some drugs, such as phenothiazines, affect the extrapyramidal tract, causing dyskinesia; others cause tetany of the jaw from hypocalcemia.

Nursing considerations

- If pain is severe, withhold food, liquids, and oral medications until diagnosis is confirmed.
- Administer an analgesic.
- Apply an ice pack if the jaw is swollen.
- Discourage the patient from talking or moving the jaw.
- Mumps causes unilateral or bilateral swelling from the lower mandible to the zygomatic arch.
- When trauma causes jaw pain in children, always consider the possibility of abuse.

Patient teaching

- Explain the disorder and the treatments that the patient needs.
- Teach the patient the proper way to insert mouth splints if indicated.
- Discuss ways to reduce stress.
- Explain the identification and avoidance of triggers.

Jugular vein distention

Jugular vein distention is the abnormal fullness and height of the pulse waves in the internal or external jugular veins. For a patient in a supine position with his head elevated 45 degrees, a pulse wave height greater than 1¼″ to 1½″ (3 to 4 cm) above the angle of Louis indicates distention. Engorged, distended veins reflect increased venous pressure in the right side of the heart, which, in turn, indicates increased central venous pressure. This common sign characteristically occurs in heart failure and other cardiovascular disorders, such as constrictive pericarditis, tricuspid stenosis, and obstruction of the superior vena cava.

QUICK ACTION ***Evaluating jugular vein distention involves visualizing and assessing venous pulsations. (See*** **Evaluating jugular vein distention.*) If you detect jugular vein distention in the patient with pale, clammy skin who suddenly appears anxious and dyspneic, take his blood pressure. If you note hypotension and a paradoxical pulse, suspect cardiac tamponade. Elevate the foot of the bed 20 to 30 degrees, give supplemental oxygen, and monitor cardiac status and rhythm, oxygen saturation, and mental status. Insert an I.V. catheter for medication administration, and keep cardiopulmonary resuscitation equipment close by. Assemble the needed equipment for emergency pericardiocentesis to relieve pressure on the heart. Throughout the procedure, monitor the patient's blood pressure, heart rhythm, respirations, and pulse oximetry.***

History

- Ask out about recent weight gain or swelling.
- Inquire about associated chest pain, shortness of breath, paroxysmal nocturnal dyspnea, anorexia, nausea, or vomiting.
- Obtain a medical history, including incidence of cancer or cardiac, pulmonary, hepatic, or renal disease; recent trauma; or surgery.
- Obtain a drug history, noting the use of diuretics.
- Inquire about diet history, especially sodium intake.

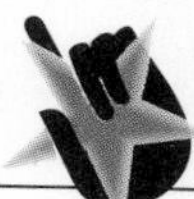

KNOW-HOW

Evaluating jugular vein distention

With the patient in a supine position, position him so that you can visualize jugular vein pulsations reflected from the right atrium. Elevate the head of the bed 45 to 90 degrees. (In the normal patient, veins distend only when the patient lies flat.)

Next, locate the angle of Louis (sternal notch)—the reference point for measuring venous pressure. To do so, palpate the clavicles where they join the sternum (the suprasternal notch). Place your first two fingers on the suprasternal notch. Then, without lifting them from the skin, slide them down the sternum until you feel a bony protuberance—this is the angle of Louis.

Find the internal jugular vein (which indicates venous pressure more reliably than the external jugular vein). Shine a flashlight across the patient's neck to create shadows that highlight his venous pulse. Be sure to distinguish jugular vein pulsations from carotid artery pulsations. One way to do this is to palpate the vessel: Arterial pulsations continue, whereas venous pulsations disappear with light finger pressure. Also, venous pulsations increase or decrease with changes in body position; arterial pulsations remain constant.

Next, locate the highest point along the vein where you can see pulsations. Using a centimeter ruler, measure the distance between that high point and the sternal notch. Record this finding as well as the angle at which the patient was lying. A finding greater than 1¼" to 1½" (3 to 4 cm) above the sternal notch, with the head of the bed at a 45-degree angle, indicates jugular vein distention.

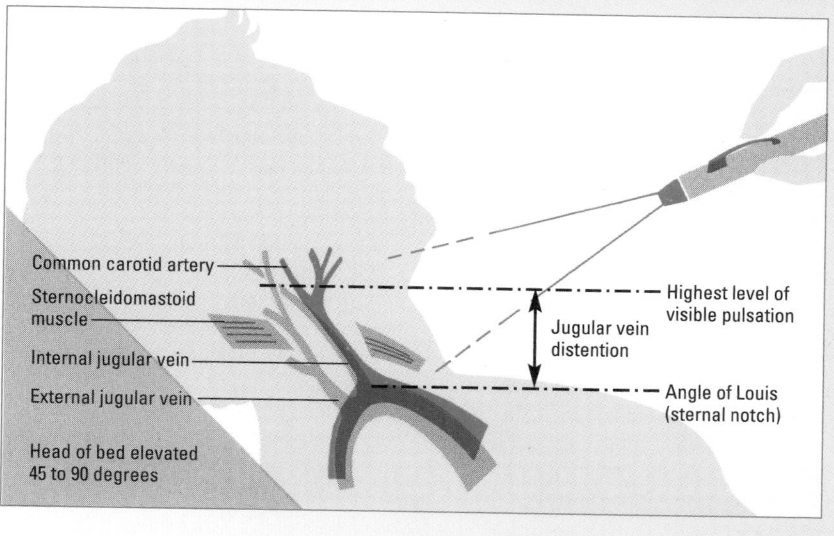

CASE CLIP

Responding to jugular vein distention

Mr. F. is a 63-year-old male patient who was admitted 2 days ago for exacerbation of heart failure. He is also a 2 pack-a-day smoker (and has been for 41 years). He has a history of arterial insufficiency in his lower extremities and hypertension. He is also a borderline diabetic. On admission, he was placed on furosemide 40 mg I.V. daily, metoprolol 20 mg P.O. b.i.d., and warfarin 5 mg P.O. daily.

On admission, Mr. F.'s vital signs were:

- temperature: 99.1° F (37.3° C)
- heart rate (HR): 88 beats/minute
- respiratory rate (RR): 28 breaths/minute
- blood pressure (BP): 140/86 mm Hg
- oxygen saturation: 91% on room air.

He had coarse crackles bilaterally in the bases of his lungs, and a chest X-ray confirmed the presence of heart failure. His vital signs have remained stable.

On hospital day 3, Mr. F.'s nurse notices that his call light is on. She arrives in the room to find him visibly short of breath despite the use of oxygen at 2 L/minute via nasal cannula. She checks his vital signs and finds the following:

- HR: 114 beats/minute and afebrile
- RR: 32 breaths/minute
- BP: 160/92 mm Hg
- oxygen saturation: 89%.

The nurse increases his oxygen to 4 L/minute and raises the head of Mr. F.'s bed to 45 degrees; at this time she notices jugular vein distention (JVD) on the right side of Mr. F.'s neck. Mr. F.'s jugular vein is visibly distended for 3″ (7.6 cm) above his sternal notch. This is a new finding.

The nurse takes a moment to review Mr. F.'s chart and sees no documentation of this prior to today. Because of the change in his vital signs, shortness of breath, and the onset of JVD, the nurse activates the rapid response team (RRT).

The team members arrive within 4 minutes. They immediately begin their assessment of Mr. F., who remains short of breath and in obvious distress despite the increased oxygen and placement in a semi-Fowler's position. A stat portable chest X-ray is ordered; while awaiting this test, an I.V. therapy nurse arrives and inserts a second I.V. line. Mr. F. is placed on a bedside cardiac monitor, which shows him to be in sinus tachycardia. An indwelling urinary catheter is placed to monitor Mr. F.'s urinary output more closely, and he is given a stat dose of furosemide 40 mg via I.V. push. He continues to exhibit shortness of breath, and the RRT discovers that he has developed coarse crackles throughout both lung fields. His oxygen saturation on 4 L/minute of nasal oxygen has only risen to 90%, so the team changes him to a 100% nonrebreather mask.

Twenty minutes into the event, Mr. F.'s urine output is 20 ml via catheter and these vital signs are noted:

- HR: 110 beats/minute
- RR: 32 breaths/minute
- BP: 162/94 mm Hg.

He's still experiencing shortness of breath and the JVD noted earlier hasn't improved. Given his past medical history, the decision is made to transfer Mr. F. to the medical intensive care unit, where his cardiac and respiratory status can be monitored more closely and he can be placed on a furosemide infusion if needed to improve his urine output, reduce his circulating fluid volume, and relieve his current symptoms.

Physical examination

- Check the patient's vital signs.
- Inspect and palpate for edema.
- Weigh the patient and compare weight to his baseline.
- Auscultate the lungs for crackles and the heart for gallops, pericardial friction rub, and muffled heart sounds.
- Inspect the abdomen for distention.
- Palpate and percuss for an enlarged liver.

Causes

Medical causes

Cardiac tamponade

- In this life-threatening condition, jugular vein distention occurs along with anxiety, restlessness, cyanosis, chest pain, dyspnea, hypotension, and clammy skin.
- Other signs and symptoms include tachycardia, tachypnea, muffled heart sounds, pericardial friction rub, weak or absent peripheral pulses that decrease during inspiration (pulsus paradoxus), and hepatomegaly.

Heart failure

- Right-sided heart failure commonly causes jugular vein distention, weakness, cyanosis, dependent edema, steady weight gain, confusion, and hepatomegaly.
- Other signs and symptoms of right-sided heart failure include nausea, vomiting, abdominal discomfort, anorexia, and ascites (a late sign).
- Jugular vein distention is a late sign in left-sided heart failure.
- Other signs and symptoms of left-sided heart failure include fatigue, dyspnea, orthopnea, paroxysmal nocturnal dyspnea, tachypnea, tachycardia, crackles, ventricular gallop, and arrhythmias.

Hypervolemia

- Jugular vein distention occurs along with rapid weight gain, elevated blood pressure, bounding pulse, peripheral edema, dyspnea, and crackles.

Pericarditis, chronic constrictive

- Jugular vein distention is a progressive sign and more prominent on inspiration (known as Kussmaul's sign).
- Other signs and symptoms include chest pain, dependent edema, hepatomegaly, ascites, and pericardial friction rub.

Superior vena cava obstruction

- Jugular vein distention may occur along with facial, neck, and upper arm edema. (See *Responding to jugular vein distention*.)

Nursing considerations

- If the patient has cardiac tamponade, prepare him for pericardiocentesis.
- Restrict fluids and monitor intake and output.
- Insert an indwelling urinary catheter if necessary.
- If the patient has heart failure, administer a diuretic as ordered.
- Routinely change the patient's position to avoid skin breakdown from peripheral edema.
- Prepare the patient for central venous or pulmonary artery catheter insertion.
- Jugular vein distention is difficult to evaluate in infants, toddlers, and children because of their short, thick necks.

Patient teaching

- Discuss the underlying condition, diagnostic tests, and treatment options.
- Explain foods or fluids the patient should avoid.
- Teach the patient to perform daily weight monitoring.
- Explain what signs and symptoms he should report.
- Explain the importance of scheduled rest periods and help him plan for them.

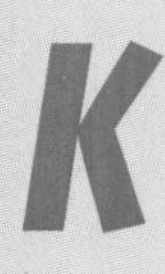

K

Kernig's sign

A reliable early indicator and tool used to diagnose meningeal irritation, Kernig's sign is hamstring stiffness and muscle pain when the examiner attempts to extend the knee while the hip and knee are flexed 90 degrees. This pain causes resistance to movement. However, when the patient's thigh isn't flexed to the abdomen, he can usually extend his leg completely. (*See Eliciting Kernig's sign.*) This sign is commonly elicited in meningitis or subarachnoid hemorrhage. With these potentially life-threatening disorders, hamstring muscle resistance results from stretching the blood- or exudate-irritated meninges surrounding spinal nerve roots.

Kernig's sign can also indicate a herniated disk or spinal tumor. With these

KNOW-HOW

Eliciting Kernig's sign

To elicit Kernig's sign, place the patient in a supine position. Flex her leg at the hip and knee, as shown here. Then try to extend the leg while you keep the hip flexed. If the patient experiences pain and possibly spasm in the hamstring muscle and resists further extension, you can assume that meningeal irritation has occurred.

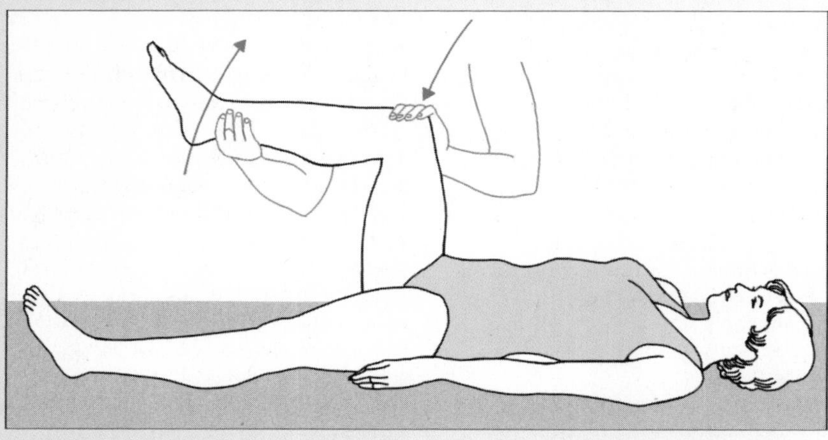

disorders, sciatic pain results from disk or tumor pressure on spinal nerve roots.

History

- Obtain medical and drug history, including use of illegal drugs.
- Ask about back pain that radiates to the legs, numbness, tingling, or weakness.
- Inquire about a history of cancer, infection, or back injury.

Physical examination

- Assess motor function by inspecting the muscles and testing muscle tone and strength.
- Perform cerebellar testing.
- Assess sensory function by checking the patient's sensations of pain, light touch, vibration, position, and discrimination.

Causes

Medical causes

Lumbosacral herniated disk

- Positive Kernig's sign may be elicited.
- Sciatic pain on the affected side or both sides is an early symptom.

Meningitis

- Positive Kernig's sign usually occurs early, along with fever and, possibly, chills.

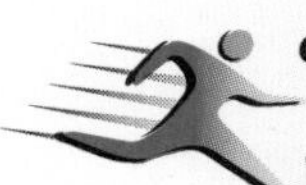

QUICK ACTION

When Kernig's sign signals CNS crisis

Because Kernig's sign may signal meningitis or subarachnoid hemorrhage—life-threatening central nervous system disorders—take the patient's vital signs at once to obtain baseline information. Then test for Brudzinski's sign to obtain further evidence of meningeal irritation. Next, ask the patient or his family to describe the onset of illness. Typically, the progressive onset of headache, fever, nuchal rigidity, and confusion suggests meningitis. Conversely, the sudden onset of severe headache, nuchal rigidity, photophobia and, possibly, loss of consciousness usually indicates subarachnoid hemorrhage.

Meningitis

If a diagnosis of meningitis is suspected, ask about recent infections, especially tooth abscesses. Ask about exposure to infected persons or places where meningitis is endemic. Meningitis is usually a complication of another bacterial infection, so draw blood for culture studies to determine the causative organism. Prepare the patient for a lumbar puncture (if a tumor or an abscess can be ruled out). Also, find out if the patient has a history of I.V. drug abuse, an open head injury, or endocarditis. Insert an I.V. catheter, and immediately begin administering an antibiotic.

Subarachnoid hemorrhage

If subarachnoid hemorrhage is the suspected diagnosis, ask about a history of hypertension, cerebral aneurysm, head trauma, or arteriovenous malformation. Also ask about sudden withdrawal of an antihypertensive.

Check the patient's pupils for dilation, and assess him for signs of increasing intracranial pressure, such as bradycardia, increased systolic blood pressure, and widened pulse pressure. Insert an I.V. catheter, and administer supplemental oxygen.

■ Other signs and symptoms include nuchal rigidity, hyperreflexia, Brudzinski's sign, opisthotonos, stupor, coma, and seizures.

Spinal cord tumor

■ Kernig's sign can be occasionally elicited.

■ The earliest symptom of spinal cord tumor is pain felt locally or along the spinal nerve, commonly in the leg.

Subarachnoid hemorrhage

■ Kernig's and Brudzinski's signs can be elicited within minutes after the initial bleeding. (See *When Kernig's sign signals CNS crisis,* page 207.)

Nursing considerations

■ Closely monitor the patient's vital signs, intracranial pressure (ICP), and cardiopulmonary and neurologic status.

■ Ensure bed rest, quiet, and minimal stress.

■ For those with subarachnoid hemorrhage, darken the room and elevate the head of the bed at least 30 degrees to reduce ICP.

■ If the patient has a herniated disk or spinal tumor, he may require pelvic traction.

■ In children, Kernig's sign is considered ominous because of the greater potential for rapid deterioration.

Patient teaching

■ Discuss the underlying condition, diagnostic tests, and treatment options.

■ Teach the patient the signs and symptoms of meningitis.

■ Discuss ways to prevent meningitis.

■ Teach the patient with a herniated disk which activities he should avoid.

■ Teach the patient how to apply his back brace or cervical collar, as needed.

L

Level of consciousness, decreased

A decrease in the patient's level of consciousness (LOC), from lethargy to stupor to coma, usually results from a neurologic disorder and may signal a life-threatening complication, such as hemorrhage, trauma, or cerebral edema. However, this sign can also result from a metabolic, GI, musculoskeletal, urologic, or cardiopulmonary disorder; severe nutritional deficiency; the effects of toxins; or drug use. LOC can deteriorate suddenly or gradually and can remain altered temporarily or permanently. (See *Responding to decreased level of consciousness,* page 210.)

Consciousness is affected by the reticular activating system (RAS), an intricate network of neurons with axons extending from the brain stem, thalamus, and hypothalamus to the cerebral cortex. A disturbance in any part of this integrated system prevents the intercommunication that makes consciousness possible. Loss of consciousness can result from a bilateral cerebral disturbance, an RAS disturbance, or both. Cerebral dysfunction characteristically produces the least dramatic decrease in a patient's LOC. In contrast, dysfunction of the RAS produces the most dramatic decrease in LOC—coma.

The most sensitive indicator of a decreased LOC is a change in the patient's mental status. The Glasgow Coma Scale, which measures a patient's ability to respond to verbal, sensory, and motor stimulation, can be used to quickly evaluate a patient's LOC. (See *Glasgow Coma Scale,* page 211.)

QUICK ACTION ***After evaluating the patient's airway, breathing, and circulation, use the Glasgow Coma Scale to quickly determine his LOC and to obtain baseline data. Insert an artificial airway, elevate the head of the bed 30 degrees and, if spinal cord injury has been ruled out, turn the patient's head to the side. Prepare to suction the patient if necessary. You may need to hyperventilate him to reduce carbon dioxide levels and decrease intracranial pressure (ICP). Then determine the rate, rhythm, and depth of spontaneous respirations. Support his breathing with a handheld resuscitation bag, if necessary. If the patient's Glasgow Coma Scale score is less than 9, intubation and resuscitation may be necessary.***

Continue to monitor the patient's vital signs, being alert for signs of increasing ICP, such as bradycardia and a widening pulse pressure. When his airway, breathing, and circulation are stabilized, perform a neurologic examination.

History

- Ask the family about headaches, dizziness, nausea, vision or hearing disturbances, weakness, and fatigue.

CASE CLIP

Responding to decreased level of consciousness

Mr. W. is an 81-year-old male nursing home resident with a 4-day history of dyspnea, productive cough, lethargy, and activity intolerance. He was transferred to the emergency department with these symptoms as well as decreased oxygen saturation and fever, to be ruled out for pneumonia. Vital signs on arrival to the emergency department were:

- temperature (rectal): 101.3° F (38.5° C)
- heart rate (HR): 112 beats/minute
- respiratory rate (RR): 32 breaths/minute and shallow
- blood pressure: 90/46 mm Hg
- oxygen saturation: 86% on room air.

An electrocardiogram was performed and sinus tachycardia was noted. Arterial blood gas (ABG) samples were drawn, and a portable chest X-ray was done, which confirmed the presence of bilateral pneumonia. Oxygen was administered at 100% via a nonrebreather mask. The patient was transferred to the hospital's respiratory care unit for treatment of pneumonia.

Two days after admission, Mr. W. continues to have a frequent congested cough, productive for large amounts of thick, tan sputum. During morning rounds, his nurse finds him with a decreased level of consciousness and mild confusion and disorientation to place and time. He's also slightly agitated. He's noted to repeatedly remove his oxygen mask; current oxygen saturation is 87%. Other vital signs include:

- HR: 126 beats/minute
- RR: 38 breaths/minute and shallow with notable sternal and costal retractions and use of accessory muscles.

During the nurse's assessment, Mr. W. becomes increasingly restless; he suddenly clutches his throat, and the nurse notices that he's developing pallor as well as circumoral cyanosis. With these changes in mind, the nurse activates the rapid response team (RRT).

The RRT arrives within 3 minutes. The senior resident orders immediate deep suctioning. The respiratory therapist preoxygenates Mr. W. and then suctions him, obtaining a large amount of thick, tan sputum. A sample is sent to the laboratory for culture and sensitivity testing. Mr. W. remains in respiratory distress, so his oxygen mask is reapplied at 100% via nonrebreather mask. However, after several minutes he doesn't appear to be experiencing any relief, and his oxygen saturation level remains below 90%. The decision is made to insert an endotracheal (ET) tube and place him on a ventilator. The ventilator is set at assist-control at a rate of 14 breaths/minute, tidal volume of 600 cc, 5 mm of positive end-expiratory pressure, and 100% oxygen. A portable chest X-ray is ordered to confirm ET tube placement and to reassess Mr. W.'s pneumonia and respiratory status and to rule out aspiration. ABG values, electrolytes, and hourly suctioning as needed are also ordered. Mr. W remains on the respiratory care unit for observation and further respiratory treatment as needed.

Glasgow Coma Scale

You've probably heard such terms as lethargic, obtunded, and stuporous used to describe a progressive decrease in a patient's level of consciousness (LOC). However, the Glasgow Coma Scale provides a more accurate, less subjective method of recording such changes, grading consciousness in relation to eye opening and motor and verbal responses.

To use the Glasgow Coma Scale, test the patient's ability to respond to verbal, motor, and sensory stimulation. The scoring system doesn't determine the exact LOC, but it does provide an easy way to describe the patient's basic status and helps to detect and interpret changes from baseline findings. A decreased reaction score in one or more categories may signal an impending neurologic crisis. A total score of less than 9 indicates severe brain damage.

TEST	REACTION	SCORE
Eye opening response	Open spontaneously	4
	Open to verbal command	3
	Open to pain	2
	No response	1
Best motor response	Obeys verbal command	6
	Localizes painful stimulus	5
	Flexion—withdrawal	4
	Flexion—abnormal (decorticate rigidity)	3
	Extension (decerebrate rigidity)	2
	No response	1
Best verbal response	Oriented and converses	5
	Disoriented and converses	4
	Inappropriate words	3
	Incomprehensible sounds	2
	No response	1
Total		3 to 15

- Determine whether the family has noticed any changes in behavior, personality, memory, or temperament.
- Obtain a medical history, including incidence of neurologic disease or cancer and recent trauma or infection.
- Obtain a history of drug and alcohol use.

Physical examination

- Perform a complete neurologic examination.
- Perform a physical assessment.

Causes

Medical causes

Adrenal crisis

- Decreased LOC, ranging from lethargy to coma, may develop within 8 to 12 hours of onset.
- Early signs and symptoms include progressive weakness, irritability, anorexia, headache, nausea, vomiting, diarrhea, abdominal pain, and fever.
- Later signs and symptoms include hypotension; rapid, thready pulse; olig-

uria; cool, clammy skin; and flaccid extremities.

Brain abscess

- Decreased LOC varies from drowsiness to deep stupor.
- Early signs and symptoms include constant intractable headache, nausea, vomiting, and seizures.
- Later signs and symptoms include vision disturbances and signs of infection.
- Other signs and symptoms include personality changes, confusion, abnormal behavior, dizziness, facial weakness, aphasia, ataxia, tremor, and hemiparesis.

Brain tumor

- The patient's LOC decreases slowly, from lethargy to coma.
- Apathy, behavior changes, memory loss, decreased attention span, morning headache, dizziness, aphasia, seizures, vision loss, ataxia, and sensorimotor disturbances may occur.
- In later stages, signs and symptoms include papilledema, vomiting, bradycardia, and widening pulse pressure.
- In the final stages, signs include decorticate or decerebrate posture.

Cerebral aneurysm, ruptured

- Somnolence, confusion and, at times, stupor characterize moderate bleeding.
- Deep coma occurs with severe bleeding, which can be fatal.
- Onset is usually abrupt with sudden, severe headache, nausea, and vomiting.
- Nuchal rigidity, back and leg pain, fever, restlessness, irritability, seizures, and blurred vision point to meningeal irritation.
- Other signs and symptoms include hemiparesis, hemisensory defects, dysphagia, and visual defects.

Cerebral contusion

- Unconscious patients may have dilated, nonreactive pupils and decorticate or decerebrate posture.
- Conscious patients may be drowsy, confused, disoriented, agitated, or violent.
- Other signs and symptoms include blurred or double vision, fever, headache, pallor, diaphoresis, seizures, impaired mental status, slight hemiparesis, tachycardia, altered respirations, aphasia, and hemiparesis.

Diabetic ketoacidosis

- A decrease in the patient's LOC is rapid and ranges from lethargy to coma.
- Polydipsia, polyphagia, and polyuria precede decreased LOC secondary to fluid shift from elevated glucose level.
- Other signs and symptoms include weakness, anorexia, abdominal pain, nausea, vomiting, orthostatic hypotension, fruity breath odor, Kussmaul's respirations, warm and dry skin, and a rapid, thready pulse.

Encephalitis

- Decreased LOC may range from lethargy to coma within 48 hours of onset.
- Other signs and symptoms may include abrupt onset of fever, headache, nuchal rigidity, nausea, vomiting, irritability, personality changes, seizures, aphasia, ataxia, hemiparesis, nystagmus, photophobia, myoclonus, and cranial nerve palsies.

Encephalomyelitis, postvaccinal

- This life-threatening disorder produces rapid deterioration in the patient's LOC, from drowsiness to coma.
- Other signs and symptoms include rapid onset of fever, headache, nuchal rigidity, back pain, vomiting, and seizures.

Encephalopathy

- Hepatic encephalopathy produces decreased LOC that ranges from slight personality changes to coma depending on the stage.
- Hypertensive encephalopathy produces LOC that progressively decreases from lethargy to stupor to coma.
- Hypoglycemic encephalopathy produces LOC that rapidly deteriorates from lethargy to coma.
- Hypoxic encephalopathy produces a sudden or gradual decrease in the patient's LOC, leading to coma and brain death.
- Uremic encephalopathy produces LOC that decreases gradually from lethargy to coma.

Epidural hemorrhage, acute

- Momentary loss of consciousness is sometimes followed by a lucid interval.
- While the patient is lucid, signs and symptoms include severe headache, nausea, vomiting, and bladder distention.
- Rapid deterioration in consciousness follows, possibly leading to coma.
- Other signs and symptoms include irregular respirations, seizures, decreased and bounding pulse, increased pulse pressure, hypertension, fixed and dilated pupils, unilateral hemiparesis or hemiplegia, decerebrate posture, and positive Babinski's reflex.

Heatstroke

- As body temperature increases, the patient's LOC gradually decreases from lethargy to coma.
- At the onset, the skin is hot, flushed, and diaphoretic with blotchy cyanosis; when body temperature exceeds 105° F (40.6° C), it's no longer diaphoretic.
- Other early signs and symptoms include irritability, anxiety, severe headache, malaise, tachycardia, tachypnea, orthostatic hypotension, muscle cramps, rigidity, and syncope.

Hypernatremia

- The patient's LOC deteriorates from lethargy to coma.
- The patient is irritable and exhibits twitches that progress to seizures.
- Other signs and symptoms include nausea, malaise, fever, thirst, flushed skin, dry mucous membranes, and a weak, thready pulse.

Hyperosmolar hyperglycemic nonketotic syndrome

- The patient's LOC decreases rapidly from lethargy to coma.
- Early signs and symptoms include polyuria, polydipsia, weight loss, and weakness.
- Later signs and symptoms include hypotension, poor skin turgor, dry skin and mucous membranes, tachycardia, tachypnea, oliguria, and seizures.

Hypokalemia

- The patient's LOC gradually decreases to lethargy.
- Other signs and symptoms include confusion, nausea, vomiting, diarrhea, polyuria, weakness, decreased reflexes, malaise, dizziness, hypotension, arrhythmias, and abnormal electrocardiogram results.

Hyponatremia

- Decreased LOC occurs in late stages.
- Early nausea and malaise may progress to behavior changes, confusion, lethargy, incoordination and, eventually, seizures and coma.

Hypothermia

- When severe, the patient's LOC decreases from lethargy to coma.
- Mild to moderate cases produce memory loss, slurred speech, shivering, weakness, fatigue, and apathy.
- Other early signs and symptoms include ataxia, muscle stiffness, hyperactive deep tendon reflexes, diuresis,

tachycardia, bradypnea, decreased blood pressure, and cold, pale skin.
- Later signs and symptoms include muscle rigidity, decreased reflexes, peripheral cyanosis, bradycardia, arrhythmias, severe hypotension, shallow respirations, oliguria and, possibly, cardiopulmonary arrest.

Intracerebral hemorrhage
- In this life-threatening disorder, rapid, steady loss of consciousness occurs within hours and is accompanied by severe headache, dizziness, nausea, and vomiting.
- Other signs and symptoms include increased blood pressure, irregular respirations, Babinski's reflex, seizures, aphasia, decreased sensations, hemiplegia, decorticate or decerebrate posture, and dilated pupils.

Listeriosis
- If listerosis spreads to the nervous system and causes menigitis, signs and symptoms include decreased LOC, fever, headache, and nuchal rigidity.
- Early signs and symptoms include fever, myalgia, abdominal pain, nausea, vomiting, and diarrhea.

Meningitis
- Confusion and irritability occur; stupor, coma, and seizures may occur in severe cases.
- Other signs and symptoms include fever, chills, severe headache, nuchal rigidity, hyperreflexia, Kernig's and Brudzinski's signs, ocular palsies, photophobia, facial weakness, hearing loss, and opisthotonos.

Myxedema crisis
- A decline in the patient's LOC may be swift due to hypothyroidism.
- Other signs and symptoms include severe hypothermia, hypoventilation, hypotension, bradycardia, hypoactive reflexes, periorbital and peripheral edema, impaired hearing and balance, and seizures.

Pontine hemorrhage
- A sudden, rapid decrease in the patient's LOC to the point of coma occurs within minutes.
- Death occurs within hours.
- Other signs and symptoms include total paralysis, decerebrate posture, Babinski's reflex, absent doll's eye sign, and bilateral miosis.

Seizure disorders
- A complex partial seizure causes decreased LOC, manifested as a blank stare, purposeless behavior, and unintelligible speech; an aura may precede the seizure, and several minutes of mental confusion may follow the seizure.
- An absence seizure involves a brief change in the patient's LOC, indicated by blinking or eye rolling, a blank stare, and slight mouth movements.
- A generalized tonic-clonic seizure typically begins with a loud cry and sudden loss of consciousness; consciousness returns after the seizure, but the patient remains confused and may fall into a deep sleep.
- An atonic seizure produces sudden unconsciousness for a few seconds.
- Status epilepticus, a life-threatening condition, involves rapidly recurring seizures.

Shock
- Decreased LOC occurs late.
- Other signs and symptoms include confusion, anxiety, restlessness, hypotension, tachycardia, weak pulse with narrowing pulse pressure, dyspnea, oliguria, and cool, clammy skin.

Stroke
- In thrombotic stroke, LOC changes may be abrupt or take several minutes, hours, or days to evolve.

■ In embolic stroke, LOC changes occur suddenly and peak immediately.
■ In hemorrhagic stroke, LOC changes develop over minutes or hours, depending on the extent of the bleeding.
■ Other signs and symptoms of stroke include disorientation, intellectual deficits, personality changes, emotional lability, dysarthria, dysphagia, ataxia, aphasia, agnosia, unilateral sensorimotor loss, vision disturbances, incontinence, and seizures.

Subdural hematoma, chronic
■ The patient's LOC deteriorates slowly.
■ Other signs and symptoms include confusion, decreased ability to concentrate, personality changes, headache, light-headedness, seizures, and a dilated ipsilateral pupil with ptosis.

Subdural hemorrhage, acute
■ In this life-threatening condition, agitation and confusion are followed by progressively decreasing LOC from somnolence to coma.
■ Other signs and symptoms include headache, fever, unilateral pupil dilation, decreased pulse and respiratory rates, widening pulse pressure, seizures, hemiparesis, and Babinski's reflex.

Thyroid storm
■ The patient's LOC decreases suddenly and can progress to coma.
■ Irritability, restlessness, confusion, and psychotic behavior precede the deterioration.
■ Other signs and symptoms include tremors, weakness, vision disturbances, tachycardia, arrhythmias, angina, acute respiratory distress, vomiting, diarrhea, and fever.

Transient ischemic attack
■ The patient's LOC decreases abruptly (with varying severity) and gradually returns to normal within 24 hours.
■ Other signs and symptoms include transient vision loss, nystagmus, aphasia, dizziness, dysarthria, unilateral hemiparesis or hemiplegia, tinnitus, paresthesia, dysphagia, and uncoordinated gait.

West Nile encephalitis
■ Stupor, disorientation, and coma occur with severe infection.
■ Skin rash and lymphadenopathy may also develop.
■ Other signs and symptoms of severe infection include high fever, headache, neck stiffness, tremors, occasional seizures, and paralysis. In rare cases, death can occur.

Other causes

Alcohol
■ Alcohol causes varying degrees of sedation, irritability, and incoordination; intoxication causes stupor.

Drugs
■ Overdose of barbiturates, other central nervous system depressants, or aspirin can cause sedation and other degrees of decreased LOC.

Poisoning
■ Toxins, such as lead, carbon monoxide, and snake venom, can cause varying degrees of decreased LOC.

Nursing considerations

■ Reassess the patient's LOC and neurologic status at least hourly.
■ Monitor ICP and intake and output.
■ Ensure airway patency and proper nutrition.
■ Keep the patient on bed rest with the side rails up.
■ Keep the head of the bed elevated at least 30 degrees.
■ Maintain seizure precautions.
■ Don't give an opioid or a sedative.
■ In children, the primary cause of decreased LOC is head trauma.

Patient teaching

- Discuss the underlying condition, diagnostic tests, and treatment options with the patient—as appropriate for the patient's mental status or LOC—and his family.
- Teach safety and seizure precautions.
- Provide referrals to sources of support.
- Discuss quality-of-life issues.

Lymphadenopathy

Lymphadenopathy is the enlargement of one or more lymph nodes. This disorder may result from increased production of lymphocytes or reticuloendothelial cells, or from infiltration of cells that aren't normally present. The signs may be generalized (involving three or more node groups) or localized. Generalized lymphadenopathy may be caused by an inflammatory process, such as a bacterial or viral infection, connective tissue disease, an endocrine disorder, or neoplasm. Localized lymphadenopathy most commonly results from infection or trauma affecting a specific area. (See *Areas of localized lymphadenopathy*. Also see *Causes of localized lymphadenopathy,* page 218.)

Normally, lymph nodes are discrete, mobile, soft, and nontender. In children, nodes are normally palpable; in adults, they may be palpable or nonpalpable. Nodes that are more than ⅜″ (1 cm) in diameter are cause for concern. They may be tender, and the skin overlying the lymph node may be erythematous, suggesting a draining lesion. Alternatively, they may be hard and fixed, tender or nontender, suggesting a malignant tumor.

History

- Ask about the onset, location, and description of swelling.
- Find out about recent infections or health problems.
- Ask about previous biopsies and a personal or family history of cancer.

Physical examination

- Note the size of any palpable lymph nodes and whether they're fixed or mobile, tender or nontender, and erythematous.
- Note the texture of palpable nodes.
- If lymph nodes are erythematous, check the area drained by that part of the lymph system for signs of infection.
- Palpate and percuss the spleen.

Causes

Medical causes

Acquired immunodeficiency syndrome

- Lymphadenopathy occurs with fatigue, night sweats, afternoon fevers, diarrhea, and weight loss; cough arises with several concurrent infections.

Anthrax, cutaneous

- Lymphadenopathy, malaise, headache, and fever may develop.
- A small, elevated itchy lesion resembling an insect bite may progress into a painless, necrotic-centered ulcer.

Chronic fatigue syndrome

- Lymphadenopathy may occur with incapacitating fatigue, sore throat, low-grade fever, myalgia, cognitive dysfunction, and sleep disturbances.
- Other signs and symptoms include arthralgia with arthritis, headache, and memory deficits.

Cytomegalovirus infection

- Generalized lymphadenopathy is accompanied by fever, malaise, and hepatosplenomegaly.
- A pruritic rash may appear, consisting of small, erythematous macules that progress to papules and then to vesicles.

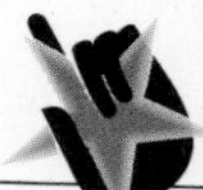

KNOW-HOW

Areas of localized lymphadenopathy

When you detect an enlarged lymph node, palpate the entire lymph node system to determine the extent of lymphadenopathy. Include the lymph nodes indicated here in your assessment.

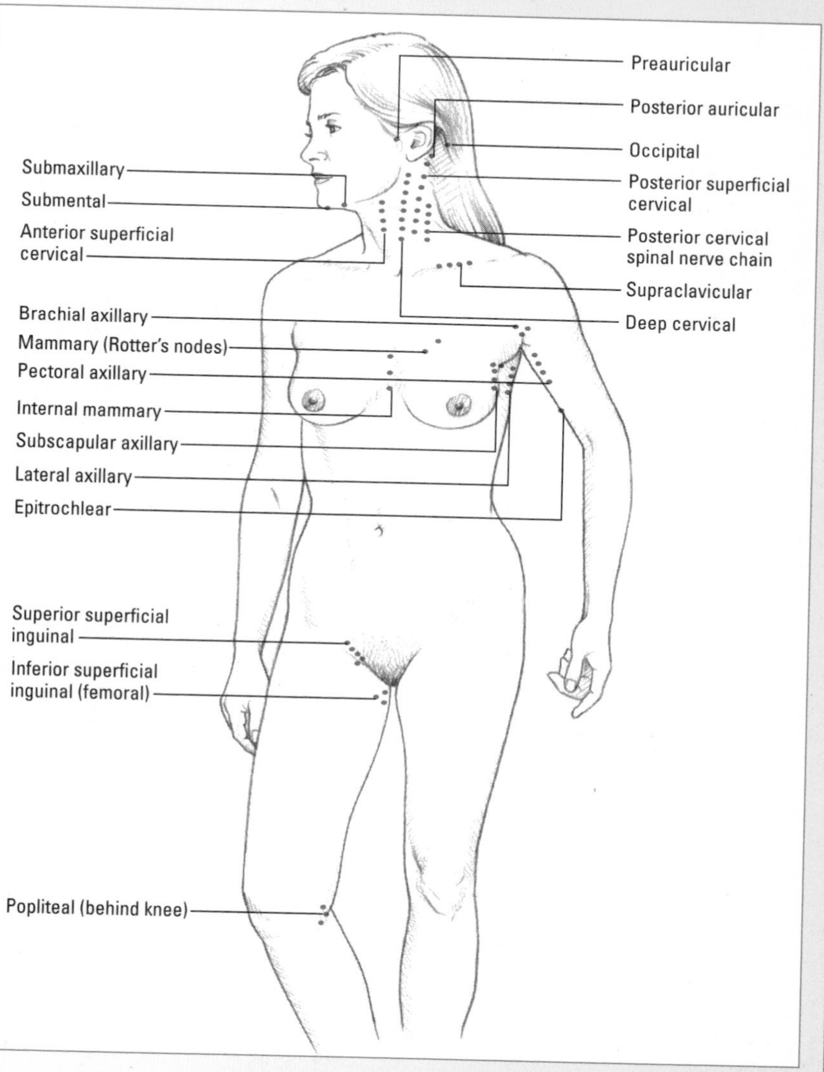

Causes of localized lymphadenopathy

Various disorders can cause localized lymphadenopathy, but this sign usually results from infection or trauma affecting the specific area. Here you'll find some common causes of lymphadenopathy listed according to the areas affected.

Auricular
- Erysipelas
- Herpes zoster ophthalmicus
- Infection
- Rubella
- Squamous cell carcinoma
- Styes or chalazion
- Tularemia

Axillary
- Breast cancer
- Infection
- Lymphoma
- Mastitis

Cervical
- Cat-scratch fever
- Facial or oral cancer
- Infection
- Mononucleosis
- Mucocutaneous lymph node syndrome
- Rubella
- Rubeola
- Thyrotoxicosis
- Tonsillitis
- Tuberculosis
- Varicella

Inguinal and femoral
- Carcinoma
- Chancroid
- Infection
- Lymphogranuloma venereum
- Syphilis

Occipital
- Infection
- Roseola
- Scalp infection
- Seborrheic dermatitis
- Tick bite
- Tinea capitis

Popliteal
- Infection

Submaxillary and submental
- Cystic fibrosis
- Dental infection
- Gingivitis
- Glossitis
- Infection

Supraclavicular
- Infection
- Neoplastic disease

Hodgkin's disease
- The extent of lymphadenopathy reflects the stage of malignancy.
- Early signs and symptoms include pruritus, fatigue, weakness, night sweats, malaise, weight loss, and fever.

Kawasaki syndrome
- Cervical lymphadenopathy is a characteristic sign.
- Other signs and symptoms include high, spiking fever, erythema, bilateral conjunctival injection, and swelling in peripheral extremities.

Leukemia
- In acute lymphocytic leukemia, generalized lymphadenopathy is accompanied by fatigue, malaise, pallor, prolonged bleeding time, swollen gums, weight loss, bone or joint pain, hepatosplenomegaly, and low-grade fever.
- In chronic lymphocytic leukemia, generalized lymphadenopathy appears early along with fatigue, malaise, and fever.
- Late signs and symptoms of the chronic form include hepatosplenomegaly, severe fatigue, weight loss, bone tenderness, edema, pallor, dyspnea, tachycardia, palpitations, bleeding, anemia, and macular or nodular lesions.

Lyme disease
- As the disease progresses, lymphadenopathy, constant malaise and fa-

tigue, and intermittent headache, fever, chills, and aches develop.

- Arthralgia and, eventually, neurologic and cardiac abnormalities may develop.

Mononucleosis, infectious

- Painful lymphadenopathy involves cervical, axillary, and inguinal nodes.
- Prodromal symptoms of headache, malaise, and fatigue appear 3 to 5 days before the appearance of the classic triad of lymphadenopathy, sore throat, and temperature fluctuations with an evening peak.
- Other signs and symptoms include hepatosplenomegaly, stomatitis, exudative tonsillitis, or pharyngitis.

Non-Hodgkin's lymphoma

- Painless enlargement of one or more peripheral lymph nodes is the most common sign.
- Generalized lymphadenopathy characterizes stage IV.
- Other signs and symptoms include dyspnea, cough, hepatosplenomegaly, fever, night sweats, fatigue, malaise, and weight loss.

Plague

- Signs and symptoms of the bubonic form include lymphadenopathy, fever, and chills.

Rheumatoid arthritis

- Lymphadenopathy is an early, nonspecific finding.
- Later signs and symptoms include joint tenderness, swelling, and warmth; joint stiffness after inactivity; subcutaneous nodules on the elbows; joint deformity; muscle weakness; and muscle atrophy.
- Other signs and symptoms include fatigue, malaise, low-grade fever, weight loss, and vague arthralgia and myalgia.

Sarcoidosis

- Generalized hilar and right paratracheal forms of lymphadenopathy with splenomegaly are common.
- Initial signs and symptoms include arthralgia, fatigue, malaise, weight loss, and pulmonary symptoms.
- Other signs and symptoms vary and may include breathlessness, cough, substernal chest pain, arrhythmias, muscle weakness and pain, phalangeal and nasal mucosal lesions, subcutaneous skin nodules, eye pain, photophobia, nonreactive pupils, seizures, and cranial or peripheral nerve palsies.

Syphilis

- Localized lymphadenopathy occurs with a painless canker that develops at the site of sexual exposure.
- In the second stage, generalized lymphadenopathy occurs along with a macular, papular, pustular, or nodular rash on the arms, trunk, palms (a diagnostic sign), soles, face, and scalp.
- Other signs and symptoms include headache, malaise, anorexia, weight loss, nausea, vomiting, sore throat, and low-grade fever.

Systemic lupus erythematosus

- Generalized lymphadenopathy accompanies butterfly rash (a hallmark sign), photosensitivity, Raynaud's phenomenon, and joint pain and stiffness.
- Other signs and symptoms include pleuritic chest pain, cough, fever, anorexia, and weight loss.

Tuberculous lymphadenitis

- Lymphadenopathy may be generalized or restricted to superficial lymph nodes.
- Lymph nodes may become fluctuant and drain to surrounding tissue.
- Other signs and symptoms include fever, chills, weakness, and fatigue.

Other causes

Drugs

- Phenytoin (Dilantin) may cause generalized lymphadenopathy.

Immunizations

- Typhoid vaccination may cause generalized lymphadenopathy.

Nursing considerations

- If the patient is uncomfortable, provide an antipyretic, a tepid sponge bath, or a hypothermia blanket.
- If diagnostic tests reveal infection, check your facility's policy regarding infection control.
- In children, infection is the most common cause of lymphadenopathy.

Patient teaching

- Teach the patient about the underlying condition, diagnostic tests, and treatment options.
- Teach the patient ways to prevent infection.
- Explain the signs and symptoms of infection that the patient should report.
- Explain the reasons for isolation as needed.
- Stress the importance of a healthy diet and rest.

M

Melena

A common sign of upper GI bleeding, melena is the passage of black, tarry stools containing digested blood. The characteristic color results from bacterial degradation and hydrochloric acid acting on the blood as it travels through the GI tract. At least 60 ml of blood in the GI tract is needed to produce this sign. (See *Comparing melena with hematochezia,* page 222.)

Severe melena can signal acute bleeding and life-threatening hypovolemic shock. Usually, melena indicates bleeding from the esophagus, stomach, or duodenum, although it can also indicate bleeding from the jejunum, ileum, or ascending colon. This sign can also result from swallowing blood, as in epistaxis; from taking certain drugs; or from ingesting alcohol. Because false melena may be caused by the ingestion of lead, iron, bismuth, or licorice (which produces black stools without the presence of blood), all black stools should be tested for occult blood.

QUICK ACTION ***If the patient is experiencing severe melena, quickly take his orthostatic vital signs to detect hypovolemic shock. A decline of 10 mm Hg or more in systolic pressure or an increase of 10 beats/minute or more in the pulse rate indicates volume depletion. Quickly examine the patient for other signs of shock, such as tachycardia, tachypnea, and cool, clammy skin. Insert a large-bore I.V. catheter to administer replacement fluids and allow for blood transfusion. Obtain hematocrit, prothrombin time, International Normalized Ratio levels, and partial thromboplastin time. Place the patient flat with his feet elevated. Administer supplemental oxygen as needed.***

History

- Ask about the onset of melena.
- Determine the frequency and quantity of bowel movements.
- Ask about hematemesis or hematochezia.
- Find out about the use of anti-inflammatory drugs, alcohol, other GI irritants, or iron supplements.
- Obtain a drug history, noting the use of warfarin (Coumadin) and other anticoagulants.

Physical examination

- Inspect the mouth and nasopharynx for bleeding.
- Auscultate, percuss, and palpate the abdomen.
- Perform a cardiovascular assessment to detect signs and symptoms of shock.

Causes

Medical causes

Colon cancer

- Early right-sided tumor growth may cause melena and abdominal aching, pressure, or cramps.
- As the right-sided tumor progresses, signs and symptoms include weakness, fatigue, anemia, diarrhea or obstipation,

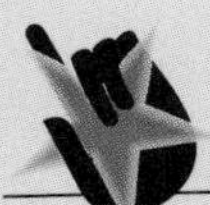

KNOW-HOW

Comparing melena with hematochezia

With GI bleeding, the site, amount, and rate of blood flow through the GI tract determine if a patient will develop melena (black, tarry stools) or hematochezia (bright red, blood stools). Usually, melena indicates *upper* GI bleeding, and hematochezia indicates *lower* GI bleeding. However, with some disorders, melena may alternate with hematochezia. This chart helps differentiate these two commonly related signs.

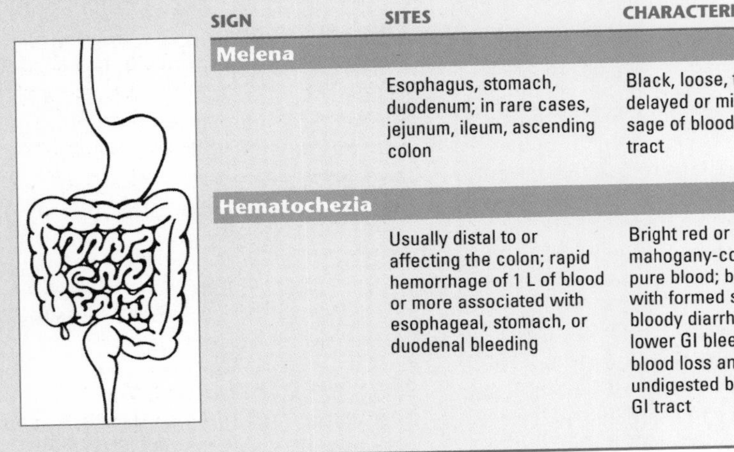

SIGN	SITES	CHARACTERISTICS
Melena		
	Esophagus, stomach, duodenum; in rare cases, jejunum, ileum, ascending colon	Black, loose, tarry stools; delayed or minimal passage of blood through GI tract
Hematochezia		
	Usually distal to or affecting the colon; rapid hemorrhage of 1 L of blood or more associated with esophageal, stomach, or duodenal bleeding	Bright red or dark, mahogany-colored stools; pure blood; blood mixed with formed stools; or bloody diarrhea; reflects lower GI bleeding or rapid blood loss and passage of undigested blood through GI tract

anorexia, weight loss, vomiting, and signs and symptoms of obstruction.

- Early left-sided tumor growth may cause rectal bleeding with intermittent abdominal fullness or cramping and rectal pressure.
- As the left-sided tumor progresses, signs and symptoms include melena (usually develops late in the disease), obstipation, diarrhea, and pencil-shaped stools.

Ebola virus

- Melena, hematemesis, and bleeding from the nose, gums, and vagina may occur late.
- The abrupt onset of headache, malaise, myalgia, high fever, diarrhea, abdominal pain, dehydration, and lethargy occurs on the 5th day of the illness.
- A maculopapular rash develops between days 5 and 7 of the illness.

Esophageal cancer

- Melena is a late sign along with painful dysphagia, anorexia, and regurgitation.
- Earlier signs and symptoms include painless dysphagia, rapid weight loss, steady chest pain with substernal fullness, nausea, vomiting, and hematemesis.

Esophageal varices, ruptured

- In this life-threatening disorder, melena, hematochezia, and hematemesis may occur.
- Melena is preceded by signs of shock.
- Agitation or confusion signals developing hepatic encephalopathy.

Gastric cancer

- Melena and altered bowel habits may occur late.
- Common signs and symptoms include the insidious onset of upper abdominal or retrosternal discomfort and chronic dyspepsia unrelieved by antacids and made worse by eating.
- Other signs and symptoms include anorexia, nausea, hematemesis, pallor, fatigue, weight loss, and a feeling of abdominal fullness.

Gastritis

- Melena and hematemesis are common signs.
- Other signs and symptoms include mild epigastric or abdominal discomfort that's made worse by eating, belching, nausea, vomiting, and malaise.

Mallory-Weiss syndrome

- Massive bleeding from the upper GI tract is characteristic, following a tear to the mucous membrane of the esophagus or esophageal gastric junction.
- Melena and hematemesis follow vomiting.
- Epigastric or back pain and signs and symptoms of shock may occur.

Mesenteric vascular occlusion

- Slight melena occurs along with 2 to 3 days of persistent, mild abdominal pain.
- Later, abdominal pain becomes severe and may be accompanied by tenderness, distention, guarding, and rigidity.
- Anorexia, vomiting, fever, and profound shock may also develop.

Peptic ulcer

- Melena may signal life-threatening hemorrhage.
- Other signs and symptoms include decreased appetite; nausea; vomiting; hematemesis; hematochezia; left epigastric pain that's gnawing, burning, or sharp; and signs and symptoms of shock.

Small-bowel tumors

- Tumors may bleed and produce melena.
- Other signs and symptoms include abdominal pain, distention, and increasing frequency and rising pitch of bowel sounds.

Thrombocytopenia

- Melena or hematochezia may accompany other manifestations of bleeding tendency.
- Malaise, fatigue, weakness, and lethargy are typical.

Other causes

Drugs and alcohol

- Aspirin, nonsteroidal anti-inflammatory drugs (NSAIDs), or alcohol can cause melena.

Nursing considerations

- Monitor the patient's vital signs, and look closely for signs of hypovolemic shock.
- Encourage bed rest.
- Keep the perianal area clean and dry to prevent skin irritation and breakdown.
- A nasogastric tube may be needed to drain gastric contents and for decompression.
- Give blood transfusions as ordered.

Patient teaching

- Explain the underlying cause of melena and its treatment.
- Explain the changes in bowel elimination that the patient needs to report.
- Stress the importance of undergoing colorectal cancer screening.
- Explain the need to avoid aspirin, NSAIDs, and alcohol.

Murmurs

Murmurs are auscultatory sounds heard within the heart chambers or major arteries. They're classified by their timing and duration in the cardiac cycle, auscultatory location, loudness, configuration, pitch, and quality.

Timing can be characterized as systolic (between S_1 and S_2), holosystolic (continuous throughout systole), diastolic (between S_2 and S_1), or continuous throughout systole and diastole. Systolic and diastolic murmurs can be further characterized as early, middle, or late.

Location refers to the area of maximum loudness, such as the apex, the lower left sternal border, or an intercostal space. *Loudness* is graded on a scale of 1 to 6. A grade 1 murmur is very faint, only detected after careful auscultation. A grade 2 murmur is a soft, evident murmur. Murmurs considered to be grade 3 are moderately loud. A grade 4 murmur is a loud murmur with a possible intermittent thrill. Grade 5 murmurs are loud and associated with a palpable precordial thrill. Grade 6 murmurs are loud and, like grade 5 murmurs, are associated with a thrill. A grade 6 murmur is audible even when the stethoscope is lifted from the thoracic wall.

Configuration, or shape, refers to the nature of loudness—crescendo (grows louder), decrescendo (grows softer), crescendo-decrescendo (first rises, then falls), decrescendo-crescendo (first falls, then rises), plateau (even intensity), or variable (uneven intensity). The murmur's *pitch* may be high or low. Its *quality* may be described as harsh, rumbling, blowing, scratching, buzzing, musical, or squeaking.

Murmurs can reflect accelerated blood flow through normal or abnormal valves; forward blood flow through a narrowed or irregular valve or into a dilated vessel; blood backflow through an incompetent valve, septal defect, or patent ductus arteriosus; or decreased blood viscosity. Commonly the result of organic heart disease, murmurs occasionally may signal an emergency—for example, a loud holosystolic murmur after an acute myocardial infarction may signal papillary muscle rupture or a ventricular septal defect. Murmurs may also result from surgical implantation of a prosthetic valve. (See *When murmurs mean emergency.*)

Some murmurs are innocent, or functional. An *innocent systolic murmur* is generally soft, medium-pitched, and loudest along the left sternal border at the second or third intercostal space. It's made worse by physical activity, excitement, fever, pregnancy, anemia, or thyrotoxicosis. Examples include Still's murmur in children and mammary souffle, commonly heard over either breast during late pregnancy and early postpartum.

History

- Ask whether the murmur is new or existing.
- Find out about other symptoms, including palpitations, dizziness, syncope, chest pain, dyspnea, and fatigue.
- Obtain a medical history, including the incidence of rheumatic fever, recent dental work, heart disease, or heart surgery.

Physical examination

- Auscultate the heart and determine the type of murmur. (See *Identifying common murmurs,* page 226.)
- Note the presence of cardiac arrhythmias, jugular vein distention, dyspnea, orthopnea, and crackles.
- Palpate the liver for enlargement or tenderness.

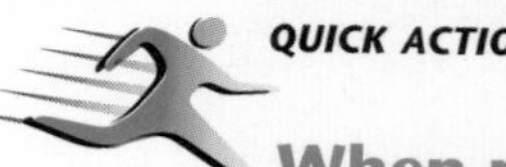

QUICK ACTION

When murmurs mean emergency

Although not usually a sign of an emergency, murmurs—especially newly developed ones—may signal a serious complication in patients with bacterial endocarditis or a recent acute myocardial infarction (MI).

When caring for a patient with known or suspected bacterial endocarditis, carefully auscultate for new murmurs. Their development, along with crackles, jugular vein distention, orthopnea, and dyspnea, may signal heart failure.

Regular auscultation is also important in a patient who has experienced an acute MI. A loud decrescendo holosystolic murmur at the apex that radiates to the axilla and left sternal border or throughout the chest is significant, particularly in association with a widely split S_2 and an atrial gallop (S_4). This murmur, when accompanied by signs of acute pulmonary edema, usually indicates the development of acute mitral insufficiency due to rupture of the chordae tendineae—a medical emergency.

Causes

Medical causes

Aortic insufficiency

- In the acute form, a soft, short diastolic murmur is heard over the left sternal border that's best heard with the patient leaning forward and at the end of a forced held expiration.
- Other acute signs and symptoms include tachycardia, dyspnea, jugular vein distention, crackles, increased fatigue, and pale, cool extremities.
- In the chronic form, a high-pitched, blowing, decrescendo diastolic murmur is heard over the second or third right intercostal space or the left sternal border; an Austin Flint murmur—a rumbling, mid-to-late diastolic murmur best heard at the apex—may also occur.
- Other chronic signs and symptoms include palpitations, tachycardia, angina, increased fatigue, dyspnea, orthopnea, and crackles.

Aortic stenosis

- The murmur is systolic, harsh and grating, medium-pitched, crescendo-decrescendo and heard loudest over the second right intercostal space with the patient leaning forward.
- Other signs and symptoms include dizziness, syncope, dyspnea on exertion, paroxysmal nocturnal dyspnea, fatigue, and angina.

Cardiomyopathy, hypertrophic

- A harsh, late systolic murmur commonly accompanies an audible S_3 or S_4.
- The murmur decreases with squatting and increases with sitting down.
- Other signs and symptoms include dyspnea, chest pain, palpitations, dizziness, and syncope.

Mitral insufficiency

- The acute form produces medium-pitched blowing, an early systolic or holosystolic decrescendo murmur at the apex along with a widely split S_2 and, commonly, S_4.
- Other acute signs and symptoms include tachycardia and signs of acute pulmonary edema.
- The chronic form produces a high-pitched, blowing, holosystolic plateau murmur that's loudest at the apex and may radiate to the axilla or back.

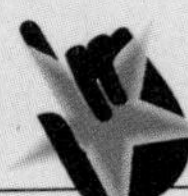

KNOW-HOW

Identifying common murmurs

The timing and configuration of a murmur can help you identify its underlying cause. Learn to recognize the characteristics of these common murmurs.

Aortic insufficiency (chronic)

Thickened valve leaflets fail to close correctly, permitting blood backflow into the left ventricle.

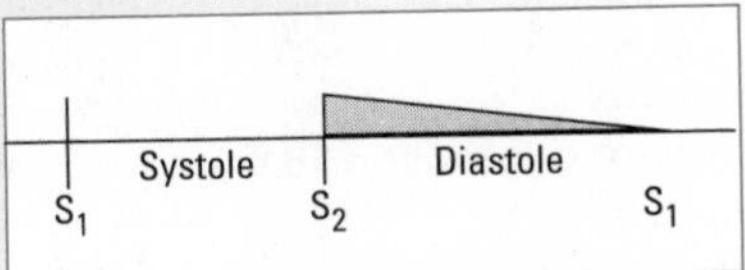

Aortic stenosis

Thickened, scarred, or calcified valve leaflets impede ventricular systolic ejection.

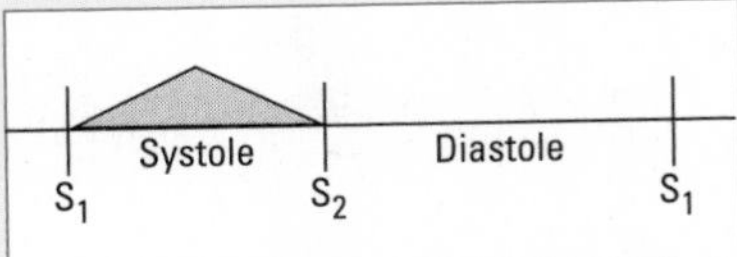

Mitral prolapse

An incompetent mitral valve bulges into the left atrium because of an enlarged posterior leaflet and elongated chordae tendineae.

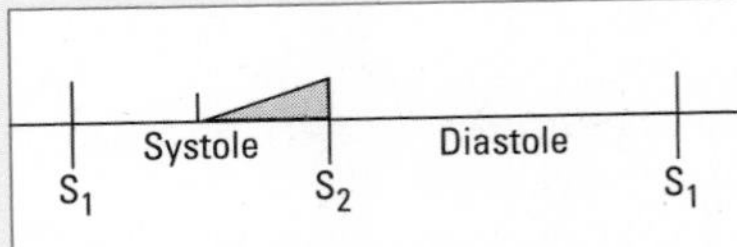

Mitral insufficiency (chronic)

Incomplete mitral valve closure permits the backflow of blood into the left atrium.

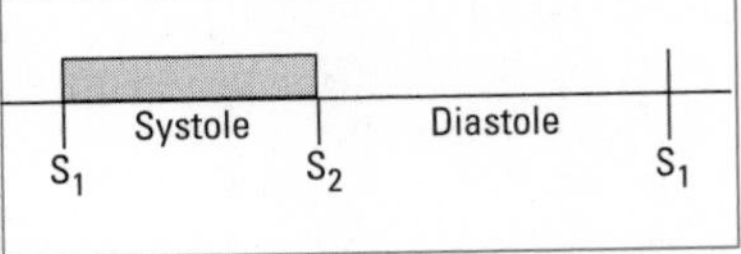

Mitral stenosis

Thickened or scarred valve leaflets cause valve stenosis and restrict blood flow.

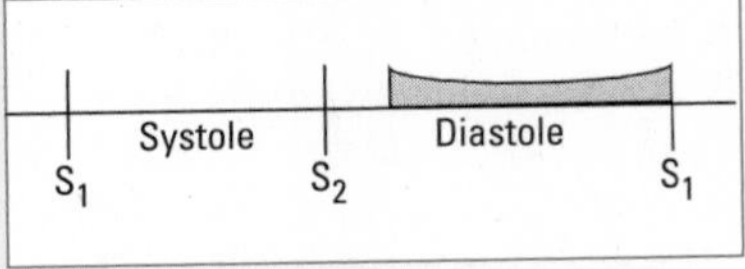

- Other chronic signs and symptoms include fatigue, dyspnea, and palpitations.

Mitral prolapse

- A midsystolic to late systolic click with a high-pitched late systolic crescendo murmur occurs, best heard at the apex.
- Other signs and symptoms include cardiac awareness, migraine headache, dizziness, weakness, syncope, palpitations, chest pain, dyspnea, severe episodic fatigue, mood swings, and anxiety.

Mitral stenosis

- The murmur is soft, low-pitched, rumbling, crescendo-decrescendo, and diastolic; is accompanied by a loud S_1 or opening snap; and is best heard with the patient lying on his left side.

- With severe stenosis, a murmur of mitral insufficiency may also be heard.
- Other signs and symptoms include hemoptysis, exertional dyspnea, fatigue, and signs of acute pulmonary edema.

Papillary muscle rupture

- In this life-threatening disorder, a loud holosystolic murmur can be auscultated at the apex.
- Other signs and symptoms include severe dyspnea, chest pain, syncope, hemoptysis, tachycardia, and hypotension.

Rheumatic fever with pericarditis

- A systolic murmur of mitral insufficiency, a midsystolic murmur from swelling of the leaflet of the mitral valve, and a diastolic murmur of aortic insufficiency are common.
- A pericardial friction rub, along with murmurs and gallops, is best heard with the patient leaning forward during forced expiration.
- Other signs and symptoms include fever, joint and sternal pain, edema, and tachypnea.

Tricuspid insufficiency

- A soft, high-pitched, holosystolic blowing murmur increases with inspiration and decreases with exhalation and Valsalva's maneuver; it's best heard over the lower left sternal border and the xiphoid area.
- Late signs and symptoms include exertional dyspnea, orthopnea, jugular vein distention, ascites, peripheral cyanosis and edema, muscle wasting, fatigue, weakness, and syncope.

Tricuspid stenosis

- A diastolic murmur is produced that's similar to that of mitral stenosis, but louder with inspiration and decreased with exhalation and Valsalva's maneuver.
- Other signs and symptoms include fatigue, syncope, peripheral edema, jugular vein distention, ascites, hepatomegaly, and dyspnea.

Other causes

Treatments

- Prosthetic valve replacement may cause variable murmurs.

Nursing considerations

- Monitor the patient's cardiovascular status if he has an acute condition.
- Give an antibiotic and anticoagulant, if needed.
- Innocent murmurs are commonly heard in young children.
- Pathognomonic heart murmurs in infants and young children usually result from congenital heart disease.
- Other murmurs can be acquired, as with rheumatic heart disease.

Patient teaching

- Discuss the underlying condition, diagnostic tests, and treatment options.
- Explain the need for prophylactic antibiotics before certain procedures such as dental work.
- Explain the signs and symptoms the patient should report.

Muscle spasticity

Spasticity is a state of excessive muscle tone manifested by increased resistance to stretching and heightened reflexes. It's commonly detected by evaluating a muscle's response to passive movement; a spastic muscle offers more resistance when the passive movement is performed quickly. Caused by an upper motor neuron lesion, spasticity usually occurs in the arm and leg muscles. Long-term spasticity results in muscle

How spasticity develops

Motor activity is controlled by pyramidal and extrapyramidal tracts that originate in the motor cortex, basal ganglia, brain stem, and spinal cord. Nerve fibers from the various tracts converge and synapse at the anterior horn in the spinal cord. Together, they maintain segmental muscle tone by modulating the stretch reflex arc. This arc, shown in simplified form below, is basically a negative feedback loop in which muscle stretch (stimulation) causes reflexive contraction (inhibition), thus maintaining muscle length and tone.

Damage to certain tracts results in a loss of inhibition and a disruption of the stretch reflex arc. Uninhibited muscle stretch produces exaggerated, uncontrolled muscle activity, accentuating the reflex arc and eventually resulting in spasticity.

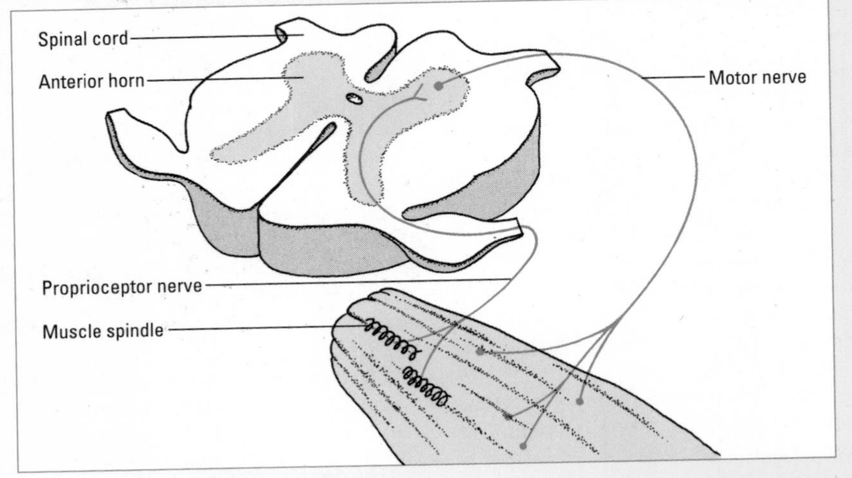

fibrosis and contractures. (See *How spasticity develops.*)

History

- Ask about the onset, duration, and progression of spasticity.
- Ask about how the spasticity started and what aggravates it.
- Find out about other muscular changes or other symptoms such as pain.
- Obtain a medical history, including the incidence of trauma or degenerative or vascular disease.

Physical examination

- Take the patient's vital signs.
- Perform a neurologic assessment.
- Test reflexes and evaluate motor and sensory function in all limbs.
- Evaluate muscles for wasting and contractures.

Causes

Medical causes

Amyotrophic lateral sclerosis

- Early signs and symptoms include progressive muscle weakness and flaccidity that typically begin in the hands

and arms and eventually spread to the trunk, neck, larynx, pharynx, and legs.
- Spasticity, spasms, coarse fasciculations, hyperactive deep tendon reflexes (DTRs), and a positive Babinski's reflex also occur.
- Other signs and symptoms include respiratory insufficiency, dysphagia, dysarthria, excessive drooling, and depression.

Epidural hemorrhage
- Limb spasticity is a late and ominous sign and may be preceded by momentary loss of consciousness after head trauma, followed by a lucid interval, and then a rapid deterioration in level of consciousness (LOC).
- Other signs and symptoms include hemiparesis or hemiplegia; seizures; fixed, dilated pupils; high fever; decreased and bounding pulse; widened pulse pressure; elevated blood pressure; irregular respiratory pattern; positive Babinski's reflex; and decerebrate posture.

Multiple sclerosis
- Muscle spasticity, hyperreflexia, and contractures may eventually develop as demyelination advances.
- Progressive weakness and atrophy occur early.
- Other signs and symptoms include diplopia, blurring or loss of vision, nystagmus, sensory loss or paresthesia, dysarthria, dysphagia, incoordination, ataxic gait, intention tremors, emotional lability, impotence, and urinary dysfunction.

Spinal cord injury
- Spastic paralysis in the affected limbs follows initial flaccid paralysis.
- Spasticity and muscle atrophy increase for up to 2 years after the injury, and then gradually regress to flaccidity.
- Other signs and symptoms vary with the level of the injury and may include respiratory insufficiency or paralysis, sensory losses, bowel and bladder dysfunction, hyperactive DTRs, positive Babinski's reflex, anhidrosis, and bradycardia.

Stroke
- Spastic paralysis may develop on the affected side following the acute stage.
- Other signs and symptoms vary and may include dysarthria, aphasia, ataxia, apraxia, agnosia, ipsilateral paresthesia or sensory loss, vision disturbances, altered LOC, personality changes, emotional lability, bowel and bladder dysfunction, and seizures.

Tetanus
- This life-threatening disease produces varying degrees of muscle spasticity.
- In generalized tetanus, signs and symptoms include painful jaw and neck stiffness, trismus, headache, irritability, restlessness, low-grade fever, chills, tachycardia, diaphoresis, and hyperactive DTRs.
- As the disease progresses, painful involuntary spasms may spread and cause boardlike abdominal rigidity, opisthotonos, and *risus sardonicus*.
- Glottal, pharyngeal, or respiratory muscle involvement can cause death by asphyxia or cardiac failure.

Nursing considerations
- Give drugs for pain and an antispasmodic.
- Passive range-of-motion exercises, splinting, traction, and application of heat may help relieve spasms and prevent contractures.
- Maintain a calm, quiet environment, and encourage bed rest.
- In cases of prolonged, uncontrollable spasticity, nerve blocks or surgical transection may be needed.

Patient teaching

- Discuss the underlying condition, diagnostic tests, and treatment options.
- Teach the patient to use assistive devices, as needed.
- Discuss ways of maintaining independence.
- Explain the prescribed medications.

Mydriasis

Mydriasis is pupillary dilation caused by contraction of the dilator of the iris. This is a normal response to decreased light, strong emotional stimuli, and the topical administration of mydriatic and cycloplegic drugs. It can also result from ocular and neurologic disorders, eye trauma, and disorders that decrease the patient's level of consciousness (LOC). In addition, mydriasis may be an adverse effect of antihistamines or other drugs.

History

- Ask about other eye problems, such as pain, blurring, diplopia, or visual field deficits.
- Obtain a health history, focusing on the incidence of eye or head trauma, glaucoma and other ocular problems, and neurologic and vascular disorders.
- Obtain a complete drug history.

Physical examination

- Inspect and compare the pupils' size, color, and shape. (See *Grading pupil size.*)
- Test each pupil for light reflex, consensual response, and accommodation.
- Perform a swinging flashlight test to evaluate a decreased response to direct light coupled with a normal consensual response.
- Check eyes for ptosis, swelling, and ecchymosis.
- Test visual acuity in both eyes with and without corrective lenses.
- Evaluate extraocular muscle function by checking the six cardinal fields of gaze.

Causes

Medical causes

Aortic arch syndrome

- Mydriasis in both eyes occurs late due to decreased circulation.
- Related ocular signs and symptoms include visual blurring, transient vision loss, and diplopia.
- Other signs and symptoms include dizziness and syncope; neck, shoulder, and chest pain; bruits; loss of radial and carotid pulses; paresthesia; intermittent claudication; and, possibly, decreased blood pressure in the arms.

Botulism

- Bilateral mydriasis usually occurs 12 to 36 hours after ingestion.
- Other early signs and symptoms include loss of pupillary reflexes, visual blurring, diplopia, ptosis, strabismus, extraocular muscle palsies, anorexia, nausea, vomiting, diarrhea, and dry mouth.
- Later signs and symptoms include vertigo, hearing loss, hoarseness, hypernasality, dysarthria, dysphagia, progressive muscle weakness, and loss of deep tendon reflexes.

Carotid artery aneurysm

- Mydriasis in one eye may be accompanied by bitemporal hemianopsia, decreased visual acuity, hemiplegia, decreased LOC, headache, aphasia, behavioral changes, and hypoesthesia.

Glaucoma, acute angle-closure

- Moderate mydriasis and loss of pupillary reflexes occur with excruciating pain, redness, decreased visual acuity, visual blurring, halo vision, conjunctival injection, a cloudy cornea and, in 2 to 5 days without treatment, permanent blindness.

Oculomotor nerve palsy

- Mydriasis in one eye is commonly the first sign.
- Other signs and symptoms include ptosis, diplopia, decreased pupillary reflexes, exotropia, and complete loss of accommodation.

Traumatic iridoplegia

- Mydriasis and loss of pupillary reflexes (caused by paralysis of sphincter of iris) are usually transient.
- Other signs and symptoms include a quivering iris, ecchymosis, pain, and swelling.

Other causes

Drugs

- Mydriasis can be caused by anesthesia induction, anticholinergics, antihistamines, sympathomimetics, barbiturates (overdose), estrogens, and tricyclic antidepressants.
- Topical mydriatic drugs and cycloplegics are given for their mydriatic effect.

Surgery

- Traumatic mydriasis commonly results from ocular surgery.

Nursing considerations

- If the patient is experiencing photophobia, darken the room, and encourage the patient to close or shade his eyes or wear sunglasses.
- Administer eyedrops or ointments as prescribed.

Patient teaching

- Discuss the effects of mydriatic drugs and ways to reduce adverse reactions.
- Teach about the underlying diagnosis and treatment plan.

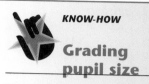

KNOW-HOW

Grading pupil size

To accurately evaluate pupil size, compare the patient's pupils with the scale shown here. Keep in mind that the maximum constriction may be less than 1 mm and the maximum dilation greater than 9 mm.

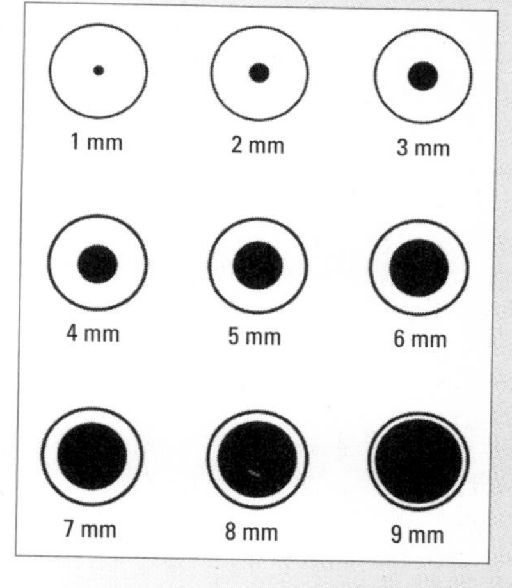

Myoclonus

Myoclonus—sudden, shocklike contractions of a single muscle or muscle group—occurs with various neurologic disorders and may precede the onset of a seizure. These contractions may be isolated or repetitive, rhythmic or arrhythmic, symmetrical or asymmetrical, synchronous or asynchronous, and generalized or focal. They may be precipitated by bright flickering lights, a loud sound, or unexpected physical contact. One type, *intention myoclonus,* is evoked by intentional muscle movement.

Normally, myoclonus may occur just before falling asleep and as part of the natural startle reaction. It also occurs with some poisonings and, in rare cases, as a complication of hemodialysis.

QUICK ACTION ***If you observe myoclonus, check for seizure activity. Take the patient's vital signs to rule out arrhythmias or an occluded airway. Have resuscitation equipment on hand.***

If the patient has a seizure, gently help him lie down. Place a pillow or a rolled-up towel under his head to prevent injury. Loosen constrictive clothing, especially around the neck, and turn his head (gently, if possible) to one side to prevent airway occlusion or aspiration of secretions or vomitus.

History

- Ask about the frequency, severity, location, and circumstances of myoclonus.
- Determine whether the patient has had previous seizures.
- Find out what causes the patient's myoclonus.

Physical examination

- Evaluate the patient's level of consciousness (LOC) and mental condition.
- Check for muscle rigidity and wasting.
- Test for deep tendon reflexes.
- Complete neurologic and musculoskeletal assessments.

Causes

Medical causes

Alzheimer's disease

- Generalized myoclonus may occur in advanced stages.
- Other late signs and symptoms include mild choreoathetoid movements, muscle rigidity, bowel and bladder incontinence, delusions, and hallucinations.

Creutzfeldt-Jakob disease

- In this progressive neurologic disease, diffuse myoclonic jerks are initially random; gradually they become rhythmic and symmetrical in response to sensory stimuli.
- Other signs and symptoms include ataxia, aphasia, hearing loss, muscle rigidity and wasting, fasciculations, hemiplegia, vision disturbances and, possibly, blindness.

Encephalitis, viral

- Myoclonus is intermittent.
- Other signs and symptoms vary but may include rapidly decreasing LOC, fever, headache, irritability, nuchal rigidity, vomiting, seizures, aphasia, ataxia, hemiparesis, facial muscle weakness, nystagmus, ocular palsies, and dysphagia.

Encephalopathy

- In hepatic encephalopathy, myoclonic jerks are produced in association with asterixis and focal or generalized seizures.
- In hypoxic encephalopathy, generalized myoclonus or seizures occur almost immediately after restoration of cardiopulmonary function.
- In uremic encephalopathy, myoclonic jerks and seizures are common.

Epilepsy

- With idiopathic epilepsy, localized myoclonus usually occurs upon awakening, in an arm or a leg, and singly or in short bursts.
- With myoclonic epilepsy, myoclonus is initially infrequent and localized, but becomes more frequent and generalized over a period of months.

Other causes

Drug withdrawal

- Myoclonus may be seen in patients with alcohol, opioid, or sedative withdrawal or alcohol withdrawal delirium.

Poisoning

- Acute intoxication with methylbromide, bismuth, or strychnine may produce an acute onset of myoclonus and confusion.

Nursing considerations

- If myoclonus is progressive, take seizure precautions.
- Keep an oral airway and suction equipment at the bedside.
- Pad the bed's side rails and remove potentially harmful objects.
- Remain with the patient while he walks.
- Give drugs that suppress myoclonus, as needed.

Patient teaching

- Discuss the underlying condition, diagnostic tests, and treatment options.
- Talk with the patient about taking safety measures and seizure precautions.
- Refer the patient to social service or community resources as needed.
- Teach the patient about prescribed medications.

N

Nasal flaring

Nasal flaring is the abnormal dilation of the nostrils. Usually occurring during inspiration, nasal flaring may occasionally occur during expiration or throughout the respiratory cycle. It indicates respiratory dysfunction, ranging from mild difficulty to potentially life-threatening respiratory distress.

QUICK ACTION ***If you note nasal flaring in the patient, quickly evaluate his respiratory status. Absent breath sounds, cyanosis, diaphoresis, and tachycardia point to complete airway obstruction. As necessary, deliver back blows or abdominal thrusts (Heimlich maneuver) to relieve the obstruction. If these don't clear the airway, emergency intubation or tracheostomy and mechanical ventilation may be needed.***

If the patient's airway isn't obstructed but he displays breathing difficulty, give oxygen by nasal cannula or face mask. Intubation and mechanical ventilation may be necessary. Insert an I.V. catheter for fluid and drug administration. Begin cardiac monitoring. Obtain a chest X-ray and samples for arterial blood gas (ABG) analysis and electrolyte studies.

History

- Obtain a pertinent history, including the incidence of cardiac and pulmonary disorders, such as asthma, allergies, respiratory tract infection, or trauma.
- Obtain a smoking and drug history.

Physical examination

- Take the patient's vital signs.
- Auscultate breath sounds.

Causes

Medical causes

Acute respiratory distress syndrome (ARDS)

- ARDS causes increased respiratory difficulty and hypoxemia, with nasal flaring, dyspnea, tachypnea, diaphoresis, cyanosis, scattered crackles, rhonchi, wheezing, and accessory muscle use. It also produces tachycardia, anxiety, and a decreased level of consciousness (LOC).

Airway obstruction

- Complete obstruction above the tracheal bifurcation causes sudden nasal flaring; absent breath sounds, despite intercostal retractions and marked accessory muscle use; tachycardia; diaphoresis; cyanosis; a decreasing LOC; and, eventually, respiratory arrest.
- Partial obstruction causes nasal flaring with inspiratory stridor, gagging, wheezing, a violent cough, marked accessory muscle use, agitation, cyanosis, and hoarseness.

Anaphylaxis

- Severe reactions can produce respiratory distress with nasal flaring, stridor, wheezing, accessory muscle use, intercostal retractions, and chest tightness.

- Associated signs and symptoms include nasal congestion, sneezing, pruritus, urticaria, erythema, diaphoresis, angioedema, weakness, hoarseness, dysphagia and, rarely, vomiting, nausea, diarrhea, urinary urgency, and incontinence.
- Cardiac arrhythmias, hypotension, and signs of shock may occur late.

Asthma, acute

- An asthma attack can cause nasal flaring, dyspnea, tachypnea, prolonged expiratory wheezing, accessory muscle use, cyanosis, and a dry or productive cough.
- Auscultation may reveal rhonchi, crackles, and decreased or absent breath sounds.
- Other signs and symptoms include anxiety, tachycardia, and increased blood pressure.

Chronic obstructive pulmonary disease

- Nasal flaring is accompanied by prolonged pursed-lip expiration; accessory muscle use; a loose, rattling, productive cough; cyanosis; reduced chest expansion; crackles; rhonchi; wheezing; and dyspnea.
- Chronic obstructive pulmonary disease can lead to acute respiratory failure secondary to pulmonary infection or edema.

Pneumonia, bacterial

- Nasal flaring occurs with dyspnea, tachypnea, high fever, sudden shaking chills, and a dry, hacking cough that progresses to a productive cough.
- Other signs and symptoms include stabbing chest pain, decreased or absent breath sounds, fine crackles, pleural friction rub, and dullness on percussion.

Pulmonary edema

- Pulmonary edema typically produces nasal flaring, severe dyspnea, wheezing, and a cough that produces frothy, pink sputum. Increased accessory muscle use may occur with tachycardia, cyanosis, hypotension, crackles, jugular vein distention, peripheral edema, and decreased LOC.

Pulmonary embolus

- In this potentially life-threatening disorder, nasal flaring may be accompanied by dyspnea, tachypnea, wheezing, cyanosis, pleural friction rub, and a productive cough (possibly hemoptysis).
- Other signs and symptoms include sudden chest tightness or pleuritic pain, tachycardia, atrial arrhythmias, hypotension, low-grade fever, syncope, marked anxiety, and restlessness.

Other causes

Diagnostic tests

- Pulmonary function tests, such as vital capacity testing, can produce nasal flaring with forced inspiration or expiration.

Treatments

- Certain respiratory treatments, such as deep breathing, can cause nasal flaring.

Nursing considerations

- To help ease breathing, place the patient in high Fowler's position.
- If the patient is at risk for aspirating secretions, place him in a modified Trendelenburg or side-lying position.
- Suction frequently to remove oropharyngeal secretions, if necessary.
- Administer humidified oxygen to thin secretions and decrease airway drying and irritation. Provide adequate hydration to liquefy secretions.
- Reposition the patient every hour, and encourage coughing and deep breathing.

- Avoid administering sedatives or opiates, which can depress the cough reflex or respirations.
- Continually assess the patient's respiratory status, and check his vital signs and oxygen saturation every 30 minutes or as necessary.
- For infants and children, the use of a croup tent may improve oxygenation and humidification.

Patient teaching

- Teach the patient about the underlying diagnosis and treatment plan.
- Prepare the patient for diagnostic tests, such as chest X-rays, a lung scan, pulmonary arteriography, sputum culture, complete blood count, ABG analysis, and 12-lead electrocardiogram.
- Explain the prescribed medications.
- Teach the importance of proper positioning.
- Teach the patient how to do coughing and deep-breathing exercises.

Nausea

Nausea is a sensation of profound revulsion to food or of impending vomiting. Typically accompanied by autonomic signs, such as hypersalivation, diaphoresis, tachycardia, pallor, and tachypnea, it's closely associated with anorexia and vomiting.

Nausea, a common symptom of GI disorders, also occurs with fluid and electrolyte imbalance; infection; metabolic, endocrine, labyrinthine, and cardiac disorders; and as a result of drug therapy, surgery, and radiation. It's common during the first trimester of pregnancy. In addition, nausea may arise from severe pain, anxiety, alcohol intoxication, overeating, or ingestion of distasteful food or liquids.

History

- Ask about the onset and description of nausea.
- Determine aggravating or alleviating factors.
- Obtain a medical history, including the incidence of GI, endocrine, and metabolic disorders, cancer, and infections.
- Ask about vomiting, abdominal pain, and changes in bowel habits.
- Ask the female patient if she could be pregnant.

Physical examination

- Inspect the skin for jaundice, bruises, and spider angiomas; assess skin turgor.
- Inspect for abdominal distention.
- Auscultate for bowel sounds and bruits.
- Palpate for abdominal rigidity and tenderness and test for rebound tenderness.
- Palpate and percuss the liver.

Causes

Medical causes

Adrenal insufficiency

- Common GI findings include nausea, vomiting, anorexia, and diarrhea.
- Other signs and symptoms include weakness, fatigue, weight loss, bronze-colored skin, hypotension, a weak, irregular pulse, vitiligo, and depression.

Anthrax, GI

- Initial signs and symptoms include nausea, vomiting, loss of appetite, and fever that may progress to abdominal pain, severe bloody diarrhea, and hematemesis.

Appendicitis

- A brief period of nausea may accompany the onset of abdominal pain.
- Other signs and symptoms include abdominal rigidity and tenderness, cu-

taneous hyperalgesia, fever, constipation or diarrhea, tachycardia, anorexia, and malaise.

Cholecystitis, acute

- Nausea typically follows severe right upper quadrant pain that may radiate to the back or shoulders, commonly after meals.
- Other signs and symptoms include vomiting, flatulence, abdominal tenderness, rigidity and distention, fever with chills, diaphoresis, and a positive Murphy's sign.

Cholelithiasis

- Nausea accompanies severe right upper quadrant or epigastric pain.
- Other signs and symptoms include vomiting, abdominal tenderness and guarding, flatulence, belching, epigastric burning, tachycardia, restlessness and, with an occluded common bile duct, jaundice, clay-colored stools, fever, and chills.

Cirrhosis

- Nausea, vomiting, anorexia, abdominal pain, and constipation or diarrhea occur.
- As the disease progresses, jaundice and hepatomegaly may occur with abdominal distention, spider angiomas, fetor hepaticus, enlarged superficial abdominal veins, mental changes, bilateral gynecomastia and testicular irregularities, or menstrual irregularities.

Diverticulitis

- Nausea, intermittent crampy abdominal pain, constipation or diarrhea, low-grade fever and, in many cases, a palpable, fixed mass occur.
- Other signs and symptoms include anorexia, bloody stools, and flatulence.

Electrolyte imbalances

- Nausea and vomiting occur with cardiac arrhythmias, tremors or seizures, anorexia, malaise, and weakness.

Escherichia coli *0157:H7*

- Nausea, watery or bloody diarrhea, vomiting, fever, and abdominal cramps occur.

Gastritis

- Nausea is common, especially after ingestion of alcohol, aspirin, spicy foods, or caffeine.
- Vomiting, epigastric pain, belching, and malaise may also occur.

Gastroenteritis

- Nausea, vomiting, diarrhea, and abdominal cramping occur.
- Other signs and symptoms include fever, malaise, hyperactive bowel sounds, abdominal pain and tenderness, and signs of dehydration and electrolyte imbalance.

Heart failure

- Heart failure may produce nausea and vomiting, particularly with right-sided heart failure.
- Associated signs and symptoms include tachycardia, ventricular gallop, profound fatigue, dyspnea, crackles, peripheral edema, jugular vein distention, ascites, nocturia, and diastolic hypertension.

Hepatitis

- Nausea is an early symptom.
- Vomiting, fatigue, myalgia, arthralgia, headache, anorexia, photophobia, pharyngitis, cough, and fever also occur early in the preicteric phase.

Hyperemesis gravidarum

- Unremitting nausea and vomiting persist beyond the first trimester of pregnancy.

■ Other signs and symptoms include weight loss, signs of dehydration, headache, and delirium.

Inflammatory bowel disease

■ Nausea, vomiting, abdominal pain, and anorexia may occur, but the most common sign is recurrent diarrhea with blood, pus, and mucus.

Intestinal obstruction

■ Nausea, vomiting, constipation, and abdominal pain occur.
■ Other signs and symptoms include abdominal distention and tenderness, visible peristaltic waves, and hyperactive (in partial obstruction) or hypoactive or absent bowel sounds (in complete obstruction).

Irritable bowel syndrome

■ Nausea, dyspepsia, and abdominal distention may occur.
■ Other signs and symptoms include lower abdominal pain and tenderness relieved by defecation, diurnal diarrhea alternating with constipation or normal bowel function, small stools with visible mucus, and a feeling of incomplete evacuation.

Labyrinthitis

■ Nausea and vomiting occur with severe vertigo, progressive hearing loss, nystagmus, tinnitus and, possibly, otorrhea.

Ménière's disease

■ Sudden, brief, recurrent attacks of nausea, vomiting, vertigo, tinnitus, nystagmus and, eventually, hearing loss occur.

Mesenteric venous thrombosis

■ Insidious or acute onset of nausea, vomiting, and abdominal pain occurs along with diarrhea or constipation, abdominal distention, hematemesis, and melena.

Metabolic acidosis

■ Nausea, vomiting, anorexia, diarrhea, Kussmaul's respirations, and decreased level of consciousness may develop.

Migraine headache

■ Nausea and vomiting may occur along with photophobia, light flashes, increased sensitivity to noise, lightheadedness, partial vision loss, and paresthesia of the lips, face, and hands.

Motion sickness

■ Nausea and vomiting occur along with possible headache, dizziness, fatigue, diaphoresis, hypersalivation, and dyspnea.

Myocardial infarction

■ Nausea and vomiting may occur, but the cardinal symptom is severe substernal chest pain that may radiate to the left arm, jaw, or neck.
■ Other signs and symptoms include dyspnea, pallor, clammy skin, diaphoresis, altered blood pressure, and arrhythmias.

Norovirus

■ Acute gastroenteritis causes individuals to experience nausea.
■ Other signs and symptoms include vomiting, diarrhea, abdominal pain or cramping, low-grade fever, headache, chills, muscle aches, and generalized tiredness.

Pancreatitis, acute

■ Nausea, usually followed by vomiting, is an early symptom.
■ Other signs and symptoms include severe upper abdominal pain that may radiate to the back, abdominal tenderness and rigidity, anorexia, diminished bowel sounds, and fever.

Peptic ulcer

■ Nausea and vomiting follow attacks of sharp or gnawing, burning epigastric pain when the stomach is empty or after ingesting alcohol, caffeine, or aspirin.

- Hematemesis and melena may occur.

Peritonitis

- Nausea and vomiting accompany acute abdominal pain.
- Other signs and symptoms include fever, chills, tachycardia, hypoactive or absent bowel sounds, abdominal rigidity and tenderness, diaphoresis, hypotension, and shallow respirations.

Preeclampsia

- Nausea and vomiting commonly occur along with rapid weight gain, epigastric pain, oliguria, severe frontal headache, hyperreflexia, and blurred or double vision.
- The classic diagnostic triad of signs includes hypertension, proteinuria, and edema.

Rhabdomyolysis

- Nausea, vomiting, fever, malaise, and dark urine are common due to renal damage or pain.
- Tenderness, swelling, and muscle weakness or pain may also develop.

Thyrotoxicosis

- Nausea and vomiting may accompany severe anxiety, heat intolerance, diaphoresis, diarrhea, tremors, tachycardia, palpitations, fatigue, and weakness.
- Other signs and symptoms include exophthalmos, ventricular or atrial gallop, and an enlarged thyroid gland.

Other causes

Drugs

- Antineoplastics, opiates, ferrous sulfate, levodopa (Larodopa), oral potassium chloride replacements, estrogens, sulfasalazine (Azulfidine), antibiotics, quinidine, anesthetics, digoxin (Lanoxin), theophylline (Elixophyllin) overdose, and nonsteroidal anti-inflammatory drugs can cause nausea.

Radiation and surgery

- Radiation therapy can cause nausea and vomiting.
- Postoperative nausea and vomiting is common.

Nursing considerations

- Provide measures such as medications to ease the patient's nausea.
- Evaluate fluid, electrolyte, and acid-base balance.
- Elevate the patient's head or position him on his side.
- Be prepared to insert a nasogastric tube, if needed.

Patient teaching

- Discuss what aggravates nausea and how to avoid it.
- Teach the patient about the underlying diagnosis and treatment plan.

Neck pain

Neck pain may originate from any neck structure, ranging from the meninges and cervical vertebrae to its blood vessels, muscles, and lymphatic tissue. This symptom can also be referred from other areas of the body. Its location, onset, and pattern help determine the origin and underlying causes. Neck pain usually results from trauma and degenerative, congenital, inflammatory, metabolic, and neoplastic disorders.

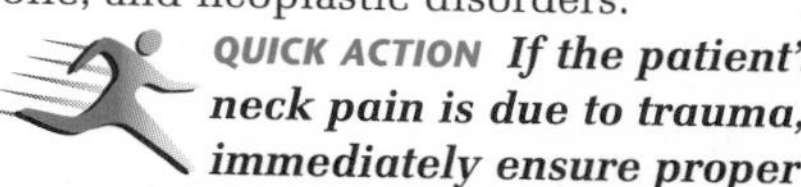

QUICK ACTION ***If the patient's neck pain is due to trauma, immediately ensure proper cervical spine immobilization, preferably with a long backboard and a Philadelphia collar. Then take his vital signs, and perform a quick neurologic examination. If he shows signs of respiratory distress, administer oxygen. Endotracheal intubation or tracheostomy and mechanical ventilation may be necessary. Ask the patient (or a family member, if the patient can't answer) how the injury occurred. Then***

examine the neck for abrasions, swelling, lacerations, erythema, and ecchymoses.

History

- Find out about the onset and description of pain.
- Ask about alleviating, aggravating, or precipitating factors.
- Find out about associated symptoms such as headache.
- Obtain a medical and drug history.

Physical examination

- Inspect the neck, shoulders, and cervical spine for swelling, masses, erythema, and ecchymoses.
- Assess active range of motion (ROM) in the neck and note any pain.
- Examine the patient's posture.
- Test and compare bilateral muscle strength and sensation.
- Assess hand grasp and arm reflexes.
- If the patient's condition permits, test for Brudzinski's and Kernig's signs.
- Palpate the cervical lymph nodes for enlargement.

Causes

Medical causes

Ankylosing spondylitis

- Intermittent, moderate to severe neck pain and stiffness with severely restricted ROM is characteristic.
- Intermittent low back pain and stiffness and arm pain are generally worse in the morning or after periods of inactivity, and are usually relieved after exercise.
- Other signs and symptoms include low-grade fever, limited chest expansion, malaise, anorexia, fatigue and, occasionally, iritis.

Cervical extension injury

- Anterior pain usually diminishes within several days after the injury.
- Posterior pain persists and may intensify.
- Other signs and symptoms include tenderness, swelling and nuchal rigidity, arm or back pain, occipital headache, muscle spasms, visual blurring, and unilateral miosis on the affected side.

Cervical spine fracture

- Severe neck pain may occur with intense occipital headache, quadriplegia, deformity, and respiratory paralysis.

Cervical spine tumor

- Metastatic tumors typically produce persistent neck pain; primary tumors cause mild to severe pain along a specific nerve root.
- Other signs and symptoms may include paresthesia, arm and leg weakness that progresses to atrophy and paralysis, and bowel and bladder incontinence.

Cervical spondylosis

- Posterior neck pain that may radiate is aggravated by and restricts movement.
- Other signs and symptoms include paresthesia, weakness, and stiffness.

Cervical stenosis

- Neck and arm pain, paresthesia, muscle weakness or paralysis, gait and balance problems, and decreased ROM may occur.

Herniated cervical disk

- Variable neck pain that's referred along a specific dermatome is aggravated by and restricts movement.
- Paresthesia and other sensory disturbances and arm weakness may also occur.

Hodgkin's disease

- Generalized pain may eventually affect the neck.
- Lymphadenopathy, the classic sign, may accompany paresthesia, muscle

weakness, fever, fatigue, weight loss, malaise, and hepatomegaly.

Laryngeal cancer

- Neck pain radiating to the ear is a late sign.
- Other signs and symptoms include dysphagia, dyspnea, hemoptysis, stridor, hoarseness, and cervical lymphadenopathy.

Lymphadenitis

- Enlarged and inflamed cervical lymph nodes cause acute pain.
- Fever, chills, and malaise may also occur.

Meningitis

- Neck pain may accompany nuchal rigidity.
- Other signs and symptoms include fever, headache, photophobia, positive Brudzinski's and Kernig's signs, and decreased level of consciousness (LOC).

Neck sprain

- Pain, slight swelling, stiffness, and restricted ROM result.
- Ligament rupture causes severe pain, marked swelling, ecchymosis, muscle spasms, and nuchal rigidity with head tilt.

Paget's disease

- Cervical vertebrae deformity may produce severe neck pain, paresthesia, and arm weakness as the disease progresses.

Rheumatoid arthritis

- Moderate to severe pain may radiate along a specific nerve root.
- Other signs and symptoms include increasingly stiff joints, paresthesia, muscle weakness, low-grade fever, anorexia, malaise, fatigue, neck deformity, and warmth, swelling, and tenderness in involved joints.

Spinous process fracture

- A fracture near the cervicothoracic junction produces acute pain that radiates to the shoulders.
- Other signs and symptoms include swelling, tenderness, restricted ROM, muscle spasm, and deformity.

Subarachnoid hemorrhage

- A life-threatening condition, moderate to severe neck pain and rigidity, headache, and decreased LOC may occur.
- Kernig's and Brudzinski's signs are present.

Torticollis

- Severe neck pain accompanies recurrent, unilateral muscle stiffness and spasms, followed by a momentary twitching or contraction that pulls the head to the affected side.

Tracheal trauma

- Torn tracheal mucosa produces mild to moderate pain and may result in airway occlusion, hemoptysis, hoarseness, and dysphagia.

Nursing considerations

- Give an anti-inflammatory and analgesic as needed.
- Apply a cervical collar as appropriate.
- Neck trauma may not initially produce a lot of pain; however, immobilization is necessary until significant injury is ruled out.
- In children, the most common causes of neck pain are meningitis and trauma.

Patient teaching

- Explain any activities the patient needs to limit.
- Teach the patient how to apply the cervical collar, if needed.
- Provide reinforcement for exercises the patient needs to perform.

Nuchal rigidity

Commonly an early sign of meningeal irritation, nuchal rigidity refers to neck stiffness that prevents flexion. To elicit this sign, attempt to passively flex the patient's neck and touch his chin to his chest. If nuchal rigidity is present, this maneuver triggers pain and muscle spasms. (Make sure that there's no cervical spinal misalignment, such as a fracture or dislocation, before testing for nuchal rigidity. Otherwise, severe spinal cord damage could result.) The patient may also notice nuchal rigidity when he attempts to flex his neck during daily activities. Be aware that this sign isn't reliable in children and infants.

Nuchal rigidity may herald life-threatening subarachnoid hemorrhage or meningitis. It may also be a late sign of cervical arthritis, in which joint mobility is gradually lost.

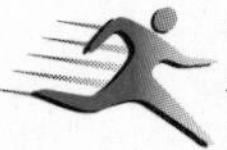

QUICK ACTION ***After eliciting nuchal rigidity, attempt to elicit Kernig's and Brudzinski's signs. Quickly evaluate the patient's level of consciousness (LOC). Take his vital signs. If you note signs of increased intracranial pressure (ICP), such as increased systolic pressure, bradycardia, and a widened pulse pressure, insert an I.V. catheter for drug and fluid administration. Administer oxygen as necessary. Don't raise the head of the bed more than 30 degrees. Draw a sample for routine blood studies such as a complete blood count with a white blood cell count and electrolyte levels.***

History

- Obtain a patient history, relying on family members if an altered LOC prevents the patient from responding. Ask about the onset and duration of neck stiffness; precipitating factors; associated signs and symptoms, such as headache, fever, and nausea and vomiting; and motor and sensory changes.
- Check for a history of hypertension, head trauma, cerebral aneurysm or arteriovenous malformation, endocarditis, recent infection (such as sinusitis or pneumonia), or recent dental work.
- Obtain a complete drug history.
- If the patient has no other signs of meningeal irritation, ask about a history of arthritis or neck trauma.

Physical examination

- Attempt to passively flex the patient's neck and touch his chin to his chest. If nuchal rigidity is present, this maneuver triggers pain and muscle spasms. Make sure that there's no cervical spine misalignment, such as a fracture or dislocation, before testing for nuchal rigidity. Severe spinal cord damage could result.
- Inspect the patient's hands for swollen, tender joints, and palpate the neck for pain or tenderness.
- Perform a complete neurologic examination.

Causes

Medical causes

Cervical arthritis

- With cervical arthritis, nuchal rigidity develops gradually. Initially, the patient may complain of neck stiffness in the early morning or after a period of inactivity. Stiffness then becomes increasingly severe and frequent and may affect other joints, especially those in the hands.
- A common sympton is pain on movement, especially with lateral motion or head turning.

Encephalitis

- Encephalitis is a viral infection that may cause nuchal rigidity accompanied by other signs of meningeal irritation, such as positive Kernig's and Brudzinski's signs.

- Usually, nuchal rigidity appears abruptly and is preceded by headache, vomiting, and fever.
- Other signs and symptoms include rapidly decreasing LOC progressing from lethargy to coma within 24 to 48 hours of onset, seizures, ataxia, hemiparesis, nystagmus, and cranial nerve palsies, such as dysphagia and ptosis.

Listeriosis

- Nuchal rigidity occurs with fever, headache, and a change in the patient's LOC.
- Initial signs and symptoms include myalgia, abdominal pain, nausea, vomiting, and diarrhea.
- If listeriosis spreads to the nervous system, meningitis may develop.
- Listeriosis infection during pregnancy may lead to premature delivery, infection of the neonate, or stillbirth.

Meningitis

- Nuchal rigidity is an early sign of meningitis and is accompanied by other signs of meningeal irritation—positive Kernig's and Brudzinski's signs, hyperreflexia and, possibly, opisthotonos.
- Other early signs and symptoms include fever with chills, confusion, headache, photophobia, irritability, and vomiting; later signs and symptoms include stupor, seizures, and coma.
- Cranial nerve involvement may cause ocular palsies, facial weakness, and hearing loss.
- An erythematous papular rash occurs in some forms of viral meningitis; a purpuric rash may occur in meningococcal meningitis.

Subarachnoid hemorrhage

- Nuchal rigidity develops immediately after bleeding into the subarachnoid space.
- Related signs and symptoms include positive Kernig's and Brudzinski's signs; an abrupt onset of severe headache; photophobia; fever; nausea and vomiting; dizziness; cranial nerve palsies; focal neurologic signs, such as hemiparesis or hemiplegia; and signs of increased ICP, such as bradycardia and altered respirations.
- The patient's LOC may deteriorate rapidly, possibly progressing to coma.

Nursing considerations

- Prepare the patient for diagnostic tests, such as computed tomography scans, magnetic resonance imaging, and cervical spinal X-rays.
- Monitor the patient's vital signs, intake and output, and neurologic status closely.
- Avoid routine administration of opioid analgesics because these may mask signs of increasing ICP.
- Enforce strict bed rest; keep the head of the bed elevated at least 30 degrees to help minimize ICP.
- Assist the patient in finding a comfortable position to obtain adequate rest.

Patient teaching

- Teach the patient about the underlying diagnosis and treatment plan.
- Orient the patient as appropriate.
- Teach family members how they can participate in the care of the patient.

Nystagmus

Nystagmus refers to the involuntary oscillations of one or, more commonly, both eyeballs. These oscillations are usually rhythmic and may be horizontal, vertical, rotary, or mixed. They may be transient or sustained and may occur spontaneously or on deviation or fixation of the eyes. Minor degrees of nystagmus at the extremes of gaze are normal. Nystagmus when the eyes are stationary and looking straight ahead is always abnormal. Although nystagmus is fairly easy to identify, the patient may be unaware of it unless it affects his vision.

Nystagmus may be classified as pendular or jerk. *Pendular nystagmus* consists of horizontal (pendular) or vertical (seesaw) oscillations that are equal in rate in both directions and resemble the movements of a clock's pendulum. *Jerk nystagmus* (convergence-retraction, downbeat, and vestibular), which is more common than pendular nystagmus, has a fast component and then a slow—perhaps unequal—corrective component in the opposite direction.

Nystagmus is considered a *supranuclear* ocular palsy—that is, it results from a disorder in the visual perceptual area, vestibular system, cerebellum, or brain stem, rather than in the extraocular muscles or cranial nerves III, IV, and VI. Its causes are varied and include brain stem or cerebellar lesions, multiple sclerosis, encephalitis, labyrinthine disease, and drug toxicity. Occasionally, nystagmus is entirely normal; it's also considered a normal response in the unconscious patient during the doll's eye test (oculocephalic stimulation) or the cold caloric water test (oculovestibular stimulation).

History

- Ask about the onset, duration, and description of nystagmus.
- Inquire about recent infection of the ear or respiratory tract.
- Note a history of head trauma or cancer.
- Find out about associated vertigo, dizziness, tinnitus, nausea or vomiting, numbness, weakness, bladder dysfunction, and fever.

Physical examination

- Evaluate the patient's level of consciousness (LOC) and vital signs.
- Be alert for signs of increased intracranial pressure (ICP), such as pupillary changes, drowsiness, elevated systolic pressure, and altered respirations.
- Test extraocular muscle function.
- Note when nystagmus occurs as well as its velocity and direction.
- Test reflexes and cranial nerves.
- Evaluate motor and sensory function.

Causes

Medical causes

Brain tumor

- The insidious onset of jerk nystagmus may occur.
- Other signs and symptoms include deafness, dysphagia, nausea and vomiting, vertigo, and ataxia.
- Brain stem compression by the tumor may cause altered LOC, bradycardia, widened pulse pressure, and elevated systolic blood pressure.

Encephalitis

- Jerk nystagmus is typically accompanied by altered LOC, ranging from lethargy to coma.
- It may be preceded by the sudden onset of fever, headache, and vomiting.
- Other signs and symptoms include nuchal rigidity, seizures, aphasia, ataxia, photophobia, and cranial nerve palsies.

Head trauma

- Brain stem injury may cause horizontal jerk nystagmus.
- Other signs and symptoms include pupillary changes, altered respiratory pattern, coma, and decerebrate posture.

Labyrinthitis, acute

- The sudden onset of jerk nystagmus is accompanied by dizziness, vertigo, tinnitus, nausea, and vomiting.
- The fast component of the fluctuating nystagmus rate is toward the unaffected ear.

■ Gradual sensorineural hearing loss may occur.

Ménière's disease

■ Acute attacks of jerk nystagmus, severe nausea, dizziness, vertigo, progressive hearing loss, and tinnitus occur.
■ The direction of jerk nystagmus varies from one attack to the next.

Multiple sclerosis

■ Jerk or pendular nystagmus may occur intermittently.
■ It may be preceded by diplopia, blurred vision, and paresthesia.
■ Other signs and symptoms include muscle weakness or paralysis, spasticity, hyperreflexia, intention tremor, gait ataxia, dysphagia, dysarthria, impotence, constipation, emotional instability, and urinary frequency, urgency, and incontinence.

Stroke

■ A stroke involving the posterior inferior cerebellar artery may cause sudden horizontal or vertical jerk nystagmus that may be gaze dependent.
■ Other signs and symptoms include dysphagia, dysarthria, loss of pain and temperature sensation in the ipsilateral face and contralateral trunk and limbs, ipsilateral Horner's syndrome, cerebellar signs, and signs of increased ICP.

Other causes

Drugs and alcohol

■ Jerk nystagmus may result from barbiturate, phenytoin (Dilantin), or carbamazepine (Tegretol) toxicity and alcohol intoxication.

Nursing considerations

■ Monitor the patient for changes in his neurologic status.
■ Provide for the patient's safety.

Patient teaching

■ Instruct the patient about safety measures.
■ Orient the patient, as appropriate.
■ Caution the patient about the importance of avoiding sudden changes in position.

O

Ocular deviation

Ocular deviation refers to abnormal eye movement that may be conjugate (both eyes move together) or disconjugate (one eye moves separately from the other). This common sign may result from ocular, neurologic, endocrine, and systemic disorders that interfere with the muscles, nerves, or brain centers governing eye movement. Occasionally, it signals a life-threatening disorder such as a ruptured cerebral aneurysm.

Normally, eye movement is directly controlled by the extraocular muscles innervated by the oculomotor, trochlear, and abducens nerves (cranial nerves III, IV, and VI). Together, these muscles and nerves direct a visual stimulus to fall on corresponding parts of the retina. Disconjugate ocular deviation may result from unequal muscle tone (nonparalytic strabismus) or muscle paralysis associated with cranial nerve damage (paralytic strabismus). Conjugate ocular deviation may result from disorders that affect the centers in the cerebral cortex and brain stem responsible for conjugate eye movement. Typically, such disorders cause gaze palsy—difficulty moving the eyes in one or more directions.

QUICK ACTION ***If the patient displays ocular deviation, take his vital signs immediately and assess him for an altered level of consciousness (LOC), pupil changes, motor or sensory dysfunction, and a severe headache. If possible, ask the patient's family about behavioral changes. Is there a history of recent head trauma? Respiratory support may be necessary. Also, prepare the patient for emergency neurologic tests such as a computed tomography scan.***

History

- Find out the duration of ocular deviation.
- Ask about associated signs and symptoms, such as double vision, eye pain, headache, motor or sensory changes, or fever.
- Obtain an ocular history, noting recent eye or head trauma or surgery.
- Obtain a medical history, including the incidence of hypertension, diabetes, allergies, and thyroid, neurologic, and muscular disorders.

Physical examination

- Perform a complete neurologic assessment, including a complete eye assessment.
- Observe for partial or complete ptosis.
- Observe for spontaneous head tilts or turns that compensate for ocular deviation.
- Check for eye redness or periorbital edema.
- Assess visual acuity.
- Evaluate extraocular muscle function by testing the six cardinal positions of gaze.

Causes

Medical causes

Brain tumor

- Ocular deviation depends on the site and extent of the tumor.
- Related signs and symptoms include headaches that are most severe in the morning, behavioral changes, memory loss, dizziness, confusion, vision loss, motor and sensory dysfunction, aphasia, signs of hormonal imbalance, and slowly deteriorating LOC from lethargy to coma.
- Other late signs and symptoms include papilledema, vomiting, increased systolic pressure, widening pulse pressure, and decorticate posture.

Cerebral aneurysm

- Typically, ocular deviation and diplopia are the first signs.
- Ptosis and a severe headache (on one side, usually in the front) are other major signs and symptoms.
- With aneurysm rupture, abrupt intensification of pain, nausea, and vomiting occur.
- With bleeding from the site, meningeal irritation, back and leg pain, fever, irritability, seizures, blurred vision, hemiparesis, dysphagia, and visual deficits may develop.

Diabetes mellitus

- Ocular deviation, ptosis, and the sudden onset of diplopia and pain occur due to nerve damage, especially in long-standing diabetes.

Encephalitis

- Ocular deviation and diplopia may occur.
- Fever, headache, and vomiting are followed by signs of meningeal irritation and neuronal damage.
- Rapid deterioration of the patient's LOC may occur within 24 to 48 hours.

Head trauma

- The nature of ocular deviation depends on the site and extent of head trauma.
- Visible soft-tissue injury, bony deformity, facial edema, and clear or bloody otorrhea or rhinorrhea may be present.
- Other signs and symptoms include blurred vision, diplopia, nystagmus, behavioral changes, headache, motor and sensory dysfunction, signs of increased intracranial pressure, and a decreased LOC that may progress to coma.

Multiple sclerosis

- Ocular deviation may be an early sign.
- Diplopia, blurred vision, and sensory dysfunction occur.
- Other signs and symptoms include nystagmus, constipation, muscle weakness, paralysis, spasticity, hyperreflexia, intention tremor, gait ataxia, dysphagia, dysarthria, impotence, emotional lability, and urinary frequency, urgency, and incontinence.

Myasthenia gravis

- Ocular deviation may accompany the more common initial signs of diplopia and ptosis.
- It may affect only the eye muscles or progress to other muscle groups, causing altered facial expression, difficulty chewing, dysphagia, weakened voice, impaired fine hand movements, and respiratory distress.

Ophthalmoplegic migraine

- Ocular deviation and diplopia persist for days after the pain subsides.
- Other signs and symptoms include headache on one side with possible ptosis on the same side; temporary hemiplegia; irritability, depression, or slight confusion; and sensory deficits.

Orbital blowout fracture

- Limited extraocular movement and ocular deviation may occur.
- Typically, upward gaze is absent.
- Other signs and symptoms include pain, diplopia, nausea, periorbital edema, and ecchymosis. In addition, the globe may be displaced downward and inward.

Orbital tumor

- Ocular deviation occurs as the tumor gradually enlarges.
- Other signs and symptoms include an edematous eyelid, proptosis, diplopia, and blurred vision.

Stroke

- Ocular deviation depends on the site and extent of the stroke.
- Related signs and symptoms vary and may include altered LOC, contralateral hemiplegia and sensory loss, dysarthria, dysphagia, homonymous hemianopsia, blurred vision, and diplopia.
- Other signs and symptoms include urine retention or urinary incontinence or both, constipation, behavioral changes, headache, vomiting, and seizures.

Thyrotoxicosis

- Exophthalmos occurs, which causes limited extraocular movement and ocular deviation.
- Usually, the upward gaze weakens first, followed by diplopia.
- Related signs and symptoms include lid retraction, a wide-eyed staring gaze, excessive tearing, edematous eyelids and, sometimes, the inability to close the eyes.
- Other signs and symptoms include tachycardia, palpitations, weight loss despite increased appetite, diarrhea, tremors, an enlarged thyroid gland, dyspnea, nervousness, diaphoresis, heat intolerance, and atrial or ventricular gallop.

Nursing considerations

- If you suspect an acute neurologic disorder, monitor the patient's vital signs and neurologic status.
- Evaluate patient areas for safety concerns, and anticipate the patient's needs due to visual deficits.

Patient teaching

- Explain the disorder and its treatment.
- Explain changes in LOC that need to be reported.
- Provide information about maintaining a safe environment.
- Teach ways of reducing environmental stress.

Oliguria

A cardinal sign of renal and urinary tract disorders, oliguria is clinically defined as urine output of less than 400 ml/24 hours. Typically, this sign occurs abruptly and may herald serious—possibly life-threatening—hemodynamic instability. Its causes can be classified as prerenal (decreased renal blood flow), intrarenal (intrinsic renal damage), or postrenal (urinary tract obstruction); the pathophysiology differs for each classification. Oliguria associated with a prerenal or postrenal cause is usually promptly reversible with treatment, although it may lead to intrarenal damage if untreated. However, oliguria associated with an intrarenal cause is usually more persistent and may be irreversible.

History

- Ask about usual voiding patterns and the onset and description of oliguria.

- Find out about pain or burning on urination, fever, loss of appetite, thirst, dyspnea, chest pain, or recent weight gain or loss.
- Record the patient's daily fluid intake.
- Obtain a medical history, including the incidence of renal, urinary tract, or cardiovascular disorders; recent traumatic injury or surgery with significant blood loss; and recent transfusions.
- Ask about use of alcohol.
- Obtain a drug history.
- Note exposure to nephrotoxic agents, such as heavy metals, organic solvents, anesthetics, or radiographic contrast media.

Physical examination

- Take the patient's vital signs, and weigh him.
- Palpate the kidneys for tenderness and enlargement.
- Percuss for costovertebral angle (CVA) tenderness.
- Inspect the flanks for edema or erythema.
- Auscultate the heart and lungs for abnormal sounds and the flank area for bruits.
- Assess for edema or signs of dehydration.
- Obtain a urine specimen, and inspect it for abnormal color, odor, or sediment; measure its specific gravity.

Causes

Medical causes

Acute tubular necrosis

- Oliguria, an early sign, may occur abruptly (in shock) or gradually (in nephrotoxicity) and persist for about 2 weeks, followed by polyuria.
- Other signs and symptoms include signs of hyperkalemia, uremia, and heart failure.

Calculi

- Oliguria or anuria may occur.
- Excruciating pain radiates from the CVA to the flank, suprapubic region, and external genitalia.
- Other signs and symptoms include urinary frequency and urgency, dysuria, hematuria or pyuria, nausea, vomiting, hypoactive bowel sounds, abdominal distention and, possibly, fever and chills.

Glomerulonephritis, acute

- Oliguria or anuria occurs.
- Other signs and symptoms include mild fever, fatigue, gross hematuria, proteinuria, generalized edema, elevated blood pressure, headache, nausea, vomiting, flank and abdominal pain, and signs of pulmonary congestion.

Heart failure

- In left-sided heart failure, oliguria occurs due to decreased renal perfusion.
- In advanced failure, orthopnea, cyanosis, clubbing, ventricular gallop, diastolic hypertension, cardiomegaly, and hemoptysis occur.
- Other signs and symptoms include dyspnea, fatigue, weakness, peripheral edema, distended neck veins, tachycardia, tachypnea, crackles, and a dry or productive cough.

Hypovolemia

- Oliguria may occur.
- Other signs and symptoms include orthostatic hypotension, apathy, lethargy, fatigue, muscle weakness, anorexia, nausea, thirst, dizziness, sunken eyeballs, poor skin turgor, and dry mucous membranes.

Pyelonephritis, acute

- Oliguria, high fever with chills, fatigue, flank pain, CVA tenderness, weakness, nocturia, dysuria, hematuria, urinary frequency and urgency, and tenesmus occur.

■ Anorexia, nausea, diarrhea, and vomiting may also develop.

Renal artery occlusion, bilateral

■ Oliguria or, more commonly, anuria may accompany severe, constant upper abdominal and flank pain, nausea and vomiting, hypoactive bowel sounds, fever, and diastolic hypertension.

Renal failure, chronic

■ Oliguria is a major sign of end-stage chronic renal failure.

■ Eventually, seizures, coma, and uremic frost develop.

■ Other signs and symptoms include fatigue, weakness, irritability, uremic fetor, ecchymoses, petechiae, peripheral edema, elevated blood pressure, confusion, emotional lability, drowsiness, coarse muscle twitching, muscle cramps, peripheral neuropathies, anorexia, metallic taste in the mouth, nausea, vomiting, constipation or diarrhea, stomatitis, pruritus, pallor, and yellow- or bronze-tinged skin.

Renal vein occlusion, bilateral

■ Occasionally, oliguria occurs with acute low back and flank pain, CVA tenderness, fever, pallor, hematuria, enlarged and palpable kidneys, edema and, possibly, signs of uremia.

Sepsis

■ Oliguria, fever, chills, restlessness, confusion, diaphoresis, anorexia, vomiting, diarrhea, pallor, hypotension, and tachycardia occur.

■ Signs of local infection may also develop.

Toxemia of pregnancy

■ Oliguria may be accompanied by elevated blood pressure, dizziness, diplopia, blurred vision, nausea and vomiting, irritability, and frontal headache.

■ Oliguria is preceded by generalized edema and sudden weight gain of more than 3 lb (1.4 kg) per week during the second trimester or more than 1 lb (0.5 kg) per week during the third trimester.

■ If the condition progresses to eclampsia, seizures and coma may occur.

Urethral stricture

■ Oliguria is accompanied by chronic urethral discharge, urinary frequency and urgency, dysuria, pyuria, and diminished urine stream.

Other causes

Diagnostic tests

■ Radiographic studies that use contract media may cause nephrotoxicity and oliguria.

Drugs

■ Oliguria may result from drugs that cause decreased renal perfusion (diuretics), nephrotoxicity (most notably aminoglycosides and chemotherapeutics), urine retention (adrenergics and anticholinergics), or urinary obstruction associated with precipitation of urinary crystals (sulfonamides and acyclovir [Zovirax]).

Nursing considerations

■ Monitor the patient's vital signs, intake and output, and daily weight.

■ Restrict fluids from 600 ml to 1 L more than the urine output for the previous day, if indicated.

■ Provide a diet low in sodium, potassium, and protein.

Patient teaching

■ Explain fluid and dietary restrictions the patient needs.

■ Teach the patient about prescribed medications.

■ Teach about the underlying diagnosis and treatment plan.

Opisthotonos

A sign of severe meningeal irritation, opisthotonos is a severe, prolonged spasm characterized by a strongly arched, rigid back; a hyperextended neck; the heels bent back; and the arms and hands flexed at the joints. Usually, this posture occurs spontaneously and continuously; however, it may be aggravated by movement. Presumably, opisthotonos represents a protective reflex because it immobilizes the spine, alleviating the pain associated with meningeal irritation.

Usually caused by meningitis, opisthotonos may also result from subarachnoid hemorrhage, Arnold-Chiari syndrome, and tetanus. Occasionally, it occurs in achondroplastic dwarfism, although not necessarily as an indicator of meningeal irritation.

Opisthotonos is far more common in children—especially infants—than in adults. It's also more exaggerated in children because of nervous system immaturity. (See *Opisthotonos: Sign of meningeal irritation*.)

QUICK ACTION ***If the patient is stuporous or comatose, immediately evaluate his vital signs. Employ resuscitative measures, as appropriate. Place the patient in bed, with the side rails raised and padded, or in a crib.***

History

- Obtain a history, noting the incidence of cerebral aneurysm, arteriovenous malformation, hypertension, or re-

Opisthotonos: Sign of meningeal irritation

In the characteristic posture, the back is severely arched with the neck hyperextended. The heels bend back on the legs, and the arms and hands flex rigidly at the joints, as shown below.

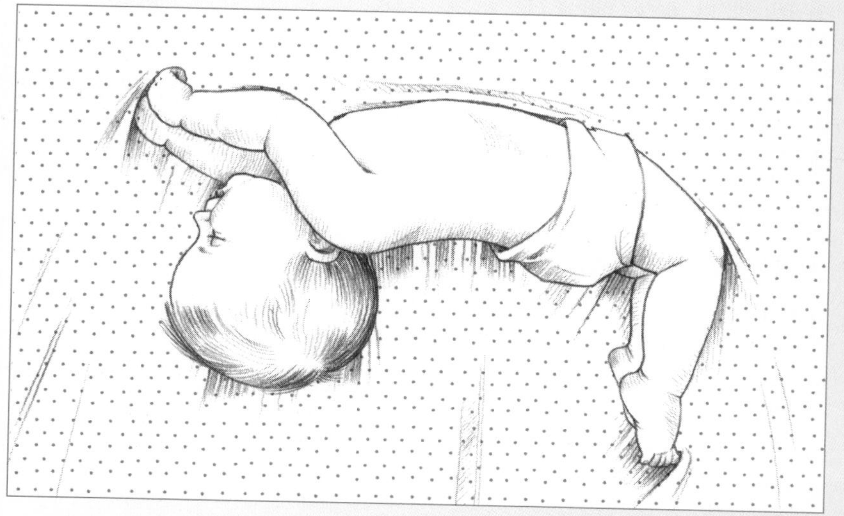

cent infection that may have spread to the nervous system.

- Explore associated signs and symptoms, such as headache, chills, and vomiting.

Physical examination

- Evaluate the patient's level of consciousness (LOC) and test sensorimotor and cranial nerve function.
- Check for Brudzinski's and Kernig's signs and for nuchal rigidity.
- Take the patient's vital signs.

Causes

Medical causes

Arnold-Chiari syndrome

- Opisthotonos typically occurs with hydrocephalus, with its characteristic enlarged head; thin, shiny scalp with distended veins; and underdeveloped neck muscles.
- Other signs and symptoms include a high-pitched cry, abnormal leg muscle tone, anorexia, vomiting, nuchal rigidity, irritability, noisy respirations, and a weak sucking reflex.

Meningitis

- Opisthotonos accompanies other signs of meningeal irritation, including nuchal rigidity, positive Brudzinski's and Kernig's signs, and hyperreflexia.
- Related cardinal signs and symptoms include moderate to high fever with chills and malaise, headache, vomiting and, eventually, papilledema.
- Other signs and symptoms include irritability; photophobia; diplopia, deafness, and other cranial nerve palsies; and decreased LOC that may progress to seizures and coma.

Subarachnoid hemorrhage

- Opisthotonos may occur along with other signs of meningeal irritation, such as nuchal rigidity and positive Kernig's and Brudzinski's signs.
- Focal signs of hemorrhage, such as severe headache, hemiplegia or hemiparesis, aphasia, and photophobia, along with other vision problems, may also occur.
- With increasing intracranial pressure, the patient may develop bradycardia, elevated blood pressure, altered respiratory pattern, seizures, and vomiting.
- The patient's LOC may rapidly deteriorate, resulting in coma; then decerebrate posture may alternate with opisthotonos.

Other causes

Drugs

- Phenothiazines and other antipsychotics may cause opisthotonos, usually as part of an acute dystonic reaction.

Nursing considerations

- Assess the patient's neurologic status, and check his vital signs frequently.
- Make the patient as comfortable as possible; place him in a side-lying position with pillows for support.
- If meningitis is suspected, institute respiratory isolation. Lumbar puncture may be ordered to identify pathogens and analyze cerebrospinal fluid.
- If subarachnoid hemorrhage is suspected, prepare the patient for a computed tomography scan or magnetic resonance imaging.
- Opisthotonos is far more common in children—especially infants—than in adults.
- It's also more exaggerated in children because of nervous system immaturity.

Patient teaching

- Teach the patient and his family about the underlying diagnosis and treatment plan.
- Teach the patient and his family about all tests and hospital procedures.
- Teach the patient and his family about prescribed medications.

Orthopnea

Orthopnea—difficulty breathing in the supine position—is a common symptom of cardiopulmonary disorders that produce dyspnea. It's usually a subtle symptom; the patient may complain that he can't catch his breath when lying down, or he may mention that he sleeps most comfortably in a reclining chair or propped up by pillows. Derived from this complaint is the common classification of two- or three-pillow orthopnea.

Orthopnea presumably results from increased hydrostatic pressure in the pulmonary vasculature related to gravitational effects in the supine position. It may be aggravated by obesity or pregnancy, which restricts diaphragmatic excursion. Sitting in an upright position relieves orthopnea by placing much of the pulmonary vasculature above the left atrium, which reduces mean hydrostatic pressure, and by enhancing diaphragmatic excursion, which increases inspiratory volume.

History

- Ask about the onset and description of orthopnea.
- Note how many pillows are used for sleeping.
- Obtain a medical history, including the incidence of cardiopulmonary disorders, such as myocardial infarction, rheumatic heart disease, heart failure, valvular disease, asthma, emphysema, or chronic bronchitis.
- Find out about smoking and alcohol habits.
- Inquire about associated cough, dyspnea, fatigue, weakness, loss of appetite, or chest pain.
- Obtain a drug history.

Physical examination

- Take the patient's vital signs.
- Check for other signs of increased respiratory effort, such as accessory muscle use, shallow respirations, and tachypnea.
- Note barrel chest.
- Inspect the skin for pallor or cyanosis, and inspect the fingers for clubbing.
- Observe and palpate for edema.
- Check jugular vein distention.
- Auscultate the lungs and heart.
- Monitor oxygen saturation.

Causes

Medical causes

Chronic obstructive pulmonary disease

- Orthopnea and other dyspneic complaints are accompanied by accessory muscle use, tachypnea, tachycardia, and paradoxical pulse.
- Related signs and symptoms include diminished breath sounds, rhonchi, crackles, and wheezing on auscultation; dry or productive cough with copious sputum; anorexia; weight loss; and edema.
- Barrel chest, cyanosis, and clubbing are late signs.

Left-sided heart failure

- If heart failure is acute, orthopnea may begin suddenly; if chronic, it may be constant.
- Early signs and symptoms include progressively severe dyspnea, Cheyne-Stokes respirations, paroxysmal nocturnal dyspnea, fatigue, weakness, a cough that may occasionally produce clear or blood-tinged sputum, tachycardia, tachypnea, and crackles.
- Late signs and symptoms include cyanosis, clubbing, ventricular gallop, and hemoptysis.

Mediastinal tumor

- Orthopnea is an early sign.
- As the tumor enlarges, signs and symptoms include retrosternal chest pain, dry cough, hoarseness, dysphagia, stertorous respirations, palpitations, cyanosis, suprasternal retractions on inspiration, tracheal deviation, dilated jugular and superficial chest veins, and edema of the face, neck, and arms.

Nursing considerations

- Place the patient in semi-Fowler's or high Fowler's position.
- Alternatively, have the patient lean over a bedside table with his chest forward.
- If needed, administer oxygen via nasal cannula.
- To reduce lung fluids, give a diuretic, as ordered.
- Monitor intake and output.
- For the patient with left-sided heart failure, give angiotensin-converting enzyme inhibitors, as ordered.
- Assist with the insertion of a central venous line or pulmonary artery catheter, as needed.
- Sleeping in an infant seat may improve symptoms for a young child.

Patient teaching

- Discuss the underlying condition, diagnostic tests, and treatment options.
- Explain the signs and symptoms the patient should report.
- Explain dietary and fluid restrictions the patient needs.
- Discuss daily weight measurement.
- Explain energy conservation measures, as appropriate.

Osler's nodes

Osler's nodes are tender, raised, pea-sized, red or purple lesions that erupt on the palms, soles, and especially the pads of fingers and toes. They're a rare but reliable sign of infective endocarditis, and are pathognomonic of the subacute form. However, the nodes usually develop after other telling signs and symptoms and disappear spontaneously within several days. How and why they develop is uncertain; they may result from bacterial emboli caught in the peripheral capillaries, or they may reflect an immunologic reaction to the causative organism. Osler's nodes must be distinguished from the even less common Janeway lesions—small, painless erythematous lesions that erupt on the palms and soles.

History

- If you discover Osler's nodes, obtain a history for clues to the cause of infective endocarditis, such as recent surgery or dental work, invasive procedures of the urinary or gynecologic tract, a prosthetic valve or an arteriovenous fistula for hemodialysis; cardiac disorders and murmurs; or recent upper respiratory, skin, or urinary tract infection.
- Find out if the patient has been using I.V. drugs and explore associated complaints, such as chills, fatigue, anorexia, and night sweats.

Physical examination

- Take the patient's vital signs, and auscultate the heart for murmurs and gallops and the lungs for crackles.
- Inspect the skin and mucous membranes for petechiae and other lesions.
- If you suspect I.V. drug abuse, inspect the patient's arms and other areas for needle tracks.

Causes

Medical causes

Acute infective endocarditis

- Osler's nodes may occur.
- Classic signs and symptoms include the acute onset of high, intermittent fever with chills and signs of heart failure, such as dyspnea, peripheral edema, and jugular vein distention.

- Janeway lesions and Roth's spots are more common in this form than in the subacute form; petechiae may also occur.
- Embolization may abruptly occur, causing organ infarction or peripheral vascular occlusion with hematuria, chest or limb pain, paralysis, blindness, and other diverse effects.

Subacute infective endocarditis

- Osler's nodes are characteristic in this form of endocarditis.
- A suddenly changing murmur or the discovery of a new murmur is another cardinal sign.
- Related signs and symptoms include intermittent fever, pallor, weakness, fatigue, arthralgia, night sweats, tachycardia, anorexia and weight loss, splenomegaly, clubbing, and petechiae.
- Occasionally, Janeway lesions, subungual splinter hemorrhages, and Roth's spots also appear. Signs of heart failure may occur with extensive valvular damage.
- Embolization may also develop, producing signs and symptoms that vary depending on the location of the emboli.

Nursing considerations

- Monitor the patient's vital signs to evaluate the effectiveness of antibiotic therapy against infective endocarditis.
- Prepare the patient for blood studies, such as a complete blood count, and procedures, such as an electrocardiogram and echocardiogram.

Patient teaching

- Discuss measures to prevent reinfection, such as prophylactic antibiotic administration before dental or invasive procedures.
- Teach the patient about the diagnosis and treatment plan.

Otorrhea

Otorrhea—drainage from the ear—may be bloody (otorrhagia), purulent, clear, or serosanguineous. Its onset, duration, and severity provide clues to the underlying cause. This sign may result from disorders that affect the external ear canal or the middle ear, including allergy, infection, neoplasms, trauma, and collagen diseases. Otorrhea may occur alone or with other symptoms such as ear pain.

History

- Ask about the onset and description of drainage.
- Find out about pain, tenderness, vertigo, or tinnitus.
- Obtain a medical history, including the incidence of recent upper respiratory infection or head trauma and a history of cancer, dermatitis, or immunosuppressant therapy.

Physical examination

- Inspect the external ear, and apply pressure on the tragus and mastoid area to elicit tenderness; then insert an otoscope.
- Observe for edema, erythema, crusts, or polyps.
- Inspect the tympanic membrane, noting color changes, perforation, absence of the normal light reflex, or a bulging membrane.
- Test hearing acuity and perform Weber's and the Rinne tests.
- Palpate the neck and preauricular, parotid, and postauricular areas for lymphadenopathy.
- Test the function of cranial nerves VII, IX, X, and XI.
- Take the patient's vital signs.

Causes

Medical causes

Allergy

- Associated tympanic membrane perforation may cause clear or cloudy otorrhea, rhinorrhea, and itchy, watery eyes.
- Other signs and symptoms include nasal congestion and an itchy nose and throat.

Aural polyps

- Foul, purulent, blood-streaked discharge may occur, possibly followed by partial hearing loss.

Basilar skull fracture

- Otorrhea may be clear and watery and show a positive reaction on a glucose test, or it may be bloody.
- Other signs and symptoms include hearing loss, cerebrospinal fluid or bloody rhinorrhea, periorbital raccoon eyes, mastoid ecchymosis (Battle's sign), cranial nerve palsies, decreased level of consciousness, and headache.

Dermatitis of the external ear canal

- With contact dermatitis, vesicles produce clear, watery otorrhea with edema and erythema of the external ear canal.
- With infectious eczematoid dermatitis, otorrhea is purulent with erythema and crusting of the external ear canal.
- With seborrheic dermatitis, otorrhea has greasy scales and flakes.

Mastoiditis

- Thick, purulent, yellow otorrhea becomes increasingly profuse.
- Related signs and symptoms include low-grade fever and dull aching and tenderness in the mastoid area.
- Conductive hearing loss may develop.

Myringitis, infectious

- Small, reddened, blood-filled blebs or blisters rupture, causing serosanguineous otorrhea.
- In the chronic form, purulent otorrhea, pruritus, and gradual hearing loss occur.
- Other signs and symptoms include severe ear pain and tenderness over the mastoid process.

Otitis externa

- The acute form usually causes purulent, yellow, sticky, foul-smelling otorrhea.
- Related acute signs and symptoms include edema, erythema, pain, and itching of the auricle and external ear; severe tenderness with movement of the mastoid, tragus, mouth, or jaw; tenderness and swelling of surrounding nodes; partial conductive hearing loss; and low-grade fever and headache ipsilateral to the affected ear.
- The chronic form usually causes scanty, intermittent otorrhea that may be serous or purulent as well as edema and slight erythema.

Otitis media

- With acute otitis media, rupture of the tympanic membrane produces bloody, purulent otorrhea and conductive hearing loss that worsens over several hours.
- With acute suppurative otitis media, otorrhea may accompany signs and symptoms of upper respiratory infection, dizziness, fever, nausea, and vomiting.
- With chronic otitis media, otorrhea is intermittent, purulent, and foul-smelling and is accompanied by gradual conductive hearing loss, pain, nausea, and vertigo.

Trauma

- Bloody otorrhea may occur and may be accompanied by partial hearing loss.

Tumor

- A benign tumor of the jugular glomus may cause bloody otorrhea.
- Related signs and symptoms include throbbing discomfort, tinnitus that resembles the sound of the patient's heartbeat, progressive stuffiness of the affected ear, vertigo, conductive hearing loss and, possibly, a reddened mass behind the tympanic membrane.
- Squamous cell carcinoma of the external ear causes purulent otorrhea with itching; deep, boring pain; hearing loss; and, in late stages, facial paralysis.
- Squamous cell carcinoma of the middle ear causes blood-tinged otorrhea that occurs early and is accompanied by hearing loss of the affected side; pain and facial paralysis are late signs.

Nursing considerations

- Apply warm, moist compresses, heating pads, or hot water bottles to the ears.
- Use cotton wicks to clean the ear or to apply topical drugs.
- Keep eardrops at room temperature; instillation of cold eardrops may cause vertigo.
- If the patient has impaired hearing, make sure he understands what's explained to him.
- Perforation of the tympanic membrane from otitis media is the most common cause of otorrhea in infants and young children.
- Children may insert foreign bodies into their ears, resulting in infection, pain, and purulent discharge.
- Because the auditory canal of a child lies horizontal, the pinna must be pulled downward and backward to examine the ear.

Patient teaching

- Discuss the underlying condition, diagnostic tests, and treatment options.
- Instruct the patient on safe ways to blow his nose and clean his ears.
- Stress the use of earplugs when swimming.
- Explain the signs and symptoms the patient needs to report.

Pq

Pallor

Pallor is abnormal paleness or loss of skin color, which may develop suddenly or gradually. Generalized pallor affects the entire body, although it's most apparent on the face, conjunctiva, oral mucosa, and nail beds. In contrast, localized pallor commonly affects a single limb.

How easily pallor is detected varies with skin color and the thickness and vascularity of underlying subcutaneous tissue. At times, it's merely a subtle lightening of skin color that may be difficult to detect in dark-skinned persons. In some cases, it's evident only on the conjunctiva and oral mucosa.

Pallor may result from decreased peripheral oxyhemoglobin or decreased total oxyhemoglobin. The former reflects diminished peripheral blood flow associated with peripheral vasoconstriction or arterial occlusion, or with low cardiac output. Transient peripheral vasoconstriction may occur with exposure to cold, causing nonpathologic pallor. Decreased total oxyhemoglobin usually results from anemia, the chief cause of pallor. (See *How pallor develops*.)

QUICK ACTION ***If generalized pallor suddenly develops, quickly look for signs of shock, such as tachycardia, hypotension, oliguria, and a decreased level of consciousness (LOC). Prepare to rapidly infuse fluids or blood. Keep emergency resuscitation equipment nearby.***

History

- Obtain a medical history, including anemia, renal failure, heart failure, or diabetes.
- Ask about diet, especially intake of green vegetables.
- Ask about the onset and description of pallor.
- Explore what aggravates and alleviates pallor.
- Inquire about dizziness, fainting, orthostasis, weakness, fatigue, dyspnea, chest pain, palpitations, menstrual irregularities, or loss of libido.

Physical examination

- Assess the patient's vital signs, checking for orthostatic hypotension.
- Auscultate the heart for murmurs or gallops.
- Auscultate the lungs for crackles.
- Check skin temperature.
- Note skin ulceration.
- Palpate peripheral pulses.
- Assess oral mucous membranes.

Causes

Medical causes

Anemia

- Pallor begins gradually; skin is gray or sallow.
- Other signs and symptoms include fatigue, dyspnea, tachycardia, bounding pulse, atrial gallop, systolic bruit over

How pallor develops

Pallor may result from decreased peripheral oxyhemoglobin or decreased total oxyhemoglobin. This flowchart illustrates the progression to pallor.

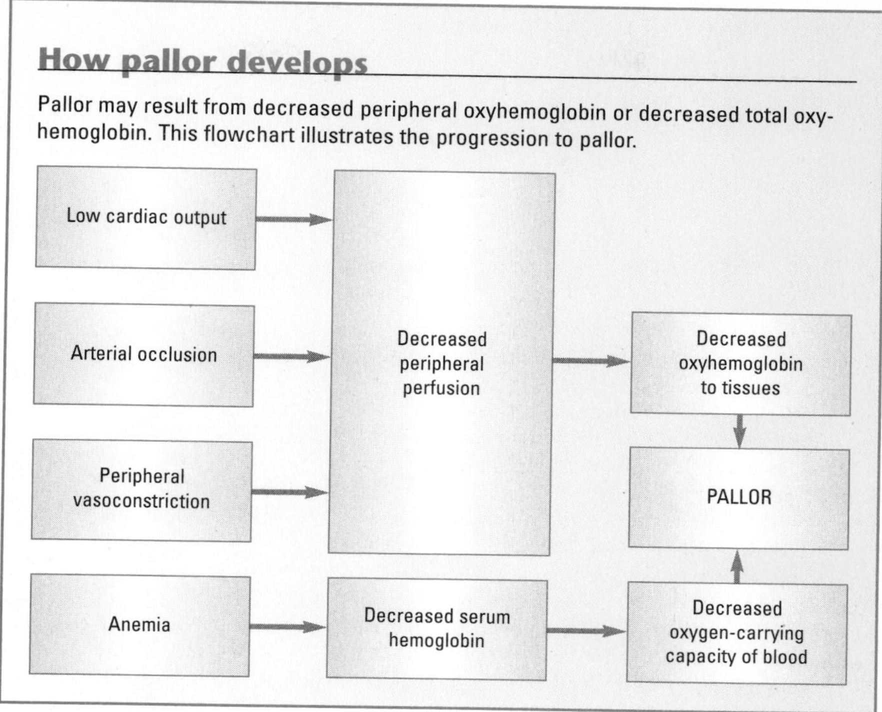

the carotid arteries and, possibly, crackles and bleeding tendencies.

Arterial occlusion, acute

- Pallor begins abruptly in the extremity with occlusion.
- A line of demarcation separates cool, pale, cyanotic, and mottled skin from normal skin.
- Other signs and symptoms include severe pain, intense intermittent claudication, paresthesia, paresis in the affected extremity, and absent pulses below the occlusion.

Arterial occlusive disease, chronic

- Pallor is specific to an extremity.
- Pallor develops gradually and is aggravated by elevating the extremity.
- Other signs and symptoms include intermittent claudication, weakness, cool skin, diminished pulses in the extremity and, possibly, ulceration and gangrene.

Cardiac arrhythmias

- Acute pallor may occur with an irregular, rapid, or slow pulse, dizziness, weakness and fatigue, hypotension, confusion, palpitations, diaphoresis, oliguria and, possibly, loss of consciousness.

Frostbite

- Pallor is localized to the frostbitten area, which feels cold, waxy and, possibly, hard; sensation may be absent.
- Skin turns purplish blue as skin thaws; if frostbite is severe, blistering and gangrene may follow.

Orthostatic hypotension

- Pallor occurs abruptly on rising from a recumbent position along with a drop

in blood pressure, tachycardia, and dizziness.
- Loss of consciousness is possible.

Raynaud's disease
- Upon exposure to cold or stress, the fingers abruptly turn pale (a classic sign) and then cyanotic in this arteriospastic disorder.
- With rewarming, fingers become red and paresthetic.
- With chronic disease, ulceration may occur.

Shock
- In hypovolemic and cardiogenic shock, acute pallor occurs early with restlessness, thirst, tachycardia, tachypnea, and cool, clammy skin.
- As shock progresses, the skin becomes increasingly clammy, the pulse becomes more rapid and thready, and hypotension develops with narrowing pulse pressure.
- Other signs and symptoms include oliguria, subnormal body temperature, and decreased LOC.

Vasovagal syncope
- Sudden pallor immediately precedes or accompanies loss of consciousness.
- These fainting spells may be triggered by emotional stress or pain and usually last for a few seconds or minutes.
- Before loss of consciousness, diaphoresis, nausea, yawning, hyperpnea, weakness, confusion, tachycardia, and dim vision may occur followed by bradycardia, hypotension, a few clonic jerks, and dilated pupils.

Nursing considerations
- Administer blood and fluids as well as a diuretic, a cardiotonic, and an antiarrhythmic, as needed.
- Frequently monitor the patient's vital signs, intake and output, electrocardiogram, and hemodynamic status.

Patient teaching
- Prepare the patient for blood studies and, possibly, bone marrow biopsy.
- For anemia, explain the importance of an iron-rich diet and rest.
- For frostbite and Raynaud's disease, discuss cold-protection measures.
- For orthostatic hypotension, explain the need to rise slowly.
- Discuss signs and symptoms the patient needs to report.

Palpitations

Defined as a conscious awareness of one's heartbeat, palpitations are usually felt over the precordium or in the throat or neck. The patient may describe them as pounding, jumping, turning, fluttering, or flopping or as missing or skipping beats. Palpitations may be regular or irregular, fast or slow, and paroxysmal or sustained.

Although usually insignificant, palpitations may result from a cardiac or metabolic disorder and from the effects of certain drugs. Nonpathologic palpitations may occur with a newly implanted prosthetic valve because the valve's clicking sound heightens the patient's awareness of his heartbeat. Transient palpitations may accompany emotional stress (such as fright, anger, or anxiety) or physical stress (such as exercise and fever). They can also accompany the use of stimulants, such as tobacco and caffeine.

To help characterize palpitations, ask the patient to simulate their rhythm by tapping his finger on a hard surface. An irregular "skipped beat" rhythm points to premature ventricular contractions, whereas an episodic racing rhythm that ends abruptly suggests paroxysmal atrial tachycardia.

QUICK ACTION ***If the patient complains of palpitations, ask him about dizziness and shortness of breath. Then, inspect***

for pale, cool, clammy skin. Take the patient's vital signs, noting hypotension and an irregular or abnormal pulse. If these signs are present, suspect cardiac arrhythmias. Place the patient on a cardiac monitor. Start an I.V. catheter to administer an antiarrhythmic if needed. Prepare for cardioversion or defibrillation, if necessary.

History

- Ask about the onset and description of palpitations.
- Inquire about aggravating and alleviating factors.
- Note associated signs and symptoms, such as dizziness, syncope, weakness, fatigue, angina, and pale, cool skin.
- Obtain a medical history, including cardiovascular or pulmonary disorders or hypoglycemia.
- Obtain a drug history, including recently prescribed digoxin (Lanoxin).
- Ask about caffeine, tobacco, and alcohol use.

Physical examination

- Perform a complete cardiac and pulmonary assessment.
- Auscultate the heart for gallops and murmurs.
- Auscultate the lungs for abnormal breath sounds.

Causes

Medical causes

Anemia

- Palpitations occur, especially on exertion, with pallor, fatigue, and dyspnea.
- Other signs and symptoms include systolic ejection murmur, bounding pulse, tachycardia, crackles, atrial gallop, and a systolic bruit over the carotid arteries.

Anxiety attack, acute

- Palpitations may be accompanied by diaphoresis, facial flushing, trembling, and an impending sense of doom.
- Hyperventilation may lead to dizziness, weakness, and syncope.
- Other signs and symptoms include tachycardia, precordial pain, shortness of breath, restlessness, and insomnia.

Cardiac arrhythmias

- Paroxysmal or sustained palpitations may be accompanied by dizziness, weakness, and fatigue.
- Other signs and symptoms include an irregular, rapid, or slow pulse rate, decreased blood pressure, confusion, pallor, chest pain, syncope, oliguria, and diaphoresis. (See *Responding to palpitations,* page 262.)

Hypertension

- Sustained palpitations may occur alone or with headache, dizziness, tinnitus, and fatigue.
- Blood pressure typically exceeds 140/90 mm Hg.
- Nausea, vomiting, seizures, and decreased level of consciousness (LOC) may also occur.

Hypocalcemia

- Palpitations occur with weakness and fatigue.
- Paresthesia progresses to muscle tension and carpopedal spasms.
- Related signs and symptoms include muscle twitching, hyperactive deep tendon reflexes, chorea, and positive Chvostek's and Trousseau's signs.

Hypoglycemia

- Sustained palpitations occur with fatigue, irritability, hunger, cold sweats, tremors, tachycardia, anxiety, and headache.
- Eventually, blurred or double vision, muscle weakness, hemiplegia, and altered LOC develop.

CASE CLIP

Responding to palpitations

Ms. J. is a 61-year-old female admitted through the emergency department (ED) 2 days ago. Her complaints included palpitations, dizziness, shortness of breath, and mild chest pain that has been relieved with sublingual nitroglycerin (Nitrostat). She has a history of hyperlipidemia and hypercholesterolemia; she's approximately 30 lb (13.6 kg) overweight and admits to a history of smoking 2 packs of cigarettes per day for the past 45 years. A myocardial infarction was ruled out in the ED. After being stabilized, she was transferred to the cardiac step-down unit for observation with an admitting diagnosis of unstable angina.

While on telemetry for the past 2 days, Ms. J.'s cardiac monitor has shown sinus tachycardia with occasional multifocal premature ventricular contractions. Her blood pressure has ranged from 134 to 152 mm Hg systolic and from 76 to 90 mm Hg diastolic. Her oxygen saturation has averaged 94% on 2 L of oxygen via nasal cannula.

During morning rounds, hospital day 3, the nurse finds Ms. J. diaphoretic, anxious, slightly tremulous, and complaining of palpitations, shortness of breath, and feeling "panicky." She also complains of mild pressure in her chest; and says she feels like something is squeezing her. Her vital signs are:

- heart rate: 156 beats/minute
- respiratory rate: 30 breaths/minute and shallow
- blood pressure: 80/46 mm Hg
- oxygen saturation: 89% on 2 L of oxygen.

Her cardiac monitor shows a rapid narrow complex rhythm. Her breath sounds are diminished bilaterally with very fine crackles in both bases. Her trachea is midline, and no jugular vein distention is noted. She remains anxious and diaphoretic and complains of feeling slightly dizzy. The head of her bed is flattened, and the rapid response team (RRT) is notified.

The RRT responds with immediate orders to obtain:

- 12-lead electrocardiogram (ECG)
- portable chest X-ray
- arterial blood gas analysis
- cardiac enzyme levels
- serum electrolyte levels
- prothrombin time
- partial thromboplastin time
- complete blood count
- blood glucose level.

The 12-lead ECG was inconclusive except to confirm the presence of a very rapid narrow complex rhythm with a rate above 150 beats/minute. The residents attempted carotid massage, which was unsuccessful. Adenosine (Adenocard) was administered via I.V. push, followed immediately by a 20 ml flush of normal saline solution. A sinus pause is noted on the cardiac monitor, and then as the rhythm reappears, atrial fibrillation is noted. The rate eventually increases back into the 150s to 160s.

Because this is a new-onset atrial fibrillation, the team decides Ms. J. needs to undergo cardioversion. The first cardioversion attempt, at 100 joules, is successful and converts her heart rhythm to sinus tachycardia with a rate of 110 to 114 beats/minute. Her oxygen saturation improves to 94% to 96% on 2 L of oxygen, and her systolic blood pressure remains in the 100 to 110 mm Hg range. Upon arousal, Ms. J. denies further palpitations, chest pressure, shortness of breath, or other symptoms.

Mitral prolapse

- Paroxysmal palpitations accompany sharp, stabbing, or aching precordial pain and midsystolic click, followed by an apical systolic murmur.
- Other signs and symptoms include dyspnea, dizziness, severe fatigue, migraine headache, anxiety, paroxysmal tachycardia, crackles, and peripheral edema.

Mitral stenosis

- Early on, sustained palpitations accompany exertional dyspnea and fatigue.
- A loud S_1 or an opening snap and a rumbling diastolic murmur at the apex are heard on auscultation.
- Other signs and symptoms include atrial gallop and, with advanced disease, orthopnea, dyspnea at rest, paroxysmal nocturnal dyspnea, peripheral edema, jugular vein distention, ascites, hepatomegaly, and atrial fibrillation.

Pheochromocytoma

- Paroxysmal palpitations occur with dramatically elevated blood pressure (the main sign of this tumor of the adrenal medulla).
- Other signs and symptoms include tachycardia, headache, chest or abdominal pain, diaphoresis, warm and pale or flushed skin, paresthesia, tremors, insomnia, nausea, vomiting, and anxiety.

Sick sinus syndrome

- Palpitations may be accompanied by bradycardia, tachycardia, chest pain, syncope, and heart failure.

Thyrotoxicosis

- Sustained palpitations may be accompanied by tachycardia, dyspnea, diarrhea, nervousness, tremors, diaphoresis, heat intolerance, weight loss despite increased appetite, atrial or ventricular gallop and, possibly, exophthalmos.

Wolff-Parkinson-White syndrome

- Seen in children and adolescents, this disease results in recurrent palpitations and frequent episodes of paroxysmal tachycardia.

Other causes

Drugs

- Drugs that may cause palpitations include atropine, beta-adrenergic blockers, calcium channel blockers, digoxin (Lanoxin), ganglionic blockers, minoxidil (Loniten), and sympathomimetics that precipitate cardiac arrhythmias or increase cardiac output.

Exercise

- Exercise can cause palpitations.

Herbal remedies

- Herbal dietary supplements, such as ginseng and ephedra (ma huang), may cause adverse reactions, including palpitations and an irregular heartbeat. (The Food and Drug Administration has banned the sale of ephedra.)

Nursing considerations

- Monitor the patient for signs of reduced cardiac output and cardiac arrhythmias.
- Prepare for procedures such as cardioversion.
- Provide supplemental oxygen.
- Provide for rest periods.

Patient teaching

- Teach the patient about the underlying disorder and treatment options.
- Explain diagnostic tests the patient will need.
- Teach the patient how to reduce anxiety.

Papular rash

A papular rash consists of small, raised, circumscribed—and perhaps discolored (red to purple)—lesions known as *papules.* Such a rash may erupt anywhere on the body in various configurations and may be acute or chronic. Papular rashes characterize many cutaneous disorders; they may also result from allergy and from infectious, neoplastic, and systemic disorders. (To compare papules with other skin lesions, see *Recognizing common skin lesions.*)

History

- Ask about the onset, course of rash, and characteristics, such as itching, burning, or tenderness.
- Inquire about fever, headache, and GI distress.
- Obtain a medical history, including allergies, previous rash and skin disorder, infection, childhood disease, sexual history, sexually transmitted disease, cancer, and exposure to chemicals and pesticides.
- Obtain a drug history.
- Ask about recent insect or rodent bites or exposure to infectious disease.

Physical examination

- Note the color, configuration, and location of rash.
- Perform a whole-body examination of skin, hair, and nails.

Causes

Medical causes

Acne vulgaris

- Inflamed papules, pustules, nodules, or cysts appear on the face, shoulders, chest, and back.
- Lesions may be painful and pruritic.

Anthrax, cutaneous

- Initially this bacterial infection appears as a small, painless, pruritic macular or papular lesion.
- A vesicle develops within 2 days and then evolves into a painless ulcer with a black necrotic center.
- Lymphadenopathy, malaise, headache, and fever may develop.

Erythema migrans

- A papular or macular rash starts as a single lesion and spreads at the margins while clearing at the center.
- A papular rash commonly appears on the thighs, trunk, or upper arms.
- Accompanying signs and symptoms include fever, chills, headache, malaise, nausea, vomiting, fatigue, backache, knee pain, and stiff neck.

Human immunodeficiency virus infection

- A generalized maculopapular rash occurs with acute infection.
- Other signs and symptoms include fever, malaise, sore throat, headache, lymphadenopathy, and hepatosplenomegaly.

Insect bites

- A papular, macular, or petechial rash may be accompanied by fever, myalgia, headache, lymphadenopathy, nausea, and vomiting.

Kaposi's sarcoma

- A cancer of the lymphatic system, Kaposi's sarcoma is the most common cancer associated with acquired immunodeficiency syndrome.
- Purple or blue papules or macules of vascular origin appear on the skin, mucous membranes, and viscera.
- Lesions decrease in size with firm pressure, and then return to their original size within 10 to 15 seconds.
- Lesions may become scaly and may ulcerate with bleeding.

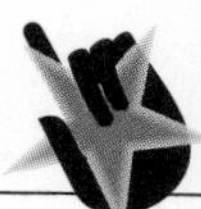

KNOW-HOW

Recognizing common skin lesions

Macule
A small (usually less than 1 cm in diameter), flat blemish or discoloration that can be brown, tan, red, or white and has the same texture as surrounding skin

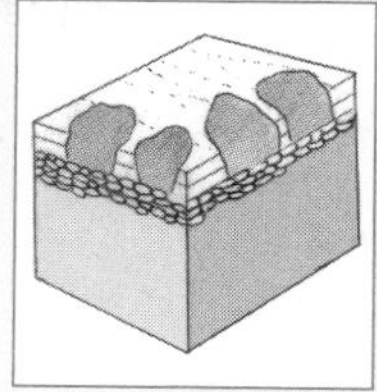

Wheal
A slightly raised, firm lesion of variable size and shape, surrounded by edema; skin may be red or pale

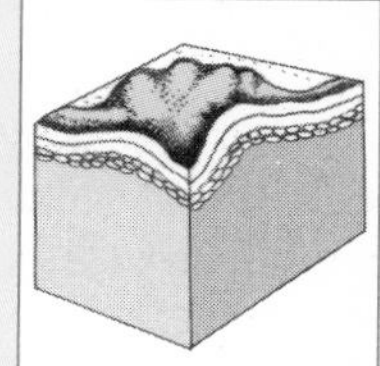

Bulla
A raised, thin-walled blister greater than 0.5 cm in diameter, containing clear or serous fluid

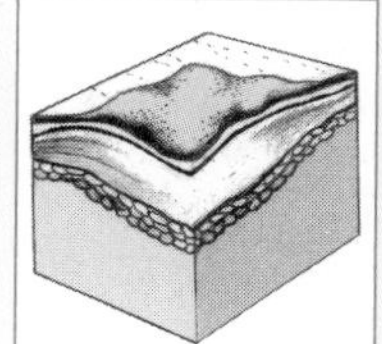

Nodule
A small, firm, circumscribed, raised lesion 1 to 2 cm in diameter, with possible skin discoloration

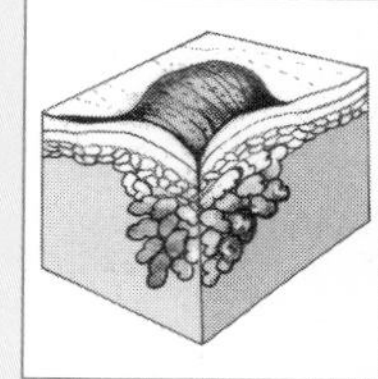

Vesicle
A small (less than 0.5 cm in diameter), thin-walled, raised blister containing clear, serous, purulent, or bloody fluid

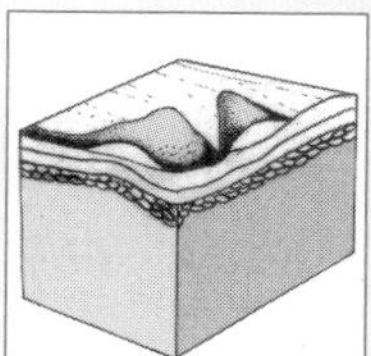

Papule
A small, solid, raised lesion less than 1 cm in diameter, with red to purple skin discoloration

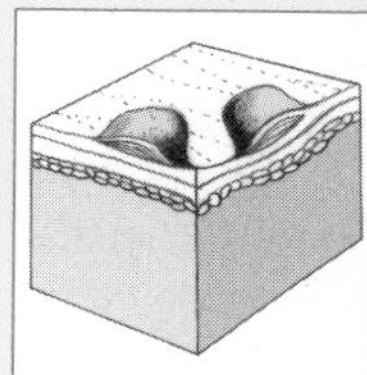

Pustule
A circumscribed, pus- or lymph-filled, raised lesion that varies in diameter and may be firm or soft and white or yellow

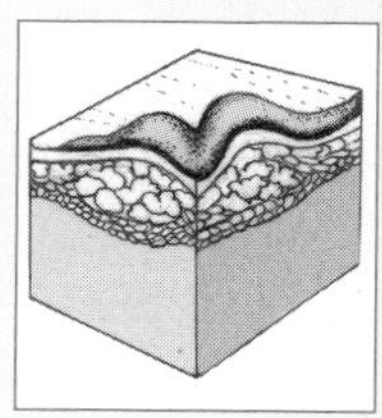

Tumor
A solid, raised mass usually larger than 2 cm in diameter, with possible skin discoloration

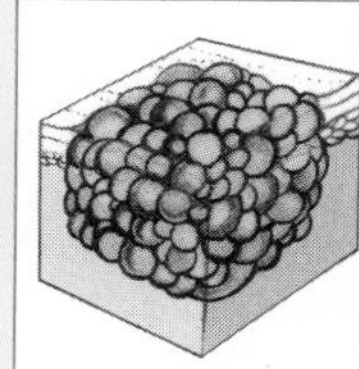

Lichen planus

- White lines or spots mark discrete, flat, angular or polygonal, violet papules.
- Papules may be linear or may coalesce into plaques and usually appear on the lumbar region, genitalia, ankles, anterior tibiae, and wrists.
- A rash usually develops first on the buccal mucosa as a lacy network of white or gray threadlike papules or plaques.

■ Other signs and symptoms include pruritus, distorted fingernails, and atrophic alopecia.

Mononucleosis, infectious

■ A maculopapular rash that resembles rubella is an early sign.
■ Headache, malaise, and fatigue typically precede the rash.
■ Other signs and symptoms include sore throat, cervical lymphadenopathy, hepatosplenomegaly, and fluctuating temperature with an evening peak of 101° to 102° F (38.3° to 38.9° C).

Necrotizing vasculitis

■ Crops of purpuric but otherwise asymptomatic papules are typical.
■ Other signs and symptoms include low-grade fever, headache, myalgia, arthralgia, and abdominal pain.

Pityriasis rosea

■ Initially, an erythematous, slightly raised, oval lesion appears anywhere on the body.
■ Later, yellow to tan or erythematous patches with scaly edges appear on the trunk, arms, and legs, commonly erupting along body cleavage lines in a pine tree–shaped pattern.

Psoriasis

■ Initially, small, erythematous, pruritic, and sometimes painful papules appear on the scalp, chest, elbows, knees, back, buttocks, and genitalia.
■ Eventually, papules enlarge and coalesce, forming elevated, red, scaly plaques covered by characteristic silver scales.
■ Other signs include pitted fingernails and arthralgia.

Rosacea

■ Persistent erythema, telangiectasia, and recurrent eruption of papules and pustules on the forehead, malar areas, nose, and chin occur.

Seborrheic keratosis

■ Benign skin tumors begin as small, yellow-brown papules on the chest, back, or abdomen, eventually enlarging and becoming deeply pigmented.

Smallpox

■ A maculopapular rash develops on the oral mucosa, pharynx, face, and forearms and then spreads to the trunk and legs.
■ Within 2 days, the rash becomes vesicular, and, later, round, firm pustules develop that are deeply embedded in the skin.
■ After 8 to 9 days, pustules form a crust; later, the scab separates from the skin, leaving a pitted scar.
■ Initial signs and symptoms include high fever, malaise, prostration, severe headache, backache, and abdominal pain.

Systemic lupus erythematosus

■ In this chronic connective tissue disease, a characteristic butterfly-shaped rash of erythematous maculopapules or discoid plaques in a malar distribution appears across the nose and cheeks.
■ Other signs and symptoms include photosensitivity, nondeforming arthritis, patchy alopecia, mucous membrane ulceration, fever, chills, lymphadenopathy, anorexia, weight loss, abdominal pain, diarrhea or constipation, dyspnea, hematuria, headache, and irritability.

Other causes

Drugs

■ Allopurinol (Zyloprim), antibiotics, benzodiazepines, gold salts, isoniazid (Nydrazid), lithium (Eskalith), and salicylates may cause transient maculopapular rashes, usually on the trunk.

Nursing considerations

■ Apply cool compresses or an antipruritic lotion.

- Administer an antihistamine for allergic reactions and an antibiotic for infection.

Patient teaching

- Teach the patient appropriate skin care measures.
- Explain ways to reduce itching.
- Discuss signs and symptoms to report.

Paralysis

Paralysis, the total loss of voluntary motor function, results from severe cortical or pyramidal tract damage. It can occur with a cerebrovascular disorder, degenerative neuromuscular disease, trauma, a tumor, or a central nervous system infection. Acute paralysis may be an early indicator of a life-threatening disorder such as Guillain-Barré syndrome.

Paralysis can be local or widespread, symmetrical or asymmetrical, transient or permanent, and spastic or flaccid. It's commonly classified according to location and severity as paraplegia (sometimes transient paralysis of the legs), quadriplegia (permanent paralysis of the arms, legs, and body below the level of the spinal lesion), or hemiplegia (unilateral paralysis of varying severity and permanence). Incomplete paralysis with profound weakness (paresis) may precede total paralysis in some patients.

QUICK ACTION ***If paralysis has developed suddenly, suspect trauma or an acute vascular insult. After ensuring that the patient's spine is properly immobilized, quickly determine his level of consciousness (LOC) and take his vital signs. Elevated systolic blood pressure, widening pulse pressure, and bradycardia may signal increasing intracranial pressure (ICP). If possible, elevate the patient's head 30 degrees to decrease ICP, and attempt to keep his head straight and facing forward.***

Evaluate the patient's respiratory status, and be prepared to administer oxygen, insert an artificial airway, or provide endotracheal intubation and mechanical ventilation as needed. To help determine the nature of the patient's injury, ask him for an account of the precipitating events. If he can't respond, try to find an eyewitness.

History

- Determine the onset (and preceding events), duration, intensity, and progression of paralysis.
- Obtain a medical history, including neurologic or neuromuscular disease, recent infectious illness, sexually transmitted disease, cancer, recent injury, or recent immunizations.
- Find out about fever, headache, vision disturbances, dysphagia, nausea and vomiting, bowel or bladder dysfunction, muscle pain or weakness, and fatigue.

Physical examination

- Perform a complete neurologic examination.
- Test cranial nerve, motor, and sensory function and deep tendon reflexes (DTRs).
- Assess strength in all major muscle groups, noting muscle atrophy.

Causes

Medical causes

Amyotrophic lateral sclerosis

- In this life-threatening progressive neurologic disorder, spastic or flaccid paralysis occurs in the major muscle groups and progresses to total paralysis.
- Early signs and symptoms include progressive muscle weakness, fasciculations, hyperreflexia, and muscle atrophy.
- Later, respiratory distress, dysarthria, drooling, choking, and difficulty chewing occur.

Bell's palsy

- Transient paralysis in muscles on one side of the face occurs.
- Increased tearing, drooling, inability to close the eyelid, and a diminished or absent corneal reflex occur.

Brain tumor

- If a tumor affects the motor cortex of the frontal lobe, contralateral hemiparesis progresses to hemiplegia.
- Early signs and symptoms include frontal headache and behavioral changes.
- Later signs and symptoms include seizures, aphasia, and signs of increased ICP.

Conversion disorder

- Loss of voluntary movement can affect any muscle group and has no obvious physical cause.
- Paralysis appears and disappears unpredictably.

Encephalitis

- Variable paralysis develops in the late stages.
- Earlier signs and symptoms include rapidly deteriorating LOC, fever, headache, photophobia, vomiting, signs of meningeal irritation, aphasia, ataxia, nystagmus, ocular palsies, myoclonus, and seizures.

Guillain-Barré syndrome

- A rapidly developing, reversible paralysis begins as leg muscle weakness and ascends symmetrically; respiratory muscle paralysis may be life-threatening.

Head trauma

- Sudden paralysis may occur; location and extent vary, depending on the injury.
- Other signs and symptoms include decreased LOC, sensory disturbances, headache, blurred or double vision, nausea, vomiting, and focal neurologic disturbances.

Migraine headache

- Hemiparesis, scotomas, paresthesia, confusion, dizziness, photophobia, and other transient symptoms may precede the onset of a throbbing unilateral headache and may persist after it subsides.

Multiple sclerosis

- Paralysis increases and decreases until the later stages, when it may become permanent; it ranges from monoplegia to quadriplegia.
- Late signs and symptoms vary and may include muscle weakness and spasticity, hyperreflexia, intention tremor, gait ataxia, dysphagia, dysarthria, impotence, constipation, and urinary frequency, urgency, and incontinence.

Myasthenia gravis

- Muscle weakness and fatigue produce paralysis of certain muscle groups.
- Paralysis is usually transient in the early stages but becomes more persistent as the disease progresses.
- Other signs and symptoms include ptosis, diplopia, lack of facial mobility, dysphagia, dyspnea, and shallow respirations.

Neurosyphilis

- Irreversible hemiplegia may occur in the late stages, accompanied by dementia, cranial nerve palsies, meningitis, personality changes, tremors, and abnormal reflexes.

Parkinson's disease

- Extreme rigidity can progress to paralysis, particularly in the extremities.
- Tremors, bradykinesia, and "lead-pipe" or "cogwheel" rigidity are the classic signs.

Peripheral nerve trauma

- Loss of motor and sensory function in the innervated area may occur.
- Muscles become flaccid and atrophied, and reflexes are lost.

Peripheral neuropathy

- Muscle weakness may lead to flaccid paralysis and atrophy.
- Related signs and symptoms include paresthesia, loss of vibration sensation, hypoactive or absent DTRs, neuralgia, and skin changes.

Rabies

- Progressive flaccid paralysis, vascular collapse, coma, and death occur within 2 weeks of contact with an infected animal.
- Early symptoms include fever, headache, hyperesthesia, photophobia, and excessive salivation, lacrimation, and perspiration.
- Within 2 to 10 days, agitation, cranial nerve dysfunction, cyclic respirations, high fever, urine retention, drooling, and hydrophobia occur.

Seizure disorder

- Transient local paralysis occurs from focal seizures, which may be preceded by an aura.

Spinal cord injury

- Complete spinal cord transection results in permanent spastic paralysis below the level of the injury; reflexes may return after spinal shock resolves.
- Partial transection causes variable paralysis and paresthesia. (See *Understanding spinal cord syndromes,* page 270.)

Spinal cord tumor

- Paresis, pain, paresthesia, and variable sensory loss may occur.
- The condition may progress to spastic paralysis with hyperactive DTRs and bladder and bowel incontinence.

Stroke

- Contralateral paresis or paralysis can result if the motor cortex is involved.
- Other signs and symptoms include headache, vomiting, seizures, decreased LOC, dysphagia, ataxia, contralateral paresthesia or sensory loss, apraxia, aphasia, vision disturbances, and bowel and bladder dysfunction.

Subarachnoid hemorrhage

- Sudden paralysis, temporary or permanent, may occur.
- Other signs and symptoms include severe headache, mydriasis, photophobia, aphasia, decreased LOC, nuchal rigidity, vomiting, and seizures.

Thoracic aortic aneurysm

- Sudden transient paralysis may occur.
- Prominent symptoms include severe chest pain radiating to the neck, shoulders, back, and abdomen and a sensation of tearing in the thorax.
- Other signs and symptoms include diaphoresis, dyspnea, tachycardia, cyanosis, diastolic heart murmur, and abrupt loss of radial and femoral pulses, or wide variations in pulses and blood pressure between the arms and legs.

Transient ischemic attack

- Transient paresis or paralysis on one side with paresthesia, blurred or double vision, dizziness, aphasia, dysarthria, and decreased LOC may occur.

West Nile encephalitis

- Paralysis may occur in more severe infections, accompanied by fever, neck stiffness, decreased LOC, seizures, headache, rash, and lymphadenopathy.

Other causes

Drugs

- Neuromuscular blockers produce paralysis.

Understanding spinal cord syndromes

When a patient's spinal cord is incompletely severed, he experiences partial motor and sensory loss. Most incomplete cord lesions fit into one of the syndromes described here.

Anterior cord syndrome, usually resulting from a flexion injury, causes motor paralysis and loss of pain and temperature sensation below the level of injury. Touch, proprioception, and vibration sensation are usually preserved.

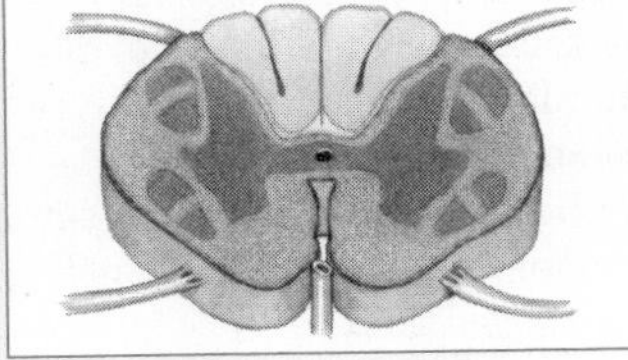

Brown-Séquard syndrome can result from flexion, rotation, or penetration injury. It's characterized by unilateral motor paralysis ipsilateral to the injury and a loss of pain and temperature sensation contralateral to the injury.

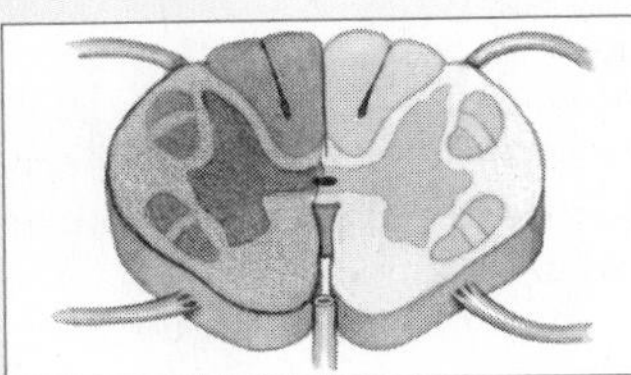

Central cord syndrome is caused by hyperextension or flexion injury. Motor loss is variable and greater in the arms than in the legs; sensory loss is usually slight.

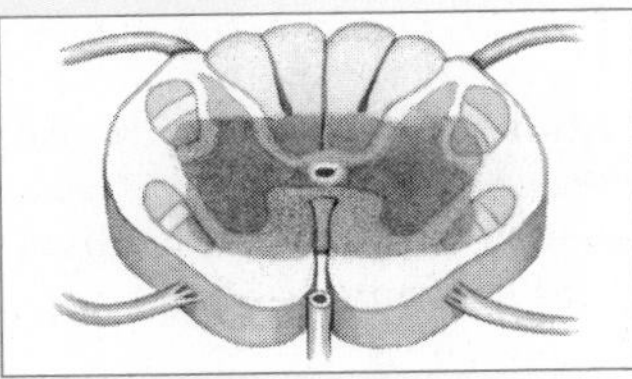

Posterior cord syndrome, produced by a cervical hyperextension injury, causes only a loss of proprioception and light touch sensation. Motor function remains intact.

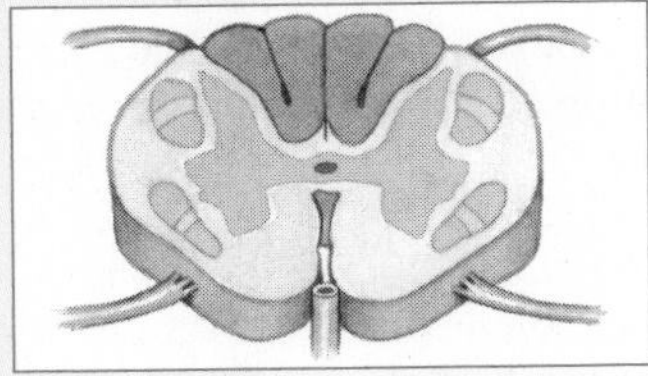

Electroconvulsive therapy

- Electroconvulsive therapy can produce acute but transient paralysis.

Nursing considerations

- Change the patient's position frequently and provide skin care to prevent breakdown.
- Administer frequent chest physiotherapy.
- Perform passive range-of-motion (ROM) exercises to maintain muscle tone.
- Apply splints to prevent contractures.
- Use footboards or other devices to prevent footdrop.
- Arrange for physical, speech, and occupational therapy as appropriate.

- Provide a thickened liquid or soft diet.
- Keep suction equipment on hand in case aspiration occurs.

Patient teaching

- Provide referrals to social and psychological services.
- Explain the underlying disorder and treatment plan.
- Teach the patient and his family or caregivers how to provide care at home, including passive ROM exercises, frequent turning, and chest physiotherapy.

Paresthesia

Paresthesia is an abnormal sensation or combination of sensations, commonly described as numbness, prickling, or tingling. These sensations, generally not painful, are felt along peripheral nerve pathways. Unpleasant or painful sensations, on the other hand, are termed *dysesthesias.* Paresthesia may develop suddenly or gradually and may be transient or permanent.

A common symptom of many neurologic disorders, paresthesia may also result from a systemic disorder or from a particular drug. It may reflect damage or irritation of the parietal lobe, thalamus, spinothalamic tract, or spinal or peripheral nerves—the neural circuit that transmits and interprets sensory stimuli.

History

- Ask about the onset and nature of abnormal sensations.
- Inquire about other symptoms, such as sensory loss and paresis.
- Find out about recent traumatic injury, surgery, or invasive procedures.
- Take a medical history, including neurologic, cardiovascular, metabolic, renal, and chronic inflammatory disorders.

Physical examination

- Assess the patient's level of consciousness (LOC) and cranial nerve function.
- Test muscle strength and deep tendon reflexes (DTRs) in affected limbs.
- Evaluate light touch, pain, temperature, vibration, and position sensation.
- Note skin color and temperature, and palpate pulses.

Causes

Medical causes

Arterial occlusion, acute

- Sudden paresthesia and coldness occur in the affected extremity; it may occur in one or both legs with a saddle embolus.
- Paresis, intermittent claudication, aching pain at rest, mottling, and absent pulses occur below the occlusion.

Arteriosclerosis obliterans

- Paresthesia may occur in the affected leg, along with intermittent claudication, pallor, paresis, coldness, and diminished or absent popliteal and pedal pulses.

Brain tumor

- Progressive contralateral paresthesia may occur with tumors of the sensory cortex.
- Other signs and symptoms include agnosia, apraxia, agraphia, homonymous hemianopsia, and loss of proprioception.

Diabetes mellitus

- Paresthesia and a burning sensation may occur in the hands and legs.
- Other signs and symptoms include anosmia, fatigue, polyuria, polydipsia, weight loss, and polyphagia.

Guillain-Barré syndrome

- Transient paresthesia may precede muscle weakness, which usually begins in the legs and ascends to the arms and facial nerves.

- Other signs and symptoms include dysarthria, dysphagia, nasal speech, orthostatic hypotension, bladder and bowel incontinence, diaphoresis, tachycardia and, possibly, life-threatening respiratory muscle paralysis.

Head trauma

- Paresthesia may occur with a concussion or contusion.
- Other signs and symptoms include variable paresis or paralysis, decreased LOC, headache, blurred or double vision, nausea, vomiting, dizziness, and seizures.

Heavy metal or solvent poisoning

- Acute or gradual paresthesia may occur.
- Mental status changes, tremors, weakness, seizures, and GI distress may occur.

Herniated disk

- Paresthesia may occur along with severe pain, muscle spasms, and weakness.

Herpes zoster

- Paresthesia occurs early in the dermatome supplied by the affected spinal nerve.
- Within several days, a pruritic, erythematous, vesicular rash associated with sharp, shooting, or burning pain occurs in the affected dermatome.

Hyperventilation syndrome

- Transient paresthesia may occur in the hands, feet, and perioral area.
- Other signs and symptoms include agitation, vertigo, syncope, pallor, muscle twitching and weakness, carpopedal spasm, and arrhythmias.

Hypocalcemia

- Asymmetrical paresthesia may occur in the fingers, toes, and circumoral area.
- Other signs and symptoms include muscle weakness, twitching, or cramps; palpitations; hyperactive DTRs; carpopedal spasm; and positive Chvostek's and Trousseau's signs.

Migraine headache

- Paresthesia in the hands, face, and perioral area may signal an impending migraine headache.
- Other early signs and symptoms include scotomas, hemiparesis, confusion, dizziness, and photophobia.

Multiple sclerosis

- An early symptom in this disease, paresthesia commonly increases and decreases until the later stages, when it becomes permanent.
- Other signs and symptoms include muscle weakness, spasticity, and hyperreflexia.

Peripheral nerve trauma

- Paresthesia and dysesthesia may occur in the area supplied by the affected nerve.
- Other signs and symptoms include flaccid paralysis or paresis, hyporeflexia, and sensory loss.

Peripheral neuropathy

- Progressive paresthesia may occur in all extremities.
- Other signs and symptoms include muscle weakness that may progress to flaccid paralysis and atrophy, loss of vibration sensation, diminished or absent DTRs, and cutaneous changes.

Rabies

- Paresthesia, coldness, and itching at the site of an animal bite may occur in the early stage.

Raynaud's disease

- Exposure to cold or stress turns fingers pale, cold, and cyanotic; with rewarming, they become red, throbbing, aching, swollen, and paresthetic.

Seizure disorder

- Paresthesia of the lips, fingers, and toes results from seizures originating in the parietal lobe.
- The paresthesia may appear as auras that precede tonic-clonic seizures.

Spinal cord injury

- Paresthesia may occur in the partial spinal cord transection at or below the level of the lesion, after spinal shock resolves.
- Sensory and motor loss varies.

Spinal cord tumor

- Paresthesia, paresis, pain, and sensory loss occur.
- Eventually, paresis may cause spastic paralysis with hyperactive DTRs and, possibly, bladder and bowel incontinence.

Thoracic outlet syndrome

- Paresthesia occurs suddenly when the affected arm is raised and abducted.
- The arm becomes pale and cool, with diminished pulses.

Transient ischemic attack

- Abrupt paresthesia limited to an isolated body part occurs.
- Other signs and symptoms include decreased LOC, dizziness, unilateral vision loss, nystagmus, aphasia, dysarthria, tinnitus, facial weakness, dysphagia, and ataxic gait.

Vitamin B deficiency

- Paresthesia and weakness may occur in the arms and legs.
- Other signs and symptoms include burning leg pain, hypoactive DTRs, variable sensory loss, changes in mental status, and impaired vision.

Other causes

Drugs

- Chemotherapeutics, chloroquine (Aralen), D-penicillamine (Depen), isoniazid (NydraZid), nitrofurantoin (Macrobid), parenteral gold therapy, and phenytoin (Dilantin) may produce transient paresthesia.

Radiation therapy

- Long-term radiation therapy may cause peripheral nerve damage, resulting in paresthesia.

Nursing considerations

- Monitor the patient's neurologic status.
- Help the patient perform daily activities as needed.
- If sensory deficits are present, protect the patient from injury.

Patient teaching

- Discuss safety measures.
- Tell the patient which signs and symptoms to report.
- Teach about the underlying diagnosis and treatment plan.

Paroxysmal nocturnal dyspnea

Dramatic and terrifying to most patients, this sign refers to an attack of dyspnea that abruptly awakens him. Common signs and symptoms include diaphoresis, coughing, wheezing, and chest discomfort. The attack abates after the patient sits up or stands for several minutes, but may recur every 2 or 3 hours.

Paroxysmal nocturnal dyspnea is a sign of left-sided heart failure. It may result from decreased respiratory drive, impaired left ventricular function, enhanced reabsorption of interstitial fluid, or increased thoracic blood volume. All of these pathophysiologic mechanisms cause dyspnea to worsen when the patient lies down.

History

- Obtain a history of the patient's dyspnea, including non-nocturnal episodes, triggers, timing, and frequency.
- Find out if the patient experiences coughing, wheezing, fatigue, or weakness during an attack.
- Ask if the patient has a history of lower extremity edema or jugular vein distention.
- Ask if the patient sleeps with his head elevated and, if so, on how many pillows; ask if he sleeps in a reclining chair.
- Obtain a cardiopulmonary history, including a history of myocardial infarction, coronary artery disease, hypertension, chronic bronchitis, emphysema, asthma, or cardiac surgery.

Physical examination

- Perform a physical examination. Begin by taking the patient's vital signs and forming an overall impression of his appearance, looking for cyanosis or edema.
- Auscultate the lungs for crackles and wheezing, and the heart for gallops and arrhythmias.

Causes

Medical causes

Left-sided heart failure

- Dyspnea—on exertion, during sleep, and eventually at rest—is an early sign of left-sided heart failure. This sign is characteristically accompanied by Cheyne-Stokes respirations, diaphoresis, weakness, wheezing, and a persistent, nonproductive cough or a cough that produces clear or blood-tinged sputum.
- As the patient's condition worsens, he develops tachycardia, tachypnea, alternating pulse (commonly initiated by a premature beat), ventricular gallop, crackles, and peripheral edema.
- With advanced left-sided heart failure, the patient may also exhibit severe orthopnea, cyanosis, clubbing, hemoptysis, and cardiac arrhythmias as well as signs and symptoms of shock, such as hypotension, a weak pulse, and cold, clammy skin.

Nursing considerations

- Prepare the patient for diagnostic tests, such as a chest X-ray, echocardiography, exercise electrocardiography, and cardiac blood pool imaging.
- If the hospitalized patient experiences paroxysmal nocturnal dyspnea, help him to sit or to walk around the room.
- If necessary, provide supplemental oxygen.
- Try to calm the patient because anxiety can worsen dyspnea.
- Help relieve dyspnea by elevating the patient's head and calming him.

Patient teaching

- Teach the patient about left-sided heart failure and its treatment plan.
- Tell about prescribed medications and their adverse effects.
- Explain to the patient what he can do during an attack to prevent worsening of dyspnea.

Peau d'orange

Usually a late sign of breast cancer, peau d'orange (orange peel skin) is the edematous thickening and pitting of breast skin. This slowly developing sign can also occur with breast or axillary lymph node infection, erysipelas, or Graves' disease. Its striking orange peel appearance stems from lymphatic edema around deepened hair follicles. (See *Recognizing peau d'orange*.)

History

- Ask when peau d'orange was first noticed.
- Inquire about lumps, pain, or other breast changes.
- Find out about associated malaise, achiness, and weight loss.
- Take a lactation history.
- Obtain a history of previous breast or axillary surgery.

Physical examination

- Estimate the extent of peau d'orange.
- Check for breast erythema and induration.
- Assess nipples for discharge, deviation, retraction, dimpling, and cracking.
- Palpate peau d'orange for warmth or induration.
- Palpate the rest of the breast for lumps.
- Palpate axillary lymph nodes, noting enlargement.
- Take the patient's temperature.

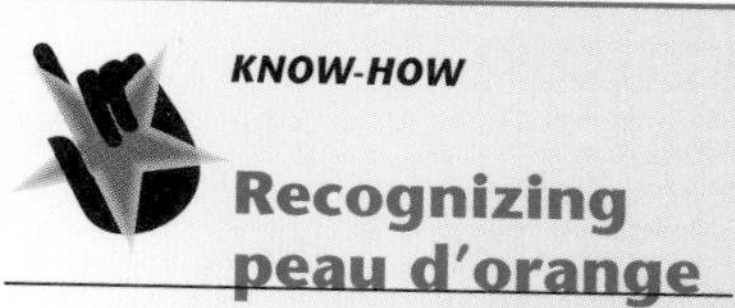

KNOW-HOW

Recognizing peau d'orange

In peau d'orange, the skin appears to be pitted (as shown below). This condition usually indicates late-stage breast cancer.

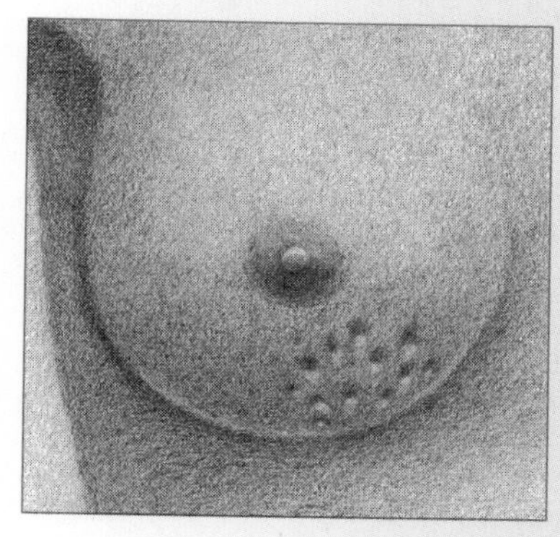

Causes

Medical causes

Breast abscess

- Peau d'orange may occur with malaise, breast tenderness and erythema, and a sudden fever with shaking chills.
- Other signs and symptoms include purulent discharge from a cracked nipple and possibly a mass.

Breast cancer

- Peau d'orange usually begins in a dependent part of the breast or areola.
- Palpation typically reveals a firm, immobile mass that adheres to the skin above the peau d'orange area.
- Other signs and symptoms may include changes in breast contour, size, or symmetry. Nipples may reveal deviation, erosion, retraction, and a thin and watery, bloody, or purulent discharge.

Erysipelas

- A well-demarcated, erythematous, elevated area, typically with a peau d'orange texture, may occur due to this streptococcal infection.
- Other signs and symptoms include pain, warmth, fever, and fatigue.

Graves' disease

- In this hyperthyroid disorder, raised, thickened, hyperpigmented, peau d'orange areas join together.
- Other signs and symptoms include weight loss, palpitations, anxiety, heat intolerance, tremor, and amenorrhea.

Nursing considerations

- Because peau d'orange usually signals advanced breast cancer, provide emotional support.

- Monitor the breast for nipple discharge and change in sensation.
- Administer prescribed pain medications as needed.

Patient teaching

- Explain diagnostic tests and treatment options.
- Teach the patient how to do monthly breast self-examinations.
- Tell the patient which signs and symptoms to report.
- Discuss skin care if nipple discharge is present.

Pericardial friction rub

Commonly transient, a pericardial friction rub is a scratching, grating, or crunching sound that occurs when two inflamed layers of the pericardium slide over one another. Ranging from faint to loud, this abnormal sound is best heard along the lower left sternal border during deep inspiration. It indicates pericarditis, which can result from an acute infection, a cardiac or renal disorder, postpericardiotomy syndrome, or the use of certain drugs.

Occasionally, a pericardial friction rub can resemble a murmur or pleural friction rub. However, the classic pericardial friction rub has three sound components, which are related to the phases of the cardiac cycle: presystolic, systolic, and early diastolic.

History

- Take a medical history, noting cancer, cardiac dysfunction, myocardial infarction, cardiac surgery, pericarditis, rheumatoid arthritis, chronic renal failure, infection, systemic lupus erythematosus, or trauma.
- Obtain a description of any chest pain, including character, location, and aggravating and alleviating factors.

Physical examination

- Take the patient's vital signs, noting hypotension, tachycardia, irregular pulse, tachypnea, and fever.
- Inspect for jugular vein distention, edema, ascites, and hepatomegaly.
- Auscultate heart sounds; to listen for a pericardial friction rub, have the patient sit upright, lean forward, and exhale.
- Auscultate the lungs for crackles.

Causes

Medical causes

Pericarditis

- Pericardial rub, the classic sign of acute pericarditis, is accompanied by sharp precordial or retrosternal pain that radiates to the left shoulder, neck, and back.
- Pain worsens with deep breathing, coughing, and lying flat.
- Pain lessens when the patient sits up and leans forward.
- Other signs and symptoms of the acute condition include fever, dyspnea, tachycardia, and arrhythmias.
- In the chronic condition, a pericardial rub develops gradually and may be accompanied by peripheral edema, ascites, Kussmaul's sign, hepatomegaly, dyspnea, orthopnea, paradoxical pulse, and chest pain.

Other causes

Drugs

- Chemotherapeutics and procainamide (Pronestyl) can cause pericarditis.

Treatments

- Cardiac surgery and high-dose radiation therapy can cause pericardial friction rub.

Nursing considerations

- Monitor the patient's cardiovascular status.
- If the pericardial rub disappears, look for signs of cardiac tamponade; if the signs develop, prepare the patient for pericardiocentesis.
- Ensure that the patient gets adequate rest.
- Give an anti-inflammatory, antiarrhythmic, diuretic, or antimicrobial, as ordered, to treat the underlying cause.
- Anticipate pericardiectomy to promote cardiac filling and contraction.
- A pericardial rub may develop with bacterial pericarditis, a life-threatening condition that usually occurs before age 6.
- A pericardial rub may occur after surgery to correct congenital cardiac anomalies.

Patient teaching

- Teach about the underlying disorder and treatments.
- Explain what the patient can do to minimize his symptoms.

Peristaltic waves, visible

With intestinal obstruction, peristalsis temporarily increases in strength and frequency as the intestine contracts to force its contents past the obstruction. As a result, visible peristaltic waves may roll across the abdomen. Typically, these waves appear suddenly and vanish quickly because increased peristalsis overcomes the obstruction or the GI tract becomes atonic. Peristaltic waves are best detected by stooping at the patient's side and inspecting his abdominal contour while he's in a supine position.

Visible peristaltic waves may also reflect normal stomach and intestinal contractions in thin patients or in malnourished patients with abdominal muscle atrophy.

History

- Obtain a medical history, including a history of pyloric ulcer, stomach cancer, chronic gastritis, intestinal obstruction, intestinal tumors or polyps, gallstones, chronic constipation, and hernia.
- Ask about recent abdominal surgery.
- Take a drug history.
- Find out about related signs and symptoms, such as abdominal pain, nausea, and vomiting.
- Obtain a description of the vomitus, including consistency, amount, and color.

Physical examination

- Inspect the abdomen for distention, surgical scars, adhesions, or visible bowel loops.
- Auscultate for bowel sounds.
- Roll the patient from side to side and then auscultate for succussion splash, which is a splashing sound in the stomach from retained secretions caused by pyloric obstruction.
- Percuss for tympany.
- Palpate the abdomen for rigidity and tenderness.
- Check the skin and mucous membranes for dryness and poor skin turgor.
- Take the patient's vital signs, noting tachycardia and hypotension.

Causes

Medical causes

Large-bowel obstruction

- Visible peristaltic waves in the upper abdomen are an early sign.
- Obstipation (severe constipation) may be the earliest sign.
- Other characteristic signs and symptoms include nausea, colicky abdominal pain, abdominal distention, and hyperactive bowel sounds.

Pyloric obstruction

- Peristaltic waves may be detected in a swollen epigastrium or in the left upper quadrant, usually beginning near

the left rib margin and rolling from left to right.
- Auscultation reveals a loud succussion splash.
- Related signs and symptoms include vague epigastric discomfort or colicky pain after eating, nausea, vomiting, anorexia, and weight loss.

Small-bowel obstruction
- Peristaltic waves rolling across the upper abdomen and intermittent, cramping, periumbilical pain are early signs, along with hyperactive bowel sounds and slight abdominal distention.
- Other signs and symptoms include nausea; vomiting of bilious or, later, fecal material; and constipation.
- With partial obstruction, diarrhea may occur.

Nursing considerations
- Withhold food and fluids.
- If obstruction is confirmed, perform nasogastric suctioning to decompress the stomach and small bowel, as ordered.
- Provide frequent oral hygiene.
- Monitor for dehydration.
- Frequently monitor the patient's vital signs and intake and output.
- In elderly patients, always check for fecal impaction, which is common in this age-group.
- Obtain a detailed drug history; antidepressants and antipsychotics can predispose the patient to constipation and bowel obstruction.

Patient teaching
- Discuss diet and fluid requirements.
- Encourage the use of stool softeners and increased intake of high-fiber foods for patients with chronic constipation.
- Discuss the underlying diagnosis and treatment plan.

Pleural friction rub

This loud, coarse, grating, creaking, or squeaking sound commonly results from a pulmonary disorder or trauma. It may be auscultated over one or both lungs during late inspiration or early expiration. It's best heard over the low axilla or the anterior, lateral, or posterior bases of the lung fields with the patient upright. Sometimes intermittent, it may resemble crackles or a pericardial friction rub.

A pleural friction rub indicates inflammation of the visceral and parietal pleural lining, which causes congestion and edema. The resultant fibrinous exudate covers both pleural surfaces, displacing the fluid that's normally between them and causing the surfaces to rub together.

QUICK ACTION ***When you detect a pleural friction rub, quickly look for signs of respiratory distress: shallow or decreased respirations; crowing, wheezing, or stridor; dyspnea; increased accessory muscle use; intercostal or suprasternal retractions; cyanosis; and nasal flaring. Check for hypotension, tachycardia, and a decreased level of consciousness.***

If you detect signs of distress, open and maintain an airway. Endotracheal intubation and supplemental oxygen may be necessary. Insert a large-bore I.V. catheter to deliver drugs and fluids. Elevate the patient's head 30 degrees. Monitor his cardiac status continually, and check his vital signs frequently.

History
- Obtain a description of chest pain, including onset, location, severity, duration, radiation, and aggravating and alleviating factors.

■ Take a medical history, including rheumatoid arthritis, a respiratory or cardiovascular disorder, recent trauma, asbestos exposure, and radiation therapy.
■ Ask about smoking history.

Physical examination

■ Auscultate the lungs with the patient sitting upright and breathing deeply and slowly through the mouth.
■ Determine whether the rub is in one lung or both.
■ Listen for absent or diminished breath sounds.
■ Palpate for decreased chest motion, and percuss for flatness or dullness.
■ Observe for clubbing and pedal edema.

Causes

Medical causes

Asbestosis

■ Pleural rub, exertional dyspnea, cough, chest pain, and crackles may occur.
■ As the disease advances, clubbing and dyspnea develop.

Lung cancer

■ A pleural rub may be heard in the area of the lung that's affected by the cancer.
■ Other signs and symptoms include cough (possibly with hemoptysis), dyspnea, chest pain, weight loss, anorexia, fatigue, clubbing, fever, and wheezing.

Pleurisy

■ A pleural rub occurs early.
■ The main symptom is sudden, intense, unilateral chest pain in the lower and lateral parts of the chest; deep breathing, coughing, and thoracic movements aggravate the pain.
■ Other signs and symptoms include decreased breath sounds, inspiratory crackles, dyspnea, tachypnea, tachycardia, cyanosis, fever, and fatigue.

Pneumonia, bacterial

■ A pleural rub occurs after a dry, painful, hacking, productive cough.
■ Other signs and symptoms include shaking chills, high fever, headache, dyspnea, pleuritic chest pain, tachypnea, tachycardia, grunting respirations, nasal flaring, dullness to percussion, decreased breath sounds, and cyanosis.

Pulmonary embolism

■ A pleural rub may occur over the affected area of the lung.
■ The first symptom is usually sudden dyspnea, which may be accompanied by angina or unilateral pleuritic chest pain.
■ Other signs and symptoms include a nonproductive cough or a cough that produces blood-tinged sputum, tachycardia, tachypnea, low-grade fever, restlessness, and diaphoresis.
■ Less common signs and symptoms include massive hemoptysis, chest splinting, leg edema, and with a large embolus, cyanosis, syncope, and jugular vein distention.

Rheumatoid arthritis

■ A unilateral pleural rub may occur.
■ Typical early signs and symptoms include fatigue, persistent low-grade fever, weight loss, and vague arthralgia and myalgia.
■ Later signs and symptoms include warm, swollen, painful joints; joint stiffness after activity; subcutaneous nodules on the elbows; joint deformity; and muscle weakness and atrophy.

Systemic lupus erythematosus

■ A pleural rub—accompanied by hemoptysis, dyspnea, pleuritic chest pain, and crackles—may occur with pulmonary involvement in this chronic inflammatory connective tissue disorder.
■ More characteristic effects include a butterfly-shaped rash, nondeforming

joint pain and stiffness, and photosensitivity.
- Fever, anorexia, weight loss, and lymphadenopathy may also occur.

Tuberculosis, pulmonary
- A pleural rub may occur over the affected part of the lung.
- Early signs and symptoms include weight loss, night sweats, low-grade fever in the afternoon, malaise, dyspnea, anorexia, and easy fatigability.
- Disease progression produces pleuritic chest pain, fine crackles over the upper lobes, and a productive cough with blood-streaked sputum.
- Advanced signs and symptoms include chest wall retraction, tracheal deviation, and dullness upon percussion.

Other causes

Treatments
- Thoracic surgery and radiation therapy can cause pleural rub.

Nursing considerations
- Monitor the patient's respiratory status and vital signs.
- If the patient has a persistent dry, hacking cough that tires him, give an antitussive.
- Administer oxygen and an antibiotic as needed.
- Follow bleeding precautions in the patient on anticoagulation therapy for pulmonary embolism.
- Auscultate for a pleural rub in a child who has grunting respirations, reports chest pain, or protects his chest.
- A pleural rub in a child is usually an early sign of pleurisy.
- Pleuritic chest pain in the elderly patient may mimic cardiac chest pain.

Patient teaching
- Prepare the patient for diagnostic tests.
- Discuss pain relief measures.
- Explain signs and symptoms the patient needs to report.
- Discuss the underlying disorder and treatment plan.

Polydipsia

Polydipsia refers to excessive thirst, a common symptom associated with endocrine disorders and certain drugs. It may reflect decreased fluid intake, increased urine output, or excessive loss of water and salt.

History
- Determine the patient's average fluid intake and output.
- Obtain a description of his urinary patterns.
- Take a personal or family history of diabetes or kidney disease.
- Take a drug history.
- Ask about recent weight loss.

Physical examination
- Obtain the patient's blood pressure and pulse when he's in the supine and standing positions.
- Check for signs of dehydration, such as poor skin turgor and dry mucous membranes.
- Obtain urine specimens and blood samples as ordered.
- Perform a complete physical assessment.

Causes
Medical causes

Diabetes insipidus
- Polydipsia, excessive voiding of dilute urine, and nocturia occur.
- Fatigue and signs of dehydration occur in severe cases.

Diabetes mellitus
- Polydipsia is a classic symptom.
- Polyuria, polyphagia, nocturia, and signs of dehydration may also occur.

Hypercalcemia

- In the later stages of this disorder, polydipsia occurs with polyuria, nocturia, constipation, paresthesia and, occasionally, hematuria and pyuria.
- If hypercalcemia is severe, vomiting, decreased level of consciousness, and renal failure develop.

Hypokalemia

- Polydipsia, polyuria, and nocturia may develop.
- Other related signs and symptoms include muscle weakness or paralysis, fatigue, decreased bowel sounds, hypoactive deep tendon reflexes, and arrhythmias.

Psychogenic polydipsia

- This psychiatric condition causes polydipsia in the absence of a physiologic stimulus to drink.
- No apparent reason for excessive thirst or fluid intake exists.
- The condition may be well-tolerated if water intoxication and hyponatremia don't occur.
- Related signs and symptoms include confusion, headache, irritability, weight gain, elevated blood pressure, stupor, and coma.

Renal disorder, chronic

- Polydipsia and polyuria signal kidney damage.
- Other signs and symptoms include nocturia, weakness, elevated blood pressure, pallor and, in later stages, oliguria.

Sickle cell anemia

- Polydipsia and polyuria occur as nephropathy develops.
- Other related signs and symptoms include abdominal pain and cramps, arthralgia and, occasionally, lower extremity skin ulcers and bone deformities such as kyphosis.

Thyrotoxicosis

- Polydipsia may occur infrequently with this disorder.
- Characteristic signs and symptoms include tachycardia, palpitations, weight loss despite increased appetite, diarrhea, tremors, nervousness, heat intolerance, and enlarged thyroid.

Other causes

Drugs

- Diuretics and demeclocycline (Declomycin) may produce polydipsia.
- Phenothiazines and anticholinergics can cause dry mouth, making the patient so thirsty that he drinks compulsively.

Nursing considerations

- Record total intake and output.
- Weigh the patient at the same time each day using the same scale.
- Check blood pressure and pulse in the supine and standing positions.
- Give the patient ample liquids if appropriate.

Patient teaching

- Explain the underlying disorder and treatments the patient will need.
- Teach about diet, exercise, and home blood-glucose monitoring.
- Stress the importance of reporting significant weight gain or loss.

Polyuria

A relatively common sign, polyuria is the daily production and excretion of more than 3 L of urine. It's usually reported by the patient as increased urination, especially when it occurs at night. Polyuria is aggravated by overhydration, consumption of caffeine or alcohol, and excessive ingestion of salt, glucose, or other hyperosmolar substances.

Polyuria usually results from the use of certain drugs, such as a diuretic, or from a psychological, neurologic, or renal disorder. It can reflect central nervous system dysfunction that diminishes or suppresses antidiuretic hormone (ADH) secretion, which regulates fluid balance. Or, when ADH levels are normal, it can reflect renal impairment. In both of these pathophysiologic mechanisms, the renal tubules fail to reabsorb sufficient water, causing polyuria.

History

- Explore the frequency and pattern of polyuria.
- Ask for a description of patterns and amounts of daily fluid intake.
- Inquire about fatigue, increased thirst, or weight loss.
- Obtain a medical history of vision deficits, headaches, head trauma, urinary tract obstruction, diabetes mellitus, a renal disorder, chronic hypokalemia or hypercalcemia, or a psychiatric disorder.
- Take a drug history.

Physical examination

- Take the patient's vital signs, noting increased body temperature, tachycardia, and orthostatic hypotension.
- Inspect for signs of dehydration.
- Perform a neurologic assessment, noting a change in the patient's level of consciousness.
- Palpate the bladder and inspect the urethral meatus.
- Obtain a urine specimen and check specific gravity.

Causes

Medical causes

Acute tubular necrosis

- During the diuretic phase, urine output of more than 8 L/day gradually subsides after about 1 week.
- Urine specific gravity (1.101 or less) increases as polyuria subsides.
- Related signs and symptoms include weight loss, decreasing edema, and nocturia.

Diabetes insipidus

- Polyuria of about 5 L/day occurs, with urine specific gravity of 1.005 or less.
- Accompanying signs and symptoms include polydipsia, nocturia, fatigue, and signs of dehydration.

Diabetes mellitus

- Polyuria is seldom more than 5 L/day, and urine specific gravity is typically more than 1.020.
- Other signs and symptoms include polydipsia, polyphagia, weight loss, frequent urinary tract infections and yeast vaginitis, fatigue, signs of dehydration, and nocturia.

Glomerulonephritis, chronic

- Polyuria gradually progresses to oliguria.
- Urine output is usually less than 4 L/day; specific gravity is about 1.010.
- Related GI signs and symptoms include anorexia, nausea, and vomiting.
- Other signs and symptoms include drowsiness, fatigue, edema, headache, elevated blood pressure, dyspnea, nocturia, hematuria, frothy or malodorous urine, and proteinuria.

Hypercalcemia

- Polyuria of more than 5 L/day occurs with a urine specific gravity of about 1.010.
- Other signs and symptoms include polydipsia, nocturia, constipation, paresthesia and, occasionally, hematuria and pyuria.
- With severe hypercalcemia, anorexia, vomiting, stupor progressing to coma, and renal failure occur.

Hypokalemia

■ Prolonged potassium depletion causes polyuria of less than 5 L/day with a urine specific gravity of about 1.010.
■ Other signs and symptoms include polydipsia, circumoral and foot paresthesia, hypoactive deep tendon reflexes, fatigue, hypoactive bowel sounds, nocturia, arrhythmias, and muscle cramping, weakness, or paralysis.

Postobstructive uropathy

■ After resolution of a urinary tract obstruction, polyuria—usually more than 5 L/day with a urine specific gravity of less than 1.010—occurs for several days before gradually subsiding.
■ Other signs and symptoms include bladder distention, edema, nocturia, and weight loss.

Pyelonephritis

■ Polyuria of less than 5 L/day with a low but variable urine specific gravity occurs in acute disease.
■ Signs and symptoms of acute pyelonephritis include persistent high fever, flank pain, hematuria, costovertebral angle tenderness, chills, weakness, dysuria, urinary frequency and urgency, tenesmus, and nocturia.
■ Chronic pyelonephritis produces polyuria of less than 5 L/day that declines as renal function worsens; urine specific gravity is usually about 1.010, but it may be higher if proteinuria is present.
■ Other effects of the chronic condition include irritability, paresthesia, fatigue, nausea, vomiting, diarrhea, drowsiness, anorexia, pyuria and, in late stages, elevated blood pressure.

Sickle cell anemia

■ Polyuria occurs with a urine output of less than 5 L/day with a specific gravity of about 1.020.
■ Additional signs and symptoms include polydipsia, fatigue, abdominal cramps, arthralgia, priapism and, occasionally, leg ulcers and bony deformities.

Other causes

Diagnostic tests

■ Radiographic tests that use contrast media may cause transient polyuria.

Drugs

■ Diuretics produce polyuria.
■ Cardiotonics, vitamin D, demeclocycline (Declomycin), phenytoin (Dilantin), and lithium (Eskalith) can also produce polyuria.

Nursing considerations

■ Record intake and output, and weigh the patient daily.
■ Monitor the patient's vital signs.
■ Encourage fluid intake to maintain adequate fluid balance.
■ Because a child's fluid balance is more delicate than an adult's, check urine specific gravity at each voiding, and be alert for signs of dehydration.

Patient teaching

■ Teach the patient about the underlying disorder.
■ Explain fluid replacement.
■ Instruct the patient on weight monitoring.
■ Discuss signs and symptoms of dehydration the patient needs to report.

Pruritus

This unpleasant itching sensation affects the skin, certain mucous membranes, and the eyes, and commonly provokes scratching to gain relief. Most severe at night, pruritus may be worsened by increased skin temperature, poor skin turgor, local vasodilation, dermatoses, and stress.

The most common symptom of dermatologic disorders, pruritus may also result from a local or systemic disorder or from drug use. Physiologic pruritus, such as pruritic urticarial papules and plaques of pregnancy, may occur in primigravidas late in the third trimester. Pruritus can also stem from emotional upset or contact with skin irritants.

History

- Ask about the onset, frequency, duration, and intensity of pruritus.
- Determine the location, whether it's localized or generalized, and what aggravates and alleviates it.
- Ask about contact with irritants.
- Obtain a description of skin care practices.
- Take a drug history.
- Obtain a medical history.
- Find out about recent travel and pets in the home.

Physical examination

- Observe for signs of scratching, such as excoriation, purpura, scabs, scars, or lichenification.
- Look for primary lesions to help confirm dermatoses.

Causes

Medical causes

Anemia, iron deficiency

- Pruritus occasionally occurs.
- Late signs and symptoms include exertional dyspnea, fatigue, listlessness, pallor, irritability, headache, tachycardia, poor muscle tone and, possibly, murmurs.
- Chronic anemia causes spoon-shaped (koilonychias) and brittle nails (cheilosis), cracked mouth corners, a smooth tongue (glossitis), and dysphagia.

Anthrax, cutaneous

- Early infection causes a small, painless or pruritic, macular or papular lesion resembling an insect bite.
- In 1 to 2 days, the lesion develops into a vesicular lesion and then a painless ulcer with a black, necrotic center.
- Other signs and symptoms include lymphadenopathy, malaise, headache, or fever.

Conjunctivitis

- All forms of conjunctivitis cause eye itching, burning, and pain along with photophobia, conjunctival injection, a foreign-body sensation, and excessive tearing.
- Allergic conjunctivitis may also cause milky redness and a stringy eye discharge.
- Bacterial conjunctivitis typically causes brilliant redness and a mucopurulent discharge that may make the eyelids stick together.
- Fungal conjunctivitis produces a thick purulent discharge, crusting, and sticking of the eyelids.
- Viral conjunctivitis may cause copious tearing but little discharge and preauricular lymph node enlargement.

Dermatitis

- Pruritus may be accompanied by a skin lesion.
- Atopic dermatitis begins with intense, severe pruritus and an erythematous rash on dry skin at flexion points.
- In chronic atopic dermatitis, lesions may progress to dry, scaly skin with white dermatographism, blanching, and lichenification.
- In contact dermatitis, itchy, small vesicles may ooze and scale, and are surrounded by redness; localized edema may occur with a severe reaction.
- Dermatitis herpetiformis initially causes intense pruritus; 8 to 12 hours later, symmetrically distributed lesions form on the buttocks, shoulders, elbows, and knees.

Enterobiasis

- Intense perianal pruritus occurs, especially at night, due to pinworm infestation.
- Other signs and symptoms include irritability, scratching, skin irritation and, sometimes, vaginitis.

Hepatobiliary disease

- Pruritus, commonly accompanied by jaundice, may be generalized or localized to the palms and soles.
- Other signs and symptoms include right upper quadrant pain, clay-colored stools, chills, fever, flatus, belching, a bloated feeling, epigastric burning, and bitter fluid regurgitation.
- Later signs and symptoms include mental changes, ascites, bleeding tendencies, spider angiomas, palmar erythema, dry skin, fetor hepaticus, enlarged superficial abdominal veins, bilateral gynecomastia, and hepatomegaly.

Herpes zoster

- Within 4 days of fever and malaise, pruritus, paresthesia or hyperesthesia, and severe, deep pain develop in a dermatome distribution.
- Up to 2 weeks after initial symptoms, red, nodular skin eruptions appear on the painful areas and become vesicular; about 10 days later, vesicles rupture and form scabs.

Lichen simplex chronicus

- Localized pruritus and a circumscribed scaling patch with sharp margins develop.
- Later, the skin thickens and papules form.

Pediculosis

- Pruritus in the area of lice infestation is a prominent symptom.
- Pediculosis capitis may cause scalp excoriation from scratching. Other signs include foul-smelling, lusterless, matted hair; occipital and cervical lymphadenopathy; and oval, gray-white nits on hair shafts.
- Pediculosis corporis initially causes red papules on the body, which become urticarial from scratching; later, rashes or wheals may develop.
- Pediculosis pubis is marked by nits or adult lice and erythematous, itching papules in pubic hair or hair around the anus, abdomen, or thighs.

Pityriasis rosea

- Pruritus that's aggravated by a hot bath or shower occasionally occurs.
- An erythematous patch forms and progresses to scaly, yellow, erythematous patches that erupt on the trunk or extremities and persist for 2 to 6 weeks.

Polycythemia vera

- Pruritus is generalized or localized to the head, neck, face, and extremities; hot baths and showers typically aggravate it.
- A deep, purplish red color develops on the oral mucosa, gingivae, and tongue.
- Related signs and symptoms include headache, dizziness, fatigue, dyspnea, paresthesia, impaired mentation, tinnitus, double or blurred vision, scotoma, hypotension, intermittent claudication, urticaria, ruddy cyanosis, hepatosplenomegaly, and ecchymosis.

Psoriasis

- Pruritus and pain commonly occur.
- Small erythematous papules enlarge or coalesce to form red, elevated plaques with silver scales on the scalp, chest, elbows, knees, back, buttocks, and genitals.

Renal failure, chronic

- Pruritus may develop gradually or suddenly.
- Other signs and symptoms include ammonia breath odor, oliguria or anuria, fatigue, decreased mental acuity,

muscle twitching and cramps, anorexia, nausea, vomiting, peripheral neuropathies, and coma.

Scabies

- Typically, localized pruritus that awakens the patient occurs.
- Threadlike lesions appear with a swollen nodule or red papule.

Tinea pedis

- Typically, severe foot pruritus occurs with scales and blisters between the toes and a dry, scaly squamous inflammation on the sole.

Urticaria

- Extreme pruritus and stinging occur as transient erythematous or whitish wheals form on the skin or mucous membranes.

Other causes

Drugs

- When mild and localized, an allergic reaction to drugs such as penicillin and sulfonamides can cause pruritus, erythema, urticaria, and edema.

Nursing considerations

- Administer a topical or oral corticosteroid, an antihistamine, or a tranquilizer.
- Many adult disorders also cause pruritus in children, but they may affect different parts of the body.
- Such childhood diseases as measles and chickenpox can also cause pruritus.

Patient teaching

- Discuss the underlying condition.
- Teach the patient ways to control pruritus.

Ptosis

Ptosis is the excessive drooping of one or both upper eyelids. This sign can be constant, progressive, or intermittent and unilateral or bilateral. When it's unilateral, it's easy to detect by comparing the eyelids' relative positions. When it's bilateral or mild, it's difficult to detect—the eyelids may be abnormally low, covering the upper part of the iris or even part of the pupil instead of merely overlapping the iris slightly. Other clues include a furrowed forehead or a tipped-back head—both of these help the patient see under his drooping lids. With severe ptosis, the patient may not be able to raise his eyelids voluntarily. Because ptosis can resemble enophthalmos, exophthalmometry may be required.

Ptosis can be classified as congenital or acquired. Classification is important for proper treatment. Congenital ptosis results from levator muscle underdevelopment or disorders of the third cranial (oculomotor) nerve. Acquired ptosis may result from trauma to or inflammation of these muscles and nerves or from certain drugs, a systemic disease, an intracranial lesion, or a life-threatening aneurysm. However, the most common cause is advanced age, which reduces muscle elasticity and produces senile ptosis.

History

- Ask about the onset of ptosis and whether the condition has worsened or improved.
- Find out about recent traumatic eye injury.
- Inquire about eye pain or headache.
- Determine whether the patient has experienced vision changes.
- Take a drug history, noting especially the use of a chemotherapeutic drug.

Physical examination

- Assess the degree of ptosis.
- Check for eyelid edema, exophthalmos, and conjunctival injection.
- Evaluate extraocular muscle function.

- Examine pupil size, color, shape, and reaction to light.
- Test visual acuity.

Causes

Medical causes

Alcoholism

- Ptosis as well as complications, such as severe weight loss, jaundice, ascites, and mental disturbances, can result from long-term alcohol abuse.

Botulism

- Cranial nerve dysfunction causes ptosis, dysarthria, dysphagia, and diplopia.
- Other signs and symptoms include dry mouth, sore throat, weakness, vomiting, diarrhea, hyporeflexia, and dyspnea.

Cerebral aneurysm

- Sudden ptosis, diplopia, a dilated pupil, and the inability to rotate the eye can occur due to compression of the oculomotor nerve and may be the first signs of this disorder.
- A ruptured aneurysm, a life-threatening condition, produces sudden severe headache, nausea, vomiting, and decreased level of consciousness (LOC).
- Other signs and symptoms include nuchal rigidity, back and leg pain, fever, restlessness, irritability, seizures, blurred vision, hemiparesis, sensory deficits, dysphagia, and visual deficits.

Hemangioma

- Ptosis may occur along with exophthalmos, limited extraocular movement, swollen periorbital tissue, and blurred vision.

Lacrimal gland tumor

- A lacrimal gland tumor commonly produces mild to severe ptosis, depending on the tumor's size and location.
- Other signs and symptoms include brow elevation, exophthalmos, eye deviation and, possibly, eye pain.

Levator muscle maldevelopment

- Ptosis results from isolated dystrophy of the levator muscle.
- Eyelid lag on downgaze is an important clue to diagnosis.

Myasthenia gravis

- Gradual ptosis in both eyes is commonly the first sign of this neuromuscular disorder.
- Ptosis is accompanied by weak eye closure and diplopia.
- Other signs and symptoms include muscle weakness and fatigue, masklike facies, difficulty chewing or swallowing, dyspnea, cyanosis and, possibly, paralysis.

Ocular muscle dystrophy

- Ptosis progresses slowly to complete closure of the eyelids.
- Other signs and symptoms include progressive external ophthalmoplegia and muscle weakness and atrophy of the upper face, neck, trunk, and limbs.

Ocular trauma

- Mild to severe ptosis can result from trauma to the nerve or muscles that control the eyelids.
- Eye pain, eyelid swelling, ecchymosis, and decreased visual acuity may also occur.

Subdural hematoma, chronic

- Ptosis may be a late sign, along with dilation of one pupil and sluggishness.
- Headache, behavioral changes, and decreased LOC commonly occur.

Other causes

Drugs

- Vinca alkaloids and chemotherapy medications can produce ptosis.

Lead poisoning

- With lead poisoning, ptosis develops over 3 to 6 months; other signs and symptoms include anorexia, nausea, vomiting, diarrhea, colicky abdominal pain, a lead line in the gums, decreased LOC, tachycardia, hypotension, irritability, and peripheral nerve weakness.

Nursing considerations

- Orient the patient with decreased visual acuity to his surroundings.
- Assist with special spectacle frames that suspend the eyelid by traction with a wire crutch.

Patient teaching

- Explain the underlying disorder and treatment options.
- Discuss self-esteem issues.
- Prepare the patient for needed diagnostic tests and surgery, if necessary.

Pulse, absent or weak

An absent or a weak pulse may be generalized or affect only one extremity. When generalized, this sign is an important indicator of such life-threatening conditions as shock and arrhythmias. (See *Managing an absent or a weak pulse,* pages 290 and 291.) Localized loss or weakness of a pulse that's normally present and strong may indicate acute arterial occlusion, which could require emergency surgery. However, the pressure of palpation may temporarily diminish or obliterate superficial pulses, such as the posterior tibial or dorsal pedal. Because of this, bilateral weakness or absence of these pulses doesn't necessarily indicate an underlying disorder.

History

- Review the medical history, including heart and vascular disease.
- Take a drug history.
- Question the patient about associated signs and symptoms, such as chest pain or dyspnea.

Physical examination

- Palpate the arterial pulses for comparison; assess the limb for color and temperature.
- Take the patient's vital signs and obtain electrocardiogram results.
- Evaluate the patient's cardiopulmonary status.

Causes

Medical causes

Aortic aneurysm, dissecting

- Weak or absent arterial pulses occur distal to the affected area when circulation to the innominate, left common carotid, subclavian, or femoral artery is affected.
- Tearing pain develops suddenly in the chest and neck, and may radiate to the back and abdomen.
- Other signs and symptoms include syncope, loss of consciousness, weakness or transient paralysis of the legs or arms, diastolic murmur of aortic insufficiency, hypotension, and mottled skin below the waist.

Aortic arch syndrome (Takayasu's arteritis)

- This syndrome produces weak or abruptly absent carotid pulses and unequal or absent radial pulses.
- These signs are usually preceded by malaise, night sweats, pallor, nausea, anorexia, weight loss, arthralgia, and Raynaud's phenomenon.
- Other signs and symptoms include neck, shoulder, and chest pain, paresthesia, intermittent claudication, bruits, vision disturbances, dizziness, and syncope.

Aortic stenosis

■ In this condition, the carotid pulse is weak.

■ Paroxysmal or exertional dyspnea, chest pain, and syncope are common.

■ Other signs and symptoms include atrial gallop, harsh systolic ejection murmur, crackles, palpitations, fatigue, and narrowed pulse pressure.

Arterial occlusion

■ With acute occlusion, arterial pulses distal to the obstruction are weak and then absent.

■ The affected limb has severe pain, varying degrees of paralysis, intermittent claudication, and paresthesia. It's cool, pale, and cyanotic, with increased capillary refill time. Furthermore, it has a line of color and temperature demarcation at the level of obstruction.

■ With chronic occlusion, pulses in the affected limb weaken gradually.

Cardiac arrhythmia

■ Generalized weak pulses may accompany cool, clammy skin.

■ Other signs and symptoms include hypotension, chest pain, dyspnea, dizziness, and decreased level of consciousness.

Cardiac tamponade

■ In this life-threatening condition, a weak rapid pulse accompanies the classic signs of paradoxical pulse, jugular vein distention, hypotension, and muffled heart sounds.

■ Other signs and symptoms include narrowed pulse pressure, pericardial friction rub, hepatomegaly, anxiety, restlessness, cyanosis, chest pain, dyspnea, tachypnea, and cold, clammy skin.

Coarctation of the aorta

■ Bounding pulses occur in the arms and neck, with decreased pulsations and systolic pulse pressure in the lower extremities.

■ Auscultation may reveal a systolic ejection click accompanied by a systolic ejection murmur.

Peripheral vascular disease

■ A weakening and loss of peripheral pulses occurs.

■ Aching pain occurs distal to the occlusion that worsens with exercise and abates with rest.

■ Other signs and symptoms include cool skin, decreased hair growth in the affected limb, and impotence with an occlusion of the descending aorta or femoral areas.

Pulmonary embolism

■ In this condition, a generalized weak, rapid pulse occurs.

■ Other symptoms include an abrupt onset of chest pain, tachycardia, apprehension, syncope, diaphoresis, and cyanosis.

■ Acute respiratory signs and symptoms include tachypnea, dyspnea, decreased breath sounds, crackles, pleural friction rub, and cough, possibly with blood-tinged sputum.

Shock

■ With anaphylactic shock, pulses become rapid and weak and then are uniformly absent within seconds or minutes after exposure to an allergen.

■ With cardiogenic shock, peripheral pulses are absent and central pulses are weak, depending on the degree of vascular collapse.

■ With hypovolemic shock, all peripheral pulses become weak and then uniformly absent, depending on the severity of hypovolemia.

■ With septic shock, all pulses in the extremities first become weak and then absent.

(Text continues on page 292.)

QUICK ACTION

Managing an absent or a weak pulse

An absent or a weak pulse can result from any one of several life-threatening disorders. Your evaluation and interventions will vary, depending on whether the weak or absent pulse is generalized or localized to one extremity. They'll also depend on associated signs and symptoms. Use this flowchart to help you establish priorities for successfully managing this emergency.

Weak or absent pulse → Localized to one extremity

↓

Generalized

↓

Patient is confused and restless and has hypotension and cool, pale, clammy skin.

↓

Patient has a history of trauma, possibly with external bleeding, and reports thirst.	Patient has a history of myocardial infarction (MI) or heart failure.	Patient has a history of recent cardiac surgery or catheterization, chest trauma, pericardial effusion, or anticoagulant therapy.	Patient has a history of MI or chronic heart or lung disease.
↓	↓	↓	↓
Check for flat jugular veins, low urine output, and narrowed pulse pressure.	Check for distended jugular veins, ventricular gallop (S_3), crackles, and narrowed pulse pressure.	Check for distended jugular veins, pulsus paradoxus, and muffled heart sounds.	Check for irregular heart rate, severe tachycardia, and bradycardia.
↓	↓	↓	↓
If your examination reveals these findings, suspect *hypovolemic shock.*	If your examination reveals these findings, suspect *cardiogenic shock.*	If your examination reveals these findings, suspect *cardiac tamponade.*	If your examination reveals these findings, suspect *arrhythmia.*

↓

Administer oxygen by nasal cannula, and insert an I.V. catheter for fluid infusion. Begin cardiac monitoring, and check the patient's vital signs every 5 to 15 minutes. A central venous pressure (CVP) line, an arterial line, or a pulmonary artery catheter (PAC) may have to be inserted. Be prepared for emergency resuscitation, if necessary.

↓

Anticipate colloid or crystalloid replacement, as well as the need for transfusion.	Anticipate administering nitroprusside, dopamine, and dobutamine.	Anticipate pericardiocentesis.	Anticipate administering antiarrhythmics, delivering cardioversion therapy, or both.

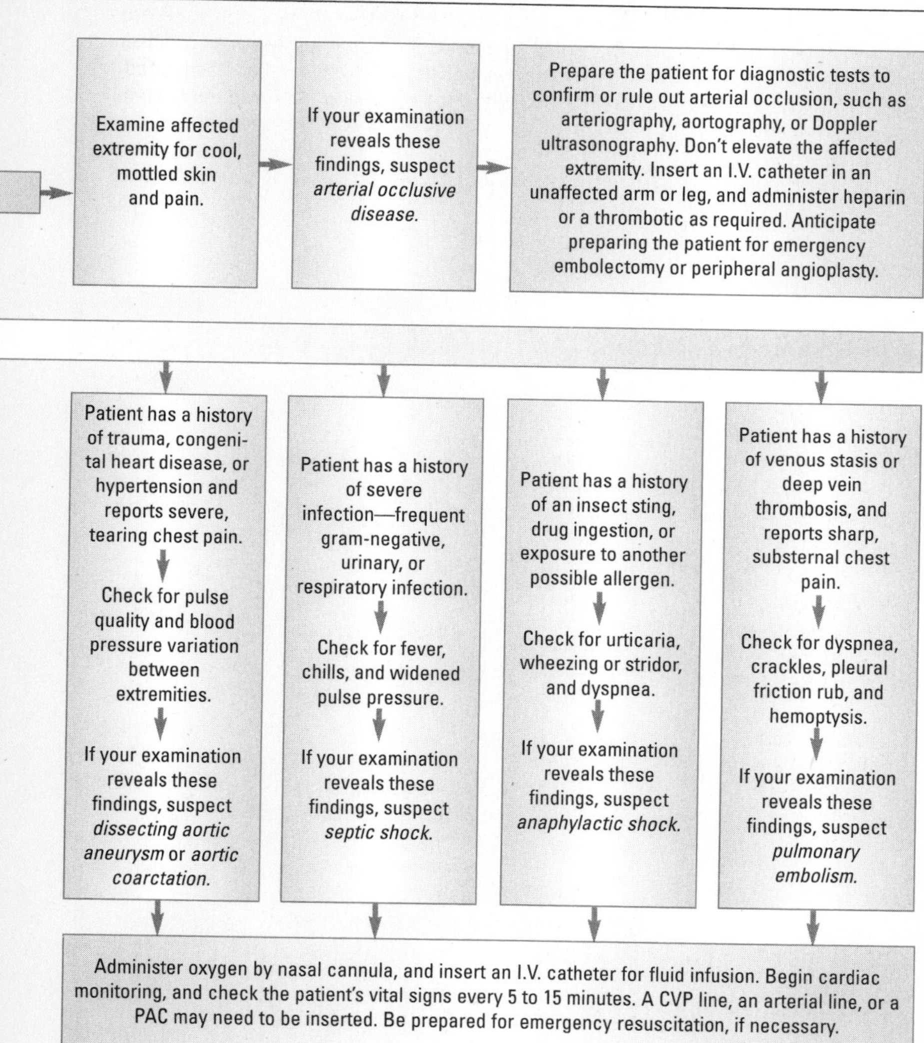
Examine affected extremity for cool, mottled skin and pain.
If your examination reveals these findings, suspect arterial occlusive disease.
Prepare the patient for diagnostic tests to confirm or rule out arterial occlusion, such as arteriography, aortography, or Doppler ultrasonography. Don't elevate the affected extremity. Insert an I.V. catheter in an unaffected arm or leg, and administer heparin or a thrombotic as required. Anticipate preparing the patient for emergency embolectomy or peripheral angioplasty.
Patient has a history of trauma, congenital heart disease, or hypertension and reports severe, tearing chest pain.
Check for pulse quality and blood pressure variation between extremities.
If your examination reveals these findings, suspect dissecting aortic aneurysm or aortic coarctation.
Patient has a history of severe infection—frequent gram-negative, urinary, or respiratory infection.
Check for fever, chills, and widened pulse pressure.
If your examination reveals these findings, suspect septic shock.
Patient has a history of an insect sting, drug ingestion, or exposure to another possible allergen.
Check for urticaria, wheezing or stridor, and dyspnea.
If your examination reveals these findings, suspect anaphylactic shock.
Patient has a history of venous stasis or deep vein thrombosis, and reports sharp, substernal chest pain.
Check for dyspnea, crackles, pleural friction rub, and hemoptysis.
If your examination reveals these findings, suspect pulmonary embolism.
Administer oxygen by nasal cannula, and insert an I.V. catheter for fluid infusion. Begin cardiac monitoring, and check the patient's vital signs every 5 to 15 minutes. A CVP line, an arterial line, or a PAC may need to be inserted. Be prepared for emergency resuscitation, if necessary.
Anticipate preparing the patient for surgery and administering an antihypertensive or nitroprusside.
Anticipate administering antibiotics and vasopressors.
Anticipate emergency endotracheal (ET) intubation or cricothyrotomy and administration of epinephrine.
Anticipate possible ET intubation and anticoagulant or thrombolytic therapy.

Thoracic outlet syndrome

- Gradual or abrupt weakness or loss of pulses in the arms occurs.
- Pulse changes commonly occur after the patient works with his hands above his shoulders, lifts a weight, or abducts his arm.
- Other signs and symptoms include paresthesia and pain along the ulnar distribution of the arm that resolves when the arm returns to a neutral position.

Other causes

Treatments

- Localized absent pulse may occur away from the arteriovenous shunts used for dialysis.

Nursing considerations

- Monitor the patient's vital signs, peripheral pulses, and limb appearances.
- Measure daily weight, intake and output, and central venous pressure.
- Maintain bleeding precautions with anticoagulation therapy.
- In children and young adults, weak or absent pulses in the legs may indicate coarctation of the aorta.

Patient teaching

- Discuss the underlying disorder and treatment options.
- Explain diagnostic tests as needed.
- Teach the techniques for checking pulse.
- Explain signs and symptoms the patient needs to report.
- Discuss foods and fluids the patient should avoid.
- Emphasize the avoidance of activities that reduce circulation.

Pulse, bounding

Produced by large waves of pressure as blood ejects from the left ventricle with each contraction, a bounding pulse is strong and easily palpable. It may even be visible over superficial peripheral arteries. It's characterized by regular, recurrent expansion and contraction of the arterial walls and isn't obliterated by the pressure of palpation. A healthy person develops a bounding pulse during exercise, pregnancy, and periods of anxiety. However, this sign also results from fever and certain endocrine, hematologic, and cardiovascular disorders that increase the basal metabolic rate.

History

- Ask about weakness, fatigue, shortness of breath, or other health changes.
- Take a medical history, noting hyperthyroidism, anemia, or a cardiovascular disorder.
- Ask about alcohol use.

Physical examination

- Check the patient's vital signs.
- Auscultate the heart and lungs for abnormal sounds, rates, or rhythms.
- Complete the cardiovascular assessment.

Causes

Medical causes

Alcoholism, acute

- A rapid, bounding pulse and flushed face result from vasodilation.
- An odor of alcohol on the breath and an ataxic gait are common.
- Other signs and symptoms include hypothermia, bradypnea, labored and loud respirations, nausea, vomiting, diuresis, decreased level of consciousness, and seizures.

Anemia

- Bounding pulse may be accompanied by systolic ejection murmur, tachycardia, atrial gallop, ventricular gallop, and a systolic bruit over the carotid artery.
- Other signs and symptoms include fatigue, pallor, dyspnea and, possibly, bleeding tendencies.

Aortic insufficiency

- Bounding pulse is characterized by rapid, forceful expansion of the arterial pulse, followed by rapid contraction.
- Widened pulse pressure also occurs.
- Other relevant signs and symptoms include weakness, severe dyspnea, hypotension, ventricular gallop, tachycardia, pallor, chest pain, strong and abrupt carotid pulsations, pulsus bisferiens, an early systolic murmur, a murmur heard over the femoral artery during systole and diastole, a high-pitched diastolic murmur that starts with S_2, and an apical diastolic rumble (Austin Flint murmur).
- With chronic aortic insufficiency, most patients are asymptomatic until age 40 or 50 when exertional dyspnea, increased fatigue, orthopnea, paroxysmal nocturnal dyspnea, angina, and syncope may develop.

Febrile disorder

- Bounding pulse may occur with fever.
- Accompanying signs and symptoms reflect the underlying disorder and may include fatigue, chills, malaise, anorexia, tachycardia, tachypnea, and diaphoresis.

Thyrotoxicosis

- A rapid, full, bounding pulse occurs.
- Other relevant signs and symptoms include tachycardia, palpitations, atrial or ventricular gallop, weight loss despite increased appetite, diarrhea, an enlarged thyroid, dyspnea, tremors, nervousness, chest pain, exophthalmos, heat intolerance, signs of cardiovascular collapse, and warm, moist, and diaphoretic skin.

Nursing considerations

- If bounding pulse is accompanied by a rapid or an irregular heartbeat, connect the patient to a cardiac monitor for further evaluation.
- Provide for rest periods to reduce metabolic demands.
- Administer iron supplements if indicated.
- Monitor intake and output.
- Weigh the patient daily.
- Restrict fluids as necessary.

Patient teaching

- Explain the underlying disorder, diagnostic tests, and treatment options.
- Discuss diet modifications and fluid restrictions the patient needs.
- Stress the need for rest periods.
- Emphasize the importance of avoiding alcohol, and refer the patient to cessation counseling as appropriate.
- Explain signs and symptoms the patient needs to report.

Pulse pressure, narrowed

Pulse pressure, the difference between systolic and diastolic blood pressures, is measured by sphygmomanometry or intra-arterial monitoring. Normally, systolic pressure exceeds diastolic pressure by about 40 mm Hg. Narrowed pressure—a difference of less than 30 mm Hg—occurs when peripheral vascular resistance increases, cardiac output declines, or intravascular volume markedly decreases.

With conditions that cause mechanical obstruction, such as aortic stenosis, pulse pressure is directly related to the severity of the underlying condition. Usually a late sign, narrowed pulse pressure alone doesn't signal an emergency, even though it commonly occurs with shock and other life-threatening disorders.

History

- Ask about specific cardiac symptoms, such as chest pain, dizziness, or syncope.
- Obtain a medical history.
- Assess risk factors for heart disease.

Physical examination

- Check for signs of heart failure, such as hypotension, tachycardia, dyspnea, jugular vein distention, pulmonary crackles, and decreased urine output.
- Check for changes in skin temperature or color.
- Palpate peripheral pulses, noting their strength.
- Evaluate the patient's level of consciousness (LOC).
- Auscultate for heart murmurs.
- Take the patient's vital signs, and weigh him.

Causes

Medical causes

Aortic stenosis

- Narrowed pulse pressure occurs late in significant stenosis.
- Other signs and symptoms include atrial or ventricular gallop, chest pain, angina, crackles, fatigue, dyspnea, paroxysmal nocturnal dyspnea, syncope, and a harsh systolic ejection murmur.

Cardiac tamponade

- In this life-threatening disorder, pulse pressure narrows by 10 to 20 mm Hg.
- Paradoxical pulse, jugular vein distention, hypotension, and muffled heart sounds are classic.
- Other signs and symptoms include anxiety, restlessness, cyanosis, clammy skin, chest pain, dyspnea, tachypnea, decreased LOC, pericardial rub, hepatomegaly, and a weak, rapid pulse.

Heart failure

- Narrowed pulse pressure occurs relatively late.
- Signs and symptoms include tachypnea, palpitations, dependent edema, steady weight gain despite nausea and anorexia, chest tightness, hypotension, diaphoresis, pallor, ventricular gallop, inspiratory crackles, oliguria and, possibly, a tender palpable liver.
- At later stages, hemoptysis, cyanosis, marked hepatomegaly, and marked pitting edema may occur.

Shock

- Narrowed pulse pressure occurs late.
- Peripheral pulses first become weak and then uniformly absent in anaphylactic, hypovolemic, and septic shock.
- In cardiogenic shock, peripheral pulses are absent and central pulses are weak.
- Anaphylactic shock may result in hypotension, anxiety, restlessness, feelings of doom, intense itching, urticaria, dyspnea, stridor, hoarseness, chest or throat tightness, skin flushing, and seizures.
- Cardiogenic shock may produce hypotension, tachycardia, tachypnea, cyanosis, oliguria, restlessness, confusion, obtundation, and cold, pale, clammy skin.
- Deepening hypovolemic shock leads to hypotension, oliguria, confusion, decreased LOC and, possibly, hypothermia.
- As septic shock progresses, the patient exhibits thirst, anxiety, restlessness, confusion, hypotension, cool and cyanotic extremities, cold and clammy skin and, eventually, severe hypotension, oliguria or anuria, respiratory failure, and coma.

Nursing considerations

- Monitor the patient closely for changes in pulse rate or quality and for hypotension.
- Assess the patient for changes in his LOC.

Patient teaching

- Explain the disorder and its treatments.
- Teach about foods and fluids the patient should avoid.

■ Stress the importance of rest periods to reduce fatigue.

Pulse pressure, widened

Pulse pressure is the difference between systolic and diastolic blood pressures. Normally, systolic pressure is about 40 mm Hg higher than diastolic pressure. Widened pulse pressure—a difference of more than 50 mm Hg—commonly occurs as a physiologic response to fever, hot weather, exercise, anxiety, anemia, or pregnancy. However, it can also result from certain neurologic disorders. Of special note is life-threatening increased intracranial pressure (ICP). Other cardiovascular disorders, such as aortic insufficiency, cause blood backflow into the heart with each contraction. Widened pulse pressure can easily be identified by monitoring arterial blood pressure and is commonly detected during routine sphygmomanometric recordings.

QUICK ACTION ***If the patient's level of consciousness (LOC) is decreased and you suspect that widened pulse pressure results from increased ICP, check his vital signs. Maintain a patent airway, and prepare to hyperventilate the patient with a handheld resuscitation bag to help reduce partial pressure of carbon dioxide levels and, thus, ICP. Perform a thorough neurologic examination to serve as a baseline for assessing subsequent changes. Use the Glasgow Coma Scale to evaluate the patient's LOC. Also, check cranial nerve function—especially in cranial nerves III, IV, and VI—and assess pupillary reactions, reflexes, and muscle tone. Insertion of an ICP monitor may be necessary. If you don't suspect increased ICP, ask about associated symptoms, such as chest pain, shortness of breath, weakness, fatigue, or syncope. Check for edema, and auscultate for murmurs.***

History

■ Obtain a medical history, including family history and trauma.
■ Take a drug history.
■ Ask about such associated signs and symptoms as chest pain, shortness of breath, weakness, fatigue, or syncope.

Physical examination

■ Assess for signs and symptoms of heart failure, such as crackles, dyspnea, and jugular vein distention.
■ Check for changes in skin temperature and color and strength of peripheral pulses.
■ Evaluate the patient's LOC.
■ Auscultate the heart for murmurs.
■ Check for peripheral edema.

Causes

Medical causes

Aortic insufficiency

■ Pulse pressure widens progressively as the valve deteriorates.
■ Other relevant signs and symptoms include bounding pulse, atrial or ventricular gallop, chest pain, palpitations, pallor, pulsus bisferiens, signs of heart failure (crackles, dyspnea, jugular vein distention), heart murmurs such as an early diastolic murmur and an apical diastolic rumble (Austin Flint murmur), and strong, abrupt carotid pulsations.

Arteriosclerosis

■ Pulse pressure widens following moderate hypertension.
■ Other symptoms include signs of vascular insufficiency, such as claudication, angina, and speech and vision disturbances.

Febrile disorders

■ Fever can cause widened pulse pressure.

- Other symptoms vary by the underlying disorder, but may include fatigue, chills, malaise, anorexia, tachycardia, tachypnea, and diaphoresis.

Increased ICP

- In this life-threatening condition, widening pulse pressure is an intermediate to late sign of increased ICP.
- Decreased LOC is the earliest and most sensitive indicator of increased ICP.
- Cushing's triad—bradycardia, hypertension, and respiratory pattern changes—is characteristic of increasing ICP.
- Other signs and symptoms include headache, vomiting, impaired or unequal motor movement, vision disturbances, and pupillary changes.

Nursing considerations

- If the patient displays increased ICP, continually reevaluate his neurologic status and vital signs.
- Be alert for restlessness, confusion, unresponsiveness, or decreased LOC.
- Watch for subtle changes in the patient's condition.

Patient teaching

- Discuss the underlying condition, diagnostic tests, and treatment options.
- Explain needed dietary modifications, such as restricting sodium and saturated fats.
- Stress the importance of planning rest periods.
- If the patient has decreased LOC, discuss specific safety measures.

Pulse rhythm, abnormal

An abnormal pulse rhythm is an irregular expansion and contraction of the peripheral arterial walls. It may be persistent or sporadic and rhythmic or arrhythmic. Detected by palpating the radial or carotid pulse, an abnormal rhythm is typically reported first by the patient, who complains of palpitations. This important finding reflects an underlying cardiac arrhythmia, which may range from benign to life-threatening. Arrhythmias are commonly associated with cardiovascular, renal, respiratory, metabolic, and neurologic disorders as well as the effects of drugs, diagnostic tests, and treatments.

QUICK ACTION ***Quickly look for signs of reduced cardiac output, such as a decreased level of consciousness (LOC), hypotension, or dizziness. Promptly obtain an electrocardiogram (ECG) and possibly a chest X-ray, and begin cardiac monitoring. Insert an I.V. catheter for administration of emergency cardiac drugs and fluids, and give oxygen by nasal cannula or mask. Closely monitor the patient's vital signs, pulse quality, and cardiac rhythm because accompanying bradycardia or tachycardia may result in deteriorating cardiac output. Keep emergency intubation, cardioversion, defibrillation, and suction equipment handy.***

History

- Ask about the onset, quality, quantity, location, and radiation of pain.
- Obtain a medical history, including heart disease and treatment for arrhythmias.
- Take a drug history and check compliance.
- Ask about caffeine or alcohol intake.

Physical examination

- Check apical and peripheral arterial pulses; check for a pulse deficit.
- Auscultate heart sounds for abnormalities.
- Count the apical beat for 60 seconds, noting the frequency of skipped peripheral beats.
- Perform a complete cardiovascular assessment.

Causes

Medical causes

Cardiac arrhythmias

- An abnormal pulse rhythm may be the only sign; pulse may be weak, rapid, or slow.
- Palpitations, a fluttering heartbeat, or weak and skipped beats may be reported by the patient.
- Dull chest pain or discomfort and hypotension may occur.
- Other signs and symptoms include decreased urine output, dyspnea, tachypnea, pallor, and diaphoresis.
- Neurologic signs and symptoms include confusion, dizziness, lightheadedness, decreased LOC and, sometimes, seizures.

Nursing considerations

- Prepare the patient for cardioversion therapy, if needed.
- Prepare the patient for transfer to a cardiac or an intensive care unit.
- Check the patient's vital signs frequently to detect bradycardia, tachycardia, hypertension or hypotension, tachypnea, or dyspnea.
- Maintain a cardiac monitor, as ordered.
- Collect blood samples for serum electrolyte, cardiac enzyme, and drug level studies.
- Obtain a 12-lead ECG and compare with previous tracings.

Patient teaching

- Tell the patient to keep a diary of activities and symptoms.
- Educate the patient on the importance of avoiding tobacco and caffeine.
- Discuss strategies to improve medication compliance.
- Teach the patient how to take his pulse rate.
- Explain the signs and symptoms the patient needs to report.

Pulsus alternans

A sign of severe left-sided heart failure, pulsus alternans (alternating pulse) is a beat-to-beat change in the size and intensity of a peripheral pulse. Although pulse rhythm remains regular, strong and weak contractions alternate. An alteration in the intensity of heart sounds and of existing heart murmurs may accompany this sign.

Pulsus alternans is thought to result from the change in stroke volume that occurs with beat-to-beat alteration in the left ventricle's contractility. Recumbency or exercise increases venous return and reduces the abnormal pulse, which typically disappears with treatment for heart failure. In rare cases, a patient with normal left ventricular function has pulsus alternans, but the abnormal pulse seldom persists for more than 10 to 12 beats.

Although most easily detected by sphygmomanometry, pulsus alternans can also be detected by palpating the brachial, radial, or femoral artery when systolic pressure varies from beat to beat by more than 20 mm Hg. Because the small changes in arterial pressure that occur during normal respirations may obscure this abnormal pulse, you'll need to have the patient hold his breath during palpation. Apply *light* pressure to avoid stamping out the weaker pulse.

When using a sphygmomanometer to detect pulsus alternans, inflate the cuff 10 to 20 mm Hg above the systolic pressure as determined by palpation, and then slowly deflate it. At first, you'll hear only the strong beats. With further deflation, all beats will become audible and palpable, and then equally intense. (The difference between this point and the peak systolic level is commonly used to determine the degree of pulsus alternans.) When the cuff is removed, pulsus alternans returns.

Occasionally, the weak beat is so small that no palpable pulse is detected at the periphery. This produces total pulsus alternans, an apparent halving of the pulse rate.

QUICK ACTION ***Pulsus alternans indicates a critical change in the patient's status. When you detect it, be sure to quickly check his other vital signs. Closely evaluate the patient's heart rate, respiratory pattern, and blood pressure. Also, auscultate for ventricular gallop and increased crackles.***

History

- Obtain a full medical history, focusing on cardiac disorders.

Physical examination

- Take the patient's vital signs.
- Assess for pulsus alternans.

Causes

Medical causes

Left-sided heart failure

- With this disorder, pulsus alternans is commonly initiated by a premature beat and is almost always associated with a ventricular gallop.
- Other signs include hypotension and cyanosis.
- Possible respiratory signs and symptoms include exertional and paroxysmal nocturnal dyspnea, orthopnea, tachypnea, Cheyne-Stokes respirations, hemoptysis, and crackles.
- Fatigue and weakness are common.

Nursing considerations

- If left-sided heart failure develops suddenly, prepare the patient for transfer to an intensive or a cardiac care unit.
- Elevate the head of the bed to promote respiratory excursion and increase oxygenation.
- Adjust the patient's current treatment plan to improve cardiac output, reduce the heart's workload, and promote diuresis.
- Monitor the patient's cardiac rhythm, vital signs, daily weight, and intake and output.
- In a child with heart failure, pulsus alternans may be difficult to assess if the child is crying or restless. Try to quiet the child by holding him, if his condition permits.

Patient teaching

- Advise the patient about prescribed medications and their adverse effects.
- Teach the patient about left-sided heart failure and its treatment plan.
- Stress the importance of follow-up care with a practitioner.

Pulsus biferiens

A biferious pulse is a hyperdynamic, double-beating pulse characterized by two systolic peaks separated by a midsystolic dip. Both peaks may be equal or either may be larger; usually, however, the first peak is taller or more forceful than the second. The first peak (percussion wave) is believed to be the pulse pressure; the second (tidal wave), reverberation from the periphery. Pulsus biferiens occurs in conditions in which a large blood volume is rapidly ejected from the left ventricle, as in aortic insufficiency. The pulse can be palpated in peripheral arteries or observed on an arterial pressure wave recording.

To detect pulsus biferiens, *lightly* palpate the carotid, brachial, radial, or femoral artery. (The pulse is easiest to palpate in the carotid artery.) At the same time, listen to the patient's heart sounds to determine if the two palpable peaks occur during systole. If they do, you'll feel the double pulse between S_1 and S_2.

History

- Obtain a medical history, including cardiac disorders.
- Take a drug history.
- Ask about associated signs and symptoms, such as dyspnea, chest pain, or fatigue.
- Find out about the onset of symptoms and aggravating or alleviating factors.

Physical examination

- Take the patient's vital signs.
- Auscultate for abnormal heart or breath sounds.
- Assess peripheral pulses.
- Complete the cardiopulmonary assessment.

Causes

Medical causes

Aortic insufficiency

- Aortic insufficiency is the most common organic cause of pulsus biferiens.
- Other signs and symptoms include exertional dyspnea, fatigue, orthopnea, paroxysmal nocturnal dyspnea, ventricular gallop, tachycardia, chest pain, palpitations, pallor, strong and abrupt carotid pulsations, widened pulse pressure, and one or more murmurs, especially an apical diastolic rumble (Austin Flint murmur).

Aortic stenosis with aortic insufficiency

- The pulse rate rises slowly, and the second wave of the double beat is the more forceful one.
- Dyspnea and fatigue are common.

High cardiac output states

- Pulsus biferiens commonly occurs with high cardiac output states, such as anemia, thyrotoxicosis, fever, and exercise.
- Other signs vary with the underlying disorder and may include tachycardia, a cervical venous hum, and widened pulse pressure.

Hypertrophic obstructive cardiomyopathy

- Pulsus biferiens occurs with the pulse rising rapidly and the first wave being the more forceful one.
- Other signs and symptoms include systolic murmur, dyspnea, angina, fatigue, and syncope.

Nursing considerations

- Prepare the patient for diagnostic tests.
- Schedule regular rest periods.
- Monitor the patient's vital signs, intake and output, and daily weight.

Patient teaching

- Discuss the disorder and its treatment.
- Explain the signs and symptoms of heart failure to report.
- Discuss the planning of rest periods.

Pulsus paradoxus

Pulsus paradoxus, or paradoxical pulse, is an exaggerated decline in blood pressure during inspiration. Normally, systolic pressure falls less than 10 mm Hg during inspiration. In pulsus paradoxus, it falls more than 10 mm Hg. When systolic pressure falls more than 20 mm Hg, the peripheral pulses may be barely palpable or may disappear during inspiration.

Pulsus paradoxus is thought to result from an exaggerated inspirational increase in negative intrathoracic pressure. Normally, systolic pressure drops during inspiration because of blood pooling in the pulmonary system. This, in turn, reduces left ventricular filling and stroke volume and transmits negative intrathoracic pressure to the aorta. Conditions associated with large intrapleural pressure swings, such as asthma, or those that reduce left-sided heart filling, such as pericardial tamponade, produce pulsus paradoxus.

To accurately detect and measure pulsus paradoxus, use a sphygmomanometer or an intra-arterial monitoring device. Inflate the blood pressure cuff 10 to 20 mm Hg beyond the peak systolic pressure. Then deflate the cuff at a rate of 2 mm Hg/second until you hear the first Korotkoff sound during expiration. Note the systolic pressure. As you continue to slowly deflate the cuff, observe the patient's respiratory pattern. If pulsus paradoxus is present, the Korotkoff sounds will disappear with inspiration and return with expiration. Continue to deflate the cuff until you hear Korotkoff sounds during inspiration and expiration and, again, note the systolic pressure. Subtract this reading from the first one to determine the degree of pulsus paradoxus. A difference of more than 10 mm Hg is abnormal.

You can also detect pulsus paradoxus by palpating the radial pulse over several cycles of slow inspiration and expiration. Marked pulse diminution during inspiration indicates pulsus paradoxus. When you check for pulsus paradoxus, remember that irregular heart rhythms and tachycardia cause variations in pulse amplitude and must be ruled out before true pulsus paradoxus can be identified.

QUICK ACTION ***Pulsus paradoxus may signal cardiac tamponade—a life-threatening complication of pericardial effusion that occurs when sufficient blood or fluid accumulates to compress the heart. When you detect pulsus paradoxus, quickly take the patient's vital signs. Check for additional signs and symptoms of cardiac tamponade, such as dyspnea, tachypnea, diaphoresis, jugular vein distention, tachycardia, narrowed pulse pressure, and hypotension. Emergency pericardiocentesis to aspirate blood or fluid from the pericardial sac may be necessary. Evaluate the effectiveness of pericardiocentesis by measuring the degree of pulsus paradoxus; it should decrease after aspiration.***

History

- Find out if the patient has a history of chronic cardiac or pulmonary disease.
- Ask about recent trauma or cardiac surgery.
- Ask about the development of associated signs and symptoms, such as a cough or chest pain.

Physical examination

- Auscultate for abnormal breath sounds.
- Take the patient's vital signs.
- Perform a cardiopulmonary assessment.
- Obtain electrocardiogram and blood samples for cardiac enzyme levels, coagulation studies, electrolyte levels, and blood count.

Causes

Medical causes

Cardiac tamponade

- Pulsus paradoxus commonly occurs with this disorder, but it may be difficult to detect if intrapericardial pressure rises abruptly and profound hypotension occurs.
- With severe tamponade, assessment also reveals these classic signs: hypotension, diminished or muffled heart sounds, and jugular vein distention.
- Related signs and symptoms include chest pain, pericardial friction rub, narrowed pulse pressure, anxiety, restlessness, clammy skin, and hepatomegaly.
- Characteristic respiratory signs and symptoms include dyspnea, tachypnea,

and cyanosis; the patient typically sits up and leans forward to facilitate breathing.

- If cardiac tamponade develops gradually, pulsus paradoxus may be accompanied by weakness, anorexia, and weight loss. The patient may also report chest pain, but he won't have muffled heart sounds or severe hypotension.

Chronic obstructive pulmonary disease

- The wide fluctuations in intrathoracic pressure that characterize this disorder produce pulsus paradoxus and possibly tachycardia.
- Other signs and symptoms may include dyspnea, tachypnea, wheezing, productive or nonproductive cough, accessory muscle use, barrel chest, and clubbing.
- The patient may show labored, pursed-lip breathing after exertion or even at rest. He typically sits up and leans forward to facilitate breathing.
- Auscultation reveals decreased breath sounds, rhonchi, and crackles.
- Weight loss, cyanosis, and edema may occur.

Pericarditis, chronic constrictive

- Pulsus paradoxus can occur in up to 50% of patients with this disorder.
- Other signs and symptoms include pericardial friction rub, chest pain, exertional dyspnea, orthopnea, hepatomegaly, and ascites.
- The patient also exhibits peripheral edema and Kussmaul's sign—jugular vein distention that becomes more prominent on inspiration.

Pulmonary embolism, massive

- Decreased left ventricular filling and stroke volume in massive pulmonary embolism produce pulsus paradoxus as well as syncope and severe apprehension, dyspnea, tachypnea, and pleuritic chest pain.
- The patient appears cyanotic, with jugular vein distention.
- The patient may succumb to circulatory collapse, with hypotension and a weak, rapid pulse.
- Pulmonary infarction may produce hemoptysis, along with decreased breath sounds and a pleural friction rub over the affected area.

Right ventricular infarction

- This infarction may produce pulsus paradoxus and elevated jugular venous or central venous pressure.
- Other signs and symptoms are similar to those of myocardial infarction.

Nursing considerations

- Prepare the patient for an echocardiogram to visualize cardiac motion and to help determine the causative disorder.
- Monitor the patient's vital signs, and frequently check the degree of paradox. An increase in the degree of paradox may indicate recurring or worsening cardiac tamponade or impending respiratory arrest in severe chronic obstructive pulmonary disease.
- Vigorous respiratory treatment, such as chest physiotherapy, may avert the need for endotracheal intubation.
- In children, pulsus paradoxus above 20 mm Hg is a reliable indicator of cardiac tamponade; a change of 10 to 20 mm Hg is equivocal.

Patient teaching

- Explain all hospital procedures and required tests.
- Explain the underlying diagnosis and treatment plan.
- Emphasize the importance of prescribed medications and explain their adverse effects.

Pupils, nonreactive

Nonreactive (fixed) pupils fail to constrict in response to light or to dilate when the light is removed. The development of a unilateral or bilateral nonreactive response indicates an important change in the patient's condition and may signal a life-threatening emergency and possibly brain death. This condition also occurs with the use of certain optic drugs.

To evaluate pupillary reaction to light, first test the patient's direct light reflex. Darken the room, and cover one of the patient's eyes while you hold open the opposite eyelid. Using a bright penlight, bring the light toward the patient from the side and shine it directly into his opened eye. If normal, the pupil will promptly constrict. Next, test the consensual light reflex. Hold the patient's eyelids open and shine the light into one eye while watching the pupil of the opposite eye. If normal, both pupils will promptly constrict. Repeat both procedures in the opposite eye. A unilateral or bilateral nonreactive response indicates dysfunction of cranial nerves II and III, which mediate the pupillary light reflex.

QUICK ACTION ***If the patient is unconscious and develops unilateral or bilateral nonreactive pupils, quickly take his vital signs. Be alert for decerebrate or decorticate posture, bradycardia, elevated systolic blood pressure, widened pulse pressure, and the development of other changes in the patient's condition. A unilateral dilated, nonreactive pupil may be an early sign of uncal brain herniation. Emergency surgery to decrease intracranial pressure (ICP) may be necessary. If the patient isn't already being treated for increased ICP, insert an I.V. catheter to administer a diuretic, an osmotic, or a corticosteroid. You may also need to start the patient on controlled hyperventilation.***

History

- Obtain a medical history, including recent infection.
- Ask about the use of eyedrops and when they were last instilled.
- Find out about pain and its location, intensity, and duration.
- Ask about recent trauma.
- Obtain information from the family if the patient can't respond.

Physical examination

- Assess the patient's neurologic status.
- Check visual acuity in both eyes.
- Test the pupillary reaction to accommodation.
- Examine the cornea and iris for abnormalities.
- Cover the affected eye with a protective metal shield.

Causes

Medical causes

Botulism

- Nonreactive pupils and mydriasis in both eyes usually appear 12 to 36 hours after ingestion of tainted food.
- Other early signs and symptoms include blurred vision, diplopia, ptosis, strabismus, extraocular muscle palsies, anorexia, nausea, vomiting, diarrhea, and dry mouth.
- Vertigo, deafness, hoarseness, nasal voice, dysarthria, and dysphagia follow.
- Progressive muscle weakness and absent deep tendon reflexes evolve over 2 to 4 days, resulting in severe constipation and paralysis of respiratory muscles with respiratory distress.

Encephalitis

- Initially, sluggish pupils become dilated and nonreactive.

■ Decreased accommodation and other symptoms of cranial nerve palsies develop.
■ A decreased level of consciousness (LOC), high fever, headache, vomiting, and nuchal rigidity occur within 48 hours.
■ Aphasia, ataxia, nystagmus, hemiparesis, and photophobia may occur with seizures.

Glaucoma, acute angle-closure
■ A moderately dilated, nonreactive pupil occurs in the affected eye in this ophthalmic emergency.
■ Sudden blurred vision occurs, followed by excruciating pain in and around the affected eye.
■ Other signs and symptoms include seeing halos around white lights at night, conjunctival injection, corneal clouding, and decreased visual acuity.
■ Nausea and vomiting occur with severely elevated intraocular pressure (IOP).

Ocular trauma
■ A transient or permanent nonreactive, dilated pupil may result from severe damage to the iris or optic nerve.
■ Eye pain, eye edema, and ecchymoses may occur.
■ A v-shaped notch in the pupillary rim, indicating a tear in the iris sphincter muscle, may be seen on slit-lamp examination.

Oculomotor nerve palsy
■ A dilated, nonreactive pupil and loss of the accommodation reaction is the first sign.
■ This sign may indicate life-threatening brain herniation.

Uveitis
■ In anterior uveitis, a small, nonreactive pupil appears suddenly and is accompanied by severe eye pain, conjunctival injection, and photophobia.
■ With posterior uveitis, similar features develop insidiously, along with blurred vision and distorted pupil shape.

Wernicke's disease
■ Nonreactive pupils occur late in this disease associated with thiamine deficiency.
■ Initial signs include an intention tremor accompanied by a sluggish pupillary reaction.
■ Other ocular signs and symptoms include diplopia, gaze paralysis, nystagmus, ptosis, decreased visual acuity, and conjunctival injection.
■ Orthostatic hypotension, tachycardia, ataxia, apathy, and confusion may also occur.

Other causes
Drugs
■ Instillation of a topical mydriatic or cycloplegic may induce a temporarily nonreactive pupil in the affected eye.
■ Opioids cause pinpoint pupils with a minimal light response that can be seen only with a magnifying glass.
■ Atropine (AtroPen) poisoning produces widely dilated, nonreactive pupils.

Nursing considerations
■ Monitor the patient's vital signs and LOC.
■ If the patient is conscious, monitor his pupillary light reflex.
■ If the patient is unconscious, close his eyes to prevent corneal exposure.

Patient teaching
■ Discuss the underlying condition, diagnostic tests, and treatment options.
■ Teach proper methods for instilling eyedrops.

- Explain methods of reducing photophobia.
- Stress the importance of follow-up care to check IOP.

Pupils, sluggish

A sluggish pupillary reaction is an abnormally slow pupillary response to light. It can occur in one pupil or both, unlike the normal reaction, which is always bilateral. A sluggish reaction accompanies degenerative disease of the central nervous system and diabetic neuropathy. It can occur normally in elderly people, whose pupils become smaller and less responsive with age.

To assess pupillary reaction to light, first test the patient's direct light reflex. Darken the room, and cover one of the patient's eyes while you hold open the opposite eyelid. Using a bright penlight, bring the light toward the patient from the side and shine it directly into his opened eye. If normal, the pupil will promptly constrict. Next, test the consensual light reflex. Hold both of the patient's eyelids open, and shine the light into one eye while watching the pupil of the opposite eye. If normal, both pupils will promptly constrict. Repeat both procedures to test light reflexes in the opposite eye. A sluggish reaction in one or both pupils indicates dysfunction of cranial nerves II and III, which mediate the pupillary light reflex.

History

- Obtain a medical history.
- Find out about the use of eyedrops and when they were last used.
- Ask about pain and other ocular symptoms.

Physical examination

- Test visual acuity.
- Assess pupillary reaction to accommodation.
- Examine the cornea and iris for irregularities, scars, and foreign bodies.
- Perform a neurologic assessment.

Causes

Medical causes

Adie's syndrome

- Sluggish pupillary response with the abrupt onset of mydriasis progresses to a nonreactive pupil in this idiopathic neurologic condition.
- Other signs and symptoms include blurred vision and hypoactive or absent deep tendon reflexes in the arms and legs.

Diabetic neuropathy

- A sluggish pupillary response occurs with long-standing disease.
- Other signs and symptoms include orthostatic hypotension, syncope, dysphagia, episodic constipation or diarrhea, painless bladder distention with overflow incontinence, retrograde ejaculation, and impotence.

Encephalitis

- A sluggish response in both pupils is an initial symptom.
- Later, dilated nonreactive pupils, decreased accommodation, and other cranial nerve palsies may occur.
- Other signs and symptoms include decreased level of consciousness, headache, high fever, vomiting, nuchal rigidity, aphasia, ataxia, nystagmus, hemiparesis, photophobia, and seizures.

Herpes zoster

- A sluggish pupillary response may occur if the nasociliary nerve is affected.
- Examination of the conjunctiva reveals follicles.
- Other ocular signs and symptoms include serous discharge, absence of tears, ptosis, and extraocular muscle palsy.

Iritis, acute

- A sluggish pupillary response and conjunctival injection occur in the affected eye.
- The pupil may remain constricted; the pupil will be irregularly shaped if posterior synechiae have formed.
- The sudden onset of eye pain, photophobia, and blurred vision may also occur.

Multiple sclerosis

- Small, irregularly shaped pupils react better to accommodation than to light in this neurologic disorder of the brain and spinal cord.
- Other signs and symptoms include ptosis, nystagmus, diplopia, and blurred vision.
- Early signs include vision problems and sensory impairment.
- Later signs and symptoms include muscle weakness and paralysis; intention tremor, spasticity, hyperreflexia, and gait ataxia; dysphagia and dysarthria; constipation; urinary urgency, frequency, and incontinence; impotence; and emotional instability.

Nursing considerations

- Treat the underlying disorder.
- If vision is affected, provide for the patient's safety.
- Monitor for eye pain and changes in vision.
- Monitor the patient's neurologic status if indicated.
- A sluggish pupillary response may occur normally in elderly people, whose pupils become smaller and less responsive with age.

Patient teaching

- Stress the importance of regular ophthalmologic examinations.
- Teach about the underlying disorder, diagnostic tests, and treatment options.
- Explain ways of reducing photophobia.
- Teach the patient self-care for diabetes if needed.

Purpura

Purpura is the extravasation of red blood cells from the blood vessels into the skin, subcutaneous tissue, or mucous membranes. It's characterized by discoloration that's easily visible through the epidermis, usually purplish or brownish red. Purpuric lesions include petechiae, ecchymoses, and hematomas. (See *Identifying purpuric lesions,* page 306.) Purpura differs from erythema in that it doesn't blanch with pressure because it involves blood in the tissues, not dilated vessels.

Purpura results from damage to the endothelium of small blood vessels, a coagulation defect, ineffective perivascular support, capillary fragility and permeability, or a combination of these factors. These faulty hemostatic factors, in turn, can result from thrombocytopenia or another hematologic disorder, an invasive procedure, or the use of an anticoagulant.

Additional causes are nonpathologic. Purpura can be a consequence of aging, when loss of collagen decreases connective tissue support of upper skin blood vessels. In an elderly or cachectic person, skin atrophy and inelasticity and loss of subcutaneous fat increase susceptibility to minor trauma, causing purpura to appear along the veins of the forearms, hands, legs, and feet. Prolonged coughing or vomiting can produce crops of petechiae in loose face and neck tissue. Violent muscle contraction, as occurs in seizures or weight lifting, sometimes results in localized ecchymoses from increased intraluminal pressure and rupture. A high fever, which increases capillary fragility, can also produce purpura.

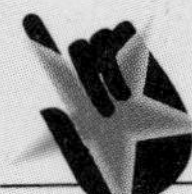

KNOW-HOW

Identifying purpuric lesions

Purpuric lesions fall into three categories: petechiae, ecchymoses, and hematomas.

Petechiae

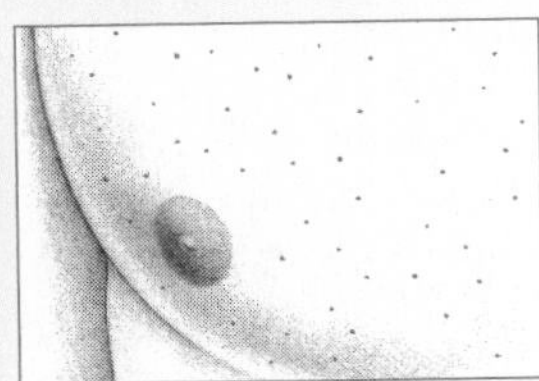

Petechiae are painless, round, pinpoint lesions, 1 to 3 mm in diameter. Caused by extravasation of red blood cells into cutaneous tissue, these red or purple lesions usually arise on dependent portions of the body. They appear and fade in crops and can group to form ecchymoses.

Ecchymoses

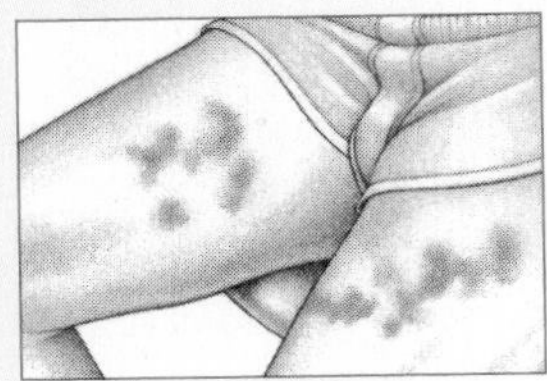

Ecchymoses, another form of blood extravasation, are larger than petechiae. These purple, blue, or yellow-green bruises vary in size and shape and can arise anywhere on the body as a result of trauma. Ecchymoses usually appear on the arms and legs of patients with bleeding disorders.

Hematomas

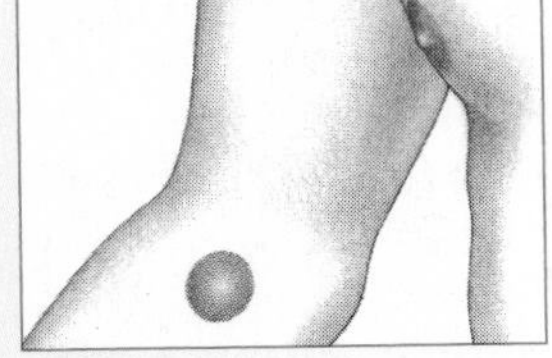

Hematomas are palpable ecchymoses that are painful and swollen. Usually the result of trauma, superficial hematomas are red, whereas deep hematomas are blue. Hematomas commonly exceed 1 cm in diameter, but their size varies widely.

History

- Ask about the onset and location of lesions.
- Take a drug and diet history.
- Find out about a personal or family history of bleeding disorders or easy bruising.
- Inquire about recent illnesses, trauma, and transfusions.
- Ask about other signs, such as epistaxis, bleeding gums, hematuria, hematochezia, fever, and heavy menstrual flow.

Physical examination

- Inspect the entire skin surface and mucous membranes to determine the type, size, location, distribution, and severity of purpuric lesions.

Causes

Medical causes

Amyloidosis

- This disorder produces purpura that appears either spontaneously on dependent areas on the skin or following minor trauma, coughing, or straining.
- Purpura commonly affects eyelid and mucous membranes.

Cholesterol emboli

- Purpura typically occurs in the lower extremities of patients with atherosclerotic vascular disease, or after anticoagulation therapy or an invasive arterial procedure.

■ Other signs and symptoms include livedo reticularis, cyanosis, gangrene, nodules, and skin ulceration.

Disseminated intravascular coagulation

■ Purpura occurs in different degrees.

■ Cutaneous oozing, hematemesis, or bleeding from incision or needle insertion sites may occur.

■ Other signs and symptoms include acrocyanosis, nausea, dyspnea, seizures, oliguria, and severe muscle, back, and abdominal pain.

Dysproteinemias

■ Petechiae and ecchymoses occur along with bleeding tendencies in multiple myeloma and cryoglobulinemia.

■ Hyperglobulinemia typically begins insidiously with occasional outbreaks of purpura over the lower legs and feet.

Ehlers-Danlos syndrome

■ This syndrome is characterized by recurrent bruising on the legs, arms, and trunk, either spontaneously or following minor trauma.

■ Bruising may be preceded by pain and is more common in women than in men, especially during menses.

Fat emboli

■ Petechiae occur on the upper body a few days after a major injury.

■ Other signs and symptoms include fever, tachycardia, tachypnea, blood-tinged sputum, cyanosis, anxiety, altered level of consciousness, seizures, coma, or rash.

Idiopathic thrombocytopenic purpura

■ Scattered petechiae on the distal arms and legs are an early sign.

■ Deep-lying ecchymoses may also occur.

■ Other signs and symptoms include epistaxis, easy bruising, hematuria, hematemesis, and menorrhagia.

Leukemia

■ Widespread persistent petechiae appear on the skin, mucous membranes, retina, and serosal surfaces.

■ Other signs and symptoms include fever, abdominal or bone pain, lymphadenopathy, splenomegaly, swollen and bleeding gums, epistaxis, and other bleeding tendencies.

Liver disease

■ Purpura, particularly ecchymoses, and other bleeding tendencies may occur.

■ Other signs and symptoms include hepatomegaly, ascites, right upper quadrant pain, jaundice, nausea, vomiting, and anorexia.

Meningococcemia

■ Cutaneous and oropharyngeal petechiae and purpura are initially discrete but become confluent, developing into hemorrhagic bullae and ulcerations.

■ Sudden severe infection results in extensive purpura and ecchymosis with irregular borders, most notably on the extremities.

■ Other signs and symptoms include spiking fever, chills, myalgia, and arthralgia progressing to headache, neck stiffness, and nuchal rigidity.

Myeloproliferative disorder

■ Hemorrhage accompanied by ecchymoses and ruddy cyanosis can occur.

■ The oral mucosa takes on a deep purplish red hue, and slight trauma causes swollen gums to bleed.

■ Other signs and symptoms include pruritus, urticaria, lethargy, fatigue, weight loss, headache, dizziness, vertigo, dyspnea, paresthesia, visual alterations, intermittent claudication, hypertension, hepatosplenomegaly, and impaired mentation.

Nutritional deficiencies

- With vitamin C deficiency, purpura patches join together to form ecchymoses on the inner thighs and lower buttocks.
- With vitamin K deficiency, abnormal bleeding tendencies, such as ecchymosis, gum bleeding, epistaxis, and hematuria, occur.
- With vitamin B_{12} and folic acid deficiencies, varying degrees of purpura occur.

Rocky Mountain spotted fever

- Initial skin lesions are small pink macules that evolve into blatant petechiae and palpable purpura; the palms and soles are particularly affected.
- Other signs and symptoms include fever, severe headache, myalgia, photophobia, nausea, and vomiting; later, shock and even death may occur.

Septicemia

- Purpura, especially petechiae, may occur with septicemia.
- Other signs and symptoms include fever, chills, headache, tachycardia, lethargy, diaphoresis, anorexia, and signs of specific infection.

Systemic lupus erythematosus

- Purpura may occur with other cutaneous signs and symptoms.
- A characteristic butterfly-shaped rash appears in the connective disorder's acute phase.
- Common signs and symptoms include nondeforming joint pain and stiffness, Raynaud's phenomenon, seizures, psychotic behavior, photosensitivity, fever, anorexia, weight loss, and lymphadenopathy.

Thrombotic thrombocytopenic purpura

- Generalized purpura, hematuria, vaginal bleeding, jaundice, and pallor are presenting signs and symptoms.
- Other signs and symptoms include fever, fatigue, weakness, headache, nausea, abdominal pain, arthralgia, hepatomegaly, and renal failure.

Trauma

- Local or widespread purpura may occur.

Other causes

Diagnostic tests and procedures

- Invasive diagnostic tests may produce local ecchymoses and hematomas.
- Procedures that disrupt circulation, coagulation, or platelet activity or production can cause purpura.

Drugs

- Anticoagulants may cause purpura.

Surgery and other procedures

- Any procedure that disrupts circulation, coagulation, or platelet activity or production can cause purpura, including cardiac surgery, radiation therapy, chemotherapy, hemodialysis, multiple blood transfusions, and the use of plasma expanders.

Nursing considerations

- Maintain bleeding precautions, as appropriate.
- Apply pressure and cold compresses to hematomas for the first 24 hours to reduce bleeding, and then apply hot compresses to speed blood absorption.
- Monitor the patient's skin condition frequently.
- When assessing a child with purpura, be alert for signs of possible child abuse.

Patient teaching

- Explain the treatment of the underlying disease.
- Reassure the patient that purpuric lesions aren't permanent and will fade if the underlying cause can be successfully treated.
- Discuss the avoidance of fade creams or other products that reduce pigmentation because they mask the rash.

Pustular rash

A pustular rash is made up of crops of pustules—a visible collection of pus within or beneath the epidermis. Commonly, pustules occur in a hair follicle or sweat pore; lesions, which vary greatly in size and shape, can either be localized to the hair follicles or sweat glands or generalized. Pustules can result from a skin or systemic disorder, the use of certain drugs, or exposure to a skin irritant. For example, people who have been swimming in salt water commonly develop a papulopustular rash under the bathing suit or elsewhere on the body from irritation by sea organisms. Although many pustular lesions are sterile, a pustular rash usually indicates an infection. A vesicular eruption, or even acute contact dermatitis, can become pustular if secondary infection occurs.

History

- Ask about the appearance, location, and onset of the first pustular lesion.
- Find out about the occurrence of different preceding lesions.
- Determine how the lesions spread.
- Take a drug history, including the use of topical medications.
- Ask about a family history of skin disorders.

Physical examination

- Assess the entire skin surface, noting if it's dry, oily, or moist.
- Record the exact location and distribution of skin lesions, noting color, shape, and size.

Causes

Medical causes

Acne vulgaris

- Pustules accompany papules, nodules, cysts, and open and closed comedones.
- Lesions commonly appear on the face, shoulders, back, and chest.
- Other signs and symptoms include pain on pressure, pruritus, burning and, if chronic, scars.

Blastomycosis

- In this fungal infection, small, painless, nonpruritic macules or papules can enlarge to well-circumscribed, verrucous, crusted, or ulcerated lesions edged by pustules.
- Other symptoms include pleuritic chest pain and a dry, hacking or productive cough with occasional hemoptysis.

Folliculitis

- Individual pustules occur, each pierced by a hair.
- Pruritus occurs with folliculitis.
- If the condition progresses, hard painful nodules of furunculosis may occur.

Furunculosis

- An acute, deep-seated, red, hot, tender abscess evolves from a staphylococcal folliculitis at the base of hair follicles.
- This condition most commonly occurs in areas prone to repeated infection, such as the face, neck, forearms, groin, axillae, buttocks, and legs.
- Pustules remain tense for 2 to 4 days and then become fluctuant.
- With rupture, pus and necrotic material are discharged and pain subsides, but erythema and edema may persist.

Impetigo contagiosa

- Vesicles form and break, and a crust forms from the exudate: a thick yellow crust in streptococcal impetigo, and a thin clear crust in staphylococcal impetigo.
- Painless itching occurs in both forms.

Nummular or annular dermatitis

- Numerous coinlike or ringed pustular lesions appear, usually on the extensor surfaces of the extremities, posterior trunk, buttocks, and lower legs.
- Lesions commonly ooze a purulent exudate, itch severely, and rapidly become crusted and scaly.

Pustular miliaria

- Pustular lesions begin as tiny erythematous papulovesicles at sweat glands.
- Diffuse erythema may radiate from the lesion.
- A rash and associated burning and pruritus worsen with sweating.

Rosacea

- Acute episodes of pustules, papules, and edema occur with telangiectasia.
- Rosacea is characterized by persistent erythema.
- It may begin as a flush covering the forehead, malar region, nose, and chin.
- Intermittent episodes gradually become more persistent, and the skin develops varying degrees of erythema.

Scabies

- Threadlike channels or burrows under the skin characterize scabies; pustules, vesicles, and excoriations may also occur.
- Lesions have a swollen nodule or red papule that contains the Sarcoptes scabiei (itch mite).

Smallpox (variola major)

- A maculopapular rash develops on the mucosa of the mouth, pharynx, face, and forearms and then spreads to the trunk and legs.
- Initial signs and symptoms include high fever, malaise, prostration, severe headache, and abdominal pain.
- Within 2 days, the rash becomes vesicular and later, pustular.
- Pustules are round, firm, and deeply embedded in the skin.
- After 8 to 9 days the pustules form a crust, and later the scab separates from the skin, leaving a pitted scar.

Varicella zoster

- Extremely painful and pruritic vesicles and pustules occur along a dermatome.
- Chronic pain may persist for months.

Other causes

Drugs

- Bromides and iodides commonly cause a pustular rash.
- Anabolic steroids, androgens, corticosteroids, dactinomycin (Cosmegen), isoniazid (Nydrazid), hormonal contraceptives, lithium (Eskalith), phenobarbital (Solfoton), and phenytoin (Dilantin) may also cause a pustular rash.

Nursing considerations

- Until infection is ruled out, follow wound and skin isolation precautions.
- If the organism is infectious, don't allow drainage to touch unaffected skin.
- Give medication to relieve pain and itching.

Patient teaching

- Discuss the underlying disorder, diagnostic tests, and treatment options.
- Explain methods to prevent the spread of infection.
- Give emotional support.
- Provide information about relieving pain and itching.

Pyrosis

Caused by reflux of gastric contents into the esophagus, pyrosis (heartburn) is a substernal burning sensation that rises in the chest and may radiate to the neck or throat. It's commonly accompanied by regurgitation, which also results from gastric reflux. Because increased intra-abdominal pressure contributes to reflux, pyrosis commonly occurs with pregnancy, ascites, or obesity. It also accompanies various GI disorders, connective tissue diseases, and the use of numerous drugs. Pyrosis usually develops after meals or when the patient lies down (especially on his right side), bends over, lifts heavy objects, or exercises vigorously. It typically worsens with swallowing and improves when the patient sits upright or takes an antacid.

A patient experiencing a myocardial infarction (MI) may mistake chest pain for pyrosis. However, he'll probably develop other signs and symptoms—such as dyspnea, tachycardia, palpitations, nausea, and vomiting—that will help distinguish an MI from pyrosis. His chest pain won't be relieved by an antacid.

History

- Ask about the patient's medical history, including diet, medication, and alcohol use.
- Find out about factors that aggravate, alleviate, or trigger heartburn.
- Determine the location of pain and whether it radiates.
- Ask about other signs and symptoms, including regurgitation.

Physical examination

- Perform an abdominal assessment.
- Examine the mouth and throat.

Causes

Medical causes

Esophageal cancer

- Painless dysphagia that progressively worsens is an early symptom.
- Regurgitation and aspiration commonly occur at night.
- Other signs and symptoms include rapid weight loss, steady pain in the front and back of the chest, hoarseness, sore throat, nausea, vomiting, and a feeling of substernal fullness.

Esophageal diverticula

- Pyrosis, regurgitation, and dysphagia may occur, although the disorder usually causes no symptoms.
- Other signs and symptoms include chronic cough, halitosis, chest pain, a bad taste in the mouth, and gurgling in the esophagus when liquids are swallowed.

Gastroesophageal reflux disease

- Pyrosis, which is typically severe, is the most common symptom.
- Pyrosis tends to be chronic, occurs 30 to 60 minutes after eating, and may be triggered by certain foods or beverages.
- Pyrosis worsens when the patient lies down or bends and abates when he sits upright or takes an antacid.
- Other signs and symptoms include postural regurgitation, dysphagia, flatulent dyspepsia, and dull retrosternal pain that may radiate.

Hiatal hernia

- Eructation after eating, with heartburn, regurgitation of sour-tasting fluid, and abdominal distention occur.
- Dull substernal or epigastric pain radiates to the shoulder.
- Other signs and symptoms include dysphagia, nausea, weight loss, dyspnea, tachypnea, cough, and halitosis.

Obesity

- Reflux and resulting pyrosis occur from increased intra-abdominal pressure.
- Other symptoms and related disorders include hypertension, cardiovascular disease, diabetes mellitus, renal disease, gallbladder disease, and psychosocial difficulties.

Peptic ulcer disease

- Pyrosis and indigestion usually signal the start of a peptic ulcer attack.
- Gnawing, burning pain in the left epigastrium may occur 2 or 3 hours after eating or when the stomach is empty—usually at night. Pain is relieved by eating or by taking an antacid or antisecretory.

Scleroderma

- In this connective tissue disease, reflux with pyrosis occurs from esophageal dysfunction.
- Other GI signs and symptoms include a sensation of food sticking behind the breastbone, odynophagia, bloating after meals, weight loss, abdominal distention, constipation or diarrhea, and malodorous floating stools.
- Early signs and symptoms include blanching, pruritus, cyanosis, and stress- or cold-induced erythema of the fingers and toes.
- Later signs and symptoms include finger and joint pain, stiffness, and swelling; skin thickening on the hands and forearms; masklike facies; and flexion contractures.
- With advanced disease, arrhythmias, dyspnea, cough, malignant hypertension, and signs of renal failure may occur.

Other causes

Drugs

- Anticholinergics, aspirin, drugs that have anticholinergic effects, and tolbutamide (Orinase) may cause or aggravate pyrosis.

Lifestyle

- Large meals or pregnancy may cause or aggravate pyrosis.

Nursing considerations

- Prepare the patient for diagnostic tests.
- Position the patient to alleviate pyrosis.
- Give antacids if needed.
- Help a child describe the sensation to help differentiate esophageal pain from pyrosis.

Patient teaching

- Explain the underlying disorder, diagnostic studies, and treatment options.
- Discuss lifestyle changes, such as eating frequent small meals and sitting upright for 2 hours after meals.
- Explain dietary restrictions and guidelines the patient needs to use.
- Discuss measures to prevent increased intra-abdominal pressure.
- Stress the importance of stopping smoking and the use of drugs that reduce sphincter control.

R

Raccoon eyes

Raccoon eyes are bilateral periorbital ecchymoses that don't result from facial soft-tissue trauma. Usually an indicator of basilar skull fracture, this sign develops when damage at the time of a fracture tears the meninges and causes the venous sinuses to bleed into the arachnoid villi and the cranial sinuses. Raccoon eyes may be the only indicator of a basilar skull fracture, which isn't always visible on skull X-rays. Their appearance signals the need for careful assessment to detect underlying trauma because a basilar skull fracture can injure cranial nerves, blood vessels, and the brain stem. Raccoon eyes can also occur after a craniotomy if the surgery causes a meningeal tear.

History

- Find out when the head injury occurred and the nature of the injury.
- Obtain a medical history.

Physical examination

- Take the patient's vital signs.
- Evaluate the patient's level of consciousness (LOC) using the Glasgow Coma Scale.
- Evaluate cranial nerve function, especially I (olfactory), III (oculomotor), IV (trochlear), VI (abducens), and VII (facial).
- Assess for signs and symptoms of increased intracranial pressure.
- Test visual acuity.
- Assess gross hearing.
- Note irregularities in the facial or skull bones.
- Observe for swelling, localized pain, Battle's sign (ecchymosis over the mastoid process or the temporal lobe), or lacerations of the face or scalp.
- Inspect for hemorrhage or cerebrospinal fluid (CSF) leakage from the nose or ears.
- Test any drainage with a sterile gauze pad and note whether a halo sign is present, indicating CSF.
- Use a glucose reagent strip to test clear drainage for glucose.

Causes

Medical causes

Basilar skull fracture

- Raccoon eyes occur after head trauma that doesn't involve the orbital area.
- Other signs and symptoms vary with the fracture site and may include pharyngeal hemorrhage, epistaxis, rhinorrhea, otorrhea, and a bulging tympanic membrane from blood or CSF.
- Additional signs and symptoms include difficulty hearing, headache, nausea, vomiting, cranial nerve palsies, positive Battle's sign, and altered LOC.

Other causes

Surgery

- Raccoon eyes occurring after craniotomy may indicate a meningeal tear and bleeding into the sinuses.

Nursing considerations

- Keep the patient on complete bed rest.

- Perform frequent neurologic evaluations to reevaluate the patient's LOC.
- Check the patient's vital signs frequently; look for such changes as bradycardia, bradypnea, hypertension, and fever.
- Instruct the patient not to blow his nose, cough vigorously, or strain to avoid worsening a dural tear.
- If rhinorrhea or otorrhea is present, don't attempt to stop the flow; instead, place a sterile loose gauze pad under the nose or ear to absorb the drainage.
- Monitor the amount of drainage and test leaking fluid with a glucose reagent strip to confirm or rule out CSF.
- To prevent infection and further tearing of the mucous membranes, never suction or pass a nasogastric tube through the patient's nose.
- Watch for signs and symptoms of meningitis, such as fever and nuchal rigidity, and expect to administer prophylactic antibiotics.
- If the dural tear doesn't heal spontaneously, contrast cisternography may be performed to locate the tear, possibly followed by corrective surgery.

Patient teaching

- Explain signs and symptoms of neurologic deterioration that the patient should report.
- Discuss activity limitations the patient needs to follow.
- Give instructions for care of a scalp wound.

Rebound tenderness

A reliable indicator of peritonitis, rebound tenderness is intense, elicited abdominal pain caused by the rebound of palpated tissue. The tenderness may be localized, as in an abscess, or generalized, as in perforation of an intra-abdominal organ. Rebound tenderness, also known as Blumberg's sign, usually occurs with abdominal pain, tenderness, and rigidity. When a patient has sudden, severe abdominal pain, this symptom is usually elicited to detect peritoneal inflammation.

QUICK ACTION ***If you elicit rebound tenderness in a patient who's experiencing constant, severe abdominal pain, quickly take his vital signs. Insert a large-bore I.V. catheter, and begin administering I.V. fluids. Also insert an indwelling urinary catheter, and monitor intake and output. Give supplemental oxygen as needed, and continue to monitor the patient for signs of shock, such as hypotension and tachycardia.***

History

- Ask about the event that led up to the tenderness.
- Inquire about what aggravates and alleviates the tenderness.
- Find out about other signs and symptoms, such as nausea, vomiting, fever, abdominal bloating or distention, or changes in bowel and bladder function.
- Take a medical history.

Physical examination

- Inspect the abdomen for distention, visible peristaltic waves, and scars.
- Auscultate for bowel sounds and characterize their motility.
- Palpate for associated rigidity or guarding, starting with light palpation and, if needed, progressing to deep palpation.
- Percuss the abdomen, noting tympany.

Causes

Medical causes

Peritonitis

- In this life-threatening disorder, rebound tenderness is accompanied by sudden and severe abdominal pain, which may be diffuse or localized.

- Pain may worsen with movement.
- Typical signs and symptoms include weakness, pallor, excessive sweating, and cold skin.
- Other signs and symptoms include hypoactive or absent bowel sounds, tachypnea, nausea, vomiting, positive psoas and obturator signs, high fever, and abdominal distention, rigidity, and guarding.
- Shoulder pain and hiccups suggest inflammation of the diaphragmatic peritoneum.

Nursing considerations

- Promote comfort by helping the patient flex his knees or assume a semi-Fowler's position.
- Know that an analgesic may mask other symptoms.
- Give an antiemetic and antipyretic.
- Withhold oral drugs and fluids because of decreased intestinal motility and the probability that the patient may require surgery.
- Give I.V. antibiotics as ordered.
- Insert a nasogastric tube if needed.
- Give continuous parenteral fluid or nutrition.
- When eliciting this symptom in children, use assessment techniques that produce minimal tenderness.
- Rebound tenderness may be diminished or absent in elderly patients.

Patient teaching

- Explain signs and symptoms the patient needs to report immediately.
- Teach the patient about required tests and procedures.
- Instruct the patient in postoperative care.

Respirations, grunting

Characterized by a deep, low-pitched grunting sound at the end of each breath, grunting respirations are a chief sign of respiratory distress in infants and children. They may be soft and heard only on auscultation, or loud and clearly audible without a stethoscope. Typically, the intensity of grunting respirations reflects the severity of respiratory distress. The grunting sound coincides with closure of the glottis, an effort to increase end-expiratory pressure in the lungs and prolong alveolar gas exchange, thereby enhancing ventilation and perfusion.

Grunting respirations indicate intrathoracic disease with lower respiratory involvement. Though most common in children, they sometimes occur in adults who are in severe respiratory distress. Whether they occur in children or adults, grunting respirations demand immediate medical attention.

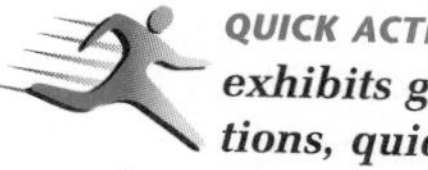

QUICK ACTION ***If the patient exhibits grunting respirations, quickly place him in a comfortable position and check for these signs and symptoms of respiratory distress:***

- ***wheezing***
- ***tachypnea (a minimum respiratory rate of 60 breaths/minute in infants, 40 breaths/minute in children ages 1 to 5, 30 breaths/minute in children older than age 5, or 20 breaths/minute in adults)***
- ***accessory muscle use***
- ***substernal, subcostal, or intercostal retractions***
- ***nasal flaring***
- ***tachycardia (a minimum of 160 beats/minute in infants, 120 to 140 beats/minute in children ages 1 to 5, 120 beats/minute in children older than age 5, or 100 beats/minute in adults)***
- ***cyanotic lips or nail beds***
- ***hypotension (less than 80/40 mm Hg in infants, less than 80/50 mm Hg in children ages 1 to 5, less than 90/55 mm Hg in children older than***

age 5, or less than 90/60 mm Hg in adults)
- ***decreased level of consciousness.***

If you detect any of these signs, monitor oxygen saturation, and administer oxygen and prescribed medications such as a bronchodilator. Have emergency equipment available and prepare to intubate the patient if necessary. Obtain arterial blood gas (ABG) analysis to determine oxygenation status.

History

- Ask about the onset of grunting respirations.
- Find out the gestational age of the infant.
- Ask if anyone in the home has recently had an upper respiratory tract infection.
- Inquire about a personal history of frequent colds or upper respiratory tract infections.
- Ask about a history of respiratory syncytial virus.
- Note changes in activity level or feeding pattern.

Physical examination

- Observe for use of accessory muscles and retractions during respiration.
- Check for cyanosis, diaphoresis, retractions, and edema.
- Auscultate the lungs, noting diminished or abnormal sounds.
- Characterize the color, amount, and consistency of any discharge or sputum.
- If the patient has a cough, note its characteristics.

Causes

Medical causes

Asthma

- Grunting respirations may be apparent during a severe attack.
- As the attack progresses, dyspnea, audible wheezing, chest tightness, and coughing occur.

Heart failure

- Grunting respirations accompany increasing pulmonary edema as a late sign of left-sided heart failure.
- Other signs and symptoms include productive cough, crackles, and chest wall retractions.
- Cyanosis may also be evident, depending on the underlying congenital cardiac defect.

Pneumonia

- Grunting respirations accompany diminished breath sounds, scattered crackles, sibilant rhonchi, high fever, tachypnea, productive cough, anorexia, and lethargy.
- As the disorder progresses, severe dyspnea, substernal and subcostal retractions, nasal flaring, cyanosis, and increasing lethargy may occur.
- GI signs, such as vomiting, diarrhea, and abdominal distention, may also be seen.

Respiratory distress syndrome

- Initially, audible expiratory grunting occurs with intercostal, subcostal, or substernal retractions, tachycardia, and tachypnea.
- With an infant, apnea or irregular respirations replace grunting as he tires.
- Cyanosis, frothy sputum, dramatic nasal flaring, lethargy, bradycardia, and hypotension characterize severe distress.

Nursing considerations

- Closely monitor the patient's condition.
- Keep emergency equipment nearby.
- Administer oxygen using an oxygen hood or tent.

- Continually monitor ABG levels and deliver the minimum amount of oxygen possible to avoid causing retinopathy of prematurity.
- Begin inhalation therapy with a bronchodilator.
- If the patient has pneumonia, give an I.V. antimicrobial.
- Perform chest physiotherapy.
- Provide emotional support to the patient and his family.
- In infants and children, grunting respirations may be a chief sign of respiratory distress.

Patient teaching

- Explain the sights and sounds of the intensive care unit.
- Teach techniques for home respiratory care and therapy.
- Give instructions on the proper use of prescribed drugs.
- Explain signs and symptoms to report.

Respirations, shallow

Respirations are shallow when a diminished volume of air enters the lungs during inspiration. In an effort to obtain enough air, the patient with shallow respirations usually breathes at an accelerated rate. However, as he tires or as his muscles weaken, this compensatory increase in respirations diminishes, leading to inadequate gas exchange and such signs as dyspnea, cyanosis, confusion, agitation, loss of consciousness, and tachycardia.

Shallow respirations may develop suddenly or gradually. They may last briefly or become chronic. They're a key sign of respiratory distress and neurologic deterioration. Causes include inadequate central respiratory control over breathing, neuromuscular disorders, increased resistance to airflow into the lungs, respiratory muscle fatigue or weakness, voluntary alterations in breathing, decreased activity from prolonged bed rest, and pain. (See *Responding to shallow respirations,* page 318.)

QUICK ACTION ***If you observe shallow respirations, be alert for impending respiratory failure or arrest. Is the patient severely dyspneic? Agitated or frightened? Look for signs of airway obstruction. If the patient is choking, perform four back blows and then four abdominal thrusts to try to expel the foreign object. Use suction if secretions occlude the patient's airway. If the patient is also wheezing, check for stridor, nasal flaring, and accessory muscle use. Administer oxygen with a face mask or handheld resuscitation bag. Attempt to calm the patient. Administer I.V. epinephrine.***

If the patient loses consciousness, insert an artificial airway and prepare for endotracheal intubation and ventilatory support. Measure his tidal volume and minute volume to determine the need for mechanical ventilation. Check arterial blood gas (ABG) levels, heart rate, blood pressure, and oxygen saturation. Tachycardia, increased or decreased blood pressure, poor minute volume, and deteriorating ABG levels or oxygen saturation signal the need for intubation and mechanical ventilation.

History

- If the patient isn't in severe respiratory distress, take a complete medical history, including chronic respiratory disorders or respiratory tract infection, neurologic or neuromuscular disease, surgery, and trauma.
- Ask if the patient has had a tetanus booster within the past 10 years.
- Ask about smoking history.

CASE CLIP

Responding to shallow respirations

Ms. A. is a 37-year-old female who underwent gastric bypass surgery 2 months ago for morbid obesity. She has done well since her surgery—until 3 days ago, when she was admitted to the surgical unit for intractable vomiting, low-grade fever, and abdominal pain. An upper endoscopy 6 weeks after surgery showed the presence of a 2 mm marginal ulcer distal to the anastomosis, but her surgeon felt that this would resolve itself over time and enforced her prescription of omeprazole (Prilosec) twice daily.

At 5:30, the nurse finds Ms. A. doubled over in bed, very pale and with shallow respirations. Ms. A. states that she has horrible belly pain that she rated as 10 on a pain scale with 10 being the worst pain she has ever felt. She's slightly diaphoretic and also complains of dizziness and nausea. Her vital signs are:

- heart rate (HR): 110 beats/minute
- respiratory rate (RR): 32 breaths/ minute and shallow
- blood pressure (BP): 94/60 mm Hg
- oxygen saturation: 90% on room air.

The nurse places Ms. A. on 2 L/ minute of oxygen via nasal cannula, and attempts to auscultate and then palpate the patient's abdomen. However, she can't complete her assessment because of the patient's continued complaints of pain and inability to remain still. The nurse's concern for the patient prompts her to initiate the rapid response team (RRT).

The RRT arrives within 2 minutes and orders:

- rectal examination and test for occult blood (patient has been receiving low-molecular-weight heparin injections twice daily)
- I.V. ketorolac (Toradol)
- additional I.V. access.

The rectal examination is negative for occult blood. Ms. A.'s pain continues to escalate, and her vital signs have continued to deteriorate:

- HR: 128 beats/minute
- RR: 36 breaths/minute and shallow
- BP: 72/40 mm Hg
- oxygen saturation: 90% on 4 L/minute of oxygen.

The patient is placed in Trendelenburg's position in an attempt to improve her BP.

Her pain continues and her vital signs continue to deteriorate. The RRT orders stat computed tomography scan of the abdomen. The scan shows a 1 cm perforated marginal ulcer in the same location as a previously noted ulcer. Free air is noted within the peritoneum, and it becomes evident that Ms. A will need surgery to repair the ulcer. She's immediately transferred to the operating room. After her recovery in the postanesthesia care unit, she's returned to the surgical unit for further care and observation.

- Take a drug history and explore the possibility of drug abuse.
- Determine the onset and duration of shallow respirations.
- Ask about factors that worsen or relieve shallow respirations.
- Note changes in appetite, weight, activity level, and behavior.

Physical examination

- Evaluate the patient's level of consciousness (LOC) and his orientation to time, place, and person.
- Observe for spontaneous movements.
- Test muscle strength and deep tendon reflexes (DTRs).
- Inspect the chest for deformities or abnormal movements.
- Inspect the extremities for cyanosis, edema, and digital clubbing.
- Palpate for expansion and diaphragmatic tactile fremitus.
- Percuss for hyperresonance or dullness.
- Auscultate for diminished, absent, or adventitious breath sounds and for abnormal or distant heart sounds.
- Examine the abdomen for distention, tenderness, or masses.

Causes

Medical causes

Acute respiratory distress syndrome

- In this life-threatening disorder, rapid, shallow respirations and dyspnea appear initially and sometimes after the patient appears stable as well.
- Other signs and symptoms include intercostal and suprasternal retractions, diaphoresis, rhonchi, crackles, restlessness, apprehension, decreased LOC, cyanosis, and tachycardia.

Amyotrophic lateral sclerosis

- Progressive degenerative respiratory muscle weakness leads to progressive shallow, ineffective respirations.
- Initial signs include upper extremity muscle weakness and wasting.
- Other signs and symptoms include muscle cramps and atrophy, hyperreflexia, slight spasticity of the legs, coarse fasciculations of the affected muscle, impaired speech, and difficulty chewing and swallowing.

Asthma

- Rapid, shallow respirations result from bronchospasm and decreased alveolar gas exchange.
- Related respiratory signs and symptoms include wheezing, rhonchi, dry cough, dyspnea, prolonged expirations, intercostal and supraclavicular retractions on inspiration, nasal flaring, chest tightness, tachycardia, diaphoresis, and accessory muscle use.

Atelectasis

- Decreased lung expansion or pleuritic pain causes the sudden onset of rapid, shallow respirations.
- Other signs and symptoms include dry cough, dyspnea, tachycardia, anxiety, cyanosis, diaphoresis, dullness to percussion, decreased breath sounds and vocal fremitus, inspiratory lag, and substernal or intercostal retractions.

Bronchiectasis

- Increased secretions obstruct airflow in the bronchi, leading to shallow respirations and a productive cough with copious, foul-smelling, mucopurulent sputum (a classic finding).
- Other signs and symptoms include hemoptysis, wheezing, rhonchi, coarse crackles during inspiration, and late-stage clubbing.

Bronchitis, chronic

- Shallow respirations result from chronic airway inflammation.
- A nonproductive, hacking cough that later becomes productive is an early sign.
- Other signs and symptoms include prolonged expirations, wheezing, dyspnea, accessory muscle use, barrel chest, cyanosis, tachypnea, scattered rhonchi, coarse crackles, and late-stage clubbing.

Emphysema

- Increased breathing effort causes muscle fatigue, leading to chronic shallow respirations.
- Other signs and symptoms include dyspnea, anorexia, malaise, tachypnea, diminished breath sounds, cyanosis, pursed-lip breathing, accessory muscle use, barrel chest, chronic productive cough, and late-stage clubbing.

Flail chest

- Decreased air movement results in rapid, shallow respirations and paradoxical chest wall motion.
- Other signs and symptoms include tachycardia, hypotension, ecchymoses, cyanosis, and pain over the affected area.

Fractured ribs

- Sharp, severe pain upon inspiration may cause shallow respirations.
- Other signs and symptoms include dyspnea, cough, splinting, and tenderness and edema at the fracture site.

Guillain-Barré syndrome

- Progressive ascending paralysis causes the rapid or progressive onset of shallow respirations.
- Muscle weakness begins in the lower limbs and extends to the face.
- Other signs and symptoms include paresthesia, dysarthria, diminished or absent corneal reflex, nasal speech, dysphagia, ipsilateral loss of facial muscle control, and flaccid paralysis.

Kyphoscoliosis

- Skeletal cage distortion causes rapid, shallow respirations from reduced lung capacity.
- Accompanying signs and symptoms include back pain, fatigue, tracheal deviation, ineffective coughing, and dyspnea.

Multiple sclerosis

- Muscle weakness causes progressive shallow respirations.
- Early signs and symptoms include diplopia, blurred vision, and paresthesia.
- Other possible signs and symptoms include nystagmus, constipation, paralysis, spasticity, hyperreflexia, intention tremor, ataxic gait, dysphagia, dysarthria, urinary dysfunction, impotence, and emotional lability.

Muscular dystrophy

- Progressive thoracic deformity and muscle weakness cause shallow respirations to occur.
- Other signs and symptoms include waddling gait, contractures, scoliosis, lordosis, and muscle atrophy or hypertrophy.

Myasthenia gravis

- Progressive respiratory muscle weakness leads to shallow respirations, dyspnea, and cyanosis.
- Other signs and symptoms include fatigue, weak eye closure, ptosis, diplopia, and difficulty chewing and swallowing.

Obesity

- Due to excess weight, the work of breathing may cause shallow respirations.

Parkinson's disease

- Fatigue and weakness lead to progressive shallow respirations.
- This disorder slowly progresses to increased rigidity, masklike facies, stooped posture, shuffling gait, dysphagia, drooling, dysarthria, and pill-rolling tremor.

Pleural effusion

- Restricted lung expansion causes shallow respirations.

■ Other signs and symptoms include nonproductive cough, weight loss, dyspnea, pleural friction rub, tachycardia, tachypnea, decreased chest motion, decreased or absent breath sounds, and pleuritic chest pain.

Pneumonia

■ Pulmonary consolidation results in rapid, shallow respirations.
■ Accompanying signs and symptoms include dyspnea, fever, shaking chills, chest pain, cough, tachycardia, decreased breath sounds, crackles, rhonchi, myalgia, fatigue, anorexia, headache, and cyanosis.

Pneumothorax

■ Shallow respirations and dyspnea begin suddenly.
■ Related signs and symptoms include tachycardia, tachypnea, nonproductive cough, cyanosis, accessory muscle use, asymmetrical chest expansion, anxiety, restlessness, subcutaneous crepitation, diminished or absent breath sounds on the affected side, and sudden, sharp, severe chest pain that worsens with movement.

Pulmonary edema

■ Pulmonary vascular congestion causes rapid, shallow respirations.
■ Early signs and symptoms include exertional dyspnea, paroxysmal nocturnal dyspnea, nonproductive cough, tachycardia, tachypnea, crackles, and ventricular gallop.
■ Severe pulmonary edema produces more rapid, labored respirations; widespread crackles; productive cough with frothy, bloody sputum; worsening tachycardia; arrhythmias; cold, clammy skin; cyanosis; hypotension; and a thready pulse.

Pulmonary embolism

■ Rapid, shallow respirations and severe dyspnea begin suddenly.
■ Other signs and symptoms include tachycardia, tachypnea, a nonproductive cough or a productive cough with blood-tinged sputum, low-grade fever, restlessness, pleural friction rub, crackles, diffuse wheezing, chest pain, and signs of circulatory collapse.

Spinal cord injury

■ Diaphragmatic breathing and shallow respirations may occur in injury to the C5 to C8 cervical vertebrae.
■ Other signs and symptoms include quadriplegia with flaccidity followed by spastic paralysis, areflexia, hypotension, sensory loss below the level of injury, and bowel and bladder incontinence.

Tetanus

■ Spasms of the intercostal muscles and diaphragm cause shallow respirations.
■ Other late signs and symptoms include jaw pain and stiffening, difficulty opening the mouth, tachycardia, profuse diaphoresis, hyperactive DTRs, and opisthotonos.

Upper airway obstruction

■ Partial airway obstruction causes acute shallow respirations with sudden gagging and dry, paroxysmal coughing, hoarseness, stridor, and tachycardia.
■ Other signs and symptoms include dyspnea, decreased breath sounds, wheezing, and cyanosis.

Other causes

Drugs

■ Anesthetics, hypnotics and sedatives, magnesium sulfate, neuromuscular blockers, opioids, and tranquilizers can produce slow, shallow respirations.

Surgery

■ After abdominal or chest surgery, pain from chest splinting and decreased chest wall motion may cause shallow respirations.

Nursing considerations

- Position the patient upright to ease his breathing.
- Ensure adequate hydration and the use of humidification, as needed.
- Give oxygen, a bronchodilator, a mucolytic, an expectorant, or an antibiotic.
- Turn the patient frequently.
- Monitor the patient for increasing lethargy, which may indicate rising carbon dioxide levels.
- Perform tracheal suctioning as needed.
- Have emergency equipment at the patient's bedside.
- In children, shallow respirations commonly indicate a life-threatening condition.
- Airway obstruction can occur rapidly because of the narrow passageways; if it does, administer back blows or chest thrusts but not abdominal thrusts, which can damage internal organs.

Patient teaching

- Explain the importance of coughing and deep breathing.
- Provide emotional support and teach the caregiver to do so as well.
- Teach the patient about the underlying diagnosis and treatment plan.

Respirations, stertorous

Characterized by a harsh, rattling, or snoring sound, stertorous respirations usually result from the vibration of relaxed oropharyngeal structures during sleep or coma, causing partial airway obstruction. Less commonly, these respirations result from retained mucus in the upper airway.

This common sign occurs in about 10% of healthy individuals; however, it's especially prevalent in middle-aged men who are obese. It may be aggravated by the use of alcohol or a sedative before bed, which increases oropharyngeal flaccidity, and by sleeping in the supine position, which allows the relaxed tongue to slip back into the airway. The major pathologic causes of stertorous respirations are obstructive sleep apnea and life-threatening upper airway obstruction associated with an oropharyngeal tumor or with uvular or palatal edema. This obstruction may also occur during the postictal phase of a generalized seizure, when mucus secretions or a relaxed tongue blocks the airway.

Occasionally, stertorous respirations are mistaken for stridor, which is another sign of upper airway obstruction. However, stridor indicates laryngeal or tracheal obstruction, whereas stertorous respirations signal higher airway obstruction.

QUICK ACTION ***If you detect stertorous respirations, check the patient's mouth and throat for edema, redness, masses, or foreign objects. If edema is marked, quickly take the patient's vital signs, including oxygen saturation. Observe him for signs and symptoms of respiratory distress, such as dyspnea, tachypnea, accessory muscle use, intercostal muscle retractions, and cyanosis. Elevate the head of the bed 30 degrees to help ease breathing and reduce edema. Then, administer supplemental oxygen by nasal cannula or face mask, and prepare to intubate the patient, perform a tracheostomy, and provide mechanical ventilation. Insert an I.V. catheter for fluid and drug access, and begin cardiac monitoring.***

If you detect stertorous respirations while the patient is sleeping, observe his breathing pattern for 3 to 4 minutes. Do noisy respirations cease when he turns on his side and recur when he assumes a supine position? Watch carefully for periods of apnea, and note their length.

History

- Ask the patient's sleeping partner about his snoring habits.
- Find out about factors that decrease snoring.
- Inquire about sleeptalking and sleepwalking.
- Ask about signs of sleep deprivation, such as personality changes, headaches, daytime somnolence, or decreased mental acuity.

Physical examination

- Perform a complete respiratory assessment.
- Examine the head, nose, and throat.
- If you detect stertorous respirations while the patient is sleeping, observe his breathing pattern for 3 to 4 minutes.
- Watch for periods of apnea, and note their length.

Causes

Medical causes

Airway obstruction

- With partial obstruction, stertorous respirations may be accompanied by wheezing, dyspnea, tachypnea, intercostal retractions, and nasal flaring.
- In complete obstruction, the patient abruptly loses the ability to talk and displays diaphoresis, tachycardia, and inspiratory chest movement but without breath sounds. Severe hypoxemia rapidly ensues, resulting in cyanosis, loss of consciousness, and cardiopulmonary collapse.

Obstructive sleep apnea

- Loud and disruptive snoring is a major characteristic, commonly affecting the obese patient.
- Snoring alternates with periods of sleep apnea, which usually end with loud gasping sounds.
- Alternating tachycardia and bradycardia may occur as well as hypertension.
- Sleep disturbances, such as somnambulism and talking during sleep, may occur.
- Other relevant signs and symptoms may include generalized headache, feeling tired and unrefreshed, daytime sleepiness, depression, hostility, and decreased mental acuity.

Other causes

Procedures

- Endotracheal intubation, suction, or surgery may cause significant palatal or uvular edema, resulting in stertorous respirations.

Nursing considerations

- Monitor the patient's respiratory status.
- Give a corticosteroid or an antibiotic.
- To reduce palatal and uvular inflammation and edema, provide cool, humidified oxygen.

Patient teaching

- Explain the disorder and treatment plan.
- Discuss the importance and methods of weight loss.
- Teach the patient how to elevate his head while sleeping.
- If the patient smokes, give information and recommend a smoking cessation program.
- Provide teaching on the use of a BiPAP or CPAP device for a patient with sleep apnea.

Retractions, costal and sternal

A cardinal sign of respiratory distress in infants and children, retractions are visible indentations of the soft tissue covering the chest wall. They may be suprasternal (directly above the sternum and clavicles), intercostal (between the ribs), subcostal (below the lower costal margin of the rib cage), or substernal (just below the xiphoid process). Retractions may be mild or severe, producing indentations that may be barely visible or deep.

Normally, infants and young children use abdominal muscles for breathing, unlike older children and adults, who use the diaphragm. When breathing requires extra effort, accessory muscles assist respiration, especially inspiration. Retractions typically accompany accessory muscle use.

QUICK ACTION ***If you detect retractions in a child, check quickly for other signs of respiratory distress, such as cyanosis, tachypnea, tachycardia, and decreased oxygen saturation. Also, prepare the child for suctioning, artificial airway insertion, and oxygen administration.***

History

- Ask the parents about the child's medical and birth history.
- Find out about recent signs of upper respiratory infection.
- Determine the frequency of respiratory problems during the past year.
- Ask about recent exposure to cold, flu, or respiratory ailment.
- Find out about aspiration of food, liquid, or a foreign body.
- Inquire about a personal or family history of allergies or asthma.

Physical examination

- If the child isn't in severe distress, complete a cardiopulmonary assessment.
- Take the child's vital signs, including his temperature.

Causes

Medical causes

Asthma attack

- Intercostal and suprasternal retractions may accompany an acute attack.
- Retractions are preceded by dyspnea, wheezing, a hacking cough, and pallor.
- Related signs and symptoms include cyanosis or flushing; crackles; rhonchi; diaphoresis; tachycardia; tachypnea; a frightened, anxious expression; and, with severe distress, nasal flaring.

Bronchiolitis

- Intercostal and subcostal retractions, nasal flaring, tachypnea, dyspnea, cough, restlessness, and a slight fever may occur, most commonly in children younger than age 2.

Croup, spasmodic

- Attacks of a barking cough, hoarseness, dyspnea, and restlessness occur.
- As distress worsens, signs and symptoms include suprasternal, substernal, and intercostal retractions; nasal flaring; tachycardia; cyanosis; and an anxious, frantic expression.

Epiglottiditis

- A life-threatening disorder, this infection may precipitate severe respiratory distress with suprasternal, substernal, and intercostal retractions.
- Early signs and symptoms include the sudden onset of a barking cough, stridor, high fever, sore throat, hoarseness, dysphagia, drooling, dyspnea, and restlessness.

Heart failure

- Intercostal and substernal retractions occur along with nasal flaring, progressive tachypnea, grunting respirations, edema, and cyanosis.
- Other signs and symptoms include productive cough, crackles, jugular vein distention, tachycardia, right upper quadrant pain, anorexia, and fatigue.

Laryngotracheobronchitis, acute

- Substernal and intercostal retractions follow low to moderate fever, runny

nose, poor appetite, barking cough, hoarseness, and inspiratory stridor.
- Other signs and symptoms include tachycardia; shallow, rapid respirations; restlessness; irritability; and pale, cyanotic skin.

Pneumonia, bacterial
- Subcostal and intercostal retractions follow signs and symptoms of acute infection.
- Other signs and symptoms include nasal flaring; dyspnea; tachypnea; grunting respirations; cyanosis; productive cough; and diminished breath sounds, crackles, and sibilant rhonchi over the affected lung.

Respiratory distress syndrome
- In this life-threatening disorder, substernal and subcostal retractions are early signs.
- Other early signs include tachypnea, tachycardia, and expiratory grunting.
- As respiratory distress worsens, intercostal and suprasternal retractions occur, and apnea or irregular respirations replace grunting.
- Other signs and symptoms include nasal flaring, cyanosis, lethargy, and eventual unresponsiveness, bradycardia, and hypotension.

Nursing considerations
- Monitor the patient's vital signs frequently.
- Keep suction equipment and an airway at the bedside.
- Place an infant who weighs less than 15 lb (6.8 kg) in an oxygen hood; if he weighs more, place him in a cool mist tent.
- Perform chest physiotherapy with postural drainage.
- Give a bronchodilator and steroid.

Patient teaching
- Explain the disorder and treatment plan.
- Instruct the patient in procedures and how to take prescribed drugs properly at home.
- Give instructions for providing a humidified environment.
- Stress the importance of ensuring adequate hydration.

Rhonchi

Rhonchi are continuous adventitious breath sounds detected by auscultation. They're usually louder and lower pitched than crackles—more like a hoarse moan or a deep snore—though they may be described as rattling, sonorous, bubbling, rumbling, or musical. However, sibilant rhonchi, or wheezes, are high-pitched.

Rhonchi are heard over large airways such as the trachea. They can occur in a patient with a pulmonary disorder when air flows through passages that have been narrowed by secretions, a tumor or foreign body, bronchospasm, or mucosal thickening. The resulting vibration of airway walls produces the rhonchi.

History
- Take a smoking history.
- Ask about a history of asthma or other pulmonary disorder.
- Obtain a drug history.

Physical examination
- Take the patient's vital signs, including oxygen saturation.
- Characterize the patient's respirations as rapid or slow, shallow or deep, and regular or irregular. (See *Differential diagnosis: Rhonchi,* pages 326 and 327.)
- Inspect the chest, noting accessory muscle use.

(Text continues on page 328.)

Differential diagnosis: Rhonchi

History of present illness
Focused physical examination: Pulmonary system

Acute respiratory distress syndrome

Signs and symptoms
- Crackles
- Rapid, shallow respirations
- Dyspnea
- Intercostal and suprasternal retractions
- Diaphoresis
- Fluid accumulation

Diagnosis: Physical examination, arterial blood gas (ABG) analysis, chest X-ray
Treatment: Oxygen therapy, treatment of underlying cause
Follow-up: Referral to pulmonologist

Common signs and symptoms
- Wheezing
- Exertional dyspnea
- Barrel chest
- Tachypnea
- Clubbing
- Decreased breath sounds

Bronchitis

Additional signs and symptoms
Acute
- Chills
- Sore throat
- Low-grade fever
- Muscle and back pain
- Substernal tightness

Chronic
- Coarse crackles
- Prolonged expiration
- Chronic productive cough
- Increased accessory muscle use
- Cyanosis
- Fluid retention

Diagnosis: Physical examination, ABG analysis, chest X-ray, pulmonary function test (PFT)
Treatment: Smoking cessation, antibiotics if indicated, nebulizer treatment, oxygen therapy, chest physiotherapy
Follow-up: Referral to pulmonologist

Emphysema

Additional signs and symptoms
- Weight loss
- Mild, chronic productive cough
- Accessory muscle use on inspiration
- Grunting expirations

Diagnosis: Physical examination, ABG analysis, serum alpha$_1$-antitrypsin level, chest X-ray, PFT
Treatment: Smoking-cessation program, medication (diuretics, bronchodilators, corticosteroids)
Follow-up: Referral to pulmonologist

Common signs and symptoms

- Tachycardia
- Tachypnea
- Dyspnea
- Cyanosis

Pneumonia

Additional signs and symptoms

- Productive cough
- Shaking chills
- Fever
- Myalgia
- Headache
- Pleuritic chest pain
- Diaphoresis
- Decreased breath sounds
- Fine crackles

Diagnosis: Physical examination, complete blood count, ABG analysis, sputum Gram stain, chest X-ray

Treatment: Antibiotics, oxygen therapy

Follow-up: Reevaluation after 7 days

Pulmonary edema

Additional signs and symptoms

- Anxiety
- Paroxysmal nocturnal dyspnea
- Nonproductive cough
- Dependent crackles
- S_3

Diagnosis: Physical examination, ABG analysis, chest X-ray, computed tomography scan, magnetic resonance imaging

Treatment: Oxygen therapy, medication (diuretics, morphine)

Follow-up: Referral to cardiologist

■ Listen for audible wheezing or gurgling.
■ Auscultate for other abnormal breath sounds and note their location.
■ Percuss the chest, and note frequency and productivity of coughing.

Causes

Medical causes

Acute respiratory distress syndrome

■ In this life-threatening disorder, initial characteristics include dyspnea, rhonchi, crackles, and rapid shallow respirations.
■ Intercostal and suprasternal retractions, diaphoresis, and fluid accumulation occur with developing hypoxemia.
■ As hypoxemia worsens, signs and symptoms include difficulty breathing, restlessness, apprehension, decreased level of consciousness, cyanosis, motor dysfunction, and tachycardia.

Aspiration of foreign body

■ Inspiratory and expiratory rhonchi and wheezing occur because of increased secretions.
■ Other signs and symptoms include diminished breath sounds over the obstructed area, fever, pain, and cough.

Asthma

■ An asthma attack can cause rhonchi, crackles and, commonly, wheezing.
■ Other signs and symptoms include apprehension, a dry cough that later becomes productive, prolonged expirations, accessory muscle use, nasal flaring, tachypnea, tachycardia, diaphoresis, flushing or cyanosis, and intercostal and supraclavicular retractions on inspiration.

Bronchiectasis

■ Lower-lobe rhonchi and crackles occur.
■ A classic sign is a cough that produces mucopurulent, foul-smelling sputum.
■ Other signs and symptoms include fever, weight loss, exertional dyspnea, fatigue, malaise, halitosis, weakness, and late-stage clubbing.

Bronchitis

■ Sonorous rhonchi and wheezing occur in acute tracheobronchitis; other features include chills, sore throat, fever, muscle and back pain, substernal tightness, and a cough that becomes productive as secretions increase.
■ Scattered rhonchi, coarse crackles, wheezing, high-pitched piping sounds, and prolonged expirations occur with chronic bronchitis. Accompanying signs and symptoms include exertional dyspnea, increased accessory muscle use, barrel chest, cyanosis, tachypnea, and late-stage clubbing.

Emphysema

■ Sonorous rhonchi may occur, but faint, high-pitched wheezing is more typical.
■ Other signs and symptoms include weight loss, anorexia, malaise, barrel chest, peripheral cyanosis, exertional dyspnea, accessory muscle use on inspiration, tachypnea, grunting expirations, late-stage clubbing, and a mild, chronic cough with scant sputum.

Pneumonia

■ Bacterial pneumonia can cause rhonchi and a dry cough that later becomes productive.
■ Related signs and symptoms include shaking chills, high fever, myalgia, headache, pleuritic chest pain, tachypnea, tachycardia, dyspnea, cyanosis, diaphoresis, decreased breath sounds, and fine crackles.

Pulmonary coccidiodomycosis

■ This disorder causes rhonchi and wheezing.
■ Other signs and symptoms include a cough with fever, occasional chills,

pleuritic chest pain, sore throat, headache, backache, malaise, marked weakness, anorexia, hemoptysis, and an itchy macular rash.

Other causes

Diagnostic tests

- Pulmonary function tests or bronchoscopy can loosen secretions and mucus, causing rhonchi.

Respiratory therapy

- Respiratory therapy may produce rhonchi from loosened secretions and mucus.

Nursing considerations

- To ease breathing, place the patient in semi-Fowler's position.
- Give an antibiotic, a bronchodilator, and an expectorant.
- Provide humidification to thin secretions, relieve inflammation, and preventing drying.
- Promote coughing, deep breathing, and incentive spirometry.
- Provide pulmonary physiotherapy with postural drainage and percussion, to loosen secretions.
- Use tracheal suctioning, if necessary, to clear secretions.

Patient teaching

- Explain deep-breathing and coughing techniques.
- Stress the need for increasing fluid intake.
- Discuss increasing activity levels. in multiple sclerosis.
- Early signs and symptoms may include vision changes, diplopia, and paresthesia.
- Other signs and symptoms include nystagmus, constipation, muscle weakness and spasticity, hyperreflexia, dysphagia, dysarthria, incontinence, urinary frequency and urgency, impotence, and emotional instability.

Romberg's sign

A positive Romberg's sign refers to a patient's inability to maintain balance when standing erect with his feet together and his eyes closed. Normally (a negative Romberg's sign), the patient should be able to stand with his feet together and his eyes closed with minimal swaying for about 20 seconds. If positive, Romberg's sign indicates a vestibular or proprioceptive disorder. Alternatively, it may signal a disorder of the spinal tracts (the posterior columns) that carry proprioceptive information—the perception of one's position in space, of joint movements, and of pressure sensations—to the brain. Insufficient vestibular or proprioceptive information causes an inability to execute precise movements and maintain balance without visual cues. Difficulty performing this maneuver with the eyes open or closed may indicate a cerebellar disorder.

History

- Obtain a medical history, including previous neurologic symptoms and disorders.
- Ask about sensory changes and their onset.

Physical examination

- Perform other neurologic screening tests, including proprioception.
- Test the patient's awareness of body part position.
- Test the patient's direction of movement.
- Test sensation and two-point discrimination in all dermatomes.
- Test and characterize the patient's deep tendon reflexes (DTRs).
- Test the patient's vibration sense.
- Assess for hearing loss.
- Observe for nystagmus.

Causes

Medical causes

Multiple sclerosis

- A positive Romberg's sign may occur in multiple sclerosis.
- Early signs and symptoms may include vision changes, diplopia, and paresthesia.
- Other signs and symptoms include nystagmus, constipation, muscle weakness and spasticity, hyperreflexia, dysphagia, dysarthria, incontinence, urinary frequency and urgency, impotence, and emotional instability.

Peripheral nerve disease

- A positive Romberg's sign may be accompanied by impotence, fatigue, and paresthesia, hyperesthesia, or anesthesia in the hands and feet.
- Related signs and symptoms include incoordination, ataxia, burning in the affected area, progressive muscle weakness and atrophy, hypoactive DTRs, and loss of vibration sense.

Pernicious anemia

- A positive Romberg's sign and loss of proprioception in the lower limbs reflect peripheral nerve and spinal cord damage.
- Gait changes (usually ataxia), muscle weakness, impaired coordination, paresthesia, and sensory loss may occur.
- Other signs and symptoms include sore tongue, positive Babinski's reflex, fatigue, blurred vision, diplopia, and light-headedness.

Spinal cerebellar degeneration

- A positive Romberg's sign accompanies decreased visual acuity, fatigue, paresthesia, loss of vibration sense, incoordination, ataxic gait, hypoactive DTRs, and muscle weakness and atrophy.

Spinal cord disease

- A positive Romberg's sign may accompany pain, fasciculations, muscle weakness and atrophy, and loss of sphincter tone, proprioception, and vibration sense.
- DTRs may be hypoactive at the level of the lesion and hyperactive above it.

Vestibular disorders

- A positive Romberg's sign may accompany vertigo, nystagmus, nausea, tinnitus, hearing loss, and vomiting.

Nursing considerations

- Help the patient with ambulation.
- Keep a night-light on and raise the side rails of the bed for safety.
- Romberg's sign can't be tested until a child can stand without support and follow commands.
- A positive sign in children commonly results from spinal cord disease.

Patient teaching

- Teach the patient about the underlying diagnosis and treatment plan.
- Provide instruction on safety measures to avoid injury.
- Discuss the proper use of assistive devices.

S

Salivation decrease

Typically a common but minor complaint, diminished production or excretion of saliva (dry mouth) usually results from mouth breathing. However, it can also result from salivary duct obstruction, Sjögren's syndrome, the use of an anticholinergic or other drug, or the effects of radiation. It can even result from vigorous exercise or autonomic stimulation—for example, fear.

History

- Ask about the onset and course of dry mouth.
- Take a drug history.
- Determine what aggravates or alleviates the condition.
- Ask about burning or itching eyes and changes in the patient's sense of smell or taste.
- Inquire about recent dental or oral procedures.

Physical examination

- Inspect the mouth for abnormalities.
- Observe the eyes for conjunctival irritation, matted lids, and corneal epithelial thickening.
- Perform simple tests of smell and taste to detect impairment.
- Check for enlarged parotid and submaxillary glands.
- Palpate for tender or enlarged areas along the neck.

Causes

Medical causes

Dehydration

- Decreased saliva production causes dry oral mucous membranes.
- Other signs and symptoms include decreased skin turgor, reduced urine output, hypotension, tachycardia, and low-grade fever.

Facial nerve paralysis

- Diminished saliva production, decreased sense of taste, and decreased facial muscle movement occur.
- The affected side of the face may sag and appear masklike.

Salivary duct obstruction

- Reduced salivation occurs with local pain and swelling of the face or neck.
- Symptoms are most noticeable when eating or drinking.

Sjögren's syndrome

- Diminished secretions from the lacrimal, parotid, and submaxillary glands produce the characteristic signs and symptoms of decreased or absent salivation and dry eyes with a persistent burning, gritty sensation.
- Dryness of the nose, respiratory tract, vagina, and skin may also occur.
- Related oral signs and symptoms include difficulty chewing, talking, and swallowing as well as ulcers and soreness of the lips and mucosa.
- Other signs and symptoms include parotid and submaxillary gland enlarge-

ment, nasal crusting, epistaxis (nasal bleeding), fatigue, lethargy, nonproductive cough, abdominal discomfort, and polyuria.

- Signs and symptoms of rheumatoid arthritis and other connective tissue disorders may also occur.

Other causes

Drugs

- Anticholinergics, antihistamines, clonidine (Catapres), opioid analgesics, phenothiazines, and tricyclic antidepressants can decrease salivation; this effect disappears after stopping therapy.

Radiation

- Excessive irradiation of the mouth or face from radiation therapy or dental X-rays may cause transient decreased salivation.

Nursing considerations

- Monitor intake and output.
- Allow the patient extra time for speaking, eating, and swallowing.

Patient teaching

- Describe ways to relieve dry mouth.
- Instruct the patient in proper oral hygiene and dental care.
- Explain the proper use of pilocarpine (Pilocar), if prescribed, for symptom relief.
- Teach the patient to chew slowly and thoroughly to help increase saliva production.

Salivation increase

Increased salivation is an uncommon symptom that can result from a GI disorder, especially of the mouth. It also accompanies certain systemic disorders and may result from the use of certain drugs or from exposure to toxins. Saliva may also accumulate because of difficulty swallowing.

History

- Ask about fatigue, fever, headache, or sore throat.
- Inquire about recent exposure to toxins.
- Take a drug history, noting the use of iodides, cholinergics, and miotics.
- Take a medical history.

Physical examination

- Test for the gag reflex.
- Observe the patient's ability to swallow and chew.
- Note any drooling.
- Inspect the mouth for lesions; note their appearance.
- Palpate mouth lesions and describe their appearance.
- Inspect the uvula, gingivae, and pharynx.
- Palpate lymph nodes, and determine if parotid glands are swollen or sore.

Causes

Medical causes

Bell's palsy

- Facial nerve paralysis causes an inability to control salivation or close the eye on the affected side.
- The affected side of the face sags and is expressionless, the nasolabial fold flattens, and the palpebral fissure (the distance between the upper and lower eyelids) widens.
- Other signs and symptoms include diminished or absent corneal reflex and partial loss of taste or abnormal taste sensation.

Motion sickness

- Hypersalivation may occur with vertigo, nausea, vomiting, and headache in response to rhythmic or erratic motions.
- Dizziness, fatigue, diaphoresis, and dyspnea may also occur.

Pregnancy

- In the early months, increased salivation, nausea, gum swelling, and breast tenderness may occur.

Rabies

- Excessive salivation occurs after initial symptoms of fever, headache, nausea, sore throat, and cough.
- Other signs and symptoms include trismus (restriction to the mouth opening), restlessness, cranial nerve dysfunction, localized pain at the bite site, and hydrophobia.
- If not promptly treated, generalized, flaccid paralysis occurs, leading to peripheral vascular collapse, coma, and death.

Stomatitis

- Mucosal ulcers may be accompanied by moderately increased salivation, mouth pain, fever, and erythema.
- Spontaneous healing usually occurs in 7 to 10 days, but scarring and recurrence are possible.

Syphilis

- With secondary syphilis, mucosal ulcers cause increased salivation that may persist for up to 1 year.
- Related signs and symptoms include fever, malaise, headache, anorexia, weight loss, nausea, vomiting, sore throat, and lymphadenopathy.
- A symmetrical rash appears on the arms, trunk, palms, soles, face, and scalp.
- Condylomata develop in the genital and perianal areas.

Tuberculosis

- Certain forms may produce solitary, irregularly shaped mouth or tongue ulcers, covered with exudate, that cause increased salivation.
- Other signs and symptoms include weight loss, anorexia, fever, fatigue, malaise, dyspnea, cough, night sweats (a common sign), and hemoptysis.

Other causes

Arsenic poisoning

- Common effects of arsenic poisoning are diarrhea, diffuse skin hyperpigmentation, and edema of the face, eyelids, and ankles; increased salivation occurs infrequently.
- Other signs and symptoms include garlicky breath odor, pruritus, headache, drowsiness, confusion, and weakness.

Drugs

- Increased salivation may occur with iodide toxicity, but the earliest symptoms are a brassy taste and a burning sensation in the mouth and throat; other signs and symptoms include sneezing, irritated eyelids, and pain in the frontal sinus.
- Pilocarpine (Pilocar) and other miotics used to treat glaucoma may be absorbed systemically, increasing salivation.
- Cholinergics, such as bethanechol (Duvoid), may cause increased salivation.

Mercury poisoning

- Stomatitis, characterized by increased salivation and a metallic taste, commonly occurs.
- Teeth may be loose with painful, swollen gums that are prone to bleeding.
- A blue line appears on the gingivae.
- Other signs and symptoms include personality changes, memory loss, abdominal cramps, diarrhea, paresthesia, and tremors of the eyelids, lips, tongue, and fingers.

Nursing considerations

- Increased salivation doesn't require treatments beyond those needed to correct the underlying disorder.

■ If the patient has difficulty swallowing, suction the mouth as needed.

Patient teaching

■ Instruct the patient in proper oral hygiene.
■ Emphasize the importance of obtaining proper dental care.
■ Teach the patient about the underlying diagnosis and treatment plan.

Salt craving

Craving salty foods is a compensatory response to the body's failure to adequately conserve sodium. Normally, the renal tubules reabsorb almost all sodium, allowing less than 1% of it to be excreted in urine. This reabsorption is regulated by aldosterone, a hormone synthesized in the adrenal gland. However, adrenal dysfunction can reduce aldosterone levels, thereby impairing reabsorption and increasing sodium excretion.

History

■ Find out how much salt the patient typically uses.
■ Ask about weakness, fatigue, anorexia, weight loss, fainting, or dizziness.
■ Check for a history of adrenal insufficiency or diabetes mellitus and for the recent onset of polydipsia or polyuria.

Physical examination

■ Inspect the patient's skin for hyperpigmentation or hypopigmentation and skin turgor.
■ Take the patient's vital signs, noting orthostatic hypotension.
■ Collect a urine specimen and test with a reagent strip for glucose and acetone.
■ Collect a serum sample for laboratory tests, such as plasma renin activity and serum aldosterone, serum electrolyte, plasma cortisol and glucose, urine 17-ketogenic steroid and 17-hydroxycorticosteroid, and corticotropin levels. Special provocative studies may include the metyrapone test and the rapid corticotropin test.
■ Obtain an electrocardiogram (ECG).

Causes

Medical causes

Adrenal insufficiency, primary

■ Commonly called *Addison's disease,* this disorder reduces aldosterone secretion. It's typically due to an autoimmune process, tuberculosis, neoplasms, or infections, such as acquired immunodeficiency syndrome and cytomegalovirus.
■ The patient may exhibit an intense craving for salty food.
■ The patient may display diffuse brown, tan, or bronze-to-black hyperpigmentation of exposed areas (such as the face, knees, and knuckles) and of nonexposed areas (such as the tongue, buccal mucosa, or palmar creases) as well as darkening of normally pigmented areas, moles, and scars.
■ Other signs and symptoms include weakness, anorexia, nausea, irritability, vomiting, decreased cold tolerance, dizziness, low blood pressure, weight loss, abdominal pain, and slowly progressive fatigue.

Adrenal insufficiency, secondary

■ Glucocorticoid deficiency can result from hypopituitarism, abrupt withdrawal of long-term corticosteroid therapy, or removal of a nonendocrine, corticotropin-secreting tumor.
■ Signs and symptoms are similar to primary insufficiency but without hyperpigmentation, hypotension, and electrolyte imbalance.

Other causes

Surgery

■ Adrenal insufficiency can develop with bilateral adrenalectomy.

Nursing considerations

- Prepare the patient for diagnostic studies.
- Monitor and record the patient's blood pressure, weight, intake and output, and skin turgor.
- Encourage the patient to drink plenty of fluids. Explain the need to follow a diet that helps maintain adequate sodium and potassium levels, and identify foods that can help with this.
- Be alert for signs of hyponatremia, such as hypotension, muscle twitching and weakness, and abdominal cramps.
- Look for signs and symptoms of hyperkalemia, such as muscle weakness, tachycardia, nausea, vomiting, and characteristic ECG changes, including tented and elevated T waves, widened QRS complex, prolonged PR interval, flattened or absent P waves, and depressed ST segment.
- If diagnostic tests confirm primary adrenal insufficiency, emphasize the importance of complying with lifelong steroid (glucocorticoid or mineralocorticoid) therapy.
- Salt craving may signal a change in the patient's condition, requiring increased steroid dosage.

Patient teaching

- For the patient is who is prescribed a steroid (usually hydrocortisone):
  - Teach the reason for taking the drug, its adverse effects, and the signs and symptoms of steroid toxicity and underdosage.
  - Tell the patient not to decrease the dose or discontinue the drug without a practitioner's order. Explain that his dosage may need to be increased during times of stress (infection, injury, even profuse sweating) to prevent adrenal crisis, and that he'll need lifelong medical supervision to monitor the steroid therapy.
  - Instruct the patient to wear a medical identification bracelet at all times, indicating his condition and the name and dosage of the drug he takes.
  - Teach the patient how to self-administer the drug parenterally in emergency situations, such as an adrenal crisis that occurs while traveling in remote areas away from medical help.
  - Urge the patient to keep a prepared syringe of the drug available for emergency use.

Scotoma

A scotoma is an area of partial or complete blindness within an otherwise normal or slightly impaired visual field. Usually located within the central 30-degree area, the defect ranges from absolute blindness to a barely detectable loss of visual acuity. Typically, the patient can pinpoint the scotoma's location in the visual field.

A scotoma can result from a retinal, choroid, or optic nerve disorder. It can be classified as absolute, relative, or scintillating. An absolute scotoma refers to the total inability to see all sizes of test objects used in mapping the visual field. A relative scotoma, in contrast, refers to the ability to see only large test objects. A scintillating scotoma refers to the flashes or bursts of light commonly seen during a migraine headache.

History

- Take a medical history, including eye disorders, vision problems, or chronic systemic disorders.
- Obtain a drug history.

Physical examination

- Test the patient's visual acuity.
- Inspect the pupils for size, equality, and reaction to light.
- Make sure an ophthalmoscopic examination is performed and intraocular pressure (IOP) is measured.
- Identify and characterize the scotoma using visual field tests.

Causes

Medical causes

Chorioretinitis

- A paracentral scotoma develops.
- Examination reveals clouding and white blood cells in the vitreous, subretinal hemorrhage, and neovascularization.
- Photophobia with blurred vision may be present.

Glaucoma

- Prolonged elevation of IOP can cause an arcuate scotoma.
- Cupping of the optic disk, loss of peripheral vision, and reduced visual acuity occur with poorly controlled glaucoma.
- Rainbow-colored halos may appear around lights.

Macular degeneration

- A central scotoma develops.
- Examination reveals changes in the macular area.
- Other signs and symptoms include changes in visual acuity and color perception and in perception of the size and shape of objects.

Migraine headache

- Transient scintillating scotomas, usually on one side, can occur during the aura.
- Other signs and symptoms include paresthesia of the lips, face, or hands, slight confusion, dizziness, nausea and vomiting, and photophobia.

Optic neuritis

- A central, circular, or centrocecal scotoma with vision loss develops in one or both eyes.
- Severe vision loss or blurring and pain—especially with eye movement—occurs.
- Other signs and symptoms include hyperemia of the optic disk, retinal vein distention, blurred disk margins, and filling of the physiologic cup.

Retinitis pigmentosa

- Annular scotoma progresses concentrically until only tunnel vision remains.
- The earliest symptom—impaired night vision—appears during adolescence.
- Other signs and symptoms include narrowing of the retinal blood vessels, pallor of the optic disk and, eventually, blindness.

Nursing considerations

- Provide safety measures.
- Give prescribed drugs.
- In young children, visual field testing is difficult and requires patience; confrontation visual field testing is the method of choice.

Patient teaching

- Emphasize the importance of compliance with drug therapy and teach the patient how to apply eyedrops correctly and safely.
- Explain the progression and complications of the disease.
- Tell the patient which signs and symptoms to report.
- Discuss which rehabilitation services and assistive devices are available.
- Stress the importance of regular eye examinations.
- Explain the use of the Amsler grid to monitor vision, if appropriate.

Scrotal swelling

Scrotal swelling occurs when a condition affecting the testicles, epididymis, or scrotal skin produces edema or a mass; the penis may be involved. Scrotal swelling can affect males of any age. It can be unilateral or bilateral and painful or painless.

The sudden onset of painful scrotal swelling suggests torsion of a testicle or testicular appendages, especially in a prepubescent male. This emergency requires immediate surgery to untwist and stabilize the spermatic cord or to remove the appendage.

QUICK ACTION ***If severe pain accompanies scrotal swelling, ask the patient when the swelling began. Using a Doppler stethoscope, evaluate blood flow to the testicle. If it's decreased or absent, suspect testicular torsion and prepare the patient for surgery. Withhold food and fluids, insert an I.V. catheter, and apply an ice pack to the scrotum to reduce pain and swelling. An attempt may be made to untwist the cord manually, but even if this is successful, the patient may still require surgery for stabilization.***

History

- Ask about a history of injury to the scrotum, urethral discharge, cloudy urine, increased urinary frequency, dysuria, sexually transmitted disease, prostate surgery, or prolonged catheterization.
- Find out about recent illness, particularly mumps.
- Obtain a history of sexual activity.
- Ask which body positions alleviate or aggravate swelling.

Physical examination

- Take the patient's vital signs, especially noting fever.
- Palpate the abdomen for tenderness and swelling.
- Examine the genital area.
- Assess the scrotum with the patient in a supine position and then standing.
- Check the testicles' position in the scrotum.
- Palpate the scrotum for a cyst or lump, and note tenderness or firmness.
- Transilluminate the scrotum to distinguish a fluid-filled cyst from a solid mass.

Causes

Medical causes

Epididymal cysts

- Painless scrotal swelling occurs.

Epididymitis

- Inflammation, pain, extreme tenderness, and swelling develop in the groin and scrotum.
- Other signs and symptoms include high fever, malaise, urethral discharge and cloudy urine, lower abdominal pain on the affected side, and hot, red, dry, flaky, and thin scrotal skin.

Hernia

- Swelling and a soft or unusually firm scrotum are produced by herniation of the bowel into the scrotum.
- Nausea, anorexia, vomiting, and reduced bowel sounds may occur if the bowel is obstructed.

Hydrocele

- Fluid accumulation produces gradual scrotal swelling that's usually painless.
- The scrotum may be soft and cystic or firm and tense.
- Palpation reveals a round, nontender scrotal mass.

Orchitis, acute

- Sudden painful swelling of one or both testicles occurs.
- Related signs and symptoms include hot and reddened scrotum, fever, chills, lower abdominal pain, nausea, vomiting, and extreme weakness.

Scrotal trauma

- Scrotal swelling, bruising, and severe pain may result.
- The scrotum may appear dark blue.

■ Nausea, vomiting, and difficult urination may also occur.

Spermatocele
■ A moveable, painless cystic mass develops that may be transilluminated.

Testicular torsion
■ Characteristics of this urologic emergency include scrotal swelling, sudden and severe pain and, possibly, elevation of the affected testicle within the scrotum.
■ Disorder occurs most commonly before puberty.
■ Other possible signs include nausea and vomiting.

Testicular tumor
■ The scrotum swells and produces a local sensation of excessive weight.
■ Typically, these tumors are painless, smooth, and firm.
■ With ureteral obstruction, urinary complaints are common.

Other causes
Surgery
■ Blood effusion from surgery can produce a hematocele, leading to scrotal swelling.

Nursing considerations
■ Place the patient on bed rest.
■ Give an antibiotic as prescribed.
■ Provide fluids, fiber, and stool softeners.
■ Place a rolled towel under the scrotum to help reduce swelling.
■ For moderate swelling, suggest a loose-fitting athletic supporter.
■ Apply heat or ice packs, and use a sitz bath to decrease inflammation.
■ Give an analgesic as needed.

Patient teaching
■ Explain the importance of performing testicular self-examinations, and teach the technique if needed.
■ Teach the patient about the underlying diagnosis and treatment plan.

Seizures, absence

Absence seizures are benign generalized seizures thought to originate subcortically. These brief episodes of unconsciousness usually last 3 to 20 seconds and can occur 100 or more times per day, causing periods of inattention. Absence seizures usually begin between ages 4 and 12. Their first sign may be deteriorating schoolwork and behavior. The cause of these seizures is unknown.

Absence seizures occur without warning. The patient suddenly stops all purposeful activity and stares blankly ahead, as if he were daydreaming. Absence seizures may produce automatisms, such as repetitive lip smacking, or mild clonic or myoclonic movements, including mild jerking of the eyelids. The patient may drop an object that he's holding, and muscle relaxation may cause him to drop his head or arms or to slump. After the attack, the patient resumes activity, typically unaware of the episode.

Absence status, a rare form of absence seizure, occurs as a prolonged absence seizure or as repeated episodes of these seizures. Usually not life-threatening, it occurs most commonly in patients who have previously experienced absence seizures.

History
■ Obtain a history from the parents as well as from the child, including how long the seizures have been occurring, how long each one is, and how far apart they are.
■ Find out if the patient has been treated for seizures in the past.
■ Ask if the family has noticed a change in behavior or deterioration of schoolwork.

Physical examination

- Evaluate absence seizure occurrence and duration by reciting a series of numbers and then asking the patient to repeat them after the attack ends. If the patient has had an absence seizure, he'll be unable to do this. Alternatively, if the seizures are occurring within minutes of each other, ask the patient to count for about 5 minutes. He'll stop counting during a seizure and resume when it's over.
- Look for accompanying automatisms (automatic repetitive behavior).

Causes

Medical causes

Idiopathic epilepsy

- Some forms of absence seizure are accompanied by learning disabilities.
- Absence seizures may produce automatisms, such as repetitive lip smacking, or mild clonic or myoclonic movements, including mild jerking of the eyelids. The patient may drop an object that he's holding, and muscle relaxation may cause him to drop his head or arms or to slump.

Nursing considerations

- Give an anticonvulsant as ordered.
- Prepare the patient for diagnostic tests, such as computed tomography scans, magnetic resonance imaging, and EEGs.
- Provide emotional support to the patient and his family.
- Ensure a safe environment for the patient.

Patient teaching

- Teach the patient and his family about these seizures and how to recognize their onset, pattern, and duration. Explain how to care for the patient.
- Include the child's teacher and school nurse in the teaching process, if possible.
- If the seizures are being controlled with drug therapy, emphasize the importance of strict compliance.
- Discuss the need to wear medical identification.

Seizures, complex partial

A complex partial seizure occurs when a focal seizure begins in the temporal lobe and causes a partial alteration of consciousness—usually confusion. Psychomotor seizures can occur at any age, but their incidence usually increases during adolescence and adulthood. Two-thirds of patients also have generalized seizures.

An aura—usually a complex hallucination, illusion, or sensation—typically precedes a psychomotor seizure. The hallucination may be audiovisual (images with sounds), auditory (abnormal or normal sounds or voices from the patient's past), or olfactory (unpleasant smells, such as rotten eggs or burning materials). Other types of auras include sensations of déjà vu, unfamiliarity with surroundings, or depersonalization. The patient may become fearful or anxious, experience lip smacking, or have an unpleasant feeling in the epigastric region that rises toward the chest and throat. The patient usually recognizes the aura and lies down before losing consciousness.

A period of unresponsiveness follows the aura. The patient may experience automatisms, appear dazed and wander aimlessly, perform inappropriate acts (such as undressing in public), be unresponsive, utter incoherent phrases or, in rare cases, go into a rage or tantrum. After the seizure, the patient is confused, drowsy, and doesn't remember the seizure. Behavioral automatisms rarely last longer than 5 minutes, but post-seizure confusion, agitation, and amnesia may persist.

Between attacks, the patient may exhibit slow and rigid thinking, outbursts of anger and aggressiveness, tedious conversation, a preoccupation with naïve philosophical ideas, a diminished libido, mood swings, and paranoid tendencies.

History

- Ask about the occurrence of an aura.
- Ask witnesses for a description of the seizure.
- Find out about previous seizures or therapies.
- Ask about a history of head trauma.

Physical examination

- Examine the patient for injury after the seizure.
- Ensure a patent airway.
- Perform a complete neurologic assessment.

Causes

Medical causes

Brain abscess

- If the temporal lobe is affected, complex partial seizures commonly occur after the abscess resolves.
- Related signs and symptoms include headache, nausea, vomiting, generalized seizures, and a decreased level of consciousness (LOC).
- Central facial weakness, auditory receptive aphasia, hemiparesis, and ocular disturbances may also occur.

Head trauma

- Trauma to the temporal lobe can produce complex partial seizures months or years later.
- Seizures may decrease in frequency and eventually stop.
- Generalized seizures may also occur, along with behavior and personality changes.

Herpes simplex encephalitis

- This disease commonly attacks the temporal lobe, resulting in complex partial seizures.
- Other signs and symptoms include fever, headache, coma, and generalized seizures.

Temporal lobe tumor

- Complex partial seizures may be the first sign.
- Other signs and symptoms include headache, pupillary changes, and mental dullness.
- Increased intracranial pressure may cause a decreased LOC, vomiting, and papilledema.

Nursing considerations

- After the seizure, reorient the patient to his surroundings and protect him from injury.
- Keep the patient in bed until he's fully alert.
- Remove harmful objects from the area.
- Provide emotional support to the patient and his family.
- Monitor for therapeutic drug levels.

Patient teaching

- Discuss methods for coping with seizures.
- Instruct the patient and his family or caregivers in safety measures to take during a seizure.
- Emphasize compliance with drug therapy.
- Tell the patient to carry medical identification.

Seizures, generalized tonic-clonic

Like other types of seizures, generalized tonic-clonic seizures are caused by the paroxysmal, uncontrolled discharge of central nervous system (CNS) neurons, leading to neurologic dysfunction. Unlike most other types of seizures, however, this cerebral hyperactivity isn't confined to the original focus or to a localized area, but extends to the entire brain.

A generalized tonic-clonic seizure may begin with or without an aura. As seizure activity spreads to the subcortical structures, the patient loses consciousness, falls, and may utter a loud cry that's precipitated by air rushing from the lungs through the vocal cords. His body stiffens (tonic phase), and then undergoes rapid, synchronous muscle jerking and hyperventilation (clonic phase). Tongue biting, incontinence, diaphoresis, profuse salivation, and signs of respiratory distress may also occur. The seizure usually stops after 2 to 5 minutes. The patient then regains consciousness but displays confusion. He may complain of a headache, fatigue, muscle soreness, and arm and leg weakness.

Generalized tonic-clonic seizures usually occur singly. The patient may be asleep or awake and active. Possible complications include respiratory arrest due to airway obstruction from secretions, status epilepticus (occurring in 5% to 8% of patients), head or spinal injuries and bruises, Todd's paralysis and, in rare cases, cardiac arrest. Life-threatening status epilepticus is marked by prolonged seizure activity or by rapidly recurring seizures with no intervening periods of recovery. It's most commonly triggered by the abrupt discontinuation of anticonvulsant therapy.

Generalized seizures may be caused by a brain tumor, vascular disorder, head trauma, infection, metabolic defect, drug or alcohol withdrawal syndrome, exposure to toxins, or a genetic defect. Generalized seizures may also result from a focal seizure. With recurring seizures, or epilepsy, the cause may be unknown. (See *Responding to generalized tonic-clonic seizures,* page 342.)

QUICK ACTION ***If you witness the beginning of the patient's seizure, first check his airway, breathing, and circulation, and ensure that the cause isn't asystole or an obstructed airway. Stay with the patient and ensure a patent airway. Focus your care on observing the seizure and protecting the patient. Place a towel under his head to prevent injury, loosen his clothing, and move any sharp or hard objects out of his way. Never try to restrain the patient or force a hard object into his mouth; you might chip his teeth or fracture his jaw. Only at the start of the seizure can you safely insert a soft object, such as a folded cloth, into his mouth.***

If possible, turn the patient to one side during the seizure to allow secretions to drain and to prevent aspiration. Otherwise, do this at the end of the clonic phase when respirations return. (If they fail to return, check for airway obstruction and suction the patient if necessary. Cardiopulmonary resuscitation, endotracheal intubation, and mechanical ventilation may be needed.)

Protect the patient after the seizure by providing a safe area in which he can rest. As he awakens, reassure and reorient him. Check his vital signs and neurologic status. Be sure to carefully record these data and your observations during the seizure.

If the seizure lasts longer than 4 minutes or if a second seizure occurs before full recovery from the first, suspect status epilepticus. Establish an airway, insert an I.V. catheter, give supplemental oxygen, and begin cardiac monitoring. Draw blood for appropriate studies. Turn the patient on his side, with his head in a semi-dependent position, to drain secretions

CASE CLIP

Responding to generalized tonic-clonic seizures

Mr. W. is a 79-year-old male admitted to the medical unit from a nursing home with fever, dehydration, weakness, and confusion; the staff wanted him checked for urinary tract infection and urosepsis. He has a history of Alzheimer's disease, congestive heart failure, and frequent urinary tract infections. His vital signs on admission were:

- temperature: 101.4° F (38.6° C)
- heart rate (HR): 116 beats/minute
- respiratory rate (RR): 28 breaths/minute
- blood pressure (BP): 92/50 mm Hg
- oxygen saturation: 90% on room air.

He was placed on 2 L/minute of oxygen via nasal cannula. Blood was drawn to check his complete blood count, electrolytes, and blood cultures, and a urine culture was obtained via straight catheterization. He was started on I.V. fluids. An initial dose of prophylactic antibiotics was given on his arrival to the medical unit.

Three days after admission, Mr. W. remains on antibiotics because his cultures are positive for a urinary tract infection and urosepsis. He still shows signs of confusion, and is frequently found trying to get out of bed. He's pulled out his I.V. twice since his arrival.

On the night shift, the nurses hear a crash down the hall. They run to investigate and find Mr. W. on the floor by his bed, conscious but mumbling incoherently. They notice a small amount of blood pooling under his head. The Rapid Response Team (RRT) is summoned immediately to Mr. W.'s room, as are the orderlies, so they can help transfer Mr. W. back to bed once he's cleared medically. Before the orderlies or RRT members arrive, however, the nurses observe Mr. W. experiencing a 10-second tonic-clonic seizure. The nurses call for the crash cart, place Mr. W. on the bedside monitor, and reapply his oxygen. The monitor shows a rapid irregular heart rate and the following vital signs:

- HR: 124 beats/ minute
- RR: 22 breaths/minute and shallow
- BP: 84/60 mm Hg.

The RRT and orderlies arrive within 3 minutes of being called. A cervical collar is applied to Mr. W's neck. He is placed on a backboard in cervical spine precautions and transferred back to his bed, at which time the team notices a small pool of fresh blood on the floor. On palpation, the resident detects a laceration on the back of Mr. W.'s head. A dry sterile dressing is applied until staples can be placed. No further seizure activity is noted, but until spinal and cranial fractures can be ruled out, the decision is made to transfer Mr. W. to the medical intensive care unit for closer observation.

and prevent aspiration. Periodically turn him to the opposite side, check his arterial blood gas levels for hypoxemia, and give oxygen by mask, increasing the flow rate if necessary. Give diazepam (Valium) or lorazepam (Ativan) by slow I.V. push, repeated two or three times at 10- to 20-minute intervals, to stop the seizures. If the patient isn't known to have epilepsy, an I.V. bolus of dextrose 50% (50 ml) with thiamine (100 mg) may be ordered. Dextrose may stop the seizures if the patient has hypoglycemia. If his

thiamine level is low, giving thiamine will protect against further damage.

History

- Obtain a description of the seizure, including onset, duration, body area affected, characteristics, and progression.
- Ask about unusual sensations before the seizure.
- Find out about a personal and family history of seizures.
- Take a drug history and determine compliance.
- Ask about head trauma, sleep deprivation, or emotional or physical stress at the time of the seizure.
- Obtain a medical history.

Physical examination

- If the patient may have sustained a head injury, observe him closely for loss of consciousness, unequal or nonreactive pupils, and focal neurologic signs.
- Examine the arms, legs, and face (including tongue) for injury, residual paralysis, or limb weakness.
- Take the patient's vital signs.
- Complete a neurologic assessment.
- Observe for adequate oxygenation.

Causes

Medical causes

Alcohol withdrawal syndrome

- Seizures as well as status epilepticus may occur 7 to 48 hours after sudden alcohol withdrawal.
- Other signs and symptoms include restlessness, hallucinations, profuse diaphoresis, and tachycardia.

Arsenic poisoning

- Generalized seizures may occur with a garlicky breath odor, increased salivation, generalized pruritus, diarrhea, nausea, vomiting, and abdominal pain.
- Related signs and symptoms include diffuse hyperpigmentation; sharply defined edema of the eyelids, face, and ankles; paresthesia of the extremities; alopecia; irritated mucous membranes; weakness; muscle aches; and peripheral neuropathy.

Brain abscess

- Generalized seizures may occur in the acute stage of abscess formation or after the abscess disappears.
- Constant headache, nausea, vomiting, and focal seizures are early signs and symptoms.
- Other signs and symptoms include decreased level of consciousness (LOC), ocular disturbances, aphasia, hemiparesis, abnormal behavior, and personality changes.

Brain tumor

- Generalized seizures may occur, depending on the tumor's location and type.
- Other signs and symptoms include a slowly decreasing LOC, morning headache, dizziness, confusion, focal seizures, vision loss, motor and sensory disturbances, aphasia, and ataxia.
- Later signs and symptoms include papilledema, vomiting, increased systolic blood pressure, widening pulse pressure and, eventually, decorticate posture.

Cerebral aneurysm

- Generalized seizures may occur.
- Onset is typically abrupt with severe headache, nausea, vomiting, and decreased LOC.
- Related signs and symptoms vary with the site and amount of bleeding, but may include nuchal rigidity, irritability, hemiparesis, hemisensory defects, dysphagia, photophobia, diplopia, ptosis, and unilateral pupil dilation.

Eclampsia

- Generalized seizures are a hallmark of this condition.
- Related signs and symptoms include severe frontal headache, nausea, vomit-

ing, vision disturbances, increased blood pressure, fever, peripheral edema, oliguria, irritability, hyperactive deep tendon reflexes (DTRs), decreased LOC, and sudden weight gain.

Encephalitis

- Seizures are an early sign, indicating a poor prognosis.
- Seizures may also occur after recovery as a result of residual damage.
- Other signs and symptoms include fever, headache, photophobia, nuchal rigidity, neck pain, vomiting, aphasia, ataxia, hemiparesis, nystagmus, irritability, cranial nerve palsies, and myoclonic jerks.

Head trauma

- Generalized seizures may occur at the time of injury; focal seizures may occur months later.
- Related signs and symptoms include decreased LOC; soft-tissue injury of the face, head, or neck; clear or bloody drainage from the mouth, nose, or ears; facial edema; bony deformity of the face, head, or neck; Battle's sign; and lack of response to oculocephalic and oculovestibular stimulation.
- Other characteristics include motor and sensory deficits, altered respirations, and signs of increasing intracranial pressure.

Hepatic encephalopathy

- Generalized seizures may occur late.
- Other signs and symptoms include fetor hepaticus, asterixis, hyperactive DTRs, and positive Babinski's sign.

Hypertensive encephalopathy

- Seizures with increased blood pressure, decreased LOC, intense headache, vomiting, transient blindness, paralysis, and Cheyne-Stokes respirations occur with this life-threatening disorder.

Hypoglycemia

- Generalized seizures usually occur in severe cases.
- Other signs and symptoms include blurred or double vision, motor weakness, hemiplegia, trembling, excessive diaphoresis, tachycardia, myoclonic twitching, and decreased LOC.

Hyponatremia

- Seizure develops when the sodium level falls below 125 mEq/L, especially if the decrease is rapid.
- Other signs and symptoms include orthostatic hypotension, headache, muscle twitching and weakness, fatigue, oliguria or anuria, cold and clammy skin, decreased skin turgor, irritability, lethargy, confusion, and stupor or coma.
- Excessive thirst, tachycardia, nausea, vomiting, and abdominal cramps may also occur.

Hypoparathyroidism

- Generalized seizures occur as a result of worsening tetany.
- Chronic hypoparathyroidism produces neuromuscular irritability, Chvostek's sign, dysphagia, tetany, and hyperactive DTRs.

Hypoxic encephalopathy

- Generalized seizures, myoclonic jerks, and coma occur.
- Later, dementia, visual agnosia, choreoathetosis, and ataxia may occur.

Neurofibromatosis

- Focal and generalized seizures occur.
- Other signs and symptoms include café-au-lait spots, multiple skin tumors, scoliosis, kyphoscoliosis, dizziness, ataxia, monocular blindness, and nystagmus.

Porphyria

- Generalized seizures are a late sign of this disorder and indicate severe CNS involvement.

■ Other related signs and symptoms include severe abdominal pain, tachycardia, muscle weakness, and psychotic behavior.

Renal failure, chronic
■ The onset of twitching, trembling, myoclonic jerks, and generalized seizures is rapid.
■ Related signs and symptoms include anuria or oliguria, fatigue, malaise, irritability, decreased mental acuity, muscle cramps, peripheral neuropathies, pruritus, uremic frost, anorexia, and constipation or diarrhea.
■ Other signs and symptoms include ammonia breath odor, nausea and vomiting, ecchymoses, petechiae, GI bleeding, mouth and gum ulcers, hypertension, and Kussmaul's respirations.

Sarcoidosis
■ Lesions may affect the brain, causing focal or generalized seizures.
■ Other related signs and symptoms include nonproductive cough with dyspnea, substernal pain, malaise, fatigue, myalgia, weight loss, tachypnea, dysphagia, skin lesions, and impaired vision.

Stroke
■ Seizures (focal more commonly than generalized) may occur within 6 months of an ischemic stroke.
■ Other signs and symptoms vary but may include decreased LOC, contralateral hemiplegia, dysarthria, dysphagia, ataxia, sensory loss on one side, apraxia, agnosia, aphasia, visual deficits, memory loss, personality changes, emotional lability, and incontinence.

Other causes
Diagnostic tests
■ Contrast agents used in radiologic tests may cause generalized seizures.

Drugs
■ In chronically intoxicated patients, barbiturate withdrawal may produce generalized seizures 2 to 4 days after the last dose.
■ Amphetamines, isoniazid (Nydrazid), phenothiazines, tricyclic antidepressants, and vincristine (Oncovin) may cause seizures in patients with preexisting epilepsy.
■ Toxic levels of some drugs, such as cimetidine (Tagamet), lidocaine (Xylocaine), meperidine (Demerol), penicillins, and theophylline (Elixophyllin), may cause generalized seizures.

Nursing considerations
■ Support the patient's respiratory status, if indicated.
■ Protect the patient from injury.
■ Monitor the patient after the seizure for recurring seizure activity.
■ Monitor for therapeutic drug levels.

Patient teaching
■ Teach the patient's family how to observe and record seizure activity and explain the reasons for doing so.
■ Emphasize the importance of compliance with drug regimen and follow-up appointments.
■ Explain the possible adverse reactions of prescribed drugs.
■ Tell the patient to carry medical identification.

Seizures, simple partial

Resulting from an irritable focus in the cerebral cortex, simple partial seizures typically last about 30 seconds and don't alter the patient's level of consciousness (LOC). The type and pattern reflect the location of the irritable focus. Simple partial seizures may be classified as motor (including jacksonian seizures and epilepsia partialis continua) or somatosensory (including visual, olfactory, and auditory seizures).

A *focal motor seizure* is a series of unilateral clonic (muscle jerking) and tonic (muscle stiffening) movements of one part of the body. The patient's head and eyes characteristically turn away from the hemispheric focus—usually the frontal lobe near the motor strip. A tonic-clonic contraction of the trunk or extremities may follow.

A *jacksonian motor seizure* typically begins with a tonic contraction of a finger, the corner of the mouth, or one foot. Clonic movements follow, spreading to other muscles on the same side of the body, moving up the arm or leg, and eventually involving the whole side. Alternatively, clonic movements may spread to the opposite side, becoming generalized and leading to loss of consciousness. In the postictal phase, the patient may experience paralysis (Todd's paralysis) in the affected limbs, usually resolving within 24 hours.

Epilepsia partialis continua causes clonic twitching of one muscle group, usually in the face, arm, or leg. Twitching occurs every few seconds and persists for hours, days, or months without spreading. Spasms usually affect the distal arm and leg muscles more than the proximal ones. In the face, spasms affect the corner of the mouth, one or both eyelids and, occasionally, the neck or trunk muscles unilaterally.

A *focal somatosensory seizure* affects a localized body area on one side. Usually, this type of seizure initially causes numbness, tingling, or crawling or "electric" sensations; occasionally, it causes pain or burning sensations in the lips, fingers, or toes. A visual seizure involves sensations of darkness or of stationary or moving lights or spots, usually red at first, then blue, green, and yellow. It can affect both visual fields or the visual field on the side opposite the lesion. The irritable focus is in the occipital lobe. In contrast, the irritable focus in an auditory or olfactory seizure is in the temporal lobe.

History

- Obtain a description of the seizure activity.
- Ask about events before the seizure.
- Ask if the patient can describe an aura or recognize its onset.
- Inquire about loss of consciousness, tonicity and clonicity, cyanosis, tongue biting, and urinary incontinence.
- Explore a history of head trauma, stroke, or infection with fever, headache, or stiff neck.

Physical examination

- Perform a complete physical assessment, focusing on the neurologic assessment.
- Check the patient's LOC.
- Test for residual deficits and sensory disturbances.

Causes

Medical causes

Brain abscess

- Seizures can occur in the acute stage of abscess formation or after resolution of the abscess.
- Decreased LOC varies from drowsiness to deep stupor.
- Early signs and symptoms reflect increased intracranial pressure, such as a constant, intractable headache, nausea, and vomiting.
- Later signs and symptoms include ocular disturbances, such as nystagmus, decreased visual acuity, and unequal pupils.
- Other signs and symptoms vary with the abscess site and may include aphasia, hemiparesis, and personality changes.

Brain tumor

- Focal seizures are commonly the earliest indicators.
- Morning headache, dizziness, confusion, vision loss, and motor and sensory disturbances may occur.
- Other signs and symptoms include aphasia, generalized seizures, ataxia, decreased LOC, papilledema, vomiting, increased systolic blood pressure, widening pulse pressure and, eventually, decorticate posture.

Head trauma

- Penetrating wounds are associated with focal seizures.
- Seizures usually begin 3 to 15 months after injury, decrease in frequency after several years, and eventually stop.
- Generalized seizures and a decreased LOC may progress to coma.

Multiple sclerosis

- Focal or generalized seizures may occur in the late stages.
- Other signs and symptoms include visual deficits, paresthesia, constipation, muscle weakness, spasticity, paralysis, hyperreflexia, intention tremor, gait ataxia, dysphagia, dysarthria, emotional lability, impotence, and urinary frequency, urgency, and incontinence.

Neurofibromatosis

- Multiple brain lesions cause focal seizures and, at times, generalized seizures.
- Other signs and symptoms include café-au-lait spots, multiple skin tumors, scoliosis, kyphoscoliosis, dizziness, ataxia, progressive monocular blindness, nystagmus, and endocrine abnormalities.

Stroke

- Focal seizures may occur up to 6 months after a stroke's onset; generalized seizures may also occur.
- Accompanying effects vary and may include decreased LOC, contralateral hemiplegia, dysarthria, dysphagia, ataxia, unilateral sensory loss, apraxia, agnosia, and aphasia.
- Other signs and symptoms include vision deficits, memory loss, poor judgment, personality changes, emotional lability, headache, urinary incontinence or urine retention, and vomiting.

Nursing considerations

- Remain with the patient during the seizure, maintain his safety, and reassure him.
- Give anticonvulsants as prescribed.
- Provide emotional support.
- Monitor for therapeutic drug levels.

Patient teaching

- Teach the patient's family how to record seizures.
- Emphasize the importance of complying with the prescribed drug regimen.
- Provide information on maintaining a safe environment.
- Tell the patient to carry medical identification.

Skin, bronze

The result of excessive circulating melanin, a bronze skin tone tends to appear at pressure points—such as the knuckles, elbows, toes, and knees—and in creases on the palms and soles. Eventually, this hyperpigmentation may extend to the buccal mucosa and gums before covering the entire body. Because bronzing develops gradually, it's sometimes mistaken for a suntan. However, the hyperpigmentation can affect the entire body, not just sun-exposed areas. Sun exposure deepens the bronze color of exposed areas, but this effect fades. In fair-skinned patients, the bronze tone can range from light to dark. The tone also varies with the disorder.

History

- Ask about the onset of bronze skin.
- Determine whether the hue has changed.
- Inquire about the last exposure to the sun or a tanning source.
- Find out about a history of infection, illness, surgery, or trauma.
- Ask about abdominal pain, weakness, fatigue, diarrhea, constipation, or weight loss.
- Ask about the patient's current maintenance therapy for adrenal insufficiency.
- Take a nutritional history.

Physical examination

- Examine the mucosa, gums, and scars for hyperpigmentation.
- Check pressure points—such as the knuckles, elbows, toes, and knees—for color changes.
- Look for signs of dehydration.
- Observe the abdomen for distention.
- Examine the entire body for loss of body hair and tissue and muscle wasting.
- Palpate for hepatosplenomegaly.

Causes

Medical causes

Adrenal hyperplasia

- A dark bronze tone develops within a few months.
- Other signs and symptoms include visual field deficits, headache, signs of masculinization in females—such as clitoral enlargement and male distribution of hair, fat, and muscle mass.

Biliary cirrhosis

- Bronze skin develops on exposed areas of jaundiced skin, including the eyelids, palms, neck, and chest or back.
- Other signs and symptoms include pruritus, weakness, fatigue, jaundice, dark urine, pale stools with steatorrhea, decreased appetite with weight loss, and hepatomegaly.

Hemochromatosis

- An early sign of this disease is progressive, generalized bronzing, accentuated by metallic gray-bronze skin on sun-exposed areas, genitalia, and scars.
- Other early associated effects include weakness, lethargy, weight loss, abdominal pain, loss of libido, polydipsia, and polyuria.

Malnutrition

- Bronzing, apathy, lethargy, anorexia, weakness, and slow pulse and respiratory rates occur.
- Other signs and symptoms include paresthesia in the extremities; dull, sparse, dry hair; brittle nails; dark, swollen cheeks; dry, flaky skin; red, swollen lips; muscle wasting; and gonadal atrophy in males.

Primary adrenal insufficiency

- Bronze skin is a classic sign.
- Other signs and symptoms include axillary and pubic hair loss, vitiligo, progressive fatigue, weakness, anorexia, nausea, vomiting, weight loss, orthostatic hypotension, weak and irregular pulse, abdominal pain, irritability, diarrhea or constipation, amenorrhea, and syncope.

Renal failure, chronic

- The skin becomes pallid, yellowish bronze, dry, and scaly.
- Other signs and symptoms include ammonia breath odor, oliguria, fatigue, decreased mental acuity, seizures, muscle cramps, peripheral neuropathy, bleeding tendencies, pruritus and, occasionally, uremic frost and hypertension.

Wilson's disease

- Kayser-Fleischer rings—rusty brown rings of pigment around the corneas—characterize this disease, which may cause skin bronzing.
- Other signs and symptoms include incoordination, dysarthria, chorea, atax-

ia, muscle spasms and rigidity, abdominal distress, fatigue, personality changes, hypotension, syncope, and seizures.

Other causes

Drugs

- Prolonged therapy with high doses of phenothiazines may cause a gradual bronzing of the skin.

Nursing considerations

- Prepare the patient for diagnostic tests.
- Encourage the patient to discuss concerns about changes in body image.
- If fatigue is a problem, encourage frequent rest periods.

Patient teaching

- Emphasize the importance of rest periods.
- Provide a referral for nutritional counseling, if appropriate.
- Discuss the underlying condition and treatment plan.

Skin, clammy

Clammy skin—moist, cool, and usually pale—is a sympathetic response to stress, which triggers release of the hormones epinephrine and norepinephrine. These hormones cause cutaneous vasoconstriction and secretion of cold sweat from eccrine glands, particularly on the palms, forehead, and soles.

Clammy skin typically accompanies shock, acute hypoglycemia, anxiety reactions, arrhythmias, and heat exhaustion. It also occurs as a vasovagal reaction to severe pain associated with nausea, anorexia, epigastric distress, hyperpnea, tachypnea, weakness, confusion, tachycardia, and pupillary dilation or a combination of these signs and symptoms. Marked bradycardia and syncope may follow.

If you detect clammy skin, remember that rapid evaluation and intervention are paramount. (See *Clammy skin: A key finding,* page 350.)

History

- Ask about a history of type 1 diabetes or cardiac disorder.
- Take a drug history, noting use of an antiarrhythmic.
- Find out about pain, chest pressure, nausea, epigastric distress, weakness, diarrhea, increased urination, or dry mouth.

Physical examination

- Take the patient's vital signs.
- Perform a cardiovascular assessment, and then complete the physical assessment.
- Examine the pupils for dilation.
- Check for abdominal distention.
- Check the blood glucose level.
- Test for increased muscle tension.

Causes

Medical causes

Anxiety

- With anxiety, clammy skin is present on the forehead, palms, and soles.
- Pallor, dry mouth, tachycardia or bradycardia, palpitations, and hypertension or hypotension also occur.
- Other signs and symptoms include possible tremors, breathlessness, headache, muscle tension, nausea, vomiting, abdominal distention, diarrhea, increased urination, and sharp chest pain.

Cardiac arrhythmias

- Generalized clammy skin occurs with mental status changes, dizziness, and hypotension.
- The pulse rate may be rapid, slow, or irregular.
- Other signs and symptoms include palpitations, chest pain, diaphoresis, light-headedness, and weakness.

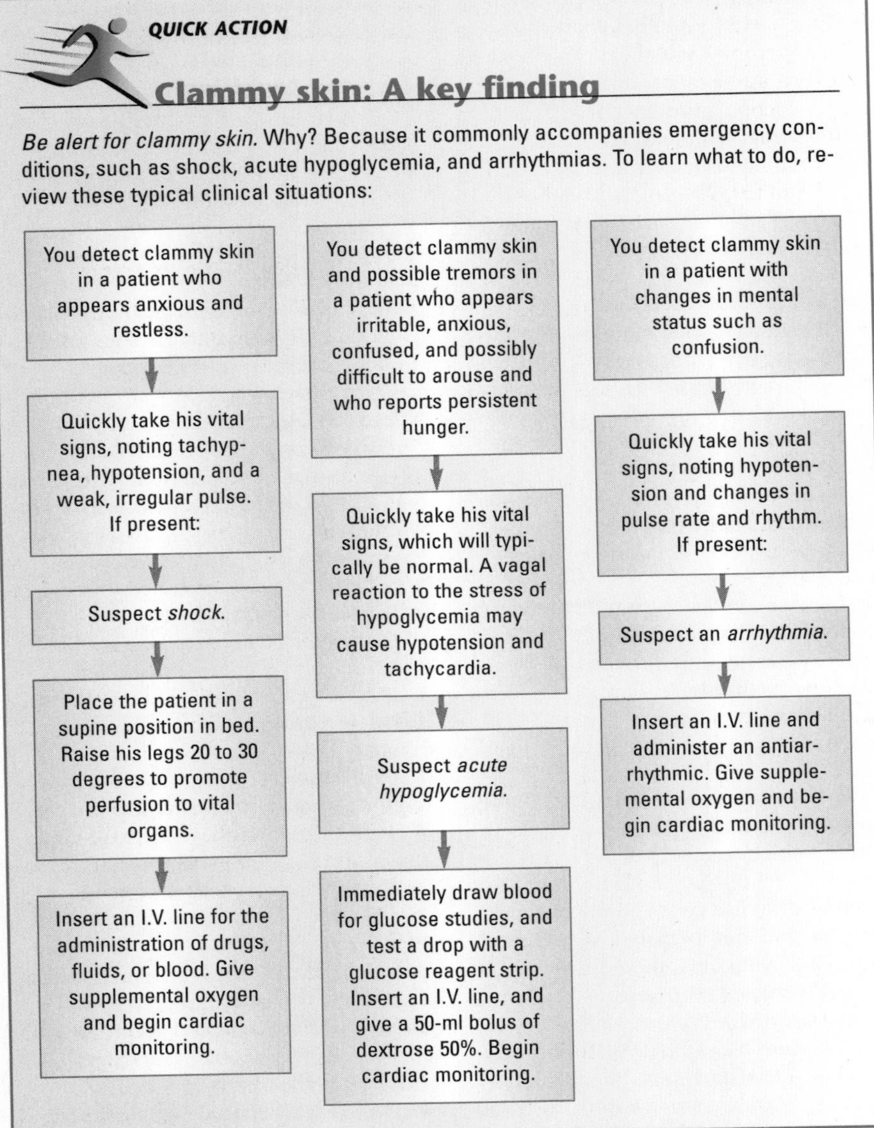

QUICK ACTION
Clammy skin: A key finding
Be alert for clammy skin. Why? Because it commonly accompanies emergency conditions, such as shock, acute hypoglycemia, and arrhythmias. To learn what to do, review these typical clinical situations:
You detect clammy skin in a patient who appears anxious and restless.
Quickly take his vital signs, noting tachypnea, hypotension, and a weak, irregular pulse. If present:
Suspect shock.
Place the patient in a supine position in bed. Raise his legs 20 to 30 degrees to promote perfusion to vital organs.
Insert an I.V. line for the administration of drugs, fluids, or blood. Give supplemental oxygen and begin cardiac monitoring.
You detect clammy skin and possible tremors in a patient who appears irritable, anxious, confused, and possibly difficult to arouse and who reports persistent hunger.
Quickly take his vital signs, which will typically be normal. A vagal reaction to the stress of hypoglycemia may cause hypotension and tachycardia.
Suspect acute hypoglycemia.
Immediately draw blood for glucose studies, and test a drop with a glucose reagent strip. Insert an I.V. line, and give a 50-ml bolus of dextrose 50%. Begin cardiac monitoring.
You detect clammy skin in a patient with changes in mental status such as confusion.
Quickly take his vital signs, noting hypotension and changes in pulse rate and rhythm. If present:
Suspect an arrhythmia.
Insert an I.V. line and administer an antiarrhythmic. Give supplemental oxygen and begin cardiac monitoring.

Cardiogenic shock

■ Generalized clammy skin accompanies confusion, restlessness, hypotension, tachycardia, tachypnea, narrowing pulse pressure, cyanosis, and oliguria.

■ Other signs and symptoms include anginal pain, dyspnea, jugular vein distention, ventricular gallop, and a bounding (early) or weak (late) pulse.

Heat exhaustion

- With mild heat exhaustion, developments include generalized clammy skin, an ashen appearance, headache, confusion, syncope, giddiness and, possibly, a subnormal temperature.
- Other signs and symptoms include a rapid and thready pulse, nausea, vomiting, tachypnea, oliguria, thirst, muscle cramps, and hypotension.

Hypoglycemia, acute

- Generalized cool, clammy skin or diaphoresis may accompany irritability, tremors, palpitations, hunger, headache, tachycardia, and anxiety.
- Central nervous system signs and symptoms include blurred vision, diplopia, confusion, motor weakness, hemiplegia, and coma.

Hypovolemic shock

- Generalized pale, cold, clammy skin accompanies subnormal body temperature, hypotension with narrowing pulse pressure, tachycardia, tachypnea, and a rapid, thready pulse.
- Other signs and symptoms are flat neck veins, increased capillary refill time, decreased urine output, poor skin turgor, confusion, and decreased level of consciousness.

Septic shock

- The cold shock stage of septic shock causes generalized cold, clammy skin.
- Other signs and symptoms include a rapid and thready pulse, severe hypotension, persistent oliguria or anuria, and respiratory failure.

Nursing considerations

- Take the patient's vital signs frequently.
- Monitor urine output.
- Provide measures to correct the underlying cause.
- Give emotional support to the patient and his family.
- Provide frequent skin care and dry bed linens, as appropriate.

Patient teaching

- Explain the underlying illness, diagnostic tests, and treatment options.
- Provide orientation to the intensive care unit, if applicable.

Skin turgor decrease

Skin turgor—the skin's elasticity—is determined by observing the time required for the skin to return to its normal position after being stretched or pinched. With decreased turgor, pinched skin "holds" for up to 30 seconds, and then slowly returns to its normal contour. Skin turgor is commonly assessed over the hand, arm, or sternum—areas normally free from wrinkles and with wide variations in tissue thickness. (See *Evaluating skin turgor,* page 352.)

Decreased skin turgor results from dehydration, or volume depletion, which moves interstitial fluid into the vascular bed to maintain circulating blood volume, leading to slackness in the skin's dermal layer. It's a normal sign in elderly patients and in people who have lost weight rapidly; it also occurs with disorders affecting the GI, renal, endocrine, and other systems.

History

- Ask about food and fluid intake and fluid loss.
- Find out about recent vomiting, diarrhea, draining wounds, fever with sweating, or increased urination.
- Take a drug history, noting the use of diuretics.
- Ask about the use of alcohol.

Physical examination

- Take the patient's vital signs, noting orthostatic hypotension and tachycardia.

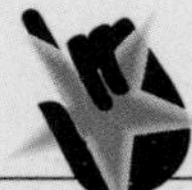

KNOW-HOW

Evaluating skin turgor

To evaluate skin turgor in an adult, pick up a fold of skin over the sternum or the arm, as shown below left. (In an infant, roll a fold of loosely adherent skin on the abdomen between your thumb and forefinger.) Then release it. Normal skin will immediately return to its previous contour. In decreased skin turgor, the skin fold will "hold," or "tent," as shown below right, for up to 30 seconds.

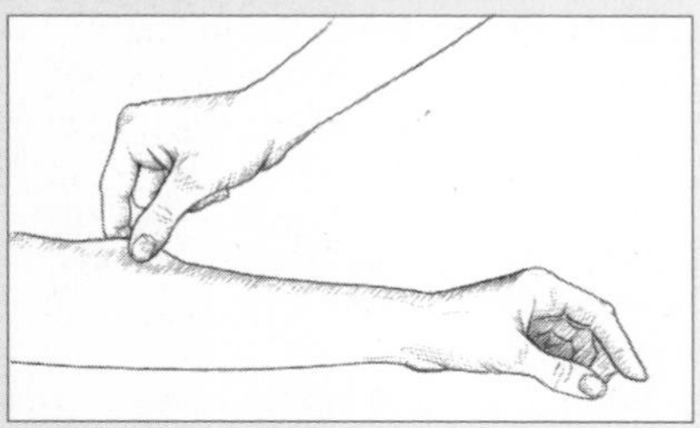

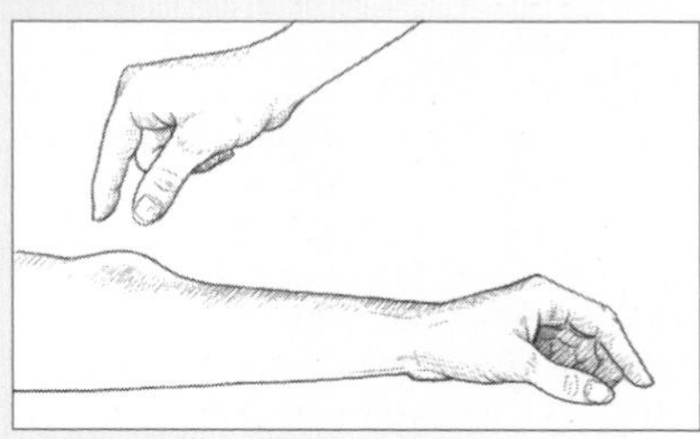

- Evaluate the patient's level of consciousness.
- Inspect the oral mucosa, the furrows of the tongue, and the axillae for dryness.
- Check jugular vein distention.
- Check capillary refill time.

Causes

Medical causes

Cholera

- Abrupt watery diarrhea and vomiting, leading to severe water and electrolyte loss that causes decreased skin turgor, characterize this disorder.
- Other signs and symptoms include intense thirst, weakness, muscle cramps, cyanosis, oliguria, tachycardia, falling blood pressure, fever, and hypoactive bowel sounds.

Dehydration

- Decreased skin turgor occurs with moderate to severe dehydration.
- Other signs and symptoms include dry oral mucosa, decreased perspiration, resting tachycardia, orthostatic hypotension, dry and furrowed tongue, increased thirst, weight loss, oliguria, fever, and fatigue.
- As dehydration worsens, signs and symptoms include enophthalmos, lethargy, weakness, confusion, delirium or obtundation, anuria, and shock.

Nursing considerations

- Monitor intake and output.
- Assess the patient's vital signs.
- Turn the patient every 2 hours to prevent skin breakdown.
- Give I.V. fluid replacement, and frequently offer oral fluids.
- Weigh the patient daily.
- Monitor electrolyte levels.

Patient teaching

- Explain the disorder and treatment.
- Explain fluid replacement and its importance.
- Tell the patient or caregiver which signs and symptoms to report.

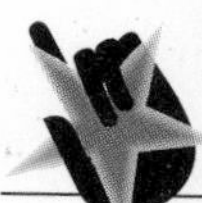

KNOW-HOW

How to palpate for splenomegaly

Detecting splenomegaly requires skillful and gentle palpation to avoid rupturing the enlarged spleen. Follow these steps carefully:

- Place the patient in the supine position and stand at her right side. Place your left hand under the left costovertebral angle and push lightly to move the spleen forward. Then press your right hand gently under the left front costal margin.
- Have the patient take a deep breath and then exhale. As she exhales, move your right hand along the tissue contours under the border of the ribs, feeling for the spleen's edge. The enlarged spleen should feel like a firm mass that bumps against your fingers. Remember to begin palpation low enough in the abdomen to catch the edge of a massive spleen.
- Grade the splenomegaly as slight (½″ to 1½″ [1 to 4 cm] below the costal margin), moderate (1½″ to 3″ [4 to 8 cm] below the costal margin), or great (3″ or more below the costal margin).
- Reposition the patient on her right side, with her hips and knees flexed slightly to move the spleen forward. Then repeat the palpation procedure.

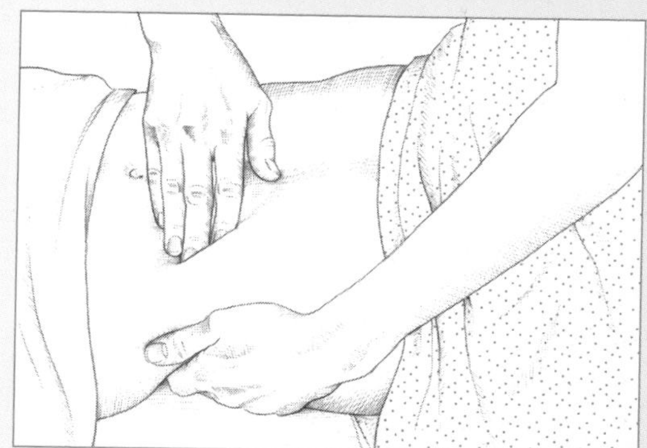

Splenomegaly

Because it occurs with various disorders and in up to 5% of normal adults, splenomegaly—an enlarged spleen—isn't a diagnostic sign by itself. Usually, however, it points to infection, trauma, or a hepatic, autoimmune, neoplastic, or hematologic disorder.

Because the spleen functions as the body's largest lymph node, splenomegaly can result from any process that triggers lymphadenopathy. For example, it may reflect reactive hyperplasia (a response to infection or inflammation), proliferation or infiltration of neoplastic cells, extramedullary hematopoiesis, phagocytic cell proliferation, increased blood cell destruction, or vascular congestion associated with portal hypertension.

Splenomegaly may be detected by light palpation under the left costal margin. (See *How to palpate for splenomegaly.*) However, because this technique isn't always advisable or effective, splenomegaly may need to be confirmed by a computed tomography or radionuclide scan.

QUICK ACTION ***If the patient has a history of abdominal or thoracic trauma, don't palpate the abdomen because this may aggravate internal bleeding. Instead, examine him for left upper quadrant pain and signs of shock, such as tachycardia and tachypnea. If these are present, suspect splenic rup-***

ture. Insert an I.V. catheter for emergency fluid and blood replacement, and give oxygen. Also, catheterize the patient to evaluate urine output, and begin cardiac monitoring. Prepare the patient for possible surgery.

History

- Inquire about fatigue; frequent colds, sore throats, or other infections; bruising; left upper quadrant pain; abdominal fullness; and early satiety.
- Obtain a complete medical history.
- Ask about recent trauma or surgery.

Physical examination

- Complete an abdominal assessment.
- Examine the skin for pallor and ecchymoses.
- Palpate the axillae, groin, and neck for lymphadenopathy.

Causes

Medical causes

Amyloidosis

- Marked splenomegaly may occur with this disorder from excessive protein deposits in the spleen.
- Associated signs and symptoms vary, depending on what organs are involved.

Cirrhosis

- Moderate to severe splenomegaly occurs with advanced cirrhosis.
- Late signs also include jaundice, hepatomegaly, leg edema, hematemesis, and ascites.
- Signs of hepatic encephalopathy may also occur, such as asterixis, fetor hepaticus, slurred speech, and decreased level of consciousness that may progress to coma.
- Other signs and symptoms include jaundice, pruritus, bleeding tendencies, menstrual irregularities or testicular atrophy, gynecomastia, and right upper abdominal pain.

Endocarditis, subacute infective

- The spleen is enlarged but nontender in this disorder.
- A suddenly changing murmur or the discovery of a new murmur in the presence of a fever is a classic sign.
- Other signs and symptoms include anorexia, pallor, weakness, fever, night sweats, fatigue, tachycardia, weight loss, arthralgia, petechiae, hematuria, Osler's nodes, and Janeway lesions.

Felty's syndrome

- Splenomegaly is characteristic of Felty's syndrome.
- Associated signs and symptoms are joint pain and deformity, sensory or motor loss, rheumatoid nodules, palmar erythema, lymphadenopathy, and leg ulcers.

Hepatitis

- Splenomegaly may occur with hepatitis.
- Characteristic signs and symptoms include dark urine, clay-colored stools, anorexia, malaise, pruritus, hepatomegaly, vomiting, jaundice, and fatigue.

Histoplasmosis

- Splenomegaly and hepatomegaly occur with this disorder.
- Other signs and symptoms include lymphadenopathy, jaundice, fever, anorexia, and signs and symptoms of anemia.

Hypersplenism, primary

- Splenomegaly accompanies anemia, neutropenia, or thrombocytopenia.
- Left-sided abdominal pain may occur.
- With anemia, symptoms include weakness, fatigue, malaise, and pallor.
- With severe neutropenia, signs include frequent infections.
- With thrombocytopenia, easy bruising or spontaneous, widespread hemorrhage may occur.

Leukemia

- Moderate to severe splenomegaly is an early sign of leukemia.
- With chronic granulocytic leukemia, signs and symptoms include hepatomegaly, lymphadenopathy, fatigue, malaise, pallor, fever, gum swelling, bleeding tendencies, weight loss, anorexia, and abdominal, bone, and joint pain.
- Acute leukemia may produce dyspnea, tachycardia, and palpitations.

Lymphoma

- Moderate to massive splenomegaly is a late sign of lymphoma.
- Other late signs and symptoms include hepatomegaly, painless lymphadenopathy, night sweats, fever, fatigue, weight loss, malaise, and scaly dermatitis with pruritus.

Mononucleosis, infectious

- Splenomegaly, a common sign, is most pronounced during the second and third weeks of illness.
- The triad includes sore throat, cervical lymphadenopathy, and fluctuating temperature with an evening peak.
- Hepatomegaly, jaundice, and a maculopapular rash may also develop.

Pancreatic cancer

- Moderate to severe splenomegaly may occur if a tumor compresses the splenic vein.
- Other characteristic signs and symptoms include abdominal or back pain, anorexia, nausea, vomiting, weight loss, GI bleeding, jaundice, pruritus, skin lesions, emotional lability, weakness, and fatigue.

Polycythemia vera

- An enlarged spleen, resulting in easy satiety, abdominal fullness, and left upper quadrant abdominal pain or pleuritic chest pain, occur late in the disease.
- Also occurring with polycythemia vera are finger and toe paresthesia, impaired mentation, tinnitus, blurred or double vision, scotoma, increased blood pressure, pruritus, epigastric distress, weight loss, hepatomegaly, bleeding tendencies, and intermittent claudication.
- Other possible signs and symptoms include deep purplish red oral mucous membranes, headache, dyspnea, dizziness, vertigo, weakness, and fatigue.

Splenic rupture

- Splenomegaly may result from massive abdominal or thoracic hemorrhage that predisposes the spleen to rupture.
- Left upper quadrant pain, abdominal rigidity, Kehr's sign, and signs of shock may also be present.

Thrombotic thrombocytopenic purpura

- This disorder may produce splenomegaly and hepatomegaly.
- Accompanying signs and symptoms include fever, generalized purpura, jaundice, pallor, vaginal bleeding, hematuria, fatigue, weakness, headache, abdominal pain, and arthralgia.
- Eventually the patient develops signs of neurologic deterioration and renal failure.

Nursing considerations

- Monitor the patient's vital signs and blood count.
- Prepare the patient for diagnostic tests.
- Provide measures to treat the underlying disorder.

Patient teaching

- Instruct the patient to avoid infection.
- Emphasize the importance of complying with drug therapy.
- Teach the patient about the underlying diagnosis and treatment plan.

Stools, clay-colored

Pale, putty-colored stools usually result from hepatic, gallbladder, or pancreatic disorders. Normally, bile pigments give stools their characteristic brown color. However, hepatocellular degeneration or biliary obstruction may interfere with the formation or release of these pigments into the intestine, resulting in clay-colored stools. These stools are commonly associated with jaundice and dark "cola-colored" urine.

History

- Ask about the onset of clay-colored stools.
- Explore associated abdominal or back pain, nausea and vomiting, fatigue, anorexia, weight loss, and dark urine.
- Inquire about difficulty digesting fatty foods or heavy meals.
- Note whether the patient bruises easily.
- Take a medical history, noting gallbladder, hepatic, or pancreatic disorders.
- Ask about recent barium studies or use of antacids.
- Note a history of alcoholism.
- Find out about exposure to toxic substances.

Physical examination

- Take the patient's vital signs.
- Check for jaundice.
- Inspect the abdomen for distention and ascites.
- Auscultate for hypoactive bowel sounds.
- Percuss and palpate for masses and rebound tenderness.

Causes

Medical causes

Bile duct cancer

- Clay-colored stools may be accompanied by jaundice, pruritus, anorexia, weight loss, bleeding tendencies, and a palpable mass in bile duct cancer.
- Pain may develop in the epigastrium or right upper quadrant.

Biliary cirrhosis

- Clay-colored stools typically follow unexplained pruritus that worsens at bedtime, weakness, fatigue, weight loss, and vague abdominal pain.
- Other signs and symptoms include jaundice; hyperpigmentation; signs of malabsorption; bone and back pain; hematemesis; ascites; edema; firm, nontender hepatomegaly; and xanthomas on the palms, soles, and elbows.

Cholangitis, sclerosing

- Clay-colored stools, chronic or intermittent jaundice, pruritus, right upper quadrant pain, weakness, fatigue, chills, and fever occur.

Cholelithiasis

- Obstruction of the common bile duct may result in clay-colored stools.
- Associated symptoms include dyspepsia and biliary colic.
- Right upper quadrant pain intensifies over several hours, may radiate to the epigastrium or shoulder blades, and is relieved by antacids.
- Pain is accompanied by tachycardia, restlessness, nausea, intolerance to certain foods, vomiting, upper abdominal tenderness, fever, chills, and jaundice.

Hepatic cancer

- Weight loss, weakness, and anorexia precede clay-colored stools in hepatic cancer.
- Later, nodular, firm hepatomegaly; jaundice; right upper quadrant pain; ascites; dependent edema; and fever develop.

Hepatitis

- Clay-colored stools signal the start of the icteric phase of hepatitis.
- Associated signs include mild weight loss, dark urine, anorexia, jaundice, and tender hepatomegaly.
- Signs and symptoms during the icteric phase include irritability, right upper quadrant pain, splenomegaly, enlarged cervical lymph nodes, and severe pruritus.

Pancreatic cancer

- Common bile duct obstruction may cause clay-colored stools in pancreatic cancer.
- Classic signs and symptoms associated with this disease include abdominal or back pain, jaundice, pruritus, nausea and vomiting, anorexia, weight loss, fatigue, weakness, and fever.
- Other signs and symptoms include diarrhea, skin lesions, emotional lability, splenomegaly, and signs of GI bleeding.

Pancreatitis, acute

- With acute pancreatitis, there may be clay-colored stools, dark urine, jaundice, and severe epigastric pain aggravated by lying down.
- Other signs and symptoms include nausea, vomiting, fever, abdominal rigidity and tenderness, hypoactive bowel sounds, and crackles at the lung bases.

Other causes

Surgery

- Biliary surgery may cause bile duct stricture, resulting in clay-colored stools.

Nursing considerations

- Prepare the patient for diagnostic tests.
- Encourage rest periods.
- Give analgesics, as prescribed.
- Give vaccines for hepatitis A and B as ordered.

Patient teaching

- Discuss the underlying disorder and treatment options.
- Explain ways to reduce abdominal pain.
- Discuss the dietary modifications the patient needs.
- Stress the need for a restful environment.
- Emphasize the importance of avoiding alcohol.

Stridor

A loud, harsh, musical respiratory sound, stridor results from a partial to near complete obstruction of the trachea or larynx. Usually heard during inspiration, this sign may also occur during expiration in severe upper airway obstruction. It may begin as low-pitched "croaking" and progress to high-pitched "crowing" as respirations become more vigorous.

Life-threatening upper airway obstruction can stem from foreign-body aspiration, increased secretions, an intraluminal tumor, localized edema or muscle spasms, and external compression by a tumor or aneurysm.

QUICK ACTION ***If you hear stridor, quickly check the patient's vital signs, including oxygen saturation. Also examine him for other signs of partial airway obstruction: choking or gagging, tachypnea, dyspnea, shallow respirations, intercostal retractions, nasal flaring, tachycardia, cyanosis, and diaphoresis. Be aware that abrupt cessation of stridor signals complete obstruction, meaning that the patient has inspiratory chest movement but absent breath sounds. Unable to talk, he quickly becomes lethargic and loses consciousness.***

If you detect signs of airway obstruction, try to clear the airway with back blows or abdominal thrusts. Next, give oxygen by nasal cannula or face mask, or prepare the patient for emergency endotracheal (ET) intubation or tracheostomy and mechanical ventilation. Have equipment ready to suction aspirated vomitus or blood through the ET or tracheostomy tube. Connect the patient to a cardiac monitor, and position him in Fowler's position to ease his breathing.

History

- Ask about the onset of stridor.
- Inquire about previous instances of stridor.
- Note any current respiratory tract infection.
- Ask about a history of allergies, tumors, or respiratory and vascular disorders.
- Note recent exposure to smoke or noxious fumes or gases.
- Inquire about associated pain or cough.

Physical examination

- Examine the mouth for excessive secretions, foreign matter, inflammation, and swelling.
- Assess the neck for swelling, masses, subcutaneous crepitation, and scars.
- Observe the chest for decreased or asymmetrical expansion.
- Auscultate for wheezes, rhonchi, crackles, rubs, and other abnormal breath sounds.
- Percuss for dullness, tympany, or flatness.
- Note burns or signs of trauma.

Causes

Medical causes

Airway trauma

- Acute airway obstruction is common and results in the sudden onset of stridor.
- Other signs and symptoms include dysphonia, dysphagia, hemoptysis, cyanosis, accessory muscle use, intercostal retractions, nasal flaring, tachypnea, progressive dyspnea, and shallow respirations.

Anaphylaxis

- Upper airway edema and laryngospasm cause stridor and other signs of respiratory distress.
- Typically, these respiratory effects are preceded by a feeling of impending doom or fear, weakness, diaphoresis, sneezing, nasal pruritus, urticaria, erythema, and angioedema.
- Other common signs and symptoms include chest or throat tightness, dysphagia and, possibly, signs of shock.

Anthrax, inhalation

- The second stage develops abruptly with rapid deterioration marked by stridor, fever, dyspnea, and hypotension generally leading to death within 24 hours.
- Initial signs and symptoms include fever, chills, weakness, cough, and chest pain.

Aspiration of foreign body

- Sudden stridor is characteristic in this life-threatening situation.
- Other signs and symptoms include the abrupt onset of dry, paroxysmal coughing, gagging, or choking; hoarseness; tachycardia; wheezing; dyspnea; tachypnea; intercostal muscle retractions; diminished breath sounds; cyanosis; anxiety; and shallow respirations.

Epiglottiditis

- Stridor, caused by an erythematous, edematous epiglottis that obstructs the upper airway, occurs along with fever, sore throat, and a croupy cough in this life-threatening situation.

■ Other signs and symptoms include cough that may progress to severe respiratory distress with sternal and intercostal retractions, nasal flaring, cyanosis, and tachycardia.

Hypocalcemia

■ Laryngospasm can cause stridor in hypocalcemia.

■ Other signs and symptoms include paresthesia, carpopedal spasm, hyperactive deep tendon reflexes, muscle twitching and cramping, and positive Chvostek's and Trousseau's signs.

Inhalation injury

■ Laryngeal edema and bronchospasms, resulting in stridor, may develop within 48 hours after the inhalation of smoke or noxious fumes.

■ Other signs and symptoms include singed nasal hairs, orofacial burns, coughing, hoarseness, sooty sputum, crackles, rhonchi, wheezes, dyspnea, accessory muscle use, intercostal retractions, and nasal flaring.

Laryngeal tumor

■ This type of tumor is a late sign, occurring with possible dysphagia, dyspnea, enlarged cervical nodes, and pain that radiates to the ear.

■ Laryngeal tumor is preceded by hoarseness, minor throat pain, and a mild, dry cough.

Laryngitis, acute

■ Severe laryngeal edema, resulting in stridor and dyspnea, may occur.

■ Mild to severe hoarseness is the chief sign.

■ Other signs and symptoms include sore throat, dysphagia, dry cough, malaise, and fever.

Mediastinal tumor

■ Compression of the trachea and bronchi results in stridor.

■ Other signs and symptoms include hoarseness, brassy cough, tracheal shift or tug, dilated neck veins, swelling of the face and neck, stertorous respirations, dyspnea, dysphagia, suprasternal retractions on inspiration, and pain in the chest, shoulder, or arm.

Thoracic aortic aneurysm

■ If the trachea is compressed, stridor, dyspnea, wheezing, and a brassy cough may result.

■ Other signs and symptoms include hoarseness or complete voice loss, dysphagia, jugular vein distention, prominent chest veins, tracheal tug, paresthesia or neuralgia, and edema of the face, neck, and arms.

Other causes

Diagnostic tests

■ Bronchoscopy or laryngoscopy may precipitate laryngospasm and stridor due to airway irritation.

Treatments

■ Neck surgery, such as thyroidectomy, may cause laryngeal paralysis and stridor.

■ After prolonged intubation, the patient may exhibit laryngeal edema and stridor when the tube is removed.

Nursing considerations

■ Continue to monitor the patient's vital signs and oxygen saturation, and watch for signs of respiratory distress.

■ Prepare the patient for diagnostic tests.

■ Offer reassurance and calm the patient.

■ Give antibiotics and respiratory treatments as ordered.

Patient teaching

■ Explain all procedures and treatments.

■ Teach about the underlying diagnosis.

Syncope

A common neurologic sign, syncope (or *fainting*) refers to a transient loss of consciousness associated with impaired cerebral blood supply or cerebral hypoxia. It usually occurs abruptly and lasts for seconds to minutes. An episode of syncope usually starts as a feeling of light-headedness. A patient can usually prevent an episode of syncope by lying down or sitting with his head between his knees. Typically, the patient lies motionless with his skeletal muscles relaxed but sphincter muscles controlled. However, the depth of unconsciousness varies—some patients can hear voices or see blurred outlines; others are unaware of their surroundings.

In many ways, syncope simulates death: The patient is strikingly pale with a slow, weak pulse, hypotension, and almost imperceptible breathing. If severe hypotension lasts for 20 seconds or longer, the patient may also develop convulsive, tonic-clonic movements.

Syncope may result from cardiac and cerebrovascular disorders, hypoxemia, and postural changes in the presence of autonomic dysfunction. It may also follow vigorous coughing (tussive syncope) and emotional stress, injury, shock, or pain (vasovagal syncope, or common fainting). Hysterical syncope may also follow emotional stress but isn't accompanied by other vasodepressor effects.

QUICK ACTION ***If you see a patient experience syncope, ensure a patent airway and the patient's safety, and take his vital signs. Then place the patient in a supine position, elevate his legs, and loosen tight clothing. Be alert for tachycardia, bradycardia, or an irregular pulse. Meanwhile, place him on a cardiac monitor to detect arrhythmias. If an arrhythmia appears, give oxygen and insert an I.V. catheter for medication or fluid administration. Be ready to begin cardiopulmonary resuscitation. Cardioversion, defibrillation, or insertion of a temporary pacemaker may be required.***

History

- Obtain a description of the syncopal episode and its duration.
- Inquire about precipitating factors.
- Ask about preceding symptoms, including weakness, light-headedness, nausea, or diaphoresis.
- Ask about associated headache.
- Obtain a history of previous syncope.

Physical examination

- Take the patient's vital signs.
- Examine the patient for any injuries from falling during syncope.
- Perform a complete cardiac and neurologic assessment.

Causes

Medical causes

Aortic arch syndrome

- Syncope may be accompanied by weak or abruptly absent carotid pulses and unequal or absent radial pulses.
- Early signs and symptoms include night sweats, pallor, nausea, anorexia, weight loss, arthralgia, and Raynaud's phenomenon.
- Other signs and symptoms include hypotension in the arms; neck, shoulder, and chest pain; paresthesia; intermittent claudication; bruits; vision disturbances; and dizziness.

Aortic stenosis

- A classic late sign, syncope is accompanied by exertional dyspnea and angina.
- Fatigue, orthopnea, paroxysmal nocturnal dyspnea, palpitations, atrial and ventricular gallops, and diminished carotid pulses occur.

■ A harsh, crescendo-decrescendo systolic ejection murmur may be heard; it will be loudest at the right sternal border of the second intercostal space.

Cardiac arrhythmias
■ Decreased cardiac output and impaired cerebral circulation may cause syncope.

Carotid sinus hypersensitivity
■ Syncope is triggered by compression of the carotid sinus.
■ Early signs and symptoms include palpitations, pallor, confusion, diaphoresis, dyspnea, and hypotension.
■ Syncope may develop without warning in Stokes-Adams syndrome; asystole during syncope may precipitate spasm and myoclonic jerks if prolonged.

Hypoxemia
■ Syncope, confusion, tachycardia, restlessness, tachypnea, dyspnea, cyanosis, and incoordination may occur.

Orthostatic hypotension
■ Syncope occurs when the patient rises quickly from a recumbent position.
■ Other signs and symptoms include tachycardia, pallor, dizziness, blurred vision, nausea, and diaphoresis.

Transient ischemic attack
■ Syncope and decreased level of consciousness may result.
■ Other signs and symptoms vary with the affected artery but may include vision loss, nystagmus, aphasia, dysarthria, unilateral numbness, hemiparesis or hemiplegia, tinnitus, facial weakness, dysphagia, and staggering or uncoordinated gait.

Vagal glossopharyngeal neuralgia
■ Localized pressure may trigger pain in the base of the tongue, pharynx, larynx, tonsils, and ear, resulting in syncope.

Other causes

Diagnostic tests
■ Tilt-table tests cause syncope to help identify a cardiogenic source of the symptom.

Drugs
■ Occasionally, griseofulvin (Grisactin), indomethacin (Indocin), and levodopa (Sinemet) can produce syncope.
■ Prazosin (Minipress) may cause severe orthostatic hypotension and syncope, usually after the first dose.
■ Other medications that cause orthostatic hypotension include antihypertensives, diuretics, levodopa (Sinemet), monamine oxidase inhibitors, morphine, nitrates, phenothiazines, spinal anesthesia, and tricyclic antidepressants.
■ Quinidine (Quinidex) may cause syncope—and possibly death—associated with ventricular fibrillation.

Nursing considerations
■ Continue to monitor the patient's vital signs, oxygenation, and heart rhythm, as appropriate.
■ Prepare the patient for diagnostic studies.

Patient teaching
■ Discuss the underlying condition.
■ Encourage the patient to pace his activities.
■ Explain that the patient should avoid standing for prolonged periods and that he should make position changes slowly.
■ Tell the patient what measures to take if he's feeling faint.
■ Discuss medications and their adverse effects.

T

Tachycardia

Easily detected by counting the apical, carotid, or radial pulse, tachycardia is a heart rate greater than 100 beats/minute. The patient with tachycardia usually complains of palpitations or a "racing" heart. Tachycardia normally occurs in response to emotional or physical stress, such as excitement, exercise, pain, anxiety, and fever. It may also result from the use of stimulants, such as caffeine and tobacco. However, tachycardia may be an early sign of a life-threatening disorder, such as cardiogenic, hypovolemic, or septic shock. It also may result from a cardiovascular, respiratory, or metabolic disorder or from the effects of certain drugs, tests, or treatments.

QUICK ACTION ***After detecting tachycardia, take the patient's other vital signs and determine his level of consciousness (LOC). If the patient has increased or decreased blood pressure and is drowsy or confused, give oxygen and begin cardiac monitoring. Perform an electrocardiogram (ECG) to examine for reduced cardiac output, which may initiate or result from tachycardia. Insert an I.V. catheter for fluid, blood product, and drug administration, and gather emergency resuscitation equipment.***

History

- Explore palpitations, dizziness, shortness of breath, weakness, fatigue, syncope, and chest pain.
- Ask about a history of trauma, diabetes, and cardiac, pulmonary, or thyroid disorders.
- Obtain an alcohol and drug history.

Physical examination

- Inspect for pallor or cyanosis.
- Assess pulses and blood pressure and note peripheral edema.
- Auscultate the heart and lungs for abnormal sounds and rhythms.

Causes

Medical causes

Acute respiratory distress syndrome

- Tachycardia, crackles, rhonchi, dyspnea, tachypnea, nasal flaring, and grunting respirations occur with this disorder.
- Other signs and symptoms include cyanosis, anxiety, and decreased LOC.

Adrenocortical insufficiency

- A rapid, weak pulse with progressive weakness and fatigue occur.
- Other signs and symptoms include abdominal pain, nausea, vomiting, altered bowel habits, weight loss, orthostatic hypotension, irritability, bronze skin, decreased libido, and syncope.

Anemia

■ Tachycardia and bounding pulse occur with anemia.
■ Related signs and symptoms include fatigue, pallor, dyspnea, bleeding tendencies, atrial gallop, crackles, and a systolic bruit over the carotid arteries.

Anxiety

■ Tachycardia, tachypnea, chest pain, cold and clammy skin, dry mouth, nausea, and light-headedness are signs and symptoms of anxiety.

Aortic insufficiency

■ Tachycardia with a bounding pulse and a large, diffuse apical heave occurs with aortic insufficiency.
■ A high-pitched, blowing diastolic murmur starting with S_2 occurs.
■ Other signs and symptoms include angina, dyspnea, palpitations, strong and abrupt carotid pulsations, pallor, syncope, and signs of heart failure.

Aortic stenosis

■ Tachycardia, a weak and thready pulse, and an atrial gallop occur with aortic stenosis.
■ Chiefly, dyspnea, angina, dizziness, and syncope occur.
■ Other signs and symptoms include palpitations, crackles, fatigue, a harsh systolic ejection murmur, and signs of heart failure or pulmonary edema.

Cardiac arrhythmias

■ Tachycardia with hypotension, dizziness, palpitations, weakness, and fatigue occur with cardiac arrhythmias.
■ Related signs and symptoms include tachypnea, decreased LOC, and pale, cool, clammy skin.

Cardiac contusion

■ With a cardiac contusion, tachycardia, substernal pain, dyspnea, hypotension, palpitations, sternal ecchymoses, and a pericardial rub or tamponade occur.

Cardiac tamponade

■ A life-threatening disorder, cardiac tamponade causes tachycardia commonly with paradoxical pulse, dyspnea, and tachypnea.
■ Other signs and symptoms include anxiety, cyanosis, clammy skin, hypotension, jugular vein distention, narrowed pulse pressure, pericardial rub, muffled heart sounds, chest pain, and hepatomegaly.

Chronic obstructive pulmonary disease

■ Tachycardia with cough, tachypnea, pursed-lip breathing, accessory muscle use, cyanosis, diminished breath sounds, rhonchi, crackles, wheezing and, in late stages, barrel chest and clubbing occur in this disorder.

Diabetic ketoacidosis

■ A rapid, thready pulse with Kussmaul's respirations is the cardinal sign of this disorder.
■ Other signs and symptoms include decreased LOC, dehydration, and oliguria with ketosis.

Febrile illness

■ Fever can cause tachycardia, chills, diaphoresis, headache, and weakness.

Heart failure

■ Tachycardia occurs, along with a ventricular gallop, fatigue, dyspnea, orthopnea, and leg edema.

Hyperosmolar hyperglycemic nonketotic syndrome

■ This syndrome causes a rapidly deteriorating LOC with tachycardia, hypotension, tachypnea, seizures, oliguria without ketosis, and severe dehydration.

Hypertensive crisis

- A life-threatening disorder, hypertensive crisis causes tachycardia with diastolic blood pressure over 120 mm Hg and systolic blood pressure that may exceed 200 mm Hg.
- Related signs and symptoms include tachypnea, signs of pulmonary edema, chest pain, oliguria, severe headache, confusion, anxiety, tinnitus, epistaxis, muscle twitching, seizures, nausea, vomiting, and progressive loss of consciousness.

Hypoglycemia

- Tachycardia with nervousness, mental confusion, weakness, headache, hunger, nausea, diaphoresis, and moist, clammy skin occur with hypoglycemia.

Hypovolemia

- With hypovolemia, tachycardia with hypotension, decreased urine output, fatigue, muscle weakness, decreased skin turgor, sunken eyeballs, thirst, syncope, and dry skin and tongue occur.

Hypoxemia

- Tachycardia with dyspnea, tachypnea, and cyanosis occur with hypoxemia.
- Other signs and symptoms include confusion, restlessness, and disorientation progressing to coma.

Myocardial infarction

- This life-threatening disorder causes tachycardia or bradycardia with crushing substernal chest pain that may radiate to the left arm, jaw, neck, or shoulder.
- Related signs and symptoms include pallor, clammy skin, dyspnea, diaphoresis, atrial gallop, a new murmur, crackles, nausea, vomiting, anxiety, restlessness, and increased or decreased blood pressure.

Orthostatic hypotension

- Tachycardia with dizziness, syncope, pallor, blurred vision, diaphoresis, and nausea occur with this disorder.
- Dim vision, spots before the eyes, and signs of dehydration may also occur.

Pneumothorax

- Pneumothorax is a life-threatening disorder that causes tachycardia and other signs and symptoms of distress, such as severe dyspnea and chest pain, tachypnea, and cyanosis.
- Other signs and symptoms include dry cough, subcutaneous crepitation, absent or decreased breath sounds, reduced or absent chest movement on the affected side, and decreased vocal fremitus.

Pulmonary embolism

- Tachycardia preceded by sudden dyspnea, angina, or pleuritic chest pain occurs with a pulmonary embolism.
- Weak peripheral pulse, tachypnea, low-grade fever, restlessness, diaphoresis, and a dry cough or a cough with blood-tinged sputum may also occur. (See *Responding to tachycardia.*)

Shock

- When the patient is in shock, he may experience tachycardia, tachypnea, skin temperature changes, hypotension, apprehension, and decreased LOC before cardiac collapse.
- Whether the source is anaphylactic, cardiac, hypovolemic, neurologic, or septic, shock can be a life-threatening disorder.

Thyrotoxicosis

- Classic signs and symptoms include tachycardia, an enlarged thyroid, nervousness, heat intolerance, weight loss despite increased appetite, diaphoresis, tremors, palpitations and, possibly, exophthalmos.

CASE CLIP

Responding to tachycardia

Mr. R. is a 63-year-old male who underwent a right total hip replacement 3 days ago and is recovering on the orthopedic unit. His medical history includes venous insufficiency, type 2 diabetes mellitus, and a history of smoking 1½ packs of cigarettes per day for the past 37 years. His surgery went well with no complications, and he's scheduled for transfer to the rehabilitation unit tomorrow. However, he's been refusing to wear his antiembolism stockings and perform his incentive spirometry, as directed, and, on occasion, to participate in physical therapy. His vital signs have been stable thus far. He has strong dorsalis pedis and posterior tibial pulses, but delayed capillary refill times of 5 to 6 seconds on the right side of his body.

This morning, Mr. R. continues to complain of fatigue and shortness of breath. His vital signs are:

- heart rate (HR): 92 beats/minute
- respiratory rate (RR): 24 breaths/minute
- blood pressure (BP): 146/78 mm Hg
- oxygen saturation: 91% on room air.

The nurse administers oxygen at 2 L/minute via nasal cannula. His breath sounds are diminished bilaterally, but no adventitious sounds are heard.

Later that evening, Mr. R.'s call light goes on. The nurse finds him sitting upright in bed clutching his chest. He's agitated, breathing heavily, and profusely diaphoretic; his color is dusky, and his nail beds are cyanotic. He's extremely restless. He says he's very anxious and short of breath. He keeps repeating, "something is wrong," and he's afraid he's going to die. His vital signs are:

- HR: 132 beats/minute
- RR: 40 breaths/minute
- BP: 178/92 mm Hg
- oxygen saturation: 86% on 2 L/minute of oxygen.

Given this remarkable change in his condition, the nurse activates the Rapid Response Team (RRT) and increases his nasal oxygen to 4 L/minute after auscultation reveals that breath sounds are absent on the right and faint on the left.

The RRT arrives within 3 minutes and initiates the following orders:

- 12-lead electrocardiogram (ECG)
- portable chest X-ray
- arterial blood gas and multiple laboratory tests.

The 12-lead ECG reveals sinus tachycardia at a rate of 140 beats/minute. The portable chest X-ray is inconclusive. Mr. R. remains in severe respiratory distress and his condition continues to deteriorate. Based on his symptoms and medical background, the team suspects a possible pulmonary embolus and orders a stat ventilation-perfusion scan, which confirms their diagnosis. Mr. R. is immediately transferred to the operating room for evacuation of the embolus.

Other causes

Diagnostic tests

- Cardiac catheterization and electrophysiologic studies may induce transient tachycardia.

Drugs and alcohol

- Acetylcholinesterase inhibitors, alpha blockers, anticholinergics, beta-adrenergic bronchodilators, nitrates, phenothiazines, sympathomimetics, and vasodilators may cause tachycardia.

■ Excessive caffeine intake and alcohol intoxication may also cause tachycardia.

Surgery and pacemakers

■ Cardiac surgery and pacemaker malfunction or wire irritation may cause tachycardia.

Nursing considerations

■ Continue to monitor the patient's cardiovascular status and vital signs.
■ Explain the ordered diagnostic tests to the patient.
■ Obtain a resting 12-lead ECG.
■ Give medications or fluids to control the heart rate.

Patient teaching

■ Explain the possibility of tachyarrhythmia recurrence and signs and symptoms to report.
■ Discuss the use of antiarrhythmics, pacemaker, internal defibrillator, or ablation therapy.
■ Teach the patient about the underlying diagnosis and treatment plan.
■ Teach the patient how to take his pulse.

Tachypnea

A common sign of cardiopulmonary disorders, tachypnea is an abnormally fast respiratory rate—greater than 20 breaths/minute. Tachypnea may reflect the need to increase minute volume—the amount of air breathed each minute. Under these circumstances, it may be accompanied by an increase in tidal volume—the volume of air inhaled or exhaled per breath—resulting in hyperventilation. Tachypnea, however, may also reflect stiff lungs or overloaded ventilatory muscles, in which case tidal volume may actually be reduced.

Tachypnea may result from reduced arterial oxygen tension or arterial oxygen content, decreased perfusion, or increased oxygen demand. The latter may be caused by fever, exertion, anxiety, and pain. Heightened oxygen demand may also occur as a compensatory response to metabolic acidosis or may result from pulmonary irritation, stretch receptor stimulation, or a neurologic disorder that upsets medullary respiratory control.

QUICK ACTION ***After detecting tachypnea, quickly evaluate the patient's cardiopulmonary status; take his vital signs with oxygen saturation; and check for cyanosis, chest pain, dyspnea, tachycardia, and hypotension. If the patient has paradoxical chest movement, suspect flail chest and immediately splint his chest with your hands or with sandbags. Then give supplemental oxygen by nasal cannula or face mask and, if possible, place him in semi-Fowler's position to help ease his breathing. Endotracheal intubation and mechanical ventilation may be necessary if respiratory failure occurs. Also, insert an I.V. catheter for fluid and drug administration and begin cardiac monitoring.***

History

■ Ask about the onset, precipitating factors, and how the patient experiences tachypnea.
■ Inquire about a history of pulmonary or cardiac conditions or anxiety attacks.
■ Find out about other signs and symptoms, such as diaphoresis, chest pain, or recent weight loss.
■ Take a drug history.

Physical examination

■ Take the patient's vital signs, including oxygen saturation. (See *Differential diagnosis: Tachypnea,* pages 368 and 369.)
■ Auscultate the chest for abnormal heart and breath sounds.

■ Record the color, amount, and consistency of sputum.
■ Check for jugular vein distention.
■ Examine the skin for pallor, cyanosis, edema, and warmth or coolness.

Causes

Medical causes

Acute respiratory distress syndrome

■ Tachypnea, an early finding, gradually worsens as fluid accumulates in the lungs.
■ Other signs and symptoms include accessory muscle use, grunting expirations, suprasternal and intercostal retractions, crackles, and rhonchi.

Anaphylactic shock

■ Tachypnea develops within minutes after exposure to an allergen.
■ Accompanying signs and symptoms include anxiety, pounding headache, skin flushing, intense pruritus and, possibly, diffuse urticaria, widespread edema, cool, clammy skin, rapid, thready pulse, cough, dyspnea, stridor, and laryngeal edema.

Anemia

■ Tachypnea may occur, depending on the disorder.
■ Other signs and symptoms include fatigue, pallor, dyspnea, tachycardia, postural hypotension, bounding pulse, atrial gallop, and a systolic bruit over the carotid arteries.

Anxiety

■ Tachypnea may occur with tachycardia, restlessness, chest pain, nausea, and light-headedness.

Aspiration of a foreign body

■ With partial obstruction, a dry, paroxysmal cough with rapid, shallow respirations develops abruptly.
■ Other signs and symptoms include dyspnea, gagging or choking, intercostal retraction, nasal flaring, cyanosis, decreased or absent breath sounds, hoarseness, and stridor or coarse wheezing.

Asthma

■ In the initial stages, tachypnea is common along with mild wheezing and a dry cough.
■ If left untreated, this disorder progresses to productive cough, prolonged expirations, intercostal and supraclavicular retractions on inspiration, severe wheezing, rhonchi, flaring nostrils, tachycardia, diaphoresis, and flushing or cyanosis.

Bronchitis, chronic

■ Mild tachypnea may occur, accompanied by a dry, hacking cough, which later produces copious amounts of sputum.
■ Other signs and symptoms include dyspnea, prolonged expirations, wheezing, scattered rhonchi, accessory muscle use, cyanosis, and late-stage clubbing and barrel chest.

Cardiac arrhythmias

■ Tachypnea may occur along with hypotension, dizziness, palpitations, weakness, fatigue and, possibly, decreased level of consciousness (LOC).

Cardiac tamponade

■ A life-threatening disorder, cardiac tamponade may cause tachypnea that's accompanied by tachycardia, dyspnea, and paradoxical pulse.
■ Related signs and symptoms include muffled heart sounds, pericardial rub, chest pain, hypotension, narrowed pulse pressure, hepatomegaly, anxiety, cyanosis, clammy skin, and neck vein distention.

Emphysema

■ Tachypnea is accompanied by exertional dyspnea.

(Text continues on page 370.)

Differential diagnosis: Tachypnea

HISTORY OF PRESENT ILLNESS

Focused physical examination: Skin, cardiovascular, and respiratory systems.

Common signs and symptoms
- Tachycardia
- Dyspnea
- Cyanosis

Pulmonary embolism

Additional signs and symptoms
- Acute dyspnea
- Sudden pleuritic chest pain
- Low-grade fever
- Nonproductive cough or productive cough with blood-tinged sputum
- Pleural friction rub
- Crackles
- Hemoptysis (possibly)
- Wheezing
- Dullness on percussion
- Decreased breath sounds
- Diaphoresis
- Restlessness
- Anxiety
- Signs of shock (possibly)

Diagnosis: Imaging studies (chest X-rays, pulmonary V scan, spiral chest computed tomography scan, pulmonary angiography), electrocardiogram (ECG)

Treatment: Oxygen therapy, medication (anticoagulants, thrombolytic therapy)

Follow-up: Return visit within first week after hospitalization

Pneumothorax

Additional signs and symptoms
- Severe, sharp, and usually unilateral chest pain that's aggravated by chest wall movement
- Accessory muscle use
- Dry cough
- Anxiety
- Restlessness

Diagnosis: Physical examination, arterial blood gas (ABG) analysis, chest X-rays

Treatment: Chest tube insertion, analgesics, oxygen therapy

Follow-up: Referral to pulmonologist

Pneumonia

Additional signs and symptoms
- Hacking, dry cough that progresses to a productive cough
- High-grade fever
- Shaking chills
- Headache
- Pleuritic chest pain
- Fatigue
- Nasal flaring

Diagnosis: Chest X-rays, sputum specimens, bronchoscopy if necessary

Treatment: Medication (antibiotics, expectorants), oxygen if necessary, intubation if warranted

Follow-up: Referral to pulmonologist, hospitalization if necessary

Asthma

Signs and symptoms

- Acute dyspneic attacks
- Audible or auscultated wheezing
- Dry cough
- Hyperpnea
- Chest tightness
- Accessory muscle use
- Nasal flaring
- Intercostal and supraclavicular retractions
- Tachycardia
- Diaphoresis
- Prolonged expiration
- Flushing or cyanosis
- Apprehension

Diagnosis: Laboratory tests (complete blood count [CBC], ABG analysis, allergy skin testing), chest X-rays, pulmonary function tests

Treatment: Avoidance of allergens, tobacco, and beta-adrenergic blockers; medication, including inhaled $beta_2$-agonists, inhaled corticosteroids, nedocromil (Tilade Inhaler) or cromolyn (Intal) if less than age 12, leukotriene receptor agonists (possibly), systemic corticosteroids during infections and exacerbations; peak expiratory flow monitoring

Follow-up: For acute conditions, return visit within 24 hours, then every 3 to 5 days, and then every 1 to 3 months; referral to pulmonologist if treatment is ineffective

Common signs and symptoms

- Gradually developing dyspnea
- Chronic paroxysmal nocturnal dyspnea
- Orthopnea
- Tachycardia
- Palpitations
- S_3
- Fatigue
- Dependent peripheral edema
- Hepatomegaly
- Dry cough
- Anorexia
- Weight gain
- Loss of mental acuity
- Hemoptysis

Acute onset heart failure

Additional signs and symptoms

- Distended jugular veins
- Bibasilar crackles
- Oliguria
- Hypotension

Diagnosis: Laboratory tests (CBC, cardiac enzymes, troponin), imaging studies (chest X-rays, echocardiogram), ECG

Treatment: Medication (angiotensin-converting enzyme inhibitors, diuretics, possibly carvedilol [Coreg], possibly digoxin [Lanoxin])

Follow-up: Return visit within 1 week after discharge, at 4 weeks, and then every 3 months; referral to cardiologist if condition is chronic

Additional differential diagnoses: abdominal pain ■ anaphylactic shock ■ anemia ■ acute respiratory distress syndrome ■ ascites ■ bronchiectasis ■ bronchitis, chronic ■ cardiac arrhythmias ■ cardiac tamponade ■ cardiogenic shock ■ chest trauma ■ chronic obstructive pulmonary disease ■ emphysema ■ febrile illness ■ flail chest ■ foreign body aspiration ■ head trauma ■ hepatic failure ■ hyperosmolar hyperglycemic nonketotic syndrome ■ hypovolemic shock ■ hypoxia ■ interstitial fibrosis ■ lung abscess ■ lung, pleural, or mediastinal tumor ■ mesothelioma, malignant ■ neurogenic shock ■ pancreatis ■ pleural effusion ■ pulmonary edema ■ pulmonary hypertension ■ septic shock

Other cause: salicylates

■ Accompanying signs and symptoms include anorexia, malaise, peripheral cyanosis, pursed-lip breathing, accessory muscle use, chronic productive cough, and late-stage clubbing and barrel chest.

Febrile illness

■ Fever can cause tachypnea, tachycardia, chills, diaphoresis, headache, and weakness.

Flail chest

■ In this life-threatening disorder, tachypnea usually appears early.
■ Other signs and symptoms include paradoxical chest wall movement, rib bruises and palpable fractures, localized chest pain, hypotension, diminished breath sounds, dyspnea, and accessory muscle use.

Head trauma

■ When trauma affects the brain stem, central neurogenic hyperventilation may produce a form of tachypnea marked by rapid, even, and deep respirations.
■ Other signs of life-threatening neurogenic dysfunction include coma, unequal and nonreactive pupils, seizures, hemiplegia, flaccidity, and hypoactive or absent deep tendon reflexes.

Hyperosmolar hyperglycemic nonketotic syndrome

■ Rapidly deteriorating LOC occurs with tachypnea, tachycardia, hypotension, seizures, oliguria, and signs of dehydration.

Hypoxia

■ Tachypnea occurs, possibly with restlessness, impaired judgment, tachycardia, dyspnea, and cyanosis.

Interstitial fibrosis

■ Tachypnea develops gradually and may become severe.
■ Other signs and symptoms include exertional dyspnea, pleuritic chest pain, a paroxysmal, dry cough, crackles, late inspiratory wheezing, cyanosis, fatigue, weight loss, and late-stage clubbing.

Lung abscess

■ Tachypnea occurs with dyspnea and worsens with fever.
■ The chief sign of lung abscess is a productive cough with copious amounts of purulent, foul-smelling, usually bloody sputum.

Neurogenic shock

■ Tachypnea is commonly accompanied by apprehension, bradycardia or tachycardia, oliguria, fluctuating body temperature, and decreased LOC that may progress to coma.
■ Other signs and symptoms include nausea, vomiting, and warm, dry, and perhaps flushed skin.

Plague

■ Plague causes tachypnea, productive cough, chest pain, dyspnea, hemoptysis, and increasing respiratory distress and cardiopulmonary insufficiency.

Pneumonia, bacterial

■ Tachypnea is usually preceded by a painful, hacking, dry cough that rapidly becomes productive.
■ Other signs and symptoms include high fever, shaking chills, headache, dyspnea, pleuritic chest pain, tachycardia, grunting respirations, nasal flaring, and cyanosis.

Pneumothorax

■ A life-threatening disorder, pneumothorax causes tachypnea and is typically accompanied by severe, sharp, one-sided chest pain.
■ Other signs and symptoms include dyspnea, tachycardia, accessory muscle use, asymmetrical chest expansion, dry

cough, cyanosis, anxiety, and restlessness.
- A deviated trachea occurs with tension pneumothorax.

Pulmonary edema
- Tachypnea, an early sign, is accompanied by exertional dyspnea, paroxysmal nocturnal dyspnea and, later, orthopnea.
- Other signs and symptoms include productive cough with pink frothy sputum, crackles, tachycardia, and ventricular gallop.

Pulmonary embolism, acute
- Sudden tachypnea occurs with dyspnea.
- Related signs and symptoms include angina or pleuritic pain, tachycardia, a dry or productive cough with blood-tinged sputum, fever, restlessness, and diaphoresis.

Septic shock
- With septic shock, the patient is likely to experience tachypnea, sudden fever, chills, flushed, warm, yet dry skin, and possibly nausea, vomiting, and diarrhea.
- Other signs and symptoms include tachycardia, hypotension, anxiety, restlessness, decreased LOC, cool, clammy sin, rapid, thready pulse, thirst, and oliguria.

Tumor
- A lung, pleural, or mediastinal tumor causes tachypnea along with exertional dyspnea, cough, hemoptysis, and pleuritic chest pain.
- Related signs and symptoms include tracheal shift, neck vein distention, weight loss, anorexia, and fatigue.

Other causes
Drugs
- Tachypnea may result from a salicylate overdose.

Nursing considerations
- Continue to monitor the patient's vital signs and oxygenation status.
- Keep suction and emergency equipment nearby.
- Prepare for intubation and mechanical ventilation if needed.

Patient teaching
- Explain that slight increases in respiratory rate may be normal.
- Teach the patient about the underlying diagnosis and treatment plan.
- Discuss the importance of compliance with drug therapy.

Throat pain

Throat pain—commonly known as a *sore throat*—refers to discomfort in any part of the pharynx: the nasopharynx, the oropharynx, or the hypopharynx. This common symptom ranges from a sensation of scratchiness to severe pain. It's commonly accompanied by ear pain because cranial nerves IX and X stimulate the pharynx as well as the middle and external ear.

Throat pain may result from infection, trauma, allergy, cancer, or a systemic disorder. It may also follow surgery and endotracheal intubation. Nonpathologic causes include dry mucous membranes associated with mouth breathing and laryngeal irritation associated with alcohol consumption, inhaling smoke or chemicals like ammonia, and vocal strain.

History
- Ask about the onset of throat pain.
- Find out about fever, ear pain, or dysphagia.
- Take a medical history, including throat problems, mouth breathing, and allergies.
- Ask about vocal strain, alcohol consumption, and inhalation of smoke or chemicals such as ammonia.

Physical examination

- Examine the pharynx, oropharynx, and nasopharynx, noting redness, exudate, and swelling.
- Observe the tonsils for redness, swelling, or exudate.
- Obtain an exudate specimen for culture.
- Examine the nose, using a nasal speculum.
- Check the ears using an otoscope.
- Palpate the neck and oropharynx for nodules or lymph node enlargement.

Causes

Medical causes

Agranulocytosis

- Sore throat occurs after progressive fatigue and weakness.
- Related signs and symptoms include nausea, vomiting, anorexia, bleeding tendencies and, possibly, rough-edged ulcers with gray or black membranes on the gums, palate, or perianal area.

Allergic rhinitis

- Sore throat occurs with nasal congestion, a thin nasal discharge, postnasal drip, paroxysmal sneezing, decreased sense of smell, frontal or temporal headache, and itchy eyes, nose, and throat.

Avian flu

- Throat pain, muscle aches, cough, and fever are common early signs and symptoms of this disorder.
- Other signs and symptoms include pneumonia and acute respiratory distress.

Bronchitis, acute

- Lower throat pain occurs with fever, chills, productive cough, and muscle and back pain.
- Other signs and symptoms include rhonchi, wheezing, and crackles on auscultation.

Chronic fatigue syndrome

- Incapacitating fatigue with sore throat, myalgia, lymphadenopathy, and cognitive dysfunction occur with this syndrome.

Common cold

- Sore throat occurs with cough, sneezing, nasal congestion, mouth breathing, rhinorrhea, fatigue, headache, myalgia, and arthralgia.
- A transient loss of taste and smell may also occur.

Contact ulcers

- Ulcers appear symmetrically on the posterior vocal cords, resulting in sore throat.
- Pain is aggravated by talking and may occur with referred ear pain and, occasionally, hemoptysis.

Foreign body

- A foreign body lodged in the palatine or lingual tonsil and pyriform sinus may produce localized throat pain.

Gastroesophageal reflux disease

- With this disease, chronic sore throat and hoarseness occur.
- Pyrosis is the most common symptom.

Glossopharyngeal neuralgia

- Knifelike throat pain occurs on one side in the tonsillar fossa, possibly radiating to the ear.
- Sore throat may also result from yawning, chewing, swallowing, or eating spicy foods.

Herpes simplex virus

- Sore throat may result from lesions on the oral mucosa.
- After causing brief discomfort, lesions erupt into erythematous vesicles that eventually rupture and leave a painful ulcer, followed by a yellowish crust.

Influenza

■ Sore throat with fever, chills, headache, weakness, malaise, cough, muscle aches and, occasionally, hoarseness and rhinorrhea may occur.

Laryngeal cancer

■ With extrinsic laryngeal cancer, the patient may experience pain or burning in the throat when drinking citrus juice or hot liquids or feel a lump in the throat.

■ With intrinsic laryngeal cancer, hoarseness lasts for longer than 3 weeks.

■ Later, during metastasis, signs and symptoms include dysphagia, dyspnea, cough, enlarged cervical lymph nodes, and pain that radiates to the ear.

Laryngitis, acute

■ Sore throat with mild to severe hoarseness is the chief sign of acute laryngitis.

■ Related signs and symptoms include malaise, fever, dysphagia, dry cough, and tender, enlarged lymph nodes.

Mononucleosis, infectious

■ Sore throat, cervical lymphadenopathy, and fluctuating temperature occur.

■ Possible signs and symptoms include hepatomegaly and splenomegaly.

Necrotizing ulcerative gingivitis, acute

■ Abrupt sore throat and gums that ulcerate and bleed occur with this disorder.

■ Gray exudate on the gums and pharyngeal tonsils also may occur.

■ Related signs and symptoms include a foul taste in the mouth, halitosis, cervical lymphadenopathy, headache, malaise, and fever.

Peritonsillar abscess

■ Severe throat pain may occur, radiating to the ear.

■ Associated signs and symptoms include dysphagia, drooling, dysarthria, halitosis, fever with chills, malaise, and nausea.

Pharyngeal burns

■ Throat pain and dysphagia occur.

■ If the larynx is involved, laryngeal edema, bronchospasm, and stridor may also occur.

Pharyngitis

■ With the bacterial form, abrupt sore throat on one side occurs.

■ With the fungal form, a diffuse, burning sore throat occurs.

■ With the viral form, a diffuse sore throat, malaise, fever, and mild erythema and edema of the posterior oropharyngeal wall occur.

Pharyngomaxillary space abscess

■ Mild throat pain occurs, with a bulge in the medial wall of the pharynx and swelling of the neck on the affected side.

■ Related signs and symptoms include fever, dysphagia, trismus and, possibly, signs of respiratory distress or toxemia.

Sinusitis, acute

■ Sore throat with purulent nasal discharge and postnasal drip occur with acute sinusitis.

■ Other signs and symptoms include halitosis, headache, malaise, cough, fever, and facial pain and swelling associated with nasal congestion.

Tongue cancer

■ Localized throat pain occurs around a white lesion or ulcer.

■ Pain radiates to the ear with dysphagia.

Tonsillar cancer

■ Throat pain may radiate to the ear.

■ A superficial ulcer occurs on the tonsil or extends to the base of the tongue.

Tonsillitis

- With acute tonsillitis, mild to severe throat pain occurs.
- With chronic tonsillitis, mild sore throat occurs.
- With lingual tonsillitis, throat pain on one or both sides just above the hyoid bone occurs.

Uvulitis

- A characteristic symptom is throat pain or a sensation of something in the throat.
- Related signs include swollen and red uvula; in allergic uvulitis, pale uvula.

Other causes

Treatments

- Endotracheal intubation and local surgery, such as tonsillectomy and adenoidectomy, may cause throat pain.
- Radiation therapy to the head and neck may cause irritation and throat pain.

Nursing considerations

- Provide analgesic sprays or lozenges to relieve throat pain.
- Prepare the patient for throat culture, blood work, and a monospot test.

Patient teaching

- Explain the importance of completing the full course of antibiotic treatment.
- Discuss ways to soothe the throat.
- Go over the underlying diagnosis and treatment plan.

Thyroid enlargement

An enlarged thyroid can result from inflammation, physiologic changes, iodine deficiency, thyroid tumors, and drugs. Depending on the medical cause, hyperfunction or hypofunction may occur with resulting excess or deficiency, respectively, of the hormone thyroxine. If no infection is present, enlargement is usually slow and progressive. An enlarged thyroid that causes visible swelling in the front of the neck is called a *goiter.*

History

- Ask about the onset of the enlargement.
- Inquire about the use of thyroid hormone replacement drugs.
- Ask about previous irradiation of the thyroid gland or neck and recent infections.
- Take a personal and family history, including thyroid disease.

Physical examination

- Inspect the trachea for midline deviation.
- Palpate the enlarged gland; note the size, shape, consistency of gland, and the presence or absence of nodules.
- Using the bell of the stethoscope, listen over the lobes of the thyroid gland for a bruit.

Causes

Medical causes

Hypothyroidism

- An enlarged thyroid occurs with weight gain despite anorexia; fatigue; cold intolerance; constipation; menorrhagia; slowed intellectual and motor activity; dry, pale, cool skin; dry, sparse hair; and thick, brittle nails.
- Eventually, the face assumes a dull expression with periorbital edema.

Thyroiditis

- Autoimmune thyroiditis may not produce symptoms other than thyroid enlargement.
- In subacute granulomatous thyroiditis, thyroid enlargement may follow an upper respiratory infection or a sore throat. Other signs and symptoms may include a painful and tender thyroid and dysphagia.

Thyrotoxicosis

- An enlarged thyroid gland is a classic sign.
- Other signs and symptoms include nervousness; heat intolerance; fatigue; weight loss despite increased appetite; diarrhea; sweating; palpitations; tremors; smooth, warm, flushed skin; fine, soft hair; exophthalmos; nausea and vomiting; and oligomenorrhea or amenorrhea.

Tumors

- An enlarged thyroid may be accompanied by hoarseness, loss of voice, and dysphagia.
- A malignant tumor usually appears as a single nodule in the neck.
- A nonmalignant tumor may appear as multiple nodules in the neck.

Other causes

Drugs

- Certain drugs, including aminosalicylic acid (Paser), lithium (Eskalith), and sulfonamides may decrease thyroxine production.

Goitrogens

- Foods that contain goitrogens include peanuts, cabbage, soybeans, strawberries, spinach, rutabagas, and radishes and may cause an enlarged thyroid.

Nursing considerations

- Prepare the patient for diagnostic tests and surgery or radiation therapy, if needed.
- Specific interventions depend on whether the patient is hypothyroid, has thyroiditis, or is recovering from a thyroidectomy.
- Provide postoperative care for the patient who has undergone thyroidectomy.

Patient teaching

- Explain the signs and symptoms of hypothyroidism or hyperthyroidism to report.
- Describe post-treatment precautions to a patient undergoing radioactive iodine therapy.
- Teach the patient about thyroid hormone replacement therapy and signs of thyroid hormone overdose.

Tics

A tic is an involuntary, repetitive movement of a specific group of muscles—usually those of the face, neck, shoulders, trunk, and hands. This sign typically occurs suddenly and intermittently. It may involve a single isolated movement, such as lip smacking, grimacing, blinking, sniffing, tongue thrusting, throat clearing, hitching up one shoulder, or protruding the chin. Or, it may involve a complex set of movements. Mild tics, such as twitching of an eyelid, are especially common. Tics differ from minor seizures in that tics aren't associated with transient loss of consciousness or amnesia.

The tics may subside as the child matures, or they may persist into adulthood. However, tics are also associated with one rare affliction—Tourette syndrome, which typically begins during childhood.

History

- Obtain a history of the tic by asking the parents how long the child has had the tic and how often he experiences it.
- Ask if there are factors that precipitate or worsen the tic, and if the patient can control them with conscious effort.
- Ask about stressors in the child's life such as difficult schoolwork.

Physical examination

- Observe the tic to find out if it's a purposeful or involuntary movement.
- Note whether it's localized or generalized, and describe it in detail.
- Complete a neurologic assessment.

Causes

Medical causes

Psychogenic causes

- Tics may be aggravated by stress or anxiety.
- Psychogenic tics typically begin between ages 5 and 10 as voluntary, coordinated, and purposeful actions that the child feels compelled to perform to decrease anxiety.
- Unless the tics are severe, the child may be unaware of them, and they may subside as the child matures or persist into adulthood.

Tourette syndrome

- Tourette syndrome is rare and thought to be a genetic disorder that typically begins between ages 2 and 15 with a tic that involves the face or neck.
- Signs and symptoms include motor and vocal tics that may involve the muscles of the shoulders, arms, trunk, and legs.
- The tics may be associated with violent movements and outbursts of obscenities (coprolalia). The patient may snort, bark, and grunt and emit explosive sounds, such as hissing, when he speaks.
- He may involuntarily repeat another person's words (echolalia) or movements (echopraxia).
- The syndrome sometimes subsides spontaneously or undergoes a prolonged remission, but it may persist throughout life.

Nursing considerations

- A tranquilizer and/or psychotherapy may provide relief.
- Offer emotional support to the patient and his family.

Patient teaching

- Explain the disorder and the treatment plan.
- Teach the patient and his family how to identify and eliminate avoidable stressors.
- Help them learn positive ways to deal with anxiety.

Tinnitus

Tinnitus literally means ringing in the ears, but the term covers many other abnormal sounds. Examples of tinnitus may be described as the sound of escaping air, running water, the inside of a seashell, or as a sizzling, buzzing, or humming noise. Occasionally, it's described as a roaring or musical sound. This common symptom may be unilateral or bilateral and constant or intermittent. Although the brain may adjust to or suppress constant tinnitus, tinnitus may be so disturbing that some patients contemplate suicide as their only source of relief.

Tinnitus can be classified in several ways. Subjective tinnitus is heard only by the patient; objective tinnitus is also heard by the observer who places a stethoscope near the patient's affected ear. Tinnitus aurium refers to noise that the patient hears in his ears; tinnitus cerebri, to noise that he hears in his head.

Tinnitus is usually associated with neural injury within the auditory pathway, resulting in altered, spontaneous firing of sensory auditory neurons. Commonly resulting from an ear disorder, tinnitus may also stem from a cardiovascular or systemic disorder or from the effects of drugs. Nonpathologic causes of tinnitus include acute anxiety

Common causes of tinnitus

Tinnitus usually results from a disorder that affects the external, middle, or inner ear. Below are some of its more common causes and their locations.

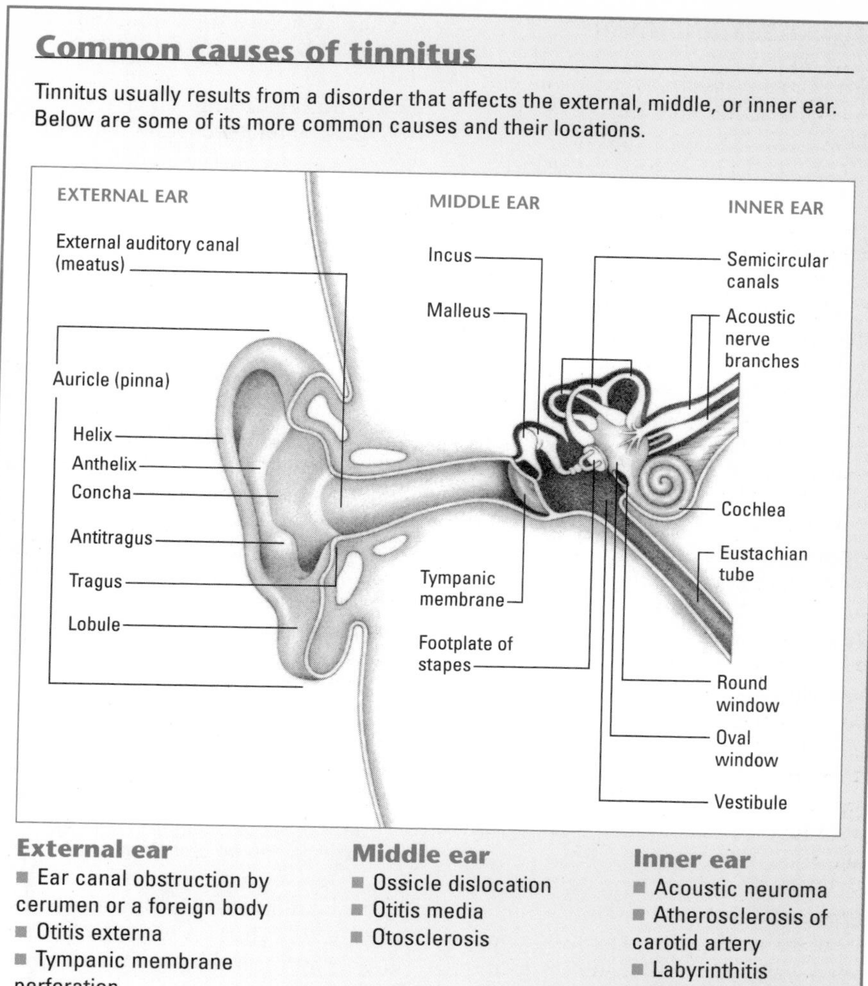

External ear

- Ear canal obstruction by cerumen or a foreign body
- Otitis externa
- Tympanic membrane perforation

Middle ear

- Ossicle dislocation
- Otitis media
- Otosclerosis

Inner ear

- Acoustic neuroma
- Atherosclerosis of carotid artery
- Labyrinthitis
- Ménière's disease

and presbycusis. (See *Common causes of tinnitus.*)

History

- Ask about the onset, location, and description of the sound.
- Inquire about other symptoms, such as vertigo, headache, or hearing loss.
- Take a health and drug history.

Physical examination

- Inspect the ears and examine the tympanic membrane, using an otoscope.
- Perform Weber's and the Rinne tests to check for hearing loss.
- Auscultate for bruits in the neck.
- Compress the jugular or carotid artery to see if this affects the tinnitus.

■ Examine the nasopharynx for masses that might cause eustachian tube dysfunction and tinnitus.

Causes

Medical causes

Acoustic neuroma

■ Tinnitus in one ear precedes sensorineural hearing loss and vertigo in the same ear.
■ Facial paralysis, headache, nausea, vomiting, and papilledema may occur.

Anemia

■ Mild tinnitus may occur if anemia is severe.
■ Other signs and symptoms include pallor, weakness, fatigue, exertional dyspnea, tachycardia, bounding pulse, atrial gallop, and a systolic bruit over the carotid arteries.

Atherosclerosis of the carotid artery

■ Constant tinnitus can be stopped by applying pressure over the carotid artery.
■ Auscultation over the upper part of the neck, on the auricle, or near the ear on the affected side may detect a bruit.
■ Palpation may reveal a weak carotid pulse.

Cervical spondylosis

■ Osteophytic growths may compress the vertebral arteries, resulting in tinnitus.
■ A stiff neck and pain aggravated by activity accompany tinnitus.
■ Other signs and symptoms include brief vertigo, nystagmus, hearing loss, paresthesia, weakness, and pain that radiates down the arms.

Ear canal obstruction

■ Tinnitus with conductive hearing loss, itching, blockage, and a feeling of fullness or pain in the ear may occur.

Eustachian tube patency

■ Tinnitus, audible breath sounds, loud and distorted voice sounds, and a sense of fullness in the ear can occur.
■ Use a pneumatic otoscope to see if the tympanic membrane moves with respiration.

Hypertension

■ High-pitched tinnitus in both ears may occur with severe hypertension.
■ Diastolic blood pressure over 120 mm Hg may also cause severe, throbbing headache, restlessness, nausea, vomiting, blurred vision, seizures, and decreased level of consciousness.

Intracranial arteriovenous malformation

■ A large malformation may cause tinnitus, accompanied by a bruit over the mastoid process.
■ Other signs and symptoms include severe headache, seizures, and progressive neurologic deficits.

Labyrinthitis, suppurative

■ Tinnitus occurs with sudden, severe attacks of vertigo, sensorineural hearing loss in one or both ears, nystagmus, dizziness, nausea, and vomiting.

Ménière's disease

■ Attacks of tinnitus occur with vertigo, a feeling of fullness or blockage in the ear, and fluctuating sensorineural hearing loss for 10 minutes to several hours.
■ Other signs and symptoms include severe nausea, vomiting, diaphoresis, and nystagmus.

Ossicle dislocation

■ Tinnitus and sensorineural hearing loss occur.
■ Possible bleeding from the middle ear may also occur.

Otitis externa, acute

- If debris in the external ear canal invades the tympanic membrane, tinnitus may result.
- More typical signs and symptoms include pruritus, foul-smelling purulent discharge, and severe ear pain aggravated by manipulation of the tragus or auricle, teeth clenching, mouth opening, and chewing.
- The external ear canal appears red and edematous and may be occluded by debris, causing partial hearing loss.

Otitis media

- Tinnitus and conductive hearing loss may occur.
- More typical signs and symptoms include ear pain, a red and bulging tympanic membrane, high fever, chills, and dizziness.

Otosclerosis

- The patient may describe ringing, roaring, or whistling tinnitus or a combination of these sounds.
- Progressive hearing loss and vertigo may occur.

Presbycusis

- Tinnitus and a progressive, symmetrical, sensorineural hearing loss in both ears, usually of high-frequency tones, occur.

Tympanic membrane perforation

- Tinnitus is usually the chief complaint in a small perforation; hearing loss, in a larger perforation.
- Other signs and symptoms include pain, vertigo, and a feeling of fullness in the ear.

Other causes

Drugs and alcohol

- Alcohol, indomethacin (Indocin), and quinine (Quinamm) may also cause reversible tinnitus.
- Common drugs that may cause irreversible tinnitus include aminoglycoside antibiotics and vancomycin (Vancocin).
- Overdose of salicylates commonly causes reversible tinnitus.

Noise

- Chronic exposure to noise, especially high-pitched sounds, can damage the ear's hair cells, causing temporary or permanent tinnitus and total hearing loss.

Nursing considerations

- Take steps to communicate clearly with patients with hearing loss.
- Address safety concerns in patients with vertigo.
- A hearing aid may be used to amplify environmental sounds, thereby obscuring tinnitus.

Patient teaching

- Educate the patient about strategies for adapting to the tinnitus, including biofeedback and masking devices.
- Coach the patient on how to avoid excessive noise, ototoxic agents, and other factors that may cause cochlear damage.
- Teach the patient about the treatment plan.
- Prepare the patient for diagnostic testing.

Tracheal deviation

Normally, the trachea is located at the midline of the neck—except at the bifurcation, where it shifts slightly toward the right. Visible deviation from its normal position signals an underlying condition that can compromise pulmonary function and possibly cause respiratory distress. A hallmark of life-threatening tension pneumothorax, tracheal deviation occurs with disorders that produce

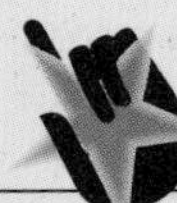

KNOW-HOW

Detecting slight tracheal deviation

Although gross tracheal deviation is visible, slight deviation can only be detected by palpation or sometimes an X-ray. Try palpation first.

With the tip of your index finger, locate the patient's trachea by palpating between the sternocleidomastoid muscles. Then compare the trachea's position to an imaginary line drawn vertically through the suprasternal notch. Any deviation from midline is usually considered abnormal.

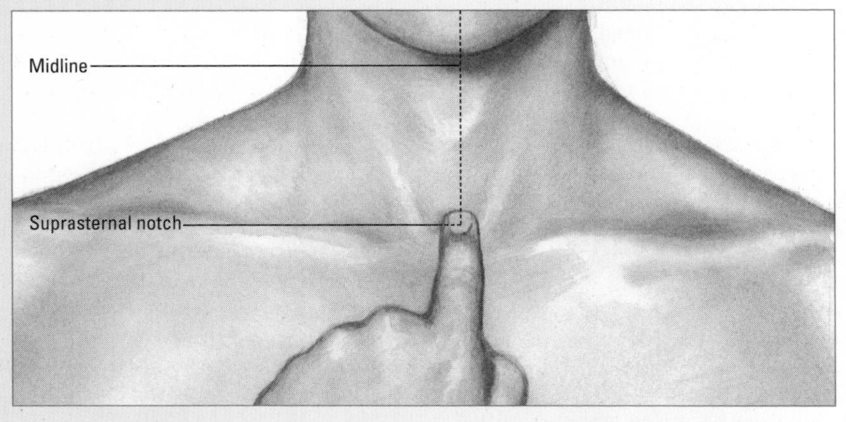

mediastinal shift due to asymmetrical thoracic volume or pressure. A nonlesion pneumothorax can produce tracheal deviation to the ipsilateral side. (See *Detecting slight tracheal deviation*.)

QUICK ACTION ***If you detect tracheal deviation, be alert for signs and symptoms of respiratory distress, such as tachypnea, dyspnea, decreased or absent breath sounds, stridor, nasal flaring, accessory muscle use, asymmetrical chest expansion, restlessness, and anxiety. If possible, place the patient in semi-Fowler's position to aid respiratory excursion and improve oxygenation. Give supplemental oxygen, and intubate the patient if necessary. Insert an I.V. catheter for fluid and drug administration. In addition, palpate for subcutaneous crepitation in the neck and chest, a sign of tension pneumothorax. Chest tube insertion may be necessary to release trapped air or fluid and to restore normal intrapleural and intrathoracic pressure gradients.***

History

- Take a history of pulmonary or cardiac disorders, surgery, trauma, or infection.
- Ask about smoking habits.
- Find out about other signs and symptoms, such as breathing difficulty, pain, and cough.

Physical examination

- Take the patient's vital signs.
- Observe for respiratory distress.

■ Perform a complete cardiopulmonary assessment.

Causes

Medical causes

Atelectasis

■ Extensive lung collapse can produce tracheal deviation toward the affected side.

■ Respiratory signs and symptoms include dyspnea, tachypnea, pleuritic chest pain, dry cough, dullness on percussion, decreased vocal fremitus and breath sounds, inspiratory lag, and substernal or intercostal retractions.

Hiatal hernia

■ Intrusion of abdominal viscera into the pleural space causes tracheal deviation toward the unaffected side.

■ Other signs and symptoms include pyrosis, regurgitation or vomiting, chest or abdominal pain, and respiratory distress.

Kyphoscoliosis

■ Rib cage distortion and mediastinal shift produce tracheal deviation toward the compressed lung.

■ Respiratory signs and symptoms include dry cough, dyspnea, asymmetrical chest expansion and, possibly, asymmetrical breath sounds.

■ Backache and fatigue are common.

Mediastinal tumor

■ If large, a mediastinal tumor can press against the trachea and nearby structures, causing tracheal deviation and dysphagia.

■ Other late signs and symptoms include stridor, dyspnea, brassy cough, hoarseness, and stertorous respirations with suprasternal retraction.

■ Shoulder, arm, or chest pain and edema of the neck, face, or arm may develop.

■ Neck and chest wall veins may be dilated.

Pleural effusion

■ If the effusion is large, the mediastinum can shift to the contralateral side, producing tracheal deviation.

■ Related signs and symptoms include dry cough, dyspnea, pleuritic pain, pleural friction rub, tachypnea, decreased chest motion, decreased or absent breath sounds, egophony, flatness on percussion, decreased tactile fremitus, fever, and weight loss.

Pulmonary fibrosis

■ Tracheal deviation occurs as the mediastinum shifts toward the affected side.

■ Other possible signs and symptoms include dyspnea, cough, clubbing, malaise, and fever.

Pulmonary tuberculosis

■ Tracheal deviation occurs toward the affected side with asymmetrical chest excursion and inspiratory crackles.

■ Insidious early signs and symptoms include anorexia, weight loss, fever, chills, and night sweats.

■ Productive cough, hemoptysis, pleuritic chest pain, and dyspnea occur as the disease progresses.

Retrosternal thyroid

■ This anatomic abnormality can displace the trachea, and the gland is felt as a movable neck mass above the suprasternal notch.

■ Other signs and symptoms include dysphagia, cough, hoarseness, and stridor.

Tension pneumothorax

■ A life-threatening disorder, tension pneumothorax causes tracheal deviation toward the unaffected side.

■ Related signs and symptoms include the sudden onset of respiratory distress, sharp chest pain, dry cough, severe dyspnea, tachycardia, wheezing, cyanosis, accessory muscle use, nasal flaring, air

CASE CLIP

Responding to tracheal deviation

Mr. M. is a 27-year-old male who arrived at the emergency department yesterday with sudden onset of shortness of breath, diminished breath sounds on the right, and slight pain on inspiration. He has a history of smoking 2 packs per day for 11 years. He says he's very physically active and denies prior incidents of this nature. A chest X-ray showed a minor (10%) pneumothorax on the right. The emergency department physician elected not to insert a chest tube; however, Mr. M. was admitted to the medical unit for observation.

In the afternoon during initial rounds, Mr. M.'s nurse enters his room to introduce herself and perform her initial assessment. She finds him sitting upright in his bed; he appears mildly short of breath. She checks his vital signs and finds:

- heart rate (HR): 92 beats/minute
- respiratory rate (RR): 28 breaths/minute and somewhat shallow
- blood pressure (BP): 132/86 mm Hg
- oxygen saturation: 92% on 2 L/minute of oxygen via nasal cannula
- diminished breath sounds on the right side (as was previously noted).

Two hours later, Mr. M.'s call light goes on. The nurse enters his room and finds him sitting upright in bed but leaning over, clutching his chest. His color is somewhat dusky, and he's very anxious. He is unable to speak in complete sentences because of increased shortness of breath. The nurse is able to discern from what he says that he suddenly felt a sharp pain in the right side of his chest when he coughed a few minutes ago, and abruptly became severely short of breath. The nurse auscultates his lungs and now finds no breath sounds at all on the right. When he's sitting straight up she also notices that his trachea no longer appears to be at the midline; rather, it seems to have shifted a bit to the left. The nurse calls for help and asks the responder to activate the rapid response team (RRT) immediately. While she waits, she checks Mr. M.'s vital signs and finds:

- HR: 132 beats/minute
- RR: 36 breaths/minute and labored but shallow
- BP: 146/100 mm Hg
- oxygen saturation level: 84%.

She immediately increases his oxygen to 4 L/minute.

The RRT arrives in 3 minutes and immediately proceeds to change Mr. M.'s oxygen delivery system to 100% nonrebreather. The residents auscultate Mr. M.'s lungs and confirm the nurse's findings of absent breath sounds on the right side. They also notice that his trachea has indeed deviated to the left, and when they lower the head of his bed to 30 degrees they note jugular vein distention as well. A stat portable chest X-ray is ordered, but recognizing that Mr. M. may have developed a sudden tension pneumothorax, they elect to perform an emergency needle decompression. Mr. M. is placed on a cardiac monitor; sinus tachycardia is noted at a rate of 147 beats/minute. The supplies are gathered for the procedure. After getting his consent, Mr. M. is prepped and the decompression takes place. Almost immediately, Mr. M. appears to experience some relief from the procedure. A chest tube is placed at the site to prevent further recurrence of the pneumothorax, and is connected to 15 cm of water pressure. Mr. M. is transferred to the respiratory intensive care unit for closer observation.

hunger, and asymmetrical chest movement.

- Other signs and symptoms include restlessness, anxiety, subcutaneous crepitation in the neck and upper chest, decreased or absent breath sounds on the affected side, jugular vein distention, and hypotension.

Thoracic aortic aneurysm

- The trachea usually deviates to the right.
- Signs and symptoms may include stridor; dyspnea; wheezing; brassy cough; hoarseness; dysphagia; edema of the face, neck, or arm; jugular vein distention; and substernal, neck, shoulder, or lower back pain. (See *Responding to tracheal deviation.*)

Nursing considerations

- Monitor the patient's respiratory and cardiac condition constantly.
- Give oxygen, if needed.
- Make sure that emergency equipment is readily available.
- Give analgesics for comfort, if needed.
- Provide emotional support.
- Assist with the insertion of a large-bore needle into the pleural space or a thoracostomy tube for tension pneumothorax.

Patient teaching

- Teach the patient how to perform coughing and deep-breathing exercises.
- Explain which signs and symptoms of respiratory difficulty the patient should report.
- Teach the patient about the underlying diagnosis and treatment plan.

Tracheal tugging

A visible recession of the larynx and trachea that occurs in synchrony with cardiac systole, tracheal tugging commonly results from an aneurysm or a tumor near the aortic arch. It may signal dangerous compression or obstruction of major airways. The tugging movement, best observed with the patient's neck hyperextended, reflects abnormal transmission of aortic pulsations because of compression and distortion of the heart, esophagus, great vessels, airways, and nerves.

QUICK ACTION ***If you observe tracheal tugging, examine the patient for signs of respiratory distress, such as tachypnea, stridor, accessory muscle use, cyanosis, and agitation. If the patient is in distress, check airway patency. Give oxygen, and prepare to intubate the patient if necessary. Insert an I.V. catheter for fluid and drug access, and begin cardiac monitoring.***

History

- Obtain a pertinent history.
- Ask about associated symptoms, especially pain, and about a history of cardiovascular disease, cancer, chest surgery, or trauma.

Physical examination

- Examine the patient's neck and chest for abnormalities.
- Palpate the neck for masses, enlarged lymph nodes, abnormal arterial pulsations, and tracheal deviation.
- Percuss and auscultate the lung fields for abnormal sounds, and auscultate the heart for murmurs.

Causes

Medical causes

Aortic arch aneurysm

- A large aneurysm can distort and compress surrounding tissues and structures, producing tracheal tugging.
- A cardinal sign is severe pain in the substernal area, sometimes radiating to the back or side of the chest.

- A sudden increase in pain may herald impending rupture—a medical emergency.
- Associated signs and symptoms may include a visible pulsatile mass in the first or second intercostal space or suprasternal notch, a diastolic murmur of aortic insufficiency, and an aortic systolic murmur and thrill without any peripheral signs of aortic stenosis.
- Dyspnea and stridor may occur with hoarseness, dysphagia, a brassy cough, and hemoptysis. Jugular vein distention may also develop along with edema of the face, neck, or arm.
- Compression of the left main bronchus can cause atelectasis of the left lung.

Hodgkin's disease

- A tumor that develops adjacent to the aortic arch can cause tracheal tugging.
- Initial signs and symptoms include usually painless cervical lymphadenopathy, sustained or remittent fever, fatigue, malaise, pruritus, night sweats, and weight loss.
- Swollen lymph nodes may become tender and painful.
- Later signs and symptoms include dyspnea and stridor; dry cough; dysphagia; jugular vein distention; edema of the face, neck, or arm; hepatosplenomegaly; hyperpigmentation, jaundice, or pallor; and neuralgia.

Malignant lymphoma

- Tracheal tugging may reflect anterior mediastinal lymphadenopathy or tumor development next to the aortic arch.
- The most common initial sign is painless peripheral lymphadenopathy.
- Other early signs and symptoms include fever, fatigue, malaise, night sweats, and weight loss.
- Later signs and symptoms include a crowing cough, dyspnea, stridor, dysphagia, jugular vein distention, neck edema, hepatomegaly, and splenomegaly.

Thymoma

- This rare tumor can cause tracheal tugging if it develops in the anterior mediastinum.
- Common signs and symptoms are cough, chest pain, dysphagia, dyspnea, hoarseness, a palpable neck mass, jugular vein distention, and edema of the face, neck, or upper arm.

Nursing considerations

- Place the patient in semi-Fowler's position to ease respiration.
- Continue to monitor the patient's respiratory status.
- Give a cough suppressant and prescribed pain medications, but be alert for signs of respiratory depression.

Patient teaching

- Prepare the patient for diagnostic procedures, which may include chest X-ray, computed tomography scan, lymphangiography, aortography, bone marrow biopsy, liver biopsy, echocardiography, and a complete blood count.
- Teach the patient about the underlying diagnosis and treatment plan.

Tremors

The most common type of involuntary muscle movement, tremors are regular rhythmic oscillations that result from alternating contraction of opposing muscle groups. They're typical signs of extrapyramidal or cerebellar disorders and can also result from certain drugs.

Tremors can be characterized by their location, amplitude, and frequency. They're classified as resting, intention, or postural. Resting tremors occur when an extremity is at rest and subside with movement. They include the classic pill-rolling tremor of Parkinson's disease. Conversely, intention tremors occur only with movement and subside with rest. Postural (or action) tremors appear when an extremity or the trunk is actively held in a particular posture or position. A common type of postural tremor is called an *essential tremor.*

Tremorlike movements may also be elicited, such as asterixis—the characteristic flapping tremor seen in hepatic failure.

Stress or emotional upset tends to aggravate a tremor. Alcohol commonly diminishes postural tremors.

History

- Ask about the onset, duration, and progression of tremors.
- Determine what aggravates or alleviates tremors.
- Find out about other symptoms, such as behavioral changes or memory loss.
- Explore personal and family history of neurologic, endocrine, or metabolic disorders.
- Obtain a drug history, especially the use of phenothiazines.
- Ask about alcohol use.

Physical assessment

- Assess the patient's overall appearance and demeanor, noting mental condition.
- Test range of motion and strength in all major muscle groups while observing for chorea, athetosis, dystonia, and other involuntary movements.
- Check deep tendon reflexes (DTRs).
- Observe the patient's gait.

Causes

Medical causes

Alcohol withdrawal syndrome

- Resting and intention tremors occur as soon as 7 hours after the last drink and progressively worsen.
- Early signs and symptoms include diaphoresis, tachycardia, elevated blood pressure, anxiety, restlessness, irritability, insomnia, headache, nausea, and vomiting.
- In severe withdrawal, profound tremors, agitation, confusion, hallucinations, and seizures occur.

Alkalosis

- A severe intention tremor occurs with twitching, carpopedal spasms, agitation, diaphoresis, and hyperventilation.
- Other signs and symptoms include dizziness, tinnitus, palpitations, and peripheral and circumoral cyanosis.

Benign familial essential tremor

- This disorder of early adulthood produces a bilateral tremor that typically begins in the fingers and hands and may spread to the head, jaw, lips, and tongue.
- Laryngeal involvement may result in a quavering voice.

Cerebellar tumor

- An intention tremor is a classic sign.
- Related signs and symptoms include ataxia, nystagmus, incoordination, muscle weakness and atrophy, and hypoactive or absent DTRs.

Graves' disease

- Fine hand tremors occur along with nervousness, weight loss, fatigue, palpitations, dyspnea, heat intolerance, an enlarged thyroid gland and, possibly, exophthalmos.

Hypercapnia

- A rapid, fine intention tremor occurs.
- Associated signs and symptoms include headache, fatigue, blurred vision, weakness, lethargy, and decreased level of consciousness (LOC).

Hypoglycemia

- A rapid, fine intention tremor occurs with confusion, weakness, tachycardia, diaphoresis, and cold, clammy skin.
- Tremors may disappear as hypoglycemia worsens and hypotonia and decreased LOC become evident.
- Early signs and symptoms include headache, profound hunger, nervousness, and blurred or double vision.

Multiple sclerosis

- An intention tremor that waxes and wanes may be an early sign, along with visual and sensory impairments.
- Other signs and symptoms may include nystagmus, muscle weakness, paralysis, spasticity, hyperreflexia, ataxic gait, dysphagia, dysarthria, constipation, urinary frequency and urgency, incontinence, impotence, and emotional lability.

Parkinson's disease

- Tremors, a classic early sign, usually begin in the fingers and may eventually affect the foot, eyelids, jaw, lips, and tongue.
- Other characteristic signs and symptoms include cogwheel rigidity, bradykinesia, propulsive gait with forward-leaning posture, monotone voice, masklike facies, drooling, dysphagia, dysarthria, and occasionally oculogyric crisis or blepharospasm.

Porphyria

- Resting tremor and rigidity with chorea and athetosis occur.
- As the disease progresses, generalized seizures with aphasia and hemiplegia occur.

Thalamic syndrome

- Contralateral ataxic tremors and other abnormal movements occur, along with Weber's syndrome; paralysis of vertical gaze and stupor or coma occur with central midbrain syndromes.
- Tremor, deep sensory loss, hemiataxia, and extrapyramidal dysfunction may occur with anteromedial-inferior syndrome.

Thyrotoxicosis

- A rapid, fine intention tremor of the hands and tongue with clonus occur as well as hyperreflexia.
- Other signs and symptoms include tachycardia, cardiac arrhythmias, palpitations, anxiety, dyspnea, diaphoresis, heat intolerance, weight loss despite increased appetite, diarrhea, an enlarged thyroid and, possibly, exophthalmos.

Wernicke's disease

- An intention tremor is an early sign of thiamine deficiency.
- Other signs and symptoms include ocular abnormalities, ataxia, apathy, confusion, orthostatic hypotension, and tachycardia.

West Nile encephalitis

- In severe infections, headache, high fever, neck stiffness, stupor, disorientation, coma, tremors, occasional seizures, and paralysis occur.

Other causes

Drugs

- Antipsychotics and phenothiazines, and infrequently metoclopramide (Reglan) and metyrosine (Demser), may cause resting and pill-rolling tremors.
- Amphetamines, lithium (Eskalith) toxicity, phenytoin (Dilantin), and sympathomimetics can cause tremors that disappear with dose reduction.

Manganese toxicity

- Early signs of manganese toxicity include resting tremor, chorea, propulsive gait, cogwheel rigidity, personality changes, amnesia, and masklike facies.

Mercury poisoning

■ Mercury poisoning is characterized by irritability, copious amounts of saliva, loose teeth, gum disease, slurred speech, and tremors.

Nursing considerations

■ Assist the patient with activities as needed.
■ Take precautions against possible injury during activities.
■ Encourage the patient to talk about changes in body image.

Patient teaching

■ Reinforce the patient's independence.
■ Instruct the patient in the use of assistive devices as needed.
■ Teach the patient about the underlying diagnosis and treatment plan.

Trismus

Commonly known as *lockjaw,* trismus is a prolonged and painful tonic spasm of the masticatory jaw muscles. This characteristic early sign of tetanus is produced by the neuromuscular effects of tetanospasmin, a potentially lethal exotoxin. It can also result from drug therapy. Occasionally, a milder form of trismus may accompany neuromuscular involvement in other disorders or infection or disease of the jaw, teeth, parotid glands, or tonsils.

History

■ Obtain a pertinent history, inquiring about a recent injury (even a slight wound), infection, animal bite or a history of epilepsy, neuromuscular disease, or endocrine or metabolic disorder.
■ Obtain a complete drug history, including self-injected drugs because the use of a contaminated needle may produce tetanus.
■ Ask about paresthesia or pain in the throat, jaw, neck, or shoulders.

Physical examination

■ Examination of the oral cavity may be difficult or impossible to perform. If possible, examine the pharynx, tonsils, oral mucosa, gingivae, and teeth.
■ Perform a neurologic assessment, evaluating cranial nerve, motor, and sensory function and deep tendon reflexes (DTRs).
■ Check the jaw jerk reflex. An extremely hyperactive response and a careful patient history usually establish the diagnosis. (See *Performing the jaw jerk test,* page 388.)

Causes

Medical causes

Hypocalcemia

■ Severe hypocalcemia can produce trismus and cramping spasms in virtually all muscle groups, except those of the eye.
■ It also causes fatigue, weakness, chorea, and palpitations.
■ Chvostek's and Trousseau's signs may be elicited.

Peritonsillar abscess

■ This disorder occurs after an episode of acute tonsillitis, when infection penetrates the tonsillar capsule and surrounding deeper tissues.
■ Symptoms include severe sore throat, trismus, odynophagia, deviation of the uvula, and fever.

Rabies

■ Trismus commonly develops after a prodromal period of fever, headache, photophobia, hyperesthesia, and increasing restlessness and agitation.
■ Other neuromuscular effects include excessive salivation, painful laryngeal and pharyngeal muscle spasms and, possibly, respiratory distress.

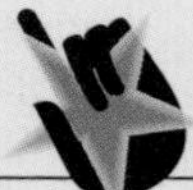

KNOW-HOW

Performing the jaw jerk test

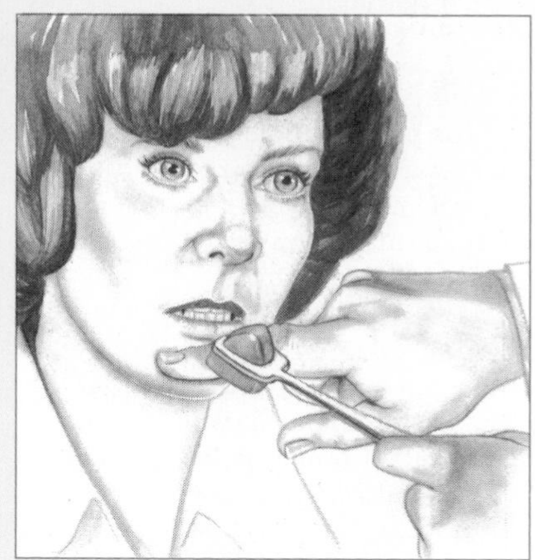

If your patient reports difficulty opening her mouth, perform the jaw jerk test. Even slight trismus may indicate an otherwise asymptomatic, mild, localized tetanus.

Here's how to elicit and interpret this important reflex: Ask the patient to relax her jaw and open her mouth slightly. Then place your index finger over the middle of her chin, and firmly tap it with a reflex hammer.

Normally, this tap produces sudden jaw closing; then an inhibitory mechanism abruptly halts motor nerve activity, and the mouth remains closed. In trismus, however, this inhibitory mechanism fails and motor activity increases, causing immediate spasm of jaw muscles.

Seizure disorder

- Trismus commonly occurs during a generalized tonic-clonic seizure along with spasms of other facial muscles, the limbs, and the trunk.

Temporomandibular joint syndrome

- This syndrome causes trismus, mandibular dysfunction, and facial pain.
- The pain may range from a severe dull ache to an intense spasm that radiates to the cheek, temple, lower jaw, ear, mastoid area, neck, or shoulders.
- Earache occurs without involvement of the tympanic membrane or external auditory canal.

Tetanus

- This acute, life-threatening infection is signaled by trismus, which typically appears within 14 days of the initial infection.
- The painful spasms increase in frequency and intensity during the initial disease stage and then gradually subside.
- Although trismus is commonly the first sign of tetanus, it occasionally follows a short prodromal period of headache, restlessness, irritability, slight fever, chills, swelling at the wound site, and dysphagia.
- As the disease progresses, painful involuntary muscle spasms spread to other areas, such as the abdomen, producing boardlike rigidity; the back, resulting in opisthotonos; the face, producing a characteristic grotesque grin (risus sardonicus); or possibly the laryngeal or chest wall muscles.
- Tachycardia, diaphoresis, hyperactive DTRs, and seizures may also develop.

Other causes

Drugs

- Phenothiazines—particularly piperazine derivatives such as fluphenazine (Prolixin)—and other antipsychotics may produce an acute dystonic reaction marked by trismus, involuntary facial movements, and tonic spasms in the limbs. These complications usually occur early in drug therapy, sometimes after the initial dose.

Strychnine poisoning

- In this potentially fatal condition, tonic seizures characterized by trismus, leg muscle rigidity, and respiratory muscle spasm follow early symptoms of irritability and twitching.

Nursing considerations

- Maintain a quiet environment for the patient with trismus; darken his room and keep all stimulation to a minimum.
- Give a sedative as needed.
- Constantly assess the patient's respiratory status and make sure that oxygen and emergency airway equipment are readily available.
- To treat tetanus, expect to administer human tetanus immune globulin, which neutralizes unbound toxin.
- Give I.V. fluids to prevent dehydration if the patient can't drink fluids.
- If trismus is prolonged enough to affect the patient's nutritional status, he may require parenteral nutrition.
- If the patient can't speak, make sure that he has a pen and paper and that his call bell is within reach at all times.

Patient teaching

- Teach the patient with tetanus about the importance of annual booster injections to ensure immunization.
- Explain the underlying diagnosis and treatment plan.

Tunnel vision

Resulting from severe constriction of the visual field that leaves only a small central area of sight, tunnel vision is typically described as the sensation of looking through a tunnel or gun barrel. It may be unilateral or bilateral and usually develops gradually. This abnormality results from chronic open-angle glaucoma and advanced retinal degeneration. Tunnel vision may also result from laser photocoagulation therapy, which aims to correct retinal detachment. A common complaint of malingerers, tunnel vision can be verified or discounted by visual field examination performed by an ophthalmologist.

History

- Ask about the onset, progression, and description of loss of peripheral vision.
- Explore personal and family history of ocular problems, especially progressive blindness that began at an early age.

Physical examination

- Test close visual acuity.
- If your assessment findings suggest tunnel vision, refer the patient to an ophthalmologist for further evaluation, including visual field testing.

Causes

Medical causes

Chronic open-angle glaucoma

- Tunnel vision in both eyes occurs late and slowly progresses to complete blindness.
- Other late signs and symptoms include mild eye pain, halo vision, and reduced visual acuity, especially at night, that isn't correctable with glasses.

Retinal pigmentary degeneration

- An annular scotoma progresses concentrically, causing tunnel vision and eventually resulting in complete blindness, usually by age 50.
- Impaired night vision, the earliest symptom, typically appears during the first or second decade of life.

- An ophthalmoscopic examination may reveal narrowed retinal blood vessels and a pale optic disk.

Nursing considerations

- Remove all potentially dangerous objects and orient the patient to his surroundings.
- Clearly explain diagnostic procedures.
- Reassure the patient.

Patient teaching

- Teach the patient how to compensate for tunnel vision and avoid bumping into objects.
- Explain the underlying diagnosis and treatment plan.
- Teach the patient about prescribed medications.

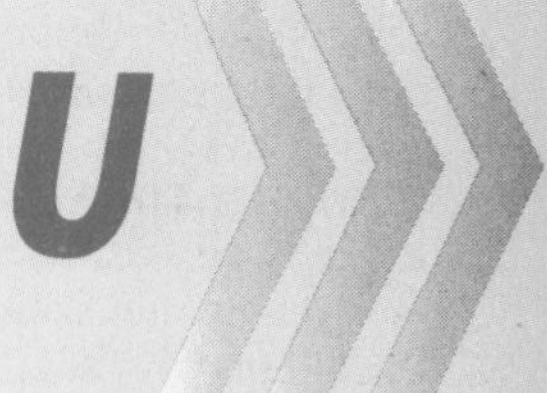

Urethral discharge

Urethral discharge is an excretion from the urinary meatus that may be purulent, mucoid, or thin; sanguineous or clear; and scant or profuse. It usually develops suddenly, most commonly in men with a prostate infection.

History

- Ask about the onset and description of the discharge.
- Inquire about other pain or burning on urination, difficulty starting a urine stream, urinary frequency, fever, chills, and perineal fullness.
- Obtain a medical history, including prostate problems, sexually transmitted disease (STD), or urinary tract infection (UTI).
- Find out about recent sexual contacts or if there is a new sex partner.

Physical examination

- Inspect the urethral meatus for inflammation and swelling.
- Obtain a culture specimen.
- Obtain a urine specimen for urinalysis and culture.

Causes

Medical causes

Prostatitis

- In the acute form, signs and symptoms include purulent urethral discharge, sudden fever, chills, lower back pain, myalgia, perineal fullness, arthralgia, frequent and urgent urination, dysuria, nocturia, and a tense, boggy, tender, and warm prostate.
- In the chronic form, signs and symptoms include a persistent urethral discharge that's thin, milky, or clear at the meatus after not voiding for a long time; dull aching in the prostate or rectum; sexual dysfunction, such as ejaculatory pain; and urinary disturbances, such as frequency, urgency, and dysuria.

Reiter's syndrome

- Urethral discharge and other signs of acute urethritis occur 1 or 2 weeks after sexual contact.
- Other signs and symptoms include asymmetrical arthritis, conjunctivitis, and ulcerations on the oral mucosa, glans penis, palms, and soles.

Urethritis

- Urethral discharge can be secondary to UTIs or STDs, such as chlamydia, gonorrhea, or trichomoniasis.
- Scant or profuse urethral discharge occurs that's thin and clear, mucoid, or thick and purulent.
- Related signs and symptoms include urinary hesitancy, urgency, and frequency and itching and burning around the meatus.

Nursing considerations

- To relieve prostatitis symptoms, suggest that the patient take hot sitz baths several times daily, increase his fluid intake, void frequently, and avoid caffeine, tea, and alcohol.

- Monitor for urine retention.

Patient teaching

- Caution the patient who has active prostatitis to avoid sexual activity until acute symptoms subside.
- Explain that chronic prostatitis symptoms can be relieved by engaging in regular sexual activity.
- Teach the patient about the importance and adverse effects of prescribed medications.
- If evaluating the patient for an STD, advise him to avoid sexual contact until test results are available.
- Teach perineal hygiene and infection control techniques, as appropriate.

Urinary frequency

Urinary frequency refers to increased incidence of the urge to void, without an increase in the total volume of urine produced. Usually resulting from decreased bladder capacity, increased frequency is a cardinal sign of urinary tract infection (UTI). However, it can also stem from another urologic disorder—neurologic dysfunction, or pressure on the bladder from a nearby tumor or from organ enlargement (as with pregnancy).

History

- Ask about current and previous voiding patterns.
- Determine the onset and duration of urinary frequency.
- Find out about fever, chills, dysuria, urgency, incontinence, hematuria, discharge, or lower abdominal pain with urination.
- Obtain a medical history, especially of UTI, other urologic problems or recent urologic procedures, and neurologic disorders.
- Inquire about a history of prostate enlargement in men.
- Ask about the possibility of pregnancy in women.

Physical examination

- Obtain a clean-catch midstream urine specimen.
- Palpate the suprapubic area, abdomen, and flanks, noting tenderness.
- Examine the urethral meatus for redness, discharge, or swelling.
- Palpate the prostate gland.
- Perform a neurologic assessment if the patient's history reveals symptoms or a history of neurologic diseases.
- Obtain a temperature reading.

Causes

Medical causes

Benign prostatic hyperplasia

- Urinary frequency with nocturia and, possibly, incontinence and hematuria occur with this disorder.
- Initial signs and symptoms include reduced caliber and force of the urine stream, urinary hesitancy, tenesmus, inability to stop the stream of urine, a feeling of incomplete voiding, and occasionally urine retention.

Bladder calculus

- Urinary frequency and urgency, dysuria, hematuria at the end of micturition, and suprapubic pain from bladder spasms occur.
- If the calculus lodges in the bladder neck, overflow incontinence occurs with greatest discomfort at the end of micturition.

Bladder cancer

- Urinary frequency, urgency, dribbling, and nocturia may develop.
- Typically, the first sign is gross, painless, intermittent hematuria (with clots).
- Suprapubic or pelvic pain commonly occurs with invasive lesions.

Multiple sclerosis

- Urinary frequency, urgency, and incontinence are common.
- Vision problems (such as diplopia and blurred vision) and sensory impairment (such as paresthesia) are the earliest symptoms.
- Other signs and symptoms include constipation, muscle weakness, paralysis, spasticity, hyperreflexia, intention tremor, ataxic gait, dysarthria, impotence, and emotional lability.

Prostate cancer

- In advanced stages, urinary frequency occurs along with hesitancy, dribbling, nocturia, dysuria, bladder distention, perineal pain, constipation, and a hard, irregularly shaped prostate.

Prostatitis

- In the acute form, urinary frequency, urgency, dysuria, nocturia, and purulent urethral discharge occur.
- Other acute signs and symptoms include fever, chills, lower back pain, myalgia, arthralgia, perineal fullness and, possibly, a tense, boggy, tender, and warm prostate.
- In the chronic form, pain on ejaculation may occur as well as the same signs and symptoms as in the acute form, but to a lesser degree.

Rectal tumor

- Pressure from the tumor on the bladder may cause urinary frequency.
- Early signs and symptoms include changed bowel habits, commonly starting with an urgent need to defecate on arising or obstipation alternating with diarrhea, blood or mucus in stools, and a sense of incomplete evacuation.

Reiter's syndrome

- Urinary frequency occurs 1 or 2 weeks after sexual contact.
- Other signs and symptoms include asymmetrical arthritis of the knees, ankles, and metatarsophalangeal joints; conjunctivitis; and small, painless ulcers on the mouth, tongue, glans penis, palms, and soles.

Reproductive tract tumor

- A tumor may compress the bladder, causing urinary frequency.
- Other signs and symptoms may include abdominal distention, menstrual disturbances, vaginal bleeding, weight loss, pelvic pain, and fatigue.

Spinal cord lesion

- Urinary frequency, continuous overflow, dribbling, urgency, urinary hesitancy, and bladder distention from incomplete spinal cord transection occur with this type of lesion.
- Other signs and symptoms below the level of the lesion may occur, such as weakness, paralysis, sensory disturbances, hyperreflexia, and impotence.

Urethral stricture

- Bladder decompensation produces urinary frequency, along with urgency and nocturia.
- Early signs include hesitancy, tenesmus, and reduced caliber and force of the urine stream.
- Overflow incontinence, urinoma, and urosepsis may also develop.

Urinary tract infection

- With UTI, urinary frequency, urgency, dysuria, hematuria, cloudy urine, and discharge occur.
- Related signs and symptoms include fever, bladder spasms, and a feeling of warmth during urination.

Uterine prolapse

- Urinary frequency, hesitancy, infection, leakage, and retention occur.
- Associated signs and symptoms include abdominal, vaginal, or lower back pain as well as dyspareunia (painful intercourse).

■ Signs and symptoms commonly occur gradually as pelvic muscles and ligaments weaken from age, childbirth, or abdominal surgery.

Other causes

Diuretics

■ Diuretics, including caffeine, reduce the body's total volume of water and salt by increasing urine excretion.

Treatments

■ Radiation therapy may cause bladder inflammation, leading to urinary frequency.

Nursing considerations

■ If mobility is impaired, keep a bedpan or commode by the bed.
■ Document the patient's daily intake and output.

Patient teaching

■ Teach the patient about diagnostic tests.
■ Emphasize safer sex practices.
■ Instruct the patient in the proper way to clean the genital area.
■ Explain the reasons for increasing fluid intake and frequency of voiding.
■ Teach the patient how to do Kegel exercises.

Urinary hesitancy

Hesitancy—difficulty starting a urine stream generally followed by a decrease in the force of the stream—can result from a urinary tract infection (UTI), a partial lower urinary tract obstruction, a neuromuscular disorder, or the use of certain drugs. Occurring at all ages and in both sexes, it's most common in older men with prostate enlargement. It also occurs in women with a gravid uterus; tumors in the reproductive system, such as uterine fibroids; or ovarian, uterine, or vaginal cancer. Hesitancy usually arises gradually, commonly going unnoticed until urine retention causes bladder distention and discomfort.

History

■ Obtain a history of the patient's urinary problems: Ask when he first noticed hesitancy and if he has ever had the problem before. Also ask about other urinary problems, especially reduced force or interruption of the urine stream.
■ If the patient is male, find out if he has ever been treated for a prostate problem. Ask patients of either sex if they've had a UTI or urinary tract obstruction.
■ Obtain a drug history.

Physical examination

■ Inspect the patient's urethral meatus for inflammation, discharge, and other abnormalities.
■ Examine the anal sphincter and test sensation in the perineum.
■ Obtain a clean-catch urine specimen for urinalysis and culture and sensitivity tests.
■ A male patient requires prostate gland palpation. A female patient requires a gynecologic examination.

Causes

Medical causes

Benign prostatic hyperplasia

■ Signs and symptoms of this disorder depend on the extent of prostate enlargement and the lobes affected.
■ Characteristic early signs and symptoms include urinary hesitancy, reduced caliber and force of the urine stream, perineal pain, a feeling of incomplete voiding, inability to stop the urine stream and, occasionally, urine retention.
■ As the obstruction increases, the patient may develop urinary frequency, nocturia, urinary overflow, inconti-

nence, bladder distention and, possibly, hematuria.

Prostate cancer

- In advanced cancer, urinary hesitancy may occur along with frequency, dribbling, nocturia, dysuria, bladder distention, perineal pain, and constipation.
- A digital rectal examination commonly reveals a hard, nodular prostate.

Spinal cord lesion

- A lesion below the micturition center that has destroyed the sacral nerve roots causes urinary hesitancy, tenesmus, and constant dribbling from urine retention and overflow incontinence.
- Associated signs and symptoms are urinary frequency and urgency, dysuria, and nocturia.

Urethral stricture

- A partial obstruction of the lower urinary tract caused by trauma or infection produces urinary hesitancy, tenesmus, and decreased force and caliber of the urine stream.
- Urinary frequency and urgency, nocturia, and eventually overflow incontinence may develop.
- Pyuria usually indicates accompanying infection. Increased obstruction may lead to urine extravasation and the formation of urinomas.

Urinary tract infection

- Urinary hesitancy may be associated with UTIs.
- Characteristic urinary changes include frequency, dysuria, nocturia, cloudy urine and, possibly, hematuria.
- Associated signs and symptoms include bladder spasms; costovertebral angle tenderness; suprapubic, low back, pelvic, or flank pain; urethral discharge in males; fever; chills; malaise; nausea; and vomiting.

Other causes

Drugs

- Anticholinergics and drugs with anticholinergic properties (such as tricyclic antidepressants and some nasal decongestants and cold remedies) may cause urinary hesitancy.
- Hesitancy also may occur in patients recovering from general anesthesia.

Nursing considerations

- Monitor the patient's voiding pattern, and palpate the abdomen frequently for bladder distention.
- Apply local heat to the perineum or the abdomen to enhance muscle relaxation and aid urination.

Patient teaching

- Teach the patient how to perform a clean, intermittent self-catheterization, if indicated.
- Prepare the patient for tests, such as cystometrography or cystourethrography.
- Explain about the underlying diagnosis and treatment plan.

Urinary incontinence

Urinary incontinence, the uncontrollable passage of urine, can result from a bladder abnormality, a neurologic disorder, or an alteration in pelvic muscle strength. A common urologic sign, incontinence may be transient or permanent, and may involve large volumes of urine or scant dribbling. It can be classified as stress, neurogenic, overflow, urge, or total incontinence. *Stress incontinence* refers to intermittent leakage resulting from a sudden physical strain, such as a cough, sneeze, laugh, or quick movement. *Neurogenic incontinence* occurs because a spinal cord injury has disrupted the process by which the patient becomes aware that he needs to void. *Overflow incontinence* is a dribble resulting from urine retention, which fills the bladder and prevents it from contracting with sufficient force to expel a urine stream. *Urge incontinence* refers to the inability to suppress a sudden urge to urinate. *Total incontinence* is continuous leakage resulting from the bladder's inability to retain urine.

History

- Ask about the onset and description of incontinence.
- Obtain a description of normal urinary pattern and fluid intake.
- Inquire about other urinary problems, such as hesitancy, frequency, urgency, nocturia, and decreased force or interruption of the urine stream.
- Ask about a history of urinary tract infections, prostate conditions, spinal injury or tumor, stroke, or surgery involving the bladder, prostate, or pelvic floor.
- Ask a female patient about the number of pregnancies and childbirths.

Physical assessment

- Have the patient empty his bladder.
- Inspect the urethral meatus for inflammation or defect.
- Have the female patient bear down; note urine leakage.
- Gently palpate the abdomen for bladder distention.
- Perform a complete neurologic assessment, noting motor and sensory function and obvious muscle atrophy.
- Assess post-void residual urine volume with a straight catheter.

Causes

Medical causes

Benign prostatic hyperplasia

- Overflow incontinence results from urethral obstruction and urine retention.
- Reduced caliber and force of the urine stream, urinary hesitancy, and a feeling of incomplete voiding constitute prostatism and are early signs and symptoms.
- Urination becomes more frequent, with nocturia and, possibly, hematuria as the obstruction increases.
- Bladder distention and an enlarged prostate are revealed by examination.

Bladder calculus

- Overflow incontinence may occur if the calculus lodges in the bladder neck.
- Other signs and symptoms may include those of an irritable bladder, such as urinary frequency and urgency, dysuria, hematuria, and suprapubic pain from bladder spasms.
- Pelvic pain may occur, along with pain referred to the tip of the penis, vulva, lower back, or heel pain.

Bladder cancer

- Urge incontinence and hematuria are early signs.
- Obstruction by a tumor may produce overflow incontinence.
- Other signs and symptoms include frequency, dysuria, nocturia, dribbling, and suprapubic pain from bladder spasms after voiding.
- A mass may be palpable on bimanual examination.

Diabetic neuropathy

- Bladder distention with overflow incontinence may occur.
- Related signs and symptoms include episodic constipation or diarrhea (which is commonly nocturnal), impotence and retrograde ejaculation, orthostatic hypotension, syncope, and dysphagia.

Guillain-Barré syndrome

- Urinary incontinence may occur early.
- Profound muscle weakness, which typically starts in the legs and extends

to the arms and facial nerves within 24 to 72 hours, is the most prominent sign.

- Other signs and symptoms include paresthesia, dysarthria, nasal speech, dysphagia, orthostatic hypotension, fecal incontinence, diaphoresis, drooling, tachycardia, and pain in the shoulders, thighs, or lumbar region.

Multiple sclerosis

- Urinary incontinence, urgency, and frequency are common to this disease.
- Early signs include vision problems and sensory impairment.
- Other signs and symptoms include constipation, muscle weakness, paralysis, spasticity, hyperreflexia, intention tremor, ataxic gait, dysarthria, impotence, and emotional lability.

Prostate cancer

- Urinary incontinence usually appears only in advanced stages.
- Other late signs and symptoms include urinary frequency and hesitancy, nocturia, dysuria, bladder distention, perineal pain, constipation, and a hard, irregularly shaped, nodular prostate.

Prostatitis, chronic

- Urinary incontinence may occur as well as urinary frequency and urgency, dysuria, hematuria, bladder distention, persistent urethral discharge, dull perineal pain that may radiate, ejaculatory pain, and decreased libido.

Spinal cord injury

- Overflow incontinence follows rapid bladder distention.
- Other signs and symptoms include paraplegia, sexual dysfunction, sensory loss, muscle atrophy, anhidrosis, and loss of reflexes far from the injury.

Stroke

- Transient or permanent urinary incontinence occurs with stroke.
- Related signs and symptoms include impaired mentation, emotional lability, behavioral changes, altered level of consciousness, and seizures.
- Other signs and symptoms include headache, vomiting, vision deficits, and decreased visual acuity.
- Sensorimotor signs and symptoms include contralateral hemiplegia, dysarthria, dysphagia, ataxia, apraxia, agnosia, aphasia, and unilateral sensory loss.

Urethral stricture

- Eventually, overflow incontinence occurs with urethral stricture.
- Urinomas and urosepsis occur as obstruction increases.

Urinary tract infection

- Incontinence, urinary urgency, dysuria, hematuria, and cloudy urine occur with UTI.
- Bladder spasms or a feeling of warmth during urination may occur.

Other causes

Surgery

- Urinary incontinence may occur after prostatectomy as a result of urethral sphincter damage.

Nursing considerations

- Obtain a urine specimen.
- Start bladder retraining.
- If incontinence is neurologic, monitor the patient for urine retention.

Patient teaching

- Explain how to perform Kegel exercises.
- Teach the patient self-catheterization techniques.
- Review drug therapy with the patient.
- Discuss the underlying disorder, diagnostic tests, and treatment plan.

Urinary urgency

A sudden compelling urge to urinate (urinary urgency), accompanied by bladder pain, is a classic symptom of a urinary tract infection (UTI). As inflammation decreases bladder capacity, discomfort results from the accumulation of even small amounts of urine. Repeated, frequent voiding in an effort to alleviate this discomfort produces urine output of only a few milliliters at each voiding.

Urgency without bladder pain may point to an upper motor neuron lesion that has disrupted bladder control.

History

- Ask about the onset and history of urgency.
- Inquire about other urologic symptoms, such as dysuria and cloudy urine.
- Ask about neurologic symptoms such as paresthesia.
- Obtain a medical history, especially of UTIs and surgery or procedures involving the urinary tract.
- Obtain a prescription and nonprescription drug history.

Physical examination

- Obtain a clean-catch specimen for urinalysis and culture.
- Note urine character, color, and odor; use a reagent strip to test for pH, glucose, and blood.
- Palpate the suprapubic area and both flanks for distention and tenderness.
- If the history or symptoms suggest neurologic dysfunction, perform a neurologic examination.

Causes

Medical causes

Bladder calculus

- Possible symptoms include urinary urgency and frequency, dysuria, chills, fever, hematuria at the end of micturition, and suprapubic pain.
- Pain may pass on to the penis, vulva, or lower back.

Multiple sclerosis

- Urinary urgency can occur with or without frequent UTIs.
- Vision and sensory impairments are the earliest signs.
- Other signs and symptoms include urinary frequency, incontinence, constipation, muscle weakness, paralysis, spasticity, intention tremor, hyperreflexia, ataxic gait, dysphagia, dysarthria, impotence, and emotional lability.

Reiter's syndrome

- Urgency occurs with other symptoms of acute urethritis 1 or 2 weeks after sexual contact, primarily in men.
- Asymmetrical arthritis of the knees, ankles, or metatarsal phalangeal joints; conjunctivitis; and ulcers on the penis or skin or in the mouth usually develop within several weeks after sexual contact.

Spinal cord lesion

- Urinary urgency can occur along with urinary frequency and difficulty initiating and inhibiting a urine stream; bladder distention and discomfort may also occur.
- Neuromuscular symptoms far from the lesion include weakness, paralysis, hyperreflexia, sensory disturbances, and impotence.

Urethral stricture

- Bladder decompensation produces urinary urgency, frequency, and nocturia.
- Early signs and symptoms include hesitancy, tenesmus, and reduced caliber and force of the urine stream.
- Eventually, overflow incontinence may occur.

Urinary tract infection

- Common signs and symptoms include urinary urgency, frequency, and hesitancy; hematuria; dysuria; nocturia; and cloudy urine.
- Related signs and symptoms include bladder spasms; costovertebral angle tenderness; suprapubic, low back, or flank pain; urethral discharge in males; fever; chills; malaise; nausea; and vomiting.

Other causes

Treatments

- Radiation therapy may irritate and inflame the bladder, causing urinary urgency.

Nursing considerations

- Increase the patient's fluid intake.
- Give the patient an antibiotic and a urinary anesthetic as prescribed.

Patient teaching

- Instruct the patient in safe sex practices.
- Explain proper genital hygiene to female patients.
- Discuss adequate fluid intake and frequent daily voiding.
- Teach the patient with a noninfective cause of urinary urgency how to do Kegel exercises.
- Discuss the underlying disorder and treatment plan.

V

Vaginal bleeding, postmenopausal

Postmenopausal vaginal bleeding—bleeding that occurs 6 or more months after menopause—is an important, albeit not a definitive, indicator of gynecologic cancer. It can also result from infection, a local pelvic disorder, estrogenic stimulation, atrophy of the endometrium, and physiologic thinning and drying of the vaginal mucous membranes. Bleeding from the vagina may also indicate bleeding from another gynecological location, such as the ovaries, fallopian tubes, uterus, cervix, or vagina. Bleeding usually occurs as slight brown (or red) spotting, which develops either spontaneously or following coitus or douching. It may also occur, however, as oozing of fresh blood or as bright red hemorrhage. Many patients—especially those with a history of heavy menstrual flow—minimize the importance of this bleeding, thus delaying diagnosis.

History

- Determine the patient's current age and age at menopause.
- Ask about the onset of bleeding.
- Obtain a thorough obstetric, gynecologic, and sexual history.
- Find out all drugs used currently or since the symptoms began, including douches and estrogen products.
- Obtain a history of sexually transmitted disease, as needed.

Physical examination

- Observe the external genitalia, noting the character of vaginal discharge and the appearance of the labia, vaginal rugae, and clitoris.
- Palpate the breasts and lymph nodes for nodules or enlargement.
- Perform pelvic and rectal examinations.

Causes

Medical causes

Atrophic vaginitis

- Bloody staining may normally follow coitus or douching, but must be evaluated to rule out cancer.
- Characteristic white, watery discharge may be accompanied by pruritus, dyspareunia, and a burning sensation in the vagina and labia.
- Sparse pubic hair, a pale vagina with decreased rugae and small hemorrhagic spots, clitoral atrophy, and shrinking of the labia minora may also occur.

Cervical cancer

- Spotting or heavier bleeding occurs early in invasive cervical cancer; bleeding may also normally follow coitus or douching.
- Related signs include persistent, pink-tinged, and foul-smelling discharge and postcoital pain.
- As the cancer spreads, back and sciatic pain, leg swelling, anorexia, weight

loss, hematuria, dysuria, rectal bleeding, and weakness may occur.

Cervical or endometrial polyps

- Spotting (possibly mucopurulent and pink) may occur after coitus, douching, or straining at stool.

Endometrial hyperplasia or cancer

- Bleeding occurs early and is brownish and scant, or red and profuse, and usually follows coitus or douching.
- Later, bleeding becomes heavier and more frequent, leading to clotting and anemia.
- Pelvic, rectal, lower back, and leg pain may accompany bleeding.
- The uterus may be enlarged.

Ovarian tumor, feminizing

- Endometrial shedding may occur and cause heavy bleeding.
- A palpable pelvic mass, increased cervical mucus, breast enlargement, and spider angiomas may be present.

Vaginal cancer

- Characteristic spotting or bleeding may be preceded by a thin, watery discharge.
- Bleeding may be spontaneous but usually follows coitus or douching.
- A firm, ulcerated vaginal lesion may be present.
- Dyspareunia, urinary frequency, bladder and pelvic pain, rectal bleeding, and vulvar lesions may develop later.

Vulvar cancer

- Bleeding, itching, groin pain, unusual lumps or sores, and abnormal urination and defecation may occur.

Other causes

Drugs

- Unopposed estrogen replacement therapy may cause abnormal vaginal bleeding, but cancer must always be ruled out.
- Antibiotics may change the normal vaginal pH and flora.

Nursing considerations

- Until a diagnosis is made, estrogen replacement should be stopped.
- Prepare the patient for diagnostic tests.

Patient teaching

- Reassure the patient that postmenopausal vaginal bleeding may be benign, but careful assessment is still needed.
- Teach the patient about the underlying diagnosis and treatment plan.

Vaginal discharge

Common in women of childbearing age, physiologic vaginal discharge is mucoid, clear or white, nonbloody, and odorless. Produced by the cervical mucosa and, to a lesser degree, by the vulvar glands, this discharge may occasionally be scant or profuse due to estrogenic stimulation and changes during the patient's menstrual cycle. However, a marked increase in discharge or a change in discharge color, odor, or consistency can signal disease. Discharge may result from infection, sexually transmitted disease, reproductive tract disease, fistulas, and certain drugs. In addition, the prolonged presence of a foreign body in the patient's vagina, such as a tampon or diaphragm, can cause irritation and an inflammatory exudate, as can frequent douching, feminine hygiene products, contraceptive products, bubble baths, and colored or perfumed toilet paper.

History

- Ask about the onset and description of the discharge.
- Find out about other symptoms, such as dysuria and perineal pruritus and burning.

Identifying causes of vaginal discharge

The color, consistency, amount, and odor of your patient's vaginal discharge provide important clues about the underlying disorder. For quick reference, use this chart to match common characteristics of vaginal discharge and their possible causes.

CHARACTERISTICS	POSSIBLE CAUSES
Thin, scant, watery, white discharge	Atrophic vaginitis
Thin, green or gray-white, foul-smelling discharge	Bacterial vaginosis
White, curdlike, profuse discharge with yeasty, sweet odor	Candidiasis
Mucopurulent, foul-smelling discharge	Chancroid
Yellow, mucopurulent, odorless or acrid discharge	Chlamydial infection
Scant, serosanguineous, or purulent discharge with foul odor	Endometritis
Copious mucoid discharge	Genital herpes
Profuse, mucopurulent discharge, possibly foul-smelling	Genital warts
Yellow or green, foul-smelling discharge from the cervix or occasionally from Bartholin's or Skene's ducts	Gonorrhea
Chronic, watery, bloody, or purulent discharge, possibly foul-smelling	Gynecologic cancer
Frothy, green-yellow, and profuse (or thin, white, and scant) foul-smelling discharge	Trichomoniasis

- Determine recent changes in sexual habits or hygiene practices.
- Ask about previous discharge or infection and the treatment used.
- Take a drug history, including the use of antibiotics, oral estrogens, and contraceptives.
- Ask about the possibility of pregnancy.

Physical examination

- Examine the external genitalia and note the character of the discharge. (See *Identifying causes of vaginal discharge.*)
- Observe vulvar and vaginal tissues for redness, edema, and excoriation.
- Palpate the inguinal nodes for tenderness or enlargement.
- Palpate the abdomen for tenderness.
- Consider that a pelvic examination may be needed.
- Obtain vaginal discharge specimens for testing.

Causes

Medical causes

Atrophic vaginitis

- A thin, scant, watery white vaginal discharge may be accompanied by pruritus, burning, and tenderness.
- Sparse pubic hair, a pale vagina with decreased rugae and small hemorrhagic spots, clitoral atrophy, and shrinking of the labia minora may also occur.

Bacterial vaginosis

- Thin, foul-smelling, green or gray-white discharge adheres to the vaginal walls and can be easily wiped away.
- Pruritus, redness, and other signs of vaginal irritation may occur.

Candidiasis

- A profuse, white, curdlike discharge with a yeasty, sweet odor is produced.
- The onset of the discharge is abrupt, usually just before menses or during a course of antibiotics.
- Exudate may be lightly attached to the labia and vaginal walls and is commonly accompanied by vulvar redness and edema.
- The inner thighs may be covered with a fine, red dermatitis and weeping erosions.
- Intense labial itching and burning and external dysuria may also occur.

Chancroid

- This condition produces a mucopurulent, foul-smelling discharge and vulvar lesions that are initially erythematous and later ulcerated.
- Within 2 to 3 weeks, inguinal lymph nodes may become tender and enlarged. In addition, pruritus, suppuration, and spontaneous drainage of nodes, headache, malaise, and fever to 102.2° F (39° C) are common.

Chlamydial infection

- A yellow, mucopurulent, odorless or acrid vaginal discharge is produced.
- Other signs and symptoms include dysuria, dyspareunia, and vaginal bleeding after douching or coitus, especially following menses.

Endometritis

- A scant, serosanguineous discharge with a foul odor can result.
- Other signs and symptoms include fever, lower back and abdominal pain, abdominal muscle spasms, malaise, dysmenorrhea, and an enlarged uterus.

Genital warts

- A profuse, mucopurulent vaginal discharge may be produced; the odor may be foul-smelling if the warts are infected.
- Mosaic, papular vulvar lesions occur, frequently with burning or paresthesia around the vaginal opening.
- Genital warts can also appear around the anus or on the cervix.

Gonorrhea

- Occasionally, yellow or green, foul-smelling discharge can be expressed from Bartholin's or Skene's ducts; however, 80% of women have no symptoms.
- Other signs and symptoms include dysuria, urinary frequency and incontinence, bleeding, vaginal redness and swelling, fever, and severe pelvic and abdominal pain.

Gynecologic cancer

- Chronic, watery, bloody, or purulent vaginal discharge may be foul-smelling.
- Other signs and symptoms include abnormal vaginal bleeding and, later, weight loss; pelvic, back, and leg pain; fatigue; urinary frequency; and abdominal distention.

Herpes simplex, genital

- Copious mucoid discharge results, but the initial complaint is painful, indurated vesicles and ulcerations on the labia, vagina, cervix, anus, thighs, or mouth.
- Erythema, marked edema, and tender inguinal lymph nodes may occur, along with fever, malaise, and dysuria.

Trichomoniasis

- A foul-smelling discharge may be produced, which may be frothy, green-yellow, and profuse or thin, white, and scant. However, about 70% of patients are asymptomatic.

- Other signs and symptoms include pruritus; a red, inflamed vagina with tiny petechiae; dysuria and urinary frequency; and dyspareunia, postcoital spotting, menorrhagia, or dysmenorrhea.

Other causes

Contraceptive creams and jellies

- Contraceptive creams and jellies can increase vaginal secretions.

Drugs

- Drugs that contain estrogen can cause increased mucoid vaginal discharge.
- Antibiotics may increase the risk of candidal vaginal infection and discharge.

Radiation therapy

- Irradiation of the reproductive tract can cause a watery, odorless, vaginal discharge.

Nursing considerations

- Obtain cultures of the discharge.
- Give antibiotics, antivirals, or other drugs if ordered.
- Observe standard precautions to prevent the spread of infection.

Patient teaching

- Explain the importance of keeping the perineum clean and dry and avoiding tight-fitting clothing.
- Suggest douching with vinegar and water to relieve discomfort, if appropriate.
- Stress compliance with prescribed drugs.
- Instruct the patient to avoid intercourse until symptoms of infection clear.
- If the vaginal discharge is the result of a sexually transmitted disease, provide information on safer sex practices.

Venous hum

A venous hum is a functional or innocent murmur heard above the clavicles throughout the cardiac cycle. Loudest during diastole, it may be low pitched, rough, or noisy. The hum commonly accompanies a thrill or, possibly, a high-pitched whine. It's best heard by applying the bell of the stethoscope to the medial aspect of the right supraclavicular area with the patient seated upright or by placing the stethoscope bell in the second or third parasternal interspace with the patient standing upright. (See *Detecting a venous hum.*)

A venous hum is a common, normal finding in children and pregnant women. However, it also occurs in hyperdynamic states, such as anemia and thyrotoxicosis. The hum results from increased blood flow through the internal jugular veins, especially on the right side, which causes audible vibrations in the tissues.

Occassionally, a venous hum may be mistaken for an intracardiac murmur or a thyroid bruit. However, a venous hum disappears with jugular vein compression and waxes and wanes with head turning. In contrast, an intracardiac murmur and a thyroid bruit persist despite jugular vein compression and head turning.

History

- Ask about a history of anemia or thyroid disorders.
- Note associated palpitations, dyspnea, nervousness, tremors, heat intolerance, weight loss, fatigue, or malaise.
- Take a drug history.

Physical examination

- Take the patient's vital signs, noting especially tachycardia, hypertension, a bounding pulse, and widened pulse pressure.

■ Auscultate the heart for gallops or murmurs.
■ Examine the skin and mucous membranes for pallor.

Causes

Medical causes

Anemia

■ In severe cases, a venous hum occurs with pale skin and mucous membranes, dyspnea, crackles, tachycardia, bounding pulse, atrial gallop, systolic bruits over the carotid arteries, bleeding tendencies, weakness, fatigue, and malaise.

Thyrotoxicosis

■ A loud venous hum may be audible whether the patient is sitting or in a supine position.
■ An atrial or ventricular gallop may be present.
■ Additional signs and symptoms include tachycardia, palpitations, weight loss despite increased appetite, diarrhea, an enlarged thyroid, dyspnea, nervousness, difficulty concentrating, tremors, diaphoresis, heat intolerance, decreased libido and, possibly, exophthalmos.
■ Women may have oligomenorrhea or amenorrhea; men may have gynecomastia.

Nursing considerations

■ Prepare the patient for diagnostic tests, such as an electrocardiogram, venous Doppler study, complete blood count, or thyroid study.

Patient teaching

■ Explain ways to manage the underlying disorder.
■ Stress the importance of rest periods.

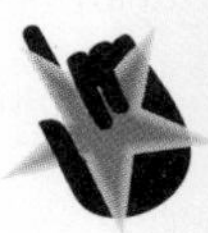

KNOW-HOW

Detecting a venous hum

To detect a venous hum, have your patient sit upright and then place the bell of the stethoscope over his right supraclavicular area. Gently lift his chin and turn his head toward the left, which increases the loudness of the hum (as shown below).

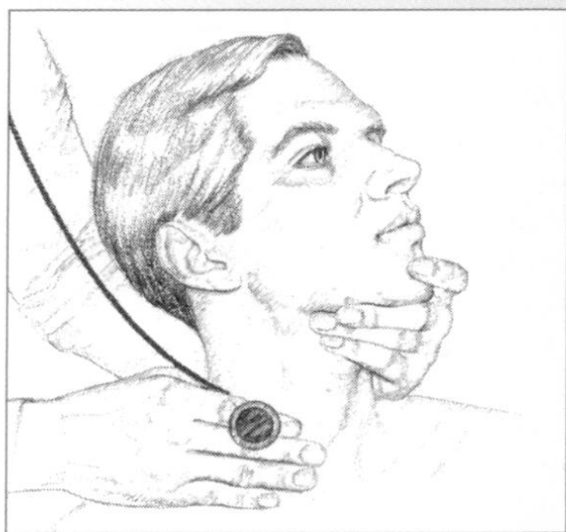

If you still can't hear the hum, press his jugular vein with your thumb (shown below). The hum will disappear with pressure but will suddenly return, temporarily louder than before, when you release your thumb—a result of the turbulence created by pressure changes.

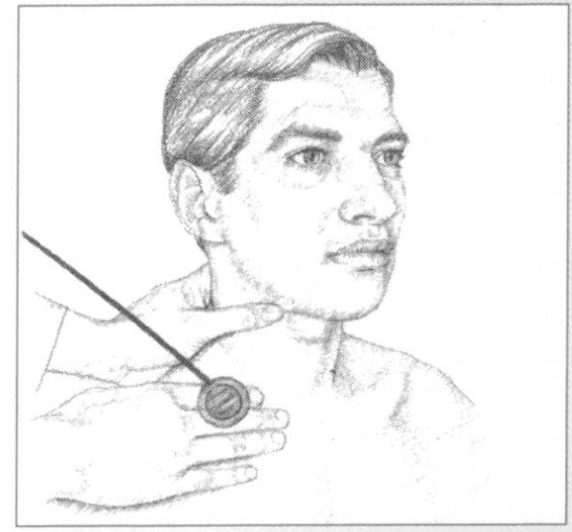

Vertigo

Vertigo is an illusion of movement in which the patient feels that he's revolving in space (subjective vertigo) or that his surroundings are revolving around him (objective vertigo). He may complain of feeling pulled sideways, as though drawn by a magnet.

A common symptom, vertigo usually begins abruptly and may be temporary or permanent and mild or severe. It may worsen when the patient moves and subside when he lies down. It's commonly confused with dizziness—a sensation of imbalance and light-headedness that's nonspecific. However, unlike dizziness, vertigo is commonly accompanied by nausea and vomiting, nystagmus, and tinnitus or hearing loss. And, although the patient's limb coordination is unaffected, vertiginous gait may occur.

Vertigo may result from a neurologic or otologic disorder that affects the equilibratory apparatus (the vestibule, semicircular canals, cranial nerve [CN] VIII, vestibular nuclei in the brain stem and their temporal lobe connections, and eyes). However, this symptom may also result from alcohol intoxication, hyperventilation, and postural changes (benign postural vertigo). It may also be an adverse effect of certain drugs, tests, or procedures.

History

- Ask about the onset and description of vertigo.
- Note what aggravates and alleviates vertigo.
- Ask about motion sickness and hearing loss.
- Obtain a recent drug history.
- Find out about alcohol use.

Physical examination

- Take the patient's vital signs.
- Perform a neurologic assessment, focusing particularly on CN VIII function.
- Observe gait and posture.
- Perform a hearing test.

Causes

Medical causes

Acoustic neuroma

- Mild, intermittent vertigo occurs with sensorineural hearing loss in one ear.
- Other signs and symptoms include tinnitus, postauricular or suboccipital pain, and—with cranial nerve compression—facial paralysis.

Benign positional vertigo

- Debris in a semicircular canal produces vertigo when the patient's head position is changed, lasting a few minutes.

Brain stem ischemia

- Sudden, severe vertigo may become episodic and later persistent.
- Other signs and symptoms include ataxia, nausea, vomiting, increased blood pressure, tachycardia, nystagmus, and lateral deviation of the eyes toward the side of the lesion.
- Hemiparesis and paresthesia may also occur.

Head trauma

- Persistent vertigo occurs soon after injury along with spontaneous or positional nystagmus and, if the temporal bone is fractured, hearing loss.
- Other signs and symptoms include headache, nausea, vomiting, and decreased level of consciousness (LOC).
- Behavioral changes, diplopia or visual blurring, seizures, motor or sensory deficits, and signs of increased intracranial pressure may also develop.

Herpes zoster

- Infection of CN VIII produces the sudden onset of vertigo, facial paralysis, hearing loss in the affected ear, and herpetic vesicular lesions in the auditory canal.

Labyrinthitis

- Severe vertigo begins abruptly and may occur in a single episode or recur over months or years.
- Associated signs and symptoms include nausea, vomiting, progressive sensorineural hearing loss, and nystagmus.

Ménière's disease

- Labyrinthine dysfunction causes the abrupt onset of vertigo, lasting minutes, hours, or days.
- Unpredictable episodes of severe vertigo and unsteady gait may cause the patient to fall.
- During an attack, any sudden motion of the head or eyes can precipitate nausea or vomiting.

Motion sickness

- Vertigo, nausea, vomiting, and headache occur in response to rhythmic or erratic motions.
- Dizziness, fatigue, diaphoresis, hypersalivation, and dyspnea may also occur.

Multiple sclerosis

- Episodic vertigo may occur early and become persistent.
- Other early signs and symptoms include diplopia, visual blurring, and paresthesia.
- Nystagmus, constipation, muscle weakness, paralysis, spasticity, hyperreflexia, intention tremor, and ataxia may also occur.

Posterior fossa tumor

- Positional vertigo occurs and lasts a few seconds.
- Other signs and symptoms include papilledema, headache, memory loss, nausea, vomiting, nystagmus, apneustic respirations, and elevated blood pressure.

Seizures

- Temporal lobe seizures may produce vertigo, usually associated with other symptoms of partial complex seizures.
- Seizures may be signaled by an aura and followed by several minutes of mental confusion.

Vestibular neuritis

- Severe vertigo usually begins abruptly and lasts several days, without tinnitus or hearing loss.
- Other signs include nausea, vomiting, and nystagmus.

Other causes

Diagnostic tests

- Caloric testing (irrigating the ears with warm or cold water) can induce vertigo.

Drugs and alcohol

- High or toxic doses of certain drugs (such as aminoglycosides, antibiotics, hormonal contraceptives, quinine, and salicylates) or alcohol may produce vertigo.

Surgery and procedures

- The use of overly warm or cold eardrops or irrigating solutions can cause vertigo.
- Ear surgery may cause vertigo that lasts for several days.

Nursing considerations

- Place the patient in a comfortable position.
- Monitor the patient's vital signs and LOC.
- Keep the bed's side rails up; if the patient is standing, help him to a chair.
- Darken the room and keep the patient calm.
- Give drugs to control nausea and vomiting and decrease labyrinthine irritability.

Patient teaching

- Explain the need to ask for assistance before moving around.
- Stress the need to avoid sudden position changes and dangerous tasks.
- Teach the patient about the underlying diagnosis and treatment plan.
- Explain prescribed medications and precautions.

Vesicular rash

A vesicular rash is a scattered or linear distribution of sharply circumscribed, blisterlike lesions that are filled with clear, cloudy, or bloody fluid. The lesions are usually less than ¼″ (0.5 cm) in diameter and may occur singly or in groups. They may also occur with bullae—fluid-filled lesions that are larger than ¼″ in diameter.

A vesicular rash may be mild or severe, temporary or permanent. It may result from infection, inflammation, or allergic reactions.

History

- Ask about the onset and characteristics of the rash.
- Take a drug history.
- Ask about other signs and symptoms.
- Find out about a family history of skin disorders.
- Ask about a history of allergies.
- Inquire about recent infections, insect bites, or exposure to allergens.

Physical examination

- Note if the skin is dry, oily, or moist.
- Observe the distribution of the lesions; record their location.
- Note the color, shape, and size of the lesions.
- Check for crusts, scales, scars, macules, papules, or wheals.
- Palpate the vesicles or bullae to determine if they're flaccid or tense.

Causes

Medical causes

Burns, second-degree

- Vesicles and bullae, erythema, swelling, pain, and moistness occur with second-degree burns.

Dermatitis

- With contact dermatitis, small vesicles are surrounded by redness and marked edema; vesicles may ooze, scale, and cause severe pruritus.
- With dermatitis herpetiformis, vesicular, papular, bullous, pustular, or erythematous lesions form; severe pruritus, burning, and stinging may also occur.
- With nummular dermatitis, groups of pinpoint vesicles and papules appear on erythematous or pustular lesions. Pustular lesions may ooze a purulent exudate, itch severely, and rapidly become crusted and scaly.

Dermatophytid

- Pruritic and tender vesicular lesions develop on the hands.
- Other signs and symptoms include fever, anorexia, generalized adenopathy, and splenomegaly.

Erythema multiforme

- This disorder is signaled by a sudden eruption of erythematous macules, papules, and occasionally vesicles and bullae.
- Vesiculobullous lesions usually appear on the mucous membranes, especially the lips and buccal mucosa—where they may rupture and ulcerate, producing thick, yellow or white exudate.
- A characteristic rash appears symmetrically over the hands, arms, feet, legs, face, and neck.

Herpes simplex

- Vesicles that are 2 to 3 mm in size and on an inflamed base most commonly appear on the lips and lower face.

- Vesicles are preceded by itching, tingling, burning, or pain.
- Eventually, vesicles rupture and form a painful ulcer, followed by a yellowish crust.

Herpes zoster

- A vesicular rash is preceded by erythema and, occasionally, by a nodular skin eruption and sharp pain along a dermatome.
- About 5 days later, lesions erupt and the pain becomes burning; vesicles dry and scab about 10 days after eruption.
- Other signs and symptoms include fever, malaise, pruritus, and paresthesia or hyperesthesia of the involved area.
- If the cranial nerves are involved, facial palsy, hearing loss, dizziness, loss of taste, eye pain, and impaired vision occur.

Insect bites

- Vesicles appear on red papules and may become hemorrhagic.
- Other signs and symptoms include fever, myalgia, headache, lymphadenopathy, nausea, and vomiting.

Pemphigus

- Groups of tiny vesicles erupt on normal skin or mucous membranes.
- Vesicles are thin-walled, flaccid, and easily broken, producing small denuded areas that eventually form crusts; itching and burning of the skin may also occur.

Pompholyx (dyshidrosis or dyshidrosis eczema)

- Symmetrical vesicular lesions that can become pustular appear on the palms and soles.
- Pruritic lesions are more common on the palms than on the soles with possible minimal erythema.

Scabies

- Small vesicles erupt on an erythematous base and may be at the end of a threadlike burrow.
- Pustules and excoriations may occur.
- Pruritus occurs and may worsen with inactivity, warmth, and nightfall.

Smallpox

- A maculopapular rash on the mucosa of the mouth, pharynx, face and forearms spreads to the trunk and legs, then turns vesicular within 2 days and later pustular.
- Initial signs and symptoms include high fever, malaise, prostration, severe headache, backache, and abdominal pain.
- After 8 to 9 days, the pustules form a crust; later, the scab separates from the skin, leaving a pitted scar.

Tinea pedis

- Vesicles and scaling develop between the toes.
- Inflammation, pruritus, and difficulty walking occur with severe infection.

Toxic epidermal necrolysis

- In this immune reaction to drugs or other toxins, vesicles and bullae are preceded by a diffuse, erythematous rash and followed by large-scale epidermal necrolysis and desquamation.
- Other signs and symptoms include a burning sensation in the conjunctivae, malaise, fever, and generalized skin tenderness.

Nursing considerations

- If skin eruptions cover a large skin surface, insert an I.V. catheter to replace fluids and electrolytes.
- Keep the environment warm and free from drafts.
- Obtain cultures to determine the causative organism.
- Look for signs of secondary infection.

- Give the patient an antibiotic and apply corticosteroid or antimicrobial ointment to the lesions as prescribed.

Patient teaching

- Explain the importance of frequent hand washing and other infection-control techniques.
- Instruct the patient to avoid touching the lesions.
- Explain the use of tepid baths or cold compresses to relieve itching and discomfort.
- Discuss the underlying condition and treatment.

Vision loss

Vision loss—the inability to perceive visual stimuli—can be sudden or gradual and temporary or permanent. The deficit can range from a slight impairment of vision to total blindness. It can result from an ocular, a neurologic, or a systemic disorder, trauma, or the use of certain drugs. The ultimate visual outcome may depend on early, accurate diagnosis and treatment.

History

- Ask about the characteristics of vision loss.
- Find out about associated photosensitivity or eye pain.
- Obtain an ocular history and family history of eye problems or systemic diseases that may lead to eye problems, such as hypertension; diabetes mellitus; thyroid, rheumatic, or vascular disease; infections; and cancer.
- Determine current medications, especially eyedrops.

Physical examination

- If the patient has perforating or penetrating ocular trauma, don't touch his eye. (See *Managing sudden vision loss.*)
- Assess visual acuity, with best available correction in each eye.
- Inspect the eyes, noting edema, foreign bodies, drainage, or conjunctival or scleral redness.
- Observe whether lid closure is complete or incomplete, and check for ptosis.
- Using a flashlight, examine the cornea and iris for scars, irregularities, and foreign bodies.
- Observe the size, shape, and color of the pupils.
- Test the direct and consensual light reflex and the effect of accommodation.

Causes

Medical causes

Amaurosis fugax

- Recurrent loss of vision in one eye may last from a few seconds to a few minutes.
- Vision is normal at other times.
- Transient one-sided weakness, hypertension, and elevated intraocular pressure (IOP) in the affected eye may also develop.

Cataract

- Painless and gradual blurring of vision precedes vision loss.
- As the disease progresses, the pupil turns milky white.
- Night blindness and halo vision may be early signs.

Concussion

- Vision may be temporarily blurred, doubled, or lost.
- Other signs and symptoms include headache, anterograde and retrograde amnesia, transient loss of consciousness, nausea, vomiting, dizziness, irritability, confusion, lethargy, and aphasia.

Diabetic retinopathy

- Retinal edema and hemorrhage lead to blurred vision, which may progress to blindness.

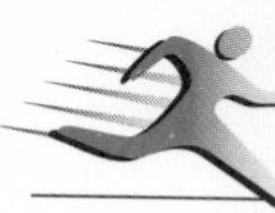

QUICK ACTION

Managing sudden vision loss

Sudden vision loss can signal central retinal artery occlusion or acute angle-closure glaucoma—ocular emergencies that require immediate intervention. If your patient reports sudden vision loss, immediately notify an ophthalmologist for an emergency examination, and perform the following interventions.

For a patient with suspected central retinal artery occlusion, perform light massage over his closed eyelid. Increase his carbon dioxide level by administering a set flow of oxygen and carbon dioxide through a Venturi mask, or have the patient breathe into a paper bag to reintroduce exhaled carbon dioxide. These steps will dilate the artery and may restore blood flow to the retina.

For a patient with suspected acute angle-closure glaucoma, measure intraocular pressure (IOP) with a tonometer. (You can also estimate IOP without a tonometer by placing your fingers over the patient's closed eyelid. A rock-hard eyeball usually indicates increased IOP.) Expect to instill timolol (Timoptic) drops and to administer I.V. acetazolamide (Dazamide) to help decrease IOP.

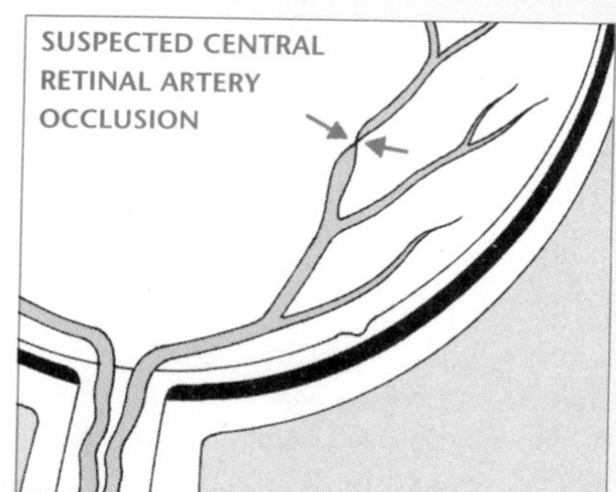

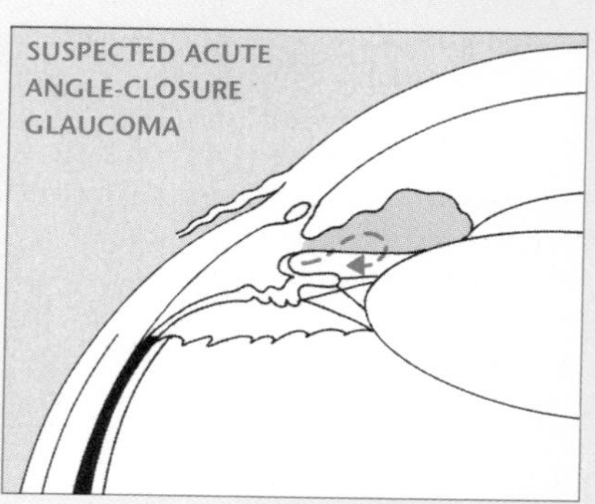

- Loss of central vision and color vision may also occur.
- This disorder is usually a sign of poorly controlled, brittle, or advanced diabetes.

Endophthalmitis

- Permanent unilateral vision loss may result as well as headache, photophobia, and ocular discharge.

Glaucoma

- Gradual blurring of vision may progress to total blindness.
- Acute angle-closure glaucoma, an ocular emergency, may produce blindness within 3 to 5 days. In addition, signs and symptoms include inflammation and pain in one eye, eye pressure, moderate pupil dilation, nonreactive pupillary response, a cloudy cornea, reduced visual acuity, photophobia, nausea, vomiting, and perception of blue or red halos around lights.
- Chronic open-angle glaucoma typically causes a slowly progressive peripheral vision loss, aching eyes, halo vision, and reduced visual acuity—especially at night.

Herpes zoster

■ When the nasociliary nerve is affected, vision loss may occur with eyelid lesions, conjunctivitis, skin lesions, and ocular muscle palsies.

Hyphema

■ Blood in the anterior chamber can reduce vision to mere light perception.
■ Other signs and symptoms include moderate pain, conjunctival injection, and eyelid edema.

Keratitis

■ Complete vision loss occurs in one eye, with an opaque cornea, increased tearing, irritation, and photophobia.

Ocular trauma

■ Vision loss is sudden, total or partial, permanent or temporary, and in one or both eyes.
■ Eyelids may be reddened, edematous, and lacerated; intraocular contents may be extruded.

Optic atrophy

■ Irreversible loss of the visual field results as well as changes in color vision.
■ Pupillary reactions are sluggish, and optic disk pallor is evident.

Optic neuritis

■ Vision loss in one eye is temporary but severe.
■ Pain around the eye occurs, especially with movement of the globe.
■ Visual field defects and a sluggish pupillary response may also occur.

Paget's disease

■ Vision loss may develop because of bony impingements on the cranial nerves.
■ Hearing loss, tinnitus, vertigo, and severe, persistent bone pain also occur.
■ Cranial enlargement may be noticeable frontally and occipitally, and headaches may occur.
■ Sites of bone involvement are warm and tender, and impaired mobility and pathologic fractures are common.

Papilledema

■ Acute papilledema may lead to momentary blurring or transiently obscured vision; chimeric papilledema may cause vision loss.

Pituitary tumor

■ Blurred vision progresses to hemianopsia and, possibly, unilateral blindness as the tumor grows.
■ Double vision, nystagmus, ptosis, limited eye movement, and headaches may also occur.

Retinal artery occlusion, central

■ In this ocular emergency, partial or complete vision loss in one eye is sudden.
■ Permanent blindness may occur within hours.
■ A sluggish direct pupillary response and a normal consensual response occur.

Retinal detachment

■ Painless vision loss may be gradual or sudden and partial or total.
■ Partial vision loss may elicit reports of visual field defects, a shadow or curtain over the visual fields, and visual floaters.
■ Total blindness occurs with macular involvement.

Retinal vein occlusion, central

■ A decrease in visual acuity in one eye may occur with variable vision loss.
■ IOP may be elevated in both eyes.

Senile macular degeneration

■ Painless blurring or loss of central vision occurs.
■ Vision loss may proceed slowly or rapidly, may eventually affect both eyes, and may be worse at night.

Temporal arteritis

■ Vision blurring and loss with a throbbing headache are characteristic signs.

■ Other signs and symptoms include malaise, anorexia, weight loss, weakness, low-grade fever, generalized muscle aches, and confusion.

Uveitis

■ Inflammation of the uveal tract may cause unilateral vision loss.

■ Anterior uveitis produces moderate to severe eye pain, severe conjunctival injection, photophobia, and a small, nonreactive pupil.

■ Posterior uveitis may produce the insidious onset of blurred vision, conjunctival injection, visual floaters, pain, and photophobia.

Vitreous hemorrhage

■ Vision loss in one eye is sudden.

■ Visual floaters and partial vision with a reddish haze may occur.

Other causes

Drugs

■ Digoxin derivatives, ethambutol, indomethacin (Indocin), methanol toxicity, and quinine may cause vision loss.

■ Chloroquine phosphate (Aralen) therapy may cause patchy retinal pigmentation that typically leads to blindness.

Nursing considerations

■ If the patient has photophobia, darken the room and suggest he wear sunglasses during the day.

■ Obtain cultures of eye drainage.

■ Announce your presence each time you approach the patient.

■ Get the patient a referral to an ophthalmologist for evaluation.

Patient teaching

■ Make sure the patient is oriented to his environment.

■ Explain safety measures to prevent injury.

■ Emphasize the importance of washing the hands frequently and *not* rubbing the eyes.

■ If vision loss is progressive or permanent, refer the patient to appropriate social service agencies for assistance with adaptation and equipment.

■ Discuss the underlying disorder, diagnostic tests, and treatment plan.

Visual blurring

Visual blurring is a common symptom that refers to the loss of visual acuity with indistinct visual details. It may result from eye injury, a neurologic or eye disorder, or a disorder with vascular complications such as diabetes mellitus. Visual blurring may also result from mucus passing over the cornea, a refractive error, improperly fitted contact lenses, or certain drugs.

History

■ Ask about eye pain, trauma, sudden vision loss, or discharge.

■ Find out about the onset of visual blurring.

■ Ask about recent accidents or injuries.

■ Obtain a medical and drug history.

Physical examination

■ Inspect the eye; note lid edema, drainage, conjunctival or scleral redness, an irregularly shaped iris, and excessive blinking.

■ Assess for pupillary changes.

■ Test visual acuity in both eyes.

■ Assess the patient's neurologic status and level of consciousness (LOC).

Causes

Medical causes

Brain tumor

■ Visual blurring occurs with decreased LOC, headache, apathy, behavioral changes, memory loss, decreased attention span, dizziness, and confusion.

- Related signs and symptoms include aphasia, seizures, ataxia, and signs of hormonal imbalance.
- Later signs and symptoms include vomiting, increased systolic blood pressure, widened pulse pressure, and decorticate posture.

Cataract

- Gradual blurring with halo vision is an early sign, followed by visual glare in bright light, progressive vision loss, and a gray pupil that turns milky white.

Concussion

- Blurred, double, or temporary vision loss occurs with a concussion.
- Related signs and symptoms include changes in the patient's LOC and behavior.

Conjunctivitis

- Visual blurring occurs with photophobia, pain, burning, tearing, itching, and a feeling of fullness around the eyes.
- Redness near the fornices (brilliant red suggests a bacterial cause; milky red, an allergic cause) and drainage occur. Copious, mucopurulent, and flaky drainage characterize bacterial conjunctivitis; stringy drainage is typical of allergic conjunctivitis.
- With viral conjunctivitis, copious tearing, minimal exudate, and an enlarged preauricular lymph node occur.

Corneal abrasions

- Visual blurring with severe eye pain occurs with corneal abrasions.
- Other signs and symptoms include photophobia, redness, and excessive tearing.

Corneal foreign bodies

- Visual blurring may accompany foreign-body sensation, excessive tearing, photophobia, intense eye pain, miosis, conjunctival injection, and a dark corneal speck.

Diabetic retinopathy

- Retinal edema and hemorrhage produce gradual blurring, which may progress to blindness.
- Loss of central vision and color vision may occur.

Eye tumor

- If the macula is involved, blurring may be the first symptom.
- Other signs and symptoms include varying visual field losses.

Glaucoma

- With acute angle-closure glaucoma, which is an ocular emergency, visual blurring and severe pain begin suddenly in one eye.
- Other acute signs and symptoms include halo vision; a moderately dilated, nonreactive pupil; conjunctival injection; a cloudy cornea; and decreased visual acuity.
- With chronic angle-closure glaucoma, transient visual blurring and halo vision may precede pain and blindness.

Hypertension

- Visual blurring and a constant morning headache occur with hypertension.
- With a diastolic blood pressure over 120 mm Hg, a severe throbbing headache occurs.
- Other signs and symptoms include restlessness, confusion, nausea, vomiting, seizures, and decreased LOC.

Hyphema

- Visual blurring from blunt eye trauma with hemorrhage into the anterior chamber causes moderate pain, diffuse conjunctival injection, visible blood in the anterior chamber, ecchymoses, eyelid edema, and a hard eye.

Iritis

■ Signs and symptoms include sudden blurring, moderate to severe eye pain, photophobia, conjunctival injection, and a constricted pupil.

Macular degeneration, dry form

■ Initially, painless visual blurring or dimming is especially noticeable with reading and worse at night.
■ Other signs and symptoms include blind spots and progressive loss of central vision.

Macular degeneration, wet form

■ Blurring with darkened vision occurs in the affected eye.
■ A blind spot occurs in the visual field, with distorted straight lines and eventual loss of central vision.

Migraine headache

■ Migraine headache is characterized by blurring and paroxysmal attacks of a severe, throbbing headache.
■ Nausea, vomiting, sensitivity to light and noise, and sensory or visual auras may also occur.

Multiple sclerosis

■ In the early stage, blurred vision, diplopia, and paresthesia occur.
■ In later stages, nystagmus, muscle weakness, paralysis, spasticity, hyperreflexia, intention tremor, and ataxic gait occur.
■ Other symptoms include urinary frequency, urgency, and incontinence.

Optic neuritis

■ With this disorder, an acute attack of blurring and vision loss occurs because of inflammation, degeneration, or demyelinization of the optic nerve.
■ Scotomas and eye pain occur.
■ Ophthalmoscopic examination reveals hyperemia of the optic disk, large vein distention, blurred disk margins, and filling of the physiologic cup.

Retinal detachment

■ Sudden visual blurring may be the first symptom, followed by visual floaters and recurring light flashes.
■ Progressive detachment increases vision loss.

Retinal vein occlusion, central

■ Gradual visual blurring and varying degrees of vision loss occur in one eye.

Stroke

■ Brief episodes of visual blurring occur before or with a stroke.
■ Associated signs and symptoms include decreased LOC, contralateral hemiplegia, dysarthria, dysphagia, ataxia, unilateral sensory loss, agnosia, aphasia, homonymous hemianopsia, diplopia, disorientation, and apraxia.
■ Other signs and symptoms include urine retention or incontinence, constipation, personality changes, emotional lability, and seizures.

Temporal arteritis

■ Sudden blurred vision with vision loss and a throbbing headache occur.
■ Early signs and symptoms include malaise, anorexia, weight loss, weakness, low-grade fever, and generalized muscle aches.
■ Later signs and symptoms include confusion; disorientation; swollen, nodular, tender temporal arteries; and erythema of overlying skin.

Uveitis, posterior

■ Blurred vision, conjunctival injection, visual floaters, pain, and photophobia occur with this disorder.

Vitreous hemorrhage

- Sudden visual blurring and varying vision loss occur in one eye.
- Associated signs and symptoms include visual floaters or dark streaks and partial vision with a reddish haze.

Other causes

Drugs

- Visual blurring can be caused by anticholinergics, antihistamines, clomiphene (Clomid), cycloplegics, guanethidine (Ismelin), phenothiazines, reserpine (Serpalan), or thiazide diuretics.

Nursing considerations

- Prepare the patient for diagnostic tests and possible surgery.
- Initiate safety measures to prevent injury.
- Provide emotional support as needed.

Patient teaching

- Teach the patient how to use eyedrops properly.
- Explain the need for orientation to his environment.
- Instruct the patient in safety measures.
- Discuss the underlying disorder.

Visual floaters

Visual floaters are particles of blood or cellular debris that move about in the vitreous. As these floaters enter the visual field, they appear as spots or dots. *Chronic* floaters may occur normally in elderly or myopic patients; however, the *sudden* onset of visual floaters commonly signals retinal detachment, an ocular emergency.

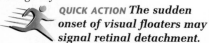

QUICK ACTION ***The sudden onset of visual floaters may signal retinal detachment. Does the patient also see flashing lights or spots in the affected eye? Is he experiencing a curtainlike loss of vision? If so, notify an ophthalmologist immediately and restrict his eye movements until the diagnosis is made.***

History

- Obtain a drug and allergy history.
- Ask about nearsightedness (a predisposing factor), use of corrective lenses, eye trauma, or other eye disorders.
- Ask about a history of granulomatous disease, diabetes mellitus, or hypertension, which may have predisposed the patient to retinal detachment, vitreous hemorrhage, or uveitis.

Physical examination

- Inspect the eyes for signs of injury, such as bruising or edema, and determine the patient's visual acuity.

Causes

Medical causes

Retinal detachment

- Floaters and light flashes appear suddenly in the portion of the visual field where the retina is detached from the choroid.
- As the retina detaches further (a painless process), the patient develops gradual vision loss, likened to a cloud or curtain falling in front of the eyes.
- Ophthalmoscopic examination reveals a gray, opaque, detached retina with an indefinite margin. Retinal vessels appear almost black.

Uveitis, posterior

- This disorder may cause visual floaters accompanied by gradual eye pain, photophobia, blurred vision, and conjunctival injection.

Vitreous hemorrhage

- Rupture of the retinal vessels produces a shower of red or black dots or a red haze across the visual field.

■ Vision suddenly becomes blurred in the affected eye, and visual acuity may be greatly reduced.

Nursing considerations

■ Encourage bed rest and provide a calm environment.

■ Depending on the cause of the floaters, the patient may require eye patches, surgery, or a corticosteroid or other drug therapy. If bilateral eye patches are necessary—as in retinal detachment—ensure the patient's safety.

■ Identify yourself when you approach the patient, and frequently orient him to time.

■ Provide sensory stimulation, such as a radio or tape player.

■ Place pillows or towels behind the patient's head to help him maintain the appropriate position.

■ Warn him not to touch or rub his eyes and to avoid straining or sudden movements.

Patient teaching

■ Teach the patient and his family about the underlying diagnosis and treatment plan.

■ Explain all hospital procedures and tests.

■ Teach the patient about prescribed medications.

Vomiting

Vomiting is the forceful expulsion of gastric contents through the mouth. Characteristically preceded by nausea, vomiting results from a coordinated sequence of abdominal muscle contractions and reverse esophageal peristalsis.

A common sign of GI disorders, vomiting also occurs with fluid and electrolyte imbalances; infections; and metabolic, endocrine, labyrinthine, central nervous system, and cardiac disorders. It can also result from drug therapy, surgery, or radiation.

Vomiting occurs normally during the first trimester of pregnancy, but its subsequent development may also signal complications. It can also result from stress, anxiety, pain, alcohol intoxication, overeating, or ingestion of distasteful foods or liquids.

QUICK ACTION ***Immediate action is required if the patient's vomiting has caused dehydration or significant blood loss. Immediate response includes instituting I.V. fluid or blood replacement. Obtain blood samples to assess electrolyte levels, renal studies, liver function tests, and a complete blood count. Assess the patient's vital signs frequently until he's stable. Give an antiemetic as ordered. Offer supportive care during vomiting episodes, and provide meticulous mouth care afterward.***

History

■ Ask about the onset, duration, and intensity of vomiting. (See *Vomitus: Characteristics and causes,* page 418.)

■ Determine aggravating or alleviating factors.

■ Ask about nausea, abdominal pain, anorexia, weight loss, changes in bowel habits, excessive belching or flatus, and bloating or fullness.

■ Obtain a medical history, including GI, endocrine, and metabolic disorders; infections; and cancer, including chemotherapy and radiation therapy.

■ Ask about current drug use and alcohol consumption.

■ Ask the female patient if she could be pregnant.

Physical examination

■ Inspect the abdomen for distention.

■ Auscultate for bowel sounds and bruits.

■ Palpate for rigidity and tenderness, and test for rebound tenderness.

Vomitus: Characteristics and causes

When you collect a specimen of the patient's vomitus, observe it carefully for clues to the underlying disorder. Listen to the patient's complaints for additional clues.

Bile-stained (greenish) vomitus
Obstruction below the pylorus, as from a duodenal lesion

Bloody vomitus
Upper GI bleeding (if bright red, may result from gastritis or a peptic ulcer; if dark red, from esophageal or gastric varices)

Brown vomitus with a fecal odor
Intestinal obstruction or infarction

Burning, bitter-tasting vomitus
Excessive hydrochloric acid in gastric contents

Coffee-ground vomitus
Digested blood from a slowly bleeding gastric or duodenal lesion

Undigested food
Gastric outlet obstruction, as from a gastric tumor or ulcer

- Palpate and percuss the liver for enlargement.
- Assess the buccal mucosa and skin for sufficient hydration.

Causes

Medical causes

Adrenal insufficiency

- Vomiting, nausea, anorexia, and diarrhea commonly occur with adrenal insufficiency.
- Other signs and symptoms include weakness, fatigue, weight loss, bronze skin, orthostatic hypotension, and a weak, irregular pulse.

Anthrax, GI

- After eating contaminated food, vomiting occurs with a loss of appetite, nausea, and fever.
- GI anthrax may progress to abdominal pain, severe bloody diarrhea, and hematemesis.

Appendicitis

- Vomiting and nausea occur after or with abdominal pain.
- Vague epigastric or periumbilical discomfort occurs and rapidly progresses to severe, stabbing pain in the right lower quadrant.
- A positive McBurney sign—severe pain and tenderness on palpation about 2″ (5 cm) from the right anterior superior spine of the ilium, on a line between that spine and the umbilicus—may also occur.
- Related signs and symptoms include abdominal rigidity and tenderness, anorexia, constipation or diarrhea, cutaneous hyperalgesia, fever, tachycardia, and malaise.

Bulimia

- Polyphagia that alternates with self-induced vomiting, fasting, or diarrhea are classic signs.
- Anorexia, a morbid fear of obesity, and calloused knuckles (from self-induced vomiting) are signs and symptoms of the disorder.

Cholecystitis, acute

- With acute cholecystitis, nausea and mild vomiting follow severe right upper quadrant pain that may radiate to the back or shoulders.
- Related signs and symptoms include abdominal tenderness and, possibly, rigidity and distention, fever, and diaphoresis.

Cholelithiasis

- Nausea and vomiting, with severe unlocalized right upper quadrant or epigastric pain, follow the ingestion of fatty foods.
- Other signs and symptoms include abdominal tenderness and guarding, flatulence, belching, epigastric burning, pyrosis, tachycardia, and restlessness.

Cholera

- Cholera causes vomiting with abrupt, watery diarrhea.
- Thirst, weakness, muscle cramps, decreased skin turgor, oliguria, tachycardia, and hypotension from severe water and electrolyte loss may also occur.

Cirrhosis

- In the early stage, nausea and vomiting, anorexia, aching abdominal pain, and constipation or diarrhea occur.
- In later stages, jaundice, hepatomegaly, and abdominal distention occur.

Escherichia coli *O157:H7*

- Vomiting occurs with watery or bloody diarrhea, nausea, fever, and abdominal cramps.
- Acute renal failure may occur in children younger than age 5 and in elderly patients.

Ectopic pregnancy

- A life-threatening disorder, ectopic pregnancy causes vomiting, nausea, vaginal bleeding, and lower abdominal pain.
- A tender abdominal mass and a 1- to 2-month history of amenorrhea is characteristic of this disorder.

Electrolyte imbalances

- Nausea and vomiting frequently occur along with arrhythmias, tremors, seizures, anorexia, malaise, and weakness.

Food poisoning

- Vomiting, diarrhea, severe and cramping abdominal pain, prostration, and fever commonly occur.

Gastritis

- Commonly, nausea and vomiting of mucus or blood occur with gastritis.
- Other signs and symptoms include epigastric pain, belching, and fever.

Gastroenteritis

- Nausea, vomiting (typically undigested food), diarrhea, and abdominal cramping occur with gastroenteritis.
- Associated signs and symptoms include fever, malaise, hyperactive bowel sounds, and abdominal pain and tenderness.

Gestational hypertension

- Nausea and vomiting occurs with rapid weight gain, epigastric pain, edema, elevated blood pressure, oliguria, severe frontal headache, and blurred or double vision.

Heart failure

- Nausea and vomiting occur, especially with right-sided heart failure.
- Tachycardia, ventricular gallop, fatigue, dyspnea, crackles, peripheral edema, and neck vein distention may also occur.

Hepatitis

- In the early stage, nausea and vomiting occur, along with fatigue, myalgia, arthralgia, headache, photophobia, anorexia, pharyngitis, cough, and fever.

Hyperemesis gravidarum

- With this disorder, unremitting nausea and vomiting last beyond the first trimester.
- Early in the disorder, undigested food, mucus, and small amounts of bile occur in the vomitus; later examination reveals a coffee-ground appearance.
- Other signs and symptoms include weight loss, headache, and delirium.

Increased intracranial pressure

- Projectile vomiting not preceded by nausea occurs with increased intracranial pressure.
- Decreased level of consciousness (LOC) and Cushing's triad (bradycardia, hypertension, and respiratory pattern changes) may also occur.
- Other signs and symptoms include headache, widened pulse pressure, impaired motor movement, vision disturbances, pupillary changes, and papilledema.

Intestinal obstruction

- Nausea and vomiting (bilious or fecal) commonly occur with intestinal obstruction.
- Usually, episodic and colicky abdominal pain occurs, possibly becoming severe and steady.
- Constipation occurs early in large intestinal obstruction and late in small intestinal obstruction.
- Obstipation occurs in complete obstruction.
- High-pitched and hyperactive bowel sounds occur in partial obstruction and hypoactive or absent bowel sounds in complete obstruction.

Labyrinthitis

- Nausea, vomiting, severe vertigo, progressive hearing loss, nystagmus and, possibly, otorrhea occur with labyrinthitis.

Listeriosis

- After ingesting food contaminated with *Listeria monocytogenes*, vomiting, fever, abdominal pain, myalgia, nausea, and diarrhea occur.

Ménière's disease

- Sudden, brief, recurrent attacks of nausea and vomiting, dizziness, vertigo, hearing loss, tinnitus, and nystagmus occur with this disease.

Mesenteric artery ischemia

- A life-threatening disorder, mesenteric artery ischemia causes nausea and vomiting and severe, cramping abdominal pain, especially after meals.
- Associated signs and symptoms include diarrhea or constipation, abdominal tenderness and bloating, anorexia, weight loss, and abdominal bruits.

Mesenteric venous thrombosis

- Nausea, vomiting, and abdominal pain with diarrhea or constipation, abdominal distention, hematemesis, and melena occur.

Metabolic acidosis

- Nausea, vomiting, anorexia, diarrhea, Kussmaul's respirations, and decreased LOC occur with this disorder.

Migraine headache

- Premonitory nausea and vomiting occur with a migraine headache.
- Other signs and symptoms include fatigue, photophobia, light flashes, increased noise sensitivity and, possibly, partial vision loss and paresthesia.

Motion sickness

- Nausea and vomiting with headache, vertigo, dizziness, fatigue, diaphoresis, and dyspnea are signs and symptoms of motion sickness.

Myocardial infarction

- Nausea and vomiting may occur with a myocardial infarction, but the main symptom is severe substernal chest pain, which may radiate to the left arm, jaw, or neck.
- Dyspnea, pallor, clammy skin, diaphoresis, and restlessness may occur.

Norovirus infection

- Violent vomiting may occur frequently and without warning.
- Additional signs and symptoms include nausea, diarrhea, and abdominal pain or cramping.

Pancreatitis, acute

- In the early stage, vomiting usually precedes nausea.
- Other signs and symptoms include steady and severe epigastric or left upper quadrant pain that may radiate to the back, abdominal tenderness and rigidity, hypoactive bowel sounds, anorexia, and fever.
- In severe cases, tachycardia, restlessness, hypotension, skin mottling, and cold, sweaty extremities may occur.

Peptic ulcer

- Nausea and vomiting may follow sharp, burning or gnawing epigastric pain.
- Pain occurs, especially when the stomach is empty or after ingestion of alcohol, caffeine, or aspirin.
- Hematemesis or melena may also occur.

Peritonitis

- Nausea and vomiting usually occur with acute abdominal pain.
- Related signs and symptoms include high fever with chills; tachycardia; hypoactive or absent bowel sounds; abdominal distention, rigidity, and tenderness; weakness; pale, cold skin; diaphoresis; hypotension; signs of dehydration; and shallow respirations.

Q fever

- In this rickettsial infection, vomiting with fever, chills, severe headache, malaise, chest pain, nausea, and diarrhea occur.

Rhabdomyolysis

- Vomiting along with muscle weakness or pain, fever, nausea, malaise, and dark urine occur.

Thyrotoxicosis

- Nausea and vomiting occur, along with the classic signs and symptoms of severe anxiety, heat intolerance, weight loss despite increased appetite, diaphoresis, diarrhea, tremors, tachycardia, and palpitations.
- Other signs include exophthalmos, ventricular or atrial gallop, and an enlarged thyroid.

Ulcerative colitis

- Vomiting, nausea, and anorexia occur, along with the common sign of recurrent diarrhea with blood, pus, and mucus.
- Related signs include fever, chills, and weight loss.

Volvulus

- Vomiting occurs with rapid, marked abdominal distention and sudden, severe abdominal pain.
- Twisting of the intestine (at least 180 degrees in its mesentery) leads to blood vessel compression and ischemia.
- In adults, volvulus is common in the sigmoid bowel; in children, the small bowel.
- Volvulus can also occur in the stomach or cecum.

Other causes

Drugs

- Anesthetics, antibiotics, antineoplastics, chloride replacements, estrogens, ferrous sulfate, levodopa (Sinemet), opiates, oral potassium, quinidine

(Quinaglute), and sulfasalazine (Azulfidine) may cause vomiting.

- Overdoses of cardiac glycosides and theophylline (Elixophyllin) may also cause vomiting.
- Syrup of ipecac may be used to induce vomiting for overdoses.

Radiation and surgery

- Radiation therapy can cause vomiting if it disrupts the gastric mucosa.
- Postoperative nausea and vomiting commonly occurs, especially after abdominal surgery.

Nursing considerations

- Draw blood to determine electrolyte and acid-base balance.
- Elevate the patient's head, or position the patient on his side to prevent aspiration of vomitus.
- Monitor the patient's vital signs and intake and output.
- Maintain hydration by giving sips of water or ice chips, if tolerated, or by I.V. fluids if the patient is hospitalized.
- Give drugs for pain promptly. If possible, give these by injection or suppository.
- If an opioid is used, monitor bowel sounds, flatus, and bowel movements.

Patient teaching

- Explain deep-breathing techniques to postoperative patients.
- Discuss how to replace fluid losses.
- Teach the patient to adjust his diet by starting with clear liquids and advancing to a bland diet.
- Discuss the underlying disorder, diagnostic tests, and treatment plan.

Wxyz

Weight gain, excessive

Weight gain occurs when ingested calories exceed body requirements for energy, causing increased adipose tissue storage. It can also occur when fluid retention causes edema. When weight gain results from overeating, emotional factors—most commonly anxiety, guilt, and depression—and social factors may be the primary causes.

Among elderly people, weight gain commonly reflects a sustained food intake in the presence of a normal, progressive fall in basal metabolic rate. Among women, a progressive weight gain occurs with pregnancy, whereas a periodic weight gain usually occurs with menstruation.

Also a primary sign of many endocrine disorders, weight gain may occur with conditions that limit activity, especially cardiovascular and pulmonary disorders. It can also result from drug therapy that increases appetite or causes fluid retention or from cardiovascular, hepatic, and renal disorders that cause edema.

History

- Ask about a previous pattern of weight gain and loss.
- Find out about a family history of obesity, thyroid disease, or diabetes mellitus.
- Note eating and activity patterns.
- Determine exercise habits.
- Ask about vision disturbances, hoarseness, paresthesia, increased urination and thirst, impotence, or menstrual irregularities.
- Take a drug history.

Physical examination

- Note the patient's mental status, memory, and response time.
- Measure skin-fold thickness.
- Note fat distribution and the presence of edema.
- Note the patient's overall nutritional status.
- Inspect for other abnormalities, such as abnormal body hair distribution or hair loss and dry skin.
- Take the patient's vital signs.
- Determine body mass index and waist circumference.

Causes

Medical causes

Acromegaly

- Moderate weight gain occurs with coarsened facial features, projecting jaw, enlarged hands and feet, increased sweating, oily skin, deep voice, back and joint pain, lethargy, sleepiness, and heat intolerance.
- Occasionally, hirsutism may occur.

Diabetes mellitus

- Increased appetite may lead to weight gain, although weight loss may also occur.
- Other signs and symptoms include fatigue, polydipsia, polyuria, polypha-

gia, nocturia, weakness, and somnolence.

Gestational hypertension

- Rapid weight gain occurs with this disorder, along with nausea and vomiting, epigastric pain, elevated blood pressure, and blurred or double vision.

Heart failure

- Weight gain from edema occurs.
- Associated signs and symptoms include paroxysmal nocturnal dyspnea, tachypnea, nausea, orthopnea, and fatigue.

Hypercortisolism

- Excessive weight gain occurs, usually over the trunk and the back of the neck (buffalo hump).
- Related signs and symptoms include slender extremities, moon face, weakness, purple striae, emotional lability, and increased susceptibility to infection.
- In men, gynecomastia occurs.
- In women, hirsutism, acne, and menstrual irregularities occur.

Hyperinsulinism

- Increased appetite leads to weight gain.
- Emotional lability, indigestion, weakness, diaphoresis, tachycardia, vision disturbances, and syncope may also occur.

Hypogonadism

- Weight gain is common.
- Prepubertal hypogonadism cause eunuchoid body proportions with relatively sparse facial and body hair and a high-pitched voice.
- Postpubertal hypogonadism causes loss of libido, impotence, and infertility.

Hypothyroidism

- Weight gain occurs despite anorexia.
- Other signs and symptoms include fatigue; cold intolerance; constipation; menorrhagia; slowed intellectual and motor activity; dry, pale, cool skin; dry, sparse hair; and thick, brittle nails.
- Other possible signs and symptoms include myalgia, hoarseness, hypoactive deep tendon reflexes, bradycardia, and abdominal distention.
- Eventually, a dull facial expression with periorbital edema occurs.

Nephrotic syndrome

- Weight gain results from edema.
- In severe cases, anasarca develops—increasing body weight as much as 50%.
- Related signs and symptoms include abdominal distention, orthostatic hypotension, and lethargy.

Pancreatic islet cell tumor

- Excessive hunger leads to weight gain.
- Other signs and symptoms include emotional lability, weakness, malaise, fatigue, restlessness, diaphoresis, palpitations, tachycardia, vision disturbances, and syncope.

Other causes

Drugs

- Corticosteroids, phenothiazines, and tricyclic antidepressants can create fluid retention and increased appetite and cause excessive weight gain.
- Cyproheptadine (Periactin) can cause increased appetite; hormonal contraceptives can cause fluid retention, and lithium (Eskalith) can trigger hypothyroidism, all of which may cause excessive weight gain.

Nursing considerations

- Psychological counseling may be necessary.
- If the patient is obese or has a cardiopulmonary disorder, exercises should be monitored closely.

■ Prepare the patient for studies to rule out possible secondary causes that include serum thyroid function studies, lipid level, glucose level, and dexamethasone suppression testing.

Patient teaching

■ Discuss the underlying disorder, if present.
■ Emphasize the importance of weight control.
■ Explain the importance of behavior modification and dietary compliance.
■ Provide guidance in appropriate exercise.

Weight loss, excessive

Weight loss can reflect decreased food intake, decreased food absorption, increased metabolic requirements, or a combination of the three. Its causes include endocrine, neoplastic, GI, and psychiatric disorders; nutritional deficiencies; infections; and neurologic lesions that cause paralysis and dysphagia. Weight loss may accompany conditions that prevent sufficient food intake, such as painful oral lesions, ill-fitting dentures, and loss of teeth. It may be the metabolic effect of poverty, fad diets, excessive exercise, or certain drugs.

Weight loss may occur as a late sign in such chronic diseases as heart failure and renal disease. In these diseases, however, weight loss is the result of anorexia.

History

■ Take a diet history, noting the use of diet pills and laxatives.
■ Question the patient about why he isn't eating properly, if applicable.
■ Ask about previous weight and if weight loss is intentional.
■ Note sources of anxiety or depression.
■ Ask about changes in bowel habits, nausea, vomiting, abdominal pain, excessive thirst, excessive urination, or heat intolerance.

Physical examination

■ Check the patient's height and weight.
■ Take the patient's vital signs and note his general appearance.
■ Examine the skin for turgor and abnormal pigmentation.
■ Look for signs of infection or irritation on the roof of the mouth; note hyperpigmentation of the buccal mucosa.
■ Check the eyes for exophthalmos and the neck for swelling.
■ Evaluate breath sounds.
■ Inspect the abdomen for wasting; palpate for masses, tenderness, and an enlarged liver.

Causes

Medical causes

Adrenal insufficiency

■ Weight loss, anorexia, weakness, fatigue, irritability, syncope, nausea, vomiting, abdominal pain, and diarrhea or constipation occur with this disorder.
■ Other signs include hyperpigmentation at the joints, belt line, palmar creases, lips, gums, tongue, and buccal mucosa.

Anorexia nervosa

■ A self-imposed weight loss of 10% to 50% of premorbid weight characterizes this disorder.
■ Signs and symptoms include a morbid fear of becoming fat, skeletal muscle atrophy, loss of fatty tissue, hypotension, constipation, dental caries, susceptibility to infection, blotchy or sallow skin, cold intolerance, hairiness on the face and body, dryness or loss of scalp hair, and amenorrhea.
■ Other related signs and symptoms include dehydration or metabolic acidosis or alkalosis from self-induced vomiting or the use of laxatives and diuretics.

Cancer

- Weight loss occurs with signs and symptoms specific to the tumor, including fatigue, pain, nausea, vomiting, anorexia, abnormal bleeding, or a palpable mass.

Crohn's disease

- Weight loss occurs with chronic cramping, abdominal pain, and anorexia.
- Associated signs and symptoms include diarrhea, nausea, fever, tachycardia, abdominal tenderness and guarding, hyperactive bowel sounds, and abdominal distention.

Cryptosporidiosis

- Weight loss occurs with profuse watery diarrhea, abdominal cramping, flatulence, anorexia, malaise, fever, nausea, vomiting, and myalgia.

Depression

- Excessive weight loss or gain occurs with insomnia or hypersomnia, anorexia, apathy, fatigue, suicidal thoughts, and feelings of worthlessness.

Diabetes mellitus

- Weight loss occurs despite increased appetite.
- Other signs and symptoms include polydipsia, polyuria, weakness, fatigue, and blurred vision.

Esophagitis

- Avoidance of eating and weight loss from painful inflammation of the esophagus occur with esophagitis.
- Associated signs and symptoms include intense pain in the mouth and anterior chest with hypersalivation, dysphagia, tachypnea, and hematemesis.

Gastroenteritis

- Malabsorption and dehydration cause sudden weight loss in acute viral infections or gradual weight loss in parasitic infections.
- Other signs and symptoms include poor skin turgor, dry mucous membranes, tachycardia, hypotension, diarrhea, abdominal pain and tenderness, hyperactive bowel sounds, nausea, vomiting, fever, and malaise.

Herpes simplex, type 1

- Painful fluid-filled blisters in and around the mouth make eating painful, causing decreased food intake and weight loss.
- Fever and pharyngitis may also occur.

Leukemia

- The acute form causes progressive weight loss; severe prostration; high fever; swollen, bleeding gums; and bleeding tendencies.
- The chronic form causes progressive weight loss, malaise, fatigue, pallor, enlarged spleen, bleeding tendencies, anemia, skin eruptions, anorexia, and fever.

Lymphoma

- Gradual weight loss occurs.
- Other signs and symptoms include fever, fatigue, night sweats, malaise, hepatosplenomegaly, and lymphadenopathy.

Pulmonary tuberculosis

- Weight loss occurs with fatigue, weakness, anorexia, night sweats, and low-grade fever.
- A cough with bloody or mucopurulent sputum, dyspnea, and pleuritic chest pain may also occur.

Stomatitis

- Weight loss occurs from the inability to eat caused by inflammation of the oral mucosa (usually red, swollen, and ulcerated).
- Related signs and symptoms include fever, increased salivation, malaise,

mouth pain, anorexia, and swollen, bleeding gums.

Thyrotoxicosis

- Increased metabolism causes weight loss.
- Other characteristics include nervousness, heat intolerance, diarrhea, increased appetite, palpitations, tachycardia, diaphoresis, fine tremor, an enlarged thyroid, and exophthalmos.

Ulcerative colitis

- Weight loss is a late sign.
- Bloody diarrhea with pus or mucus is an initial, characteristic sign.
- Weakness, crampy lower abdominal pain, tenesmus, anorexia, low-grade fever, and nausea and vomiting may also occur.

Other causes

Drugs

- Amphetamines and the inappropriate dosage of thyroid preparations commonly lead to weight loss.
- Chemotherapeutics cause stomatitis, which, when severe, causes weight loss.
- Laxative abuse may cause a malabsorptive state that leads to weight loss.

Surgery

- Intestinal and stomach surgeries that remove or bypass portions of the digestive tract may cause weight loss due to decreased absorption or intake capacity.

Nursing considerations

- Take daily calorie counts and weigh the patient weekly.
- Consult a nutritionist to determine an appropriate diet with adequate calories.
- Give hyperalimentation or tube feedings to maintain nutrition.

Patient teaching

- Provide guidance in proper diet and suggest keeping a food diary.
- Instruct the patient in good oral hygiene.
- Provide a referral to nutritional and psychological counseling if appropriate.
- Discuss the underlying disorder and treatment plan.

Wheezing

Wheezes are adventitious breath sounds with a high-pitched, musical, squealing, creaking, or groaning quality. They're caused by air flowing at a high velocity through a narrowed airway. When they originate in the large airways, they can be heard by placing an unaided ear over the chest wall or at the mouth. When they originate in smaller airways, they can be heard by placing a stethoscope over the anterior or posterior chest. Unlike crackles and rhonchi, wheezes can't be cleared by coughing.

Usually, prolonged wheezing occurs during expiration when bronchi are shortened and narrowed. Causes of airway narrowing include bronchospasm; mucosal thickening or edema; partial obstruction from a tumor, a foreign body, or secretions; and extrinsic pressure, as in tension pneumothorax or goiter. With airway obstruction, wheezing occurs during inspiration.

QUICK ACTION ***Examine the degree of the patient's respiratory distress. Is he responsive? Is he restless, confused, anxious, or afraid? Are his respirations abnormally fast, slow, shallow, or deep? Are they irregular? Can you hear wheezing through his mouth? Does he exhibit increased use of accessory muscles; increased chest wall motion; intercostal, suprasternal, or supraclavicular retractions; stridor; or nasal flaring? Take his other vital signs, noting hypotension or hypertension, decreased oxygen saturation, or an irregular, weak, rapid, or slow pulse.***

Help the patient relax, give humidified oxygen by face mask, and encourage him to take slow, deep breaths. Have endotracheal intubation and emergency resuscitation equipment readily available. Provide intermittent positive-pressure breathing and nebulization treatments with bronchodilators, if ordered. Insert an I.V. catheter for the administration of drugs, such as diuretics, steroids, bronchodilators, and sedatives. Perform the abdominal thrust maneuver, as indicated, for airway obstruction.

History

- Ask what triggers the wheezing.
- Ask about smoking habits.
- Find out about the onset, productivity, and frequency of coughing; obtain a description of any sputum.
- Ask about a history of asthma, allergies, cancer, or pulmonary or cardiac disorders.
- Find out about recent surgery, illness, or trauma or changes in appetite, weight, exercise tolerance, or sleep patterns.
- Obtain a drug history.
- Ask about exposure to irritants and toxic fumes.
- Ask about chest pain: the onset, quality, duration, intensity, aggravating or alleviating factors, and where the pain radiates.

Physical assessment

- Examine the nose and mouth for congestion, drainage, or signs of infection.
- If coughing produces sputum, obtain a sample for examination.
- Check for cyanosis, pallor, clamminess, masses, tenderness, swelling, distended neck veins, and enlarged lymph nodes.
- Inspect the chest for abnormal configuration and asymmetrical motion.
- Determine if the trachea is midline.
- Auscultate for crackles, rhonchi, or pleural friction rubs.
- Percuss for dullness or hyperresonance.
- Auscultate for heart and breath sounds.

Causes

Medical causes

Anaphylaxis

- Tracheal edema or bronchospasm can result in severe wheezing and stridor.
- Initial signs and symptoms include fright, weakness, sneezing, dyspnea, nasal pruritus, urticaria, erythema, angioedema, and signs of respiratory distress.
- Other signs and symptoms include nasal edema and congestion; profuse, watery rhinorrhea; chest or throat tightness; and dysphagia.
- Arrhythmias and hypotension may also occur.

Aspiration of foreign body

- Partial obstruction produces the sudden onset of wheezing and possibly stridor; a dry, paroxysmal cough; gagging; and hoarseness.
- Other signs and symptoms include tachycardia, dyspnea, decreased breath sounds, and possibly cyanosis.
- Fever, pain, and swelling may be caused by a retained foreign body.

Aspiration pneumonitis

- Wheezing with tachypnea, marked dyspnea, cyanosis, tachycardia, fever, productive (eventually purulent) cough, and pink, frothy sputum occur with this disorder.

Asthma

- Wheezing heard at the mouth during expiration is an initial and classic sign.
- An initially dry cough later becomes productive with thick mucus.

■ Other signs and symptoms include apprehension, prolonged expiration, intercostal and supraclavicular retractions, rhonchi, accessory muscle use, nasal flaring, and tachypnea.
■ Tachycardia, diaphoresis, and flushing or cyanosis may also occur.

Blast lung injury
■ Wheezing is a common symptom and is characterized by hypoxia and respiratory difficulty.
■ Additional signs and symptoms include hemorrhage, contusion, edema and tearing of the lung, chest pain, dyspnea, cyanosis, hemoptysis, and a classic "butterfly" pattern on chest X-ray.

Bronchial adenoma
■ Severe wheezing with chronic cough and recurring hemoptysis occurs.
■ In later stages, signs and symptoms of airway obstruction occur.

Bronchiectasis
■ Excessive mucus causes intermittent and localized or diffuse wheezing.
■ A copious, foul-smelling, mucopurulent cough is a classic finding and is accompanied by hemoptysis, rhonchi, and coarse crackles.
■ Weight loss, fatigue, weakness, exertional dyspnea, fever, malaise, halitosis, and late-stage clubbing may also occur.

Bronchiolitis
■ An upper respiratory infection causes inflammation and partial obstruction of the bronchioles that produces wheezing.
■ Other signs and symptoms include excessive mucus production, crackles, cough, dyspnea, tachypnea, nasal flaring, and retraction.

Bronchitis, chronic
■ Wheezing varies in severity, location, and intensity.
■ Signs and symptoms include prolonged expiration, coarse crackles, scattered rhonchi, and a hacking cough that later becomes productive.
■ Other signs and symptoms include dyspnea, accessory muscle use, barrel chest, tachypnea, clubbing, edema, weight gain, and cyanosis.

Bronchogenic carcinoma
■ Obstruction may cause localized wheezing.
■ Typical signs and symptoms include productive cough, dyspnea, hemoptysis (initially blood-tinged sputum, possibly leading to massive hemorrhage), anorexia, and weight loss.
■ Upper extremity edema and chest pain may also occur.

Chemical pneumonitis, acute
■ Mucosal injury causes increased secretions and edema, leading to wheezing, dyspnea, orthopnea, crackles, malaise, fever, and a productive cough with purulent sputum.
■ Signs of conjunctivitis, pharyngitis, laryngitis, and rhinitis may also occur.

Emphysema
■ Mild to moderate wheezing occurs.
■ Other signs and symptoms include dyspnea, malaise, tachypnea, diminished breath sounds, peripheral cyanosis, pursed-lip breathing, accessory muscle use, barrel chest, a chronic productive cough, clubbing, anorexia, and malaise.

Inhalation injury
■ Wheezing occurs after the initial signs and symptoms of hoarseness and coughing, singed nasal hairs, orofacial burns, and soot-stained sputum.
■ In later stages, crackles, rhonchi, and respiratory distress occur.

Pneumothorax, tension

- A life-threatening disorder, tension pneumothorax causes wheezing, dyspnea, tachycardia, tachypnea, and sudden, severe, sharp chest pain (usually one-sided).
- Other signs and symptoms include dry cough, cyanosis, accessory muscle use, asymmetrical chest wall movement, anxiety, and restlessness.

Pulmonary coccidioidomycosis

- Wheezing and rhonchi occur with cough, fever, chills, pleuritic chest pain, headache, weakness, fatigue, sore throat, backache, malaise, anorexia, and an itchy, macular rash.

Pulmonary edema

- A life-threatening disorder, pulmonary edema causes wheezing with coughing, exertional and paroxysmal nocturnal dyspnea and, later, orthopnea.
- Other signs and symptoms include tachycardia, tachypnea, crackles, and a diastolic gallop.
- In severe pulmonary edema, rapid, labored respirations; diffuse crackles; a productive cough and frothy, bloody sputum; arrhythmias; cold, clammy, cyanotic skin; hypotension; and thready pulse may occur.

Pulmonary tuberculosis

- Fibrosis causes wheezing in the late stages.
- Common signs and symptoms include a mild to severe productive cough with pleuritic chest pain and fine crackles, night sweats, anorexia, weight loss, fever, malaise, dyspnea, and fatigue.

Thyroid goiter

- Wheezing, dysphagia, and respiratory difficulty are caused by a compressed airway due to thyroid goiter.
- Other signs and symptoms include a swollen and distended neck.

Tracheobronchitis

- Wheezing, rhonchi, and moist or coarse crackles may be auscultated.
- Related signs and symptoms include cough, fever, sudden chills, muscle and back pain, and substernal tightness.

Nursing considerations

- Place the patient in semi-Fowler's position to ease breathing.
- Perform pulmonary physiotherapy as necessary.
- Give an antibiotic to treat infection, a bronchodilator to relieve bronchospasm and maintain a patent airway, a steroid to reduce inflammation, and a mucolytic or expectorant to increase the flow of secretions, as prescribed.
- Provide humidification to thin secretions.

Patient teaching

- Tell the patient how to promote drainage and prevent pooling of secretions, if needed.
- Explain deep-breathing and coughing techniques.
- Emphasize the importance of increasing fluid intake.
- Provide information about taking prescribed drugs.
- Discuss infection control techniques as appropriate.
- Explain the underlying disorder, diagnostic studies, and treatment plan.

Selected references
Index

Selected references

Anatomy & Physiology Made Incredibly Easy, 3rd ed. Philadelphia: Lippincott Williams & Wilkins, 2008.

Baranoski, S., and Ayello, E.A. *Wound Care Essentials: Practice Principles,* 2nd ed. Philadelphia: Lippincott Williams & Wilkins, 2008.

Berman, A., et al. *Kozier & Erb's Fundamentals of Nursing Concepts, Process, and Practice,* 8th ed. Upper Saddle River, N.J.: Prentice Hall Health, 2008.

Bickley, L., and Szilagyi, P. *Bates' Guide to Physical Examination and History Taking,* 9th ed. Philadelphia: Lippincott Williams & Wilkins, 2007.

Clark, J.W. *Clinical Neurology from the Classroom to the Exam Room* Philadelphia: Lippincott Williams & Wilkins, 2007.

Craven, R., and Hirnle, C. *Fundamentals of Nursing Human Health and Function,* 5th ed. Philadelphia: Lippincott Williams & Wilkins, 2007.

Dacey, M.J., et al. "The Effect of a Rapid Response Team on Major Clinical Outcome Measures in a Community Hospital," *Critical Care Medicine* 35(9):2076-82, September 2007.

ECG Interpretation Made Incredibly Easy, 4th ed. Philadelphia: Lippincott Williams & Wilkins, 2008.

Ferri, F. *Ferri's Clinical Advisor: Instant Diagnosis and Treatment.* St. Louis: Mosby–Year Book, Inc., 2008.

Handbook of Signs & Symptoms. Philadelphia: Lippincott Williams & Wilkins, 2005.

Jamison, J.R. *Differential Diagnosis for Primary Care: A Handbook for Healthcare Professionals,* 2nd ed. New York: Churchill Livingstone, 2007.

Kasper, D.L., et al., eds. *Harrison's Principles of Internal Medicine,* 17th ed. New York: McGraw-Hill Book Co., 2008.

McFarlan, S.J., and Hensley, S. "Implementation and Outcomes of a Rapid Response Team," *Journal of Nursing Care Quality* 22(4): 314-15, October-December 2007.

Nurse's 5-Minute Clinical Consult: Signs & Symptoms. Philadelphia: Lippincott Williams & Wilkins, 2007.

Nurse's Quick Check, Diseases, 2nd ed. Philadelphia: Lippincott Williams & Wilkins, 2009.

Nurse's Quick Check, Signs & Symptoms. Philadelphia: Lippincott Williams & Wilkins, 2006.

Nursing2008 Drug Handbook, 28th ed. Philadelphia: Lippincott Williams & Wilkins, 2008.

Nutrition Made Incredibly Easy, 2nd ed. Philadelphia: Lippincott Williams & Wilkins, 2007.

Porth, C.M. *Pathophysiology Concepts of Altered Health States,* 7th ed. Philadelphia: Lippincott Williams & Wilkins, 2005.

Rubin, E., and Reisner, H.W. *Essentials of Rubin's Pathology,* 5th ed. Philadelphia: Lippincott Williams & Wilkins, 2008.

Shives, L. *Basic Concepts of Psychiatric-Mental Health Nursing,* 7th ed. Philadelphia: Lippincott Williams & Wilkins, 2007.

Smeltzer, S.C., and Bare, B.G. *Brunner and Suddarth's Textbook of Medical-Surgical Nursing,* 11th ed. Philadelphia: Lippincott Williams & Wilkins, 2008.

Tierney, L., et al. *Current Medical Diagnosis and Treatment,* 47th ed. New York: McGraw-Hill Book Co., 2008.

Waldman, S. *Physical Diagnosis of Pain: An Atlas of Signs and Symptoms.* Philadelphia: Elsevier, 2006.

Woods, S.L., et al. *Cardiac Nursing,* 5th ed. Philadelphia: Lippincott Williams & Wilkins, 2005.

Index

D

i refers to an illustration; t refers to a table.

i refers to an illustration; t refers to a table.

i refers to an illustration; t refers to a table.

i refers to an illustration; t refers to a table.

i refers to an illustration; t refers to a table.

PQ

R

i refers to an illustration; t refers to a table.

S

i refers to an illustration; t refers to a table.